801 PRESCRIPTION DRUGS

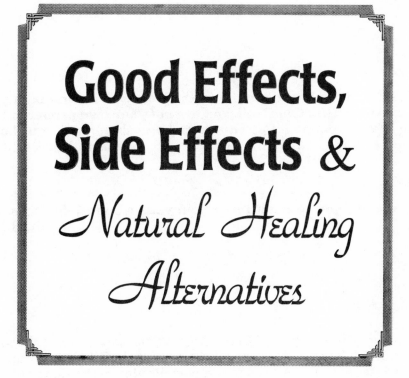

Good Effects, Side Effects & *Natural Healing Alternatives*

By the Editors of FC&A

PUBLISHER'S NOTE

The authors have worked diligently to provide up-to-date and accurate information in this book. However, since pharmacology — the science of drugs — is such a rapidly expanding field, the publisher cannot be responsible for the results of any drug therapy program undertaken by anyone who has consulted this book for information. This publication does not constitute medical practice or advice. Its only intent is to provide the consumer with easy-to-understand information. Please consult carefully with your doctor before taking any drugs or discontinuing any medication.

Your body, you know, is the temple of the Holy Spirit, who is in you since you received Him from God. You are not your own property. You have been bought and paid for. This is why you should use your body for the glory of God.   **1 Corinthians 6:19-20**

But I will restore you to health and heal your wounds, declares the Lord.   **Jeremiah 30:17a**

TABLE OF CONTENTS

Heart and Blood Vessel Disorders 139

Prescription Drug Index

DRUGS LISTED IN CAPITAL LETTERS ARE GENERIC DRUGS

DRUGS LISTED IN CAPITAL LETTERS ARE GENERIC DRUGS

DRUGS LISTED IN CAPITAL LETTERS ARE GENERIC DRUGS

DRUGS LISTED IN CAPITAL LETTERS ARE GENERIC DRUGS

DRUGS LISTED IN CAPITAL LETTERS ARE GENERIC DRUGS

DRUGS LISTED IN CAPITAL LETTERS ARE GENERIC DRUGS

THE DANGERS OF
PRESCRIPTION DRUGS

About 15 years ago, when a doctor prescribed a drug, most people took it and asked no questions. Unfortunately, that accepting and trusting attitude led to a new disease — illness caused by prescription drugs.

Prescription drugs can harm instead of help when you take them in ignorance. You should be able to recognize when your doctor has misprescribed a drug for you, or when you're having an allergic reaction to a drug, or when two drugs you take may be interacting, or when you're having drug side effects that could be dangerous.

Over 18,000 people in the United States die every year from drug side effects. Last year alone, 32,000 hip fractures occurred because of side effects from prescription drugs. (Many drugs result in hip fractures because they make you drowsy, unable to concentrate, dizzy, and unsteady on your feet. Drugs with these side effects include some blood pressure medicines, antihistamines, and arthritis drugs.)

Even if the drugs you take don't harm you, you may not get the full benefit from them — almost half of the people taking drugs don't get the maximum benefit. For instance, if a drug should be taken with food to help your body absorb it better, you need to know that.

This book should answer many of your questions, and should give you some questions to ask your doctor and some information you need to share with him. Here's a list of questions you should ask your doctor when he prescribes a drug:

What is this drug supposed to do for me?

How long will it take to work?

How often will I need to take it? If I am supposed to take my medicine several times a day, does that mean during my waking hours or at regular intervals, even at night?

What are the drug's side effects? Older people should ask if there are any side effects that may be more dangerous to them, such as dizziness that may cause falls, drowsiness that may make driving dangerous, and mental confusion that may affect memory.

Also, the older you become, the less efficient your liver and kidneys are at eliminating drugs from your bloodstream. That means drugs stay in your body longer and build up to higher levels than they would in the body of a younger person. (See chart, page 4.)

Be sure to note any side effects you experience, no matter how minor they seem. Some side effects won't seem minor at all. For example:

- Antibiotics can cause diarrhea and even colitis. Colitis is inflammation of the colon; signs are bloody diarrhea, stomach cramps, and fever.
- Nonsteroidal anti-inflammatory drugs, such as ibuprofen, can cause intestinal bleeding and kidney failure — two very serious conditions that

require medical treatment.

- The antidepressants sertraline (Zoloft) and fluoxetine (Prozac) may cause ejaculation problems for men or a loss of sexual desire.
- Tranquilizers can cause muscle tremors and rigid muscles. You might think you're developing Parkinson's disease when you're really just reacting to the drug.

When you experience side effects, your doctor may decide to change the dose, try another drug, stop the medication, or decide the benefits of the drug outweigh the bad effects you are feeling. But you should never make that decision for yourself. Just as you should never take a drug without your doctor's consent, you should never stop taking medication without consulting him.

Could this drug aggravate other medical conditions that I already have? For example:

- An asthma drug called a bronchodilator can worsen existing high blood pressure or prostate problems.
- A thiazide diuretic, such as chlorothiazide, can cause high blood sugar, and uncontrollable blood sugar is very dangerous for a diabetic.

Are there other drugs that may interact with my prescription? Let your doctor know about all other drugs you take, even over-the-counter cough and cold remedies. Many drugs interact with each other, increasing or decreasing the desired effects. Interactions may be visible changes, or they may be measurable only by laboratory tests.

For instance:

- Antihistamines and tranquilizers both have sedative effects. Taking the two drugs together may slow your breathing, cause you to faint, or even cause you to lose consciousness.
- The cholesterol-lowering drug colestipol can lessen your body's absorption of the anticoagulant warfarin. You need the proper amount of warfarin to prevent clotting problems.

Any foods I shouldn't eat? Some drugs can interact with vitamin supplements, foods, and beverages.

Iron supplements are particularly troublesome because they can interfere with a number of drugs, including the antibiotics penicillamine and tetracycline, the antibacterial drugs called quinolones, the thyroid drug thyroxine, and the blood pressure drug methyldopa. Do not take vitamin or mineral supplements at the same time you take your medicine.

Milk can decrease your body's absorption of some drugs, including laxatives with enteric coatings (that make them easier to swallow).

Alcohol can slow your breathing and even cause you to lose consciousness if you drink it while taking nausea drugs, antihistamines, or sleeping pills.

How should I store the drug? Most drugs need to be stored in a cool, dry place. Some must be kept cold, and some must be kept away from light. Get specific instructions from your pharmacist.

Should I take my prescription with or without food or water? Some pills are best taken on an empty stomach, such as asthma drugs and antibiotics. Most pills can be taken with a glass of water to help wash them all the way down your throat and to aid in absorption. Some pills are better taken with food to help avoid stomach irritation, such as the nonsteroidal anti-inflammatory drugs (NSAIDs) ibuprofen and naproxen.

Never take your medicine with hot drinks like tea or coffee because heat can destroy the drug's effectiveness.

What about missed doses? You should normally take all of your prescription, down to the last pill or dose. With some drugs, such as antibiotics, you

More prescription drug dangers

Pharmacist errors. As soon as you get your prescription filled, read the label. Then repeat back to the pharmacist the name of the drug and the condition it was prescribed to treat, just to clarify that no mistake has been made.

For example, "So, I've been prescribed Zantac to treat my ulcer, right?" Get the pharmacist to acknowledge that your statement is correct. Then read the instructions for taking the drug. If anything differs from your doctor's instructions to you, or if there is anything you don't understand, ask the pharmacist or call your doctor immediately.

Taking drugs prescribed for someone else. When a doctor prescribes a drug and a certain dosage, he takes into consideration other drugs being taken, the person's age, weight, and medical history. Exchanging medicine is extremely dangerous.

Because some drugs can be very dangerous in the wrong hands, be aware of who in your household may have access to your prescription. There are many drugs with very similar names but dramatically different effects.

If you have children or if children visit you often, you must lock all drugs away from their curious eyes and hands. Something as seemingly harmless as aspirin can be very dangerous to children.

Overdoses. Never take more than the recommended dosage of any drug. You may just need to give the drug time to accumulate in your body before you notice any good effects. Many drugs can cause dangerous, even fatal, side effects if you take too much.

If you overdose accidentally, contact your doctor immediately. If you need hospital or ambulance emergency care, give the medical personnel the medicine bottle so they'll know exactly how to treat you. If the bottle is not available, tell them the exact name and dosage of the drug and the name of the doctor who prescribed it.

Emergencies. One final precaution: Tell someone in your household or a nearby friend exactly what drugs you are taking, in case of emergency. If you were to faint or collapse, you would need someone to communicate for you with emergency personnel or doctors. This could prevent any dangerous interactions with drugs you may receive during emergency treatment.

Try to find a pharmacist you like and stick with him. He will become an ally who knows some of your medical history. A good relationship with your pharmacist may mean extra attention to your needs and less chance of mix-ups.

Dangerous drugs for older people

According to a new study, 70 percent of doctors recently flunked a test on prescribing drugs to older people. One in four older people takes a drug from the following list, but these drugs cause harmful side effects and have been labeled inappropriate for older adults by the American Medical Association. Ask your doctor about alternative medications, but don't stop taking any drug without getting your doctor's permission.

Drug	Generic Names	Brand Names
Sedative or Hypnotic Agents *Used to treat anxiety, insomnia.*	Diazepam Chlordiazepoxide Flurazepam Meprobamate Pentobarbital Secobarbital	Valium® Limbitrol®,Librium® Dalmane® Equanil®, Equagesic® Nembutal® Seconal®
Antidepressants *Used to treat depression.*	Amitriptyline	Elavil®, Endep®
NSAIDS *Nonsteroidal anti-inflammatory drugs used to treat arthritis and pain.*	Indomethacin Phenylbutazone	Indocin® Butazolidin®
Oral Hypoglycemics *Used for diabetes.*	Chlorpropamide	Diabinese®
Analgesics *Used to relieve pain.*	Propoxyphene Pentazocine	Darvon® Talwin®
Dementia Treatments *Used to improve circulation and slow dementia.*	Isoxsuprine Cyclandelate	Vasodilan® Cyclospasmol®
Platelet Inhibitors *Used to prevent stroke.*	Dipyridamole	Persantine®
Muscle Relaxants or Antispasmodic Agents *Used to relax muscles or relieve spasms.*	Cyclobenzaprine Methocarbamol Carisoprodol Orphenadrine	Flexeril® Robaxin® Soma® Disipal®
Antiemetic Agents *Used for nausea.*	Trimethobenzamide	Tigan®
Antihypertensives *Used to treat high blood pressure.*	Propranolol Methyldopa Reserpine	Inderal®, Inderide® Aldoclor®, Aldomet® Diupres®, Hydropres®

may start to feel better in a day or two, but that doesn't mean the illness is completely gone.

Find out what you should do if you miss a dose of your medication. Sometimes you should make up a missed dose, but sometimes it is safer to skip it and resume your schedule at the next dose time.

What if I'm pregnant or nursing, or trying to become pregnant? Don't forget to mention your pregnancy to your doctor. Many drugs can affect a developing baby, and some can cause serious birth defects. Most doctors recommend that pregnant or nursing women avoid prescription and over-the-counter drugs because of the possible harmful effects on their babies. But there may be times when the mother's health depends on her taking certain drugs.

Sources —
The Journal of the American Medical Association (272,4:292)
Physicians' Desk Reference, Medical Economics Data Production Co., Montvale, N.J., 1994
The Pill Book, Bantam Books, New York, 1992

INSIDERS GUIDE TO PRESCRIPTION DRUGS

Save money on prescriptions

Many people will drive a hard bargain for a pair of shoes but pay whatever the nearest drugstore charges to get a prescription filled. There are several ways you can cut your prescription drug costs, but you will need to do a little research on your own to find the best deals in your area.

Comparison shop. Neighborhood drugstores usually base their prices on what sells the most in their area. Prices may vary by as much as 25 percent, so it might be worth the drive to another pharmacy to get a better price.

Look for senior-citizen discounts. Many drugstores give good discounts to senior citizens.

Buy generic. Let's say you develop an ear infection and your doctor prescribes an antibiotic drug for you. He may prescribe a brand-name drug, such as EryPed, or he may not specify a brand name and let the pharmacist give you a "generic" equivalent. Erythromycin is the generic form of EryPed.

"Generic" is simply one stage a drug goes through in its development. When a drug company develops a new drug, it gives it a chemical name, a generic name and, when the drug goes to market, a brand name.

The cost of developing a new drug can be millions of dollars. No other company is allowed to sell the drug for 17 years so that the drug company can regain its cost of development. After 17 years, the patent expires and other companies can then make copies of the original chemical formulation, which are called "generics." The companies must prove that their generic is equivalent to the original drug. They can then sell the generic under the chemical name or give it a new brand name.

Some generic drugs may not be of the same quality as the brand-name equivalents. You can ask your pharmacist to check on a drug's equivalency status in a publication called the Orange Book. He can tell you how much a particular generic varies, if any, from the equivalent brand-name drugs.

Generic drugs are usually cheaper than the brand-name forms. The generic form of your prescription may cost 10 to 50 percent less than the brand-name version.

Caution: Before you ask the pharmacist to switch you to generics, talk with your doctor. Even though generics are usually just as safe and effective as brand names, there's a chance that you'll react differently to the generic because of small differences in the formulation.

Buy in bulk. You can often save money by buying drugs that you use all the time in larger quantities.

Ask for free samples. Find out if your doctor has any free samples of your new prescription so that you can try it without investing any money. If there are no free samples, ask for a smaller prescription. That will allow you to be sure that you tolerate the drug well before you pay for a large prescription.

If you can't afford your prescription, you may qualify for free medicine under a special prescription drug program. Check with your doctor.

Fill your prescriptions by mail order. This popular new idea is gaining acceptance. The service is usually available through health-care programs from your employer. By purchasing in large quantities, mail-order companies are able to get volume discounts. You are the winner, as long as you use the system carefully.

You need to be aware that no one will be monitoring you the way your local pharmacist would. It will take a lot longer to get your medications, sometimes over a week. But if you are a careful consumer, mindful of drug interactions and precautions to observe, you might be able to get a good discount this way without undue risk.

Protect yourself against drug tampering

You should always be aware of the possibility of drug tampering. Several brands of over-the-counter drugs have been tampered with in the past. Although over-the-counter drugs are strictly regulated by the federal government and carefully packaged by the manufacturer, there is no foolproof way to keep the drugs 100 percent safe. To protect yourself and your family, follow these guidelines:

Before you buy, consider what form the product is available in and buy the form that is the least likely to be sabotaged. A tablet or caplet is more difficult to tamper with than a capsule or liquid.

- Carefully inspect the outer packaging of the product. Don't purchase it if it looks at all unusual.
- Compare the box or container with others of the same product. Make sure there is nothing different about the package you buy.

When opening the package, watch for holes, tears, cracks, or breaks in the outer wrapping, cover, or protective seal.
- Check to see if the outer covering has been changed, unwrapped, or replaced.
- Read the lot number and information on the box or outer covering and make sure that it matches the information on the product label or container.
- Inspect the shrinkband seal around the top of the container to see if it has been stretched, distorted, or opened and retaped.
- Check that the bottle is filled properly and not overfilled or underfilled.
- Look at the cotton plug or filler at the top of the container. Make sure it hasn't been disturbed.
- Inspect the inside rim of the container for bits of paper or glue. They could be a sign that the protective seal under the cap has been replaced.

While taking the medicine, make sure the color, smell, consistency, and moistness of the product are what you're used to.
- Take the medicine in good lighting so you can double-check that it has not been tampered with and that it is the proper drug for your ailment.
- Do not take any drug that doesn't seem just right. If you are suspicious about a drug or find any evidence of tampering, contact your local office of the FDA or call your pharmacist immediately.

Store your drugs correctly

These days, most people have several different drugs in the house at any one time. You probably have one or two different kinds of pain relievers, an antihistamine, a cough suppressant, something to reduce a fever, and perhaps some prescription drugs.

Most people tend to store all their medicines in the bathroom cabinet. But drugs are chemicals that can be harmed or changed by the way they are stored. Here are a few important things to remember about storing your medicines.

Drugs should always be kept in the container the pharmacist supplies. Some medicines must be protected from light, and others may be damaged by contact with air or moisture. If the bottle or container the pharmacist gives you is too big, just ask for another container that is more convenient for you. Some drug manufacturers will provide pill containers. Use these if they are available.

Do not put different kinds of pills in the same container. It may be tempting to put your pills in little plastic boxes that have separate compartments for each day of the week. But putting different types of pills together can cause chemical reactions. The drugs can form harmful substances or become inactive.

Also, you may forget which pill is which. For example, the most popular dosages of two common drugs, digoxin and furosemide, are both little white pills of almost the same size. Without the original bottle, you may forget dosage instructions, too.

Watch for changes in color, smell, or consistency in your drugs. If you notice any such changes, take them to your pharmacist. He will be able to tell you whether they are still safe to take. For example, when aspirin develops a vinegary odor, it has probably lost its potency and should not be used.

Take note of the expiration date. This date is good only when the bottle has not been opened. Many drugs decompose when they are exposed to air. Once the seal is broken on a bottle, the expiration date is no longer in effect. Ask your pharmacist or doctor how long the drug will last after the bottle is opened. Then when you open it, write your own expiration date on the bottle.

If possible, avoid storing medicines in the bathroom. Since moisture and heat can harm the potency of your drugs, the medicine cabinet in the family bathroom is not the best place to store them. Try to choose a safe, dry, and cool place to store all your drugs.

Ask for easy-to-open containers. Many over-the-counter drugs come in childproof containers that are sometimes "adultproof," especially if you have arthritis. If you are sure that children will not be near your drugs, ask your pharmacist for a container that is easy to open.

Get the package insert. Each time you have a prescription filled, ask the pharmacist for the package insert for that medication. This leaflet describes in detail all the known side effects of that drug. If it is not available, find out the name of the drug manufacturer and request the information.

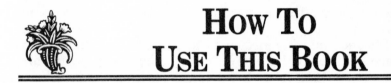

How To Use This Book

The purpose of this book is to provide you with up-to-date, easy-to-understand information. We have listed the most frequently prescribed drugs, including their intended good effects and possible harmful side effects, the possible hazards to unborn or nursing babies, precautions for people who have certain conditions that could make them more susceptible to the harmful effects of some drugs, and helpful hints on how to best use the drugs.

You'll find 15 categories, from Breathing Problems to Smoking and Alcohol Addiction, followed by a section on natural ways to treat your condition. You should use these natural alternatives in addition to any drug your doctor prescribes for you.

Each drug entry has seven sections (if one of the sections isn't used, it's because there was no information available on that topic):

Brand names: Here we list most of the common brand names of each drug. Sometimes you know your drug's brand name but you don't know its generic name. That's why we included both brand names and generic names in the big index at the front of the book. You'll also find here whether the drug is available in the generic form.

What this drug does for you: This tells you what the medication is designed to treat and what action it will take in the body. The type of drug (such as thiazide diuretic) is usually given here. You can use the drug type to look up more information from other sources.

Possible side effects of this drug: This lists the side effects that may occur with the drug. They are listed from most common or frequent to least common and rare. Don't be concerned if there are a lot of side effects listed. Some side effects are natural, expected, and unavoidable. Most of them are unusual, unexpected, and infrequent. Some may depend on the size of the dose, and they will often go away if the dose is lowered. But don't stop taking your medication or change the dosage without your doctor's approval.

Special warnings: This section will tell you when you should not take the drug, when you should take it with caution, and other important information. Notify your doctor if any of the warnings apply to you.

Pregnancy and nursing mothers: This section gives the FDA's pregnancy code for this drug. The FDA assigns a code to each drug that lets you know how safe it is to take while you are pregnant. See the FDA's pregnancy categories below for the full descriptions of the pregnancy categories. You'll also find whether mothers who are breast-feeding can take the drug safely.

Possible food and drug interactions: This section tells you the foods and other drugs that may interact with the medicine you are taking.

Helpful hints: This section is included for most drugs and will give information on topics such as storage and timing of dose with food.

At the very end, you will find a glossary of medical terms used in the book. The definitions are brief and general, but they contain information that will help you understand the drug descriptions.

It's your health

When it comes to your health and the drugs your doctor prescribes to maintain it, you need to know as much as possible. Don't be afraid to take an active role in your health care by working closely with your doctor and pharmacist. It's your responsibility to know what drugs you are taking and how to use them appropriately. We hope that the information in this book will encourage you to communicate openly with your doctor and pharmacist.

Key to FDA pregnancy categories

The Food and Drug Administration uses human studies as well as animal studies to determine the risk of prescription drugs to a developing human baby. The FDA has assigned one of the following five Pregnancy Categories to each drug. The categories rank each drug's potential to cause birth defects.

Pregnancy Category A. Studies of pregnant women have not shown a risk to the developing baby.

Pregnancy Category B. This category can mean two things: (1) Animal studies have not shown a risk to the developing baby, but studies haven't been done in pregnant women, or (2) Animal studies have shown a risk to the developing fetus, but studies in pregnant women have not shown a risk.

Pregnancy Category C. This middle category can mean two things: (1) Animal studies have shown a risk, and human studies are inconclusive because not enough have been done. The mother may gain enough benefit from the drug to make the risk to the developing baby acceptable, or (2) We really don't know the risk to the developing baby because there are no animal studies and not enough human studies.

Pregnancy Category D. Studies in pregnant women have shown evidence of a risk to the developing baby. However, the mother may gain enough benefit from the drug to make the risk to the baby acceptable.

Pregnancy Category X. Studies in animals or pregnant women have shown a definite risk to the developing baby. The drug has either caused birth defects or the developing baby has reacted badly to the drug in some way. The risk to the baby clearly outweighs any benefit the mother may gain from taking the drug.

BRAIN AND NERVOUS SYSTEM DISORDERS

Prescription Drugs

Natural Alternatives

Prescription Drugs

DRUGS TO PREVENT SEIZURES, CONVULSIONS

Carbamazepine

Brand name: *Tegretol* **(Generic available)**

What this drug does for you:

This drug is used by people with epilepsy to control certain types of seizures.

It also controls the pain associated with a facial nerve disorder called trigeminal neuralgia.

Possible side effects of this drug:

- Even though it is very rare, the riskiest side effect of carbamazepine is that it can depress your bone marrow. The bone marrow makes most of your blood cells. If you don't have enough white blood cells, your immunity is down, and you can get a fever, sore throat, or pneumonia. If you are lacking red blood cells, you can become anemic, and that makes you tired and weak. Not having enough blood platelets makes you bruise easily and keeps your blood from clotting properly when you're injured. Be on the lookout for any of these symptoms of bone marrow depression. You should have blood tests done before you begin taking the drug.
- Serious skin disorders in which dark red rings or raised spots erupt on your skin (Stevens-Johnson syndrome) or parts of your skin die are another very rare reaction.
- The most common side effects, particularly when you first start taking the drug, are dizziness, drowsiness, unsteadiness, and nausea.
- Other less common side effects are rashes, hives, flaking skin, hair loss, urinary frequency or difficulty urinating, impotence, headache, fatigue, blurred vision, hallucinations, speech disturbances, ringing in the ears, stomachache, diarrhea, dry mouth, vision changes, fever, and chills. Heart problems, such as blood pressure problems and heart attack, are a rare but dangerous side effect.

Special warnings:

- People who have a history of bone marrow depression or who have had allergic reactions to tricyclic antidepressants should not use this drug.
- Your doctor should prescribe carbamazepine to you very cautiously if you have increased pressure within the eye, if you have had bone marrow depression as a reaction to medication in the past, or if you have heart problems or kidney or liver damage. Even if you haven't had liver or kidney problems in the past, you should have your liver and kidney function tested regularly while you take carbamazepine.

Pregnancy and nursing mothers:

Category C. See page 9 for description of categories. Drug is present in mother's milk. You should not take carbamazepine if you plan to breast-feed.

Possible food and drug interactions:

- Don't take carbamazepine and the antidepressant drugs called monoamine oxidase (MAO) inhibitors at the same time. You should quit taking MAO inhibitors for at least two weeks before you begin taking carbamazepine.
- The sedative phenobarbital and the seizure drugs phenytoin and primidone may lower your levels of carbamazepine.
- This drug may decrease the effects of the seizure drug phenytoin, the anticoagulant warfarin, the antibiotic doxycycline, the asthma drug theophylline, the antipsychotic drug haloperidol, and the anticonvulsant valproic acid.

The antibiotic erythromycin, the ulcer drug cimetidine, the painkiller propoxyphene, the tuberculosis drug isoniazid, the antihistamine terfenadine, the antidepressant fluoxetine, and calcium channel blockers may increase blood levels of carbamazepine.

- Taking carbamazepine and the antipsychotic drug lithium at the same time can cause toxic side effects.
- If carbamazepine is combined with other anticonvulsants, your thyroid function can be affected.
- Carbamazepine can make birth control pills unreliable, and can cause breakthrough bleeding if you're taking the pill.

Helpful hints:

- This drug can make you dizzy and drowsy. Be careful if you plan to drive or use dangerous machinery.
- Never stop taking this drug without your doctor's permission. Quitting suddenly can cause seizures.

Clonazepam

Brand name: *Klonopin*

What this drug does for you:

Clonazepam treats certain types of seizures. In some studies, up to 30 percent of the people taking this drug quit having seizures, often within three months. Like some of the drugs for anxiety and insomnia, clonazepam is a benzodiazepine.

Possible side effects of this drug:

- Half the people taking clonazepam will have drowsiness as a side effect. Thirty percent will also feel a lack of coordination.
- One out of four people taking the drug may have behavior problems as a side effect. These include depression, hysteria, attempts at suicide, and other mental disorders. People who already have mental disturbances are more likely to have them as a side effect of the drug.
- Clonazepam can also cause respiratory problems such as stuffy sinuses or trouble breathing. It depresses your respiratory system and causes many people to produce extra saliva and mucus.
- Other side effects are abnormal eye movements, double vision, difficulty talking, headache, shakiness, dizziness, confusion, temporary memory loss, increased sex drive, insomnia, heart palpitations, hair loss or extra hair growth, rash, swelling of ankles and face, coated tongue, constipation, diarrhea, dry mouth, sore gums, nausea, urinary problems, change in appetite, and fever. Low red or white blood cell counts are a rare side effect.

Special warnings:

- People with a certain type of glaucoma (acute narrow angle glaucoma) and people with severe liver disease shouldn't use clonazepam.
- People with poor kidney function and people with chronic respiratory diseases should use clonazepam cautiously.

- You can become dependent on clonazepam. To avoid seizures and other less severe withdrawal symptoms such as heightened senses, muscle cramps, diarrhea, and blurred vision, you should quit taking the drug gradually under your doctor's supervision. Never stop abruptly, and never increase or decrease your dosage without your doctor's approval.

Pregnancy and nursing mothers:
The effects of clonazepam in pregnancy are not known. Some reports suggest that clonazepam may cause birth defects. Women taking clonazepam should not nurse.

Possible food and drug interactions:
- If you take clonazepam along with a drug that depresses your nervous system, such as tranquilizers, alcohol, antihistamines, muscle relaxers, monoamine oxidase (MAO) inhibitors and the tricyclic antidepressants, and other anticonvulsant drugs, the combination may dangerously depress your nervous system.

Helpful hints:
- You shouldn't drive a car or operate heavy machinery until you are sure the medicine isn't making you drowsy or less than alert.
- You should have regular blood counts and liver function tests while you're taking clonazepam.
- For adults, the maximum starting dosage is 1.5 mg a day divided into three doses. Your doctor may increase your dosage by 0.5 to 1 mg every three days until you reach the most effective level. The maximum recommended daily dose is 20 mg.

Divalproex Sodium

Brand name: *Depakote*

What this drug does for you:
Divalproex sodium is used alone or along with other anticonvulsant drugs to treat certain types of seizures.

Possible side effects of this drug:
- The riskiest side effect of divalproex sodium is liver failure, which can be fatal. This side effect is most common in children under the age of 2 and very rare for adults. You should have regular liver tests, and you should look for side effects such as fatigue, weakness, swelling of the face, loss of appetite, and vomiting. Usually, liver failure occurs in the first six months you take divalproex sodium.
- Another serious side effect is a low blood platelet count. This means your blood may not clot properly. Look for unusual bruising, and have regular blood tests. Low red or white blood cell counts are also a rare side effect.
- The most common side effects are sleepiness, nausea, and indigestion. These side effects usually go away after you've been taking the drug for a while.

- Other possible side effects are diarrhea, stomach cramps, constipation, increased or decreased appetite, tremor, hallucinations, loss of coordination, headache, double vision, dizziness, some hair loss at first, rash, increased sensitivity to light, emotional upset, depression, aggression, hyperactivity, irregular menstrual periods, and breast enlargement.
- Serious skin disorders in which dark red rings or raised spots erupt on your skin (Stevens-Johnson syndrome) or parts of your skin deteriorate are another very rare reaction.

Special warning:
- People with liver disease or poor liver function should not take this drug.

Pregnancy and nursing mothers:
Category D. See page 9 for a description of categories. This drug may cause birth defects. This drug is present in mother's milk.

Possible food and drug interactions:
- If you take divalproex sodium along with a drug that depresses your nervous system, such as tranquilizers, alcohol, antihistamines, muscle relaxers, and other anticonvulsant drugs, the combination may dangerously depress your nervous system. Barbiturates combined with divalproex sodium can be especially dangerous. Your doctor should carefully monitor the levels of these drugs in your body.
- Taking divalproex sodium and aspirin, carbamazepine, dicumarol, or phenytoin at the same time can increase or decrease the levels of any of these drugs in your body.
- Drugs that affect blood clotting (aspirin and warfarin, for instance) should be used cautiously with divalproex sodium.
- Divalproex sodium may make birth control pills less effective.

Helpful hints:
- You shouldn't drive a car or operate heavy machinery until you are sure the medicine isn't making you drowsy or less than alert.
- You can swallow the capsules whole or open them and sprinkle the contents on a teaspoonful of soft food such as applesauce. Swallow the mixture immediately. Don't chew it, or store the mixture to use later.
- If your medicine upsets your stomach, make sure you take it with food.

Ethosuximide

Brand name: *Zarontin*

What this drug does for you:
Ethosuximide controls petit mal seizures for people with epilepsy.

Possible side effects of this drug:
- Upset stomach, nausea, cramps, diarrhea and loss of appetite are common side effects. Less common are drowsiness, headache, dizziness, hiccups, irritability, hyperactivity, tiredness, weakness, rash, hives, hair growth, nearsightedness, and vaginal bleeding. Some people experience mental disturbances such as night terrors, aggressiveness, inability to

concentrate, increased sex drive, paranoia, and depression.

- Even though it is rare, one risky side effect of ethosuximide is that it can cause your blood cell count to be low. If you don't have enough white blood cells, your immunity is down, and you can get a fever, sore throat, or pneumonia. If you are lacking red blood cells, you can become anemic, and that makes you tired and weak. Not having enough blood platelets makes you bruise easily and keeps your blood from clotting properly when you're injured. Be on the lookout for any of these symptoms. You should have blood tests done before you begin taking the drug.
- Ethosuximide can also cause liver and kidney damage. You should have regular liver and kidney tests while you're taking this drug.

Special warning:
- You should use this drug very cautiously if you have liver or kidney problems.

Pregnancy:
This drug may cause birth defects.

Possible food and drug interaction:
- Ethosuximide may increase levels of the seizure drug phenytoin.

Helpful hints:
- You should never stop taking your medicine or change your dosage without talking to your doctor. Any sudden change could cause a seizure.
- You shouldn't drive a car or operate heavy machinery until you are sure the medicine isn't making you drowsy or less than alert.

Mephobarbital

Brand name: *Mebaral*

What this drug does for you:
This drug is a barbiturate like many of the drugs for insomnia. It is used to treat seizures for people with epilepsy, and it's used to relieve apprehension, anxiety, and tension. You can use the drug alone or in combination with other drugs that prevent seizures.

Possible side effects of this drug:
- The most common side effect is daytime sleepiness.
- Rarer side effects are agitation, confusion, nightmares, nervousness, dizziness, very slow breathing, low blood pressure, nausea, constipation, headache, skin rash, and fever.

Special warnings:
- You can become addicted to this drug. You must not increase your dose without talking to your doctor. Some symptoms of intoxication with barbiturates are walking unsteadily, slurred speech, confusion, and irritability.
- You should withdraw from mephobarbital slowly, over four or five days. If you quit taking the drug suddenly, you may have nightmares, insom-

nia, anxiety, dizziness, or nausea. If you're addicted to the drug and you quit taking it suddenly, you may have delirium, seizures, or death.

- People with a group of disorders called porphyria should not use barbiturates.
- Your doctor should adjust your dosage carefully and watch you closely for side effects if you have poor kidney function, a heart disorder, respiratory problems, the nerve/muscle disorder called myasthenia gravis, poor thyroid function, or a liver disorder.
- You may need extra vitamin D and vitamin K while you take a barbiturate.

Pregnancy and nursing mothers:

Category D. See page 9 for description of categories. This drug may cause birth defects. Drug is present in mother's milk.

Possible food and drug interactions:

- If you take mephobarbital along with a drug that depresses your nervous system, such as tranquilizers, alcohol, antihistamines, or muscle relaxers, the combination may dangerously depress your nervous system.
- Mephobarbital may increase the effects of corticosteroids.
- Mephobarbital may decrease the effectiveness of anti-clotting drugs like warfarin, the antifungal drug griseofulvin, birth control pills, and doxycycline.
- If you take mephobarbital and phenytoin together, your doctor may need to adjust your dosages of both drugs. They can affect the levels of each other.
- Sodium valproate, valproic acid, and monoamine oxidase (MAO) inhibitors may increase the depressant effects of mephobarbital.

Helpful hints:

- You shouldn't drive a car or operate heavy machinery until you are sure the medicine isn't making you drowsy or less than alert.
- You should have regular blood, liver, and kidney tests if you take this drug for a long time.
- If you take birth control pills, you should use another type of contraception while you're taking mephobarbital.
- The average dose for adults with epilepsy is 400 mg to 600 mg. You should take your dose at bedtime if you usually have seizures during the night. If you usually have seizures during the day, then you should take your medicine during the day.

Phenytoin

Brand name: *Dilantin*

What this drug does for you:

Phenytoin is used by people with epilepsy to treat and prevent certain types of seizures.

Possible side effects of this drug:

- The most common side effects are lack of coordination, slurred speech, confusion, and rolling eye movements. These side effects often mean you need a lower dose.
- Other side effects you may experience are dizziness, insomnia, nervousness, twitching muscles, headache, nausea, constipation, damage to liver, enlarged and tender gums, extra hair growth, widening of nose tip, fever, and aching muscles.
- Phenytoin may cause some lymph node diseases. Signs to look for are enlarged glands in your neck or underarms. You may also have a fever or a rash.
- Tell your doctor right away if you develop a skin rash. Your doctor may need to take you off the drug. If the rash is a mild, measles-like rash, you'll be able to take phenytoin again once the rash has cleared up. Serious skin disorders in which dark red rings or raised spots erupt on your skin (Stevens-Johnson syndrome) or parts of your skin deteriorate are a very rare reaction.
- For people with diabetes, phenytoin may raise your blood sugar levels.
- Even though it is very rare, phenytoin can lower the number of blood cells you have. If you don't have enough white blood cells, your immunity is down, and you can get a fever, sore throat, or pneumonia. If you are lacking red blood cells, you can become anemic, and that makes you tired and weak. Not having enough blood platelets makes you bruise easily and keeps your blood from clotting properly when you're injured. Be on the lookout for any of these symptoms of bone marrow depression.

Special warnings:

- People with a group of disorders called porphyria should take phenytoin very cautiously.
- Like many drugs, phenytoin can reach toxic levels more quickly if you have poor liver function and if you are an older adult.

Pregnancy and nursing mothers:

Category D. See page 9 for description of categories. Drug is present in mother's milk.

Possible food and drug interactions:

- A large amount of alcohol can increase levels of phenytoin in your body. However, chronic alcohol abuse can decrease phenytoin levels.
- The following drugs may increase the effects of phenytoin: the heart rhythm drug amiodarone, the antibiotic chloramphenicol, the anti-anxiety drugs chlordiazepoxide and diazepam, the anticoagulant dicumarol, the anti-alcoholic drug disulfiram, estrogens, the tuberculosis drug isoniazid, phenothiazine tranquilizers, the nonsteroidal anti-inflammatory drug phenylbutazone, salicylates such as aspirin, sulfonamide antibacterials, the antidiabetic drug tolbutamide, and the antidepressant trazodone.
- The following drugs may decrease effects of phenytoin: antacids, the seizure drug carbamazepine, the blood pressure drug reserpine, the ulcer

drug sucralfate, the antipsychotic drug molindone.

- If you take phenytoin and phenobarbital, valproic acid, or sodium valproate together, your doctor may need to adjust your dosages of both drugs. They can affect the levels of each other.
- Certain drugs may not work as well when you are also taking phenytoin: birth control pills, corticosteroids, anticoagulants, the heart drug digitoxin, the antibiotic doxycycline, the diuretic furosemide, the heartbeat regulator quinidine, the tuberculosis drug rifampin, and the asthma drug theophylline.

Helpful hints:

- Unless you're having an allergic reaction to the drug and under your doctor's supervision, you should never quit taking phenytoin suddenly. You could bring on a seizure. You should also stick with the exact dosage schedule your doctor advises.
- You shouldn't drive a car or operate heavy machinery until you are sure the medicine isn't making you drowsy or less than alert.
- You may need vitamin D and vitamin K supplements. Some people taking phenytoin may need folic acid supplements to help prevent anemia.
- This drug can cause gum problems, so it is very important to keep your teeth and gums clean and flossed. You should also visit your dentist regularly.
- You shouldn't take antacids containing calcium within two to three hours of taking phenytoin. The antacids could keep you from absorbing the phenytoin properly.
- Most adults take three to four 100 mg capsules a day.

Primidone

Brand name: *Mysoline*

What this drug does for you:

People with epilepsy use primidone to control many types of seizures.

Possible side effects of this drug:

- The most common side effects are lack of coordination and dizziness. These side effects usually go away after you've been taking the drug for a while.
- Other side effects are nausea, loss of appetite, tiredness, irritability, emotional disturbances, impotence, double vision, rolling movements of the eyeballs, drowsiness, and rashes. Some blood disorders such as anemia are rare side effects.

Special warnings:

- People with a group of disorders called porphyria should not use primidone.
- Don't stop taking anticonvulsants suddenly or change the dose without consulting your doctor.
- You shouldn't drive a car or operate heavy machinery until you are sure

the medicine isn't making you drowsy or less than alert.

Pregnancy and nursing mothers:

The effects of this drug during pregnancy are not known, but some reports suggest that the drug may cause birth defects. Drug is present in mother's milk.

Possible food and drug interaction:

- Primidone is partly converted to phenobarbital in the body. See the entry for phenobarbital for possible interactions with other drugs.

Helpful hints:

- The usual adult dose is three to four 250 mg tablets taken three or four times a day. You will start out on a much lower dose. Two grams is the maximum total daily dosage.
- You may need folic acid to treat anemia, a rare side effect of primidone.

Valproic Acid

Brand name: *Depakene* **(Generic available)**

What this drug does for you:

Valproic acid is used alone or along with other anticonvulsant drugs to treat certain types of seizures.

Possible side effects of this drug:

- The riskiest side effect of valproic acid is liver failure, which can be fatal. This side effect is most common in children under the age of 2 and very rare for adults. You should have regular liver tests, and you should look for side effects such as fatigue, weakness, swelling of the face, loss of appetite, and vomiting. Usually, liver failure occurs in the first six months you take valproic acid.
- Another serious side effect is a low blood platelet count. This means your blood may not clot properly. Look for unusual bruising, and have regular blood tests. Low red or white blood cell counts are also a rare side effect.
- The most common side effects are sleepiness, nausea, and indigestion. These side effects usually go away after you've been taking the drug for a while.
- Other possible side effects are diarrhea, stomach cramps, constipation, increased or decreased appetite, tremor, hallucinations, loss of coordination, headache, double vision, dizziness, some hair loss at first, rash, increased sensitivity to light, emotional upset, depression, aggression, hyperactivity, irregular menstrual periods, and breast enlargement.
- Serious skin disorders in which dark red rings or raised spots erupt on your skin (Stevens-Johnson syndrome) or parts of your skin deteriorate are another very rare reaction.

Special warning:

- People with liver disease or poor liver function should not take this drug.

Pregnancy and nursing mothers:

Category D. See page 9 for a description of categories. This drug may cause birth defects. This drug is present in mother's milk.

Possible food and drug interactions:

- If you take valproic acid along with a drug that depresses your nervous system, such as tranquilizers, alcohol, antihistamines, muscle relaxers, and other anticonvulsant drugs, the combination may dangerously depress your nervous system. Barbiturates combined with valproic acid can be especially dangerous. Your doctor should carefully monitor the levels of these drugs in your body.
- Taking valproic acid and aspirin, carbamazepine, dicumarol, or phenytoin at the same time can increase or decrease the levels of any of these drugs in your body.
- Drugs that affect blood clotting (aspirin and warfarin, for instance) should be used cautiously with valproic acid.
- Valproic acid may make birth control pills less effective.

Helpful hints:

- You shouldn't drive a car or operate heavy machinery until you are sure the medicine isn't making you drowsy or less than alert.
- If your medicine upsets your stomach, make sure you take it with food.
- Don't chew the capsules. They will irritate your mouth and throat.

DRUGS FOR ATTENTION DEFICIT DISORDER

Methylphenidate

Brand names: *Ritalin, Ritalin-SR*

What this drug does for you:

Methylphenidate is a mild stimulant. It is most often used to treat children with attention deficit disorder (ADD). It increases attention and decreases restlessness in children who are overactive and can't concentrate. Not all children with ADD should be given this drug, and your doctor should do a complete evaluation and history before he prescribes it.

Methylphenidate also helps people with narcolepsy (an uncontrollable desire for sleep or sudden attacks of deep sleep).

Possible side effects of this drug:

- For children, the most common side effects are loss of appetite, nervousness, trouble sleeping, stomach pain, and a fast heartbeat. Nervousness and trouble sleeping are common for adults too.
- Other side effects are nausea, dizziness, headache, drowsiness, chest pain, and blood pressure and pulse changes. Tourette's syndrome (uncontrollable movements and speech) may be a rare side effect. If you are allergic to the drug, you may develop a rash, hives, fever, or aching muscles.

- When children take methylphenidate for a long time, the drug can slow their growth rates.
- Visual disturbances such as blurred vision have been reported as a side effect.

Special warnings:
- People who are very anxious, tense, agitated, or emotionally unstable should not take this drug.
- If you have glaucoma, involuntary muscle movements known as "tics," or Tourette's syndrome (or a family history of it), you should not use this drug.
- Methylphenidate may increase the risk of seizures, and you should use it cautiously if you have a history of seizures. If you have a seizure, your doctor should stop your methylphenidate treatment.
- People with high blood pressure should use this drug very cautiously. You should have your blood pressure checked regularly while you're taking methylphenidate.

Pregnancy and nursing mothers:
Not known if it's safe to use this drug while you're pregnant. It's best to avoid taking it during pregnancy. Not known if drug is safe to use while nursing.

Possible food and drug interactions:
- Methylphenidate may keep the blood pressure drug guanethidine from working well.
- Methylphenidate may increase levels or effects of anticlotting drugs like warfarin, the anti-inflammatory phenylbutazone, tricyclic antidepressants, and the anticonvulsants phenobarbital, diphenylhydantoin, and primidone.
- If you take antidepressant drugs called monoamine oxidase (MAO) inhibitors, you should take methylphenidate very cautiously.

Helpful hints:
- You should have regular blood tests while you're taking this drug.
- If you're having trouble sleeping, you should try to take your last dose before 6 p.m.
- The average dosage for adults is 20 to 30 mg a day. You should take your medicine in two or three divided doses, preferably 30 to 45 minutes before meals. If you take the extended-release tablets, make sure you swallow them whole instead of chewing or crushing them.

DRUGS FOR PARKINSON'S DISEASE

Amantadine

Brand names: *None available* **(Generic available)**

What this drug does for you:

Amantadine reduces stiffness and improves muscle control for people with Parkinson's disease. In treating Parkinson's disease, it is not as effective as the drug levodopa.

Amantadine also works as an antiviral to treat and prevent certain types of flu by blocking penetration of viruses into cells. Your first weapon against the flu should be a vaccination — a "flu shot." But if you didn't get a flu shot early enough, amantadine can help you fight the flu.

Amantadine is also used to treat stiffness and shaking caused by some medicines.

Possible side effects of this drug:

- Five to 10 percent of the people taking amantadine have nausea, dizziness, or insomnia. One to five percent of people taking amantadine have depression, anxiety, irritability, hallucinations, confusion, loss of appetite, dry mouth and nose, constipation, swelling, low blood pressure upon standing, headache, drowsiness, strange dreams, diarrhea, or fatigue. Some people also get skin rashes or a bluish mottling on their legs and hands.
- Less common side effects are congestive heart failure, difficulty urinating, slurred speech, decreased sex drive, and low white blood cell count. If you don't have enough white blood cells, your immunity is lowered, and you're more likely to get infections.

Special warnings:

- People with a history of mental problems are sometimes made worse by amantadine.
- People with a history of seizures sometimes have more seizures while taking amantadine.
- People with congestive heart failure, low blood pressure upon standing, a certain type of rash, or liver problems should take this drug cautiously.

Pregnancy and nursing mothers:

Category C. See page 9 for description of categories. Drug is present in mother's milk.

Possible food and drug interactions:

- You can take amantadine along with other drugs to treat Parkinson's disease.
- You should be watched very closely by your doctor if you take other drugs that stimulate your central nervous system along with amantadine.

Helpful hints:

- If you notice any blurred vision or sleepiness as a side effect of the drug, be very careful when you drive or are in situations that could be dangerous.
- You should never stop taking this drug suddenly. Stopping suddenly could bring on neuroleptic malignant syndrome (NMS) or "parkinsonian crisis." Some signs of NMS are rigid muscles, uncontrollable movements, a rapid heartbeat, and high or low blood pressure.
- The usual adult dose of amantadine is 100 mg twice a day.
- Amantadine can lose its effectiveness for treating Parkinson's disease after you've taken it for several months.

Benztropine

Brand name: *Cogentin* **(Generic available)**

What this drug does for you:

Benztropine is similar to many antihistamines, but it is used to treat Parkinson's disease. It is also used to treat stiffness and shaking caused by some medicines.

Possible side effects of this drug:

- Difficulty urinating and weak muscles are common side effects.
- Other side effects are constipation, nausea, dry mouth, confusion, memory loss, hallucinations, nervousness, depression, numb fingers, blurred vision, dilated pupils, heatstroke, and fever. If you are having a lot of trouble with nausea and dry mouth, you may need a lower dose. Talk to your doctor.

Special warnings:

- This drug has drying side effects (for instance, it can keep you from sweating properly). You should be very careful in hot weather, and watch yourself for signs of heatstroke.
- People with certain kinds of glaucoma, a rapid heartbeat, or prostate problems should use this drug very carefully.
- This drug may cause or aggravate symptoms of tardive dyskinesia.

Pregnancy and nursing mothers:

Not known whether it is safe to use during pregnancy.

Possible food and drug interactions:

- If you also take phenothiazines, haloperidol, tricyclic antidepressants, or other drugs that have drying side effects, make sure you report to your doctor any signs of fever or stomach complaints or any signs that you can't tolerate heat.

Helpful hints:

- You shouldn't drive a car or operate heavy machinery until you are sure the medicine isn't making you drowsy or less than alert.
- The usual daily dose is 1 to 2 mg, taken at bedtime.

Bromocriptine

Brand name: *Parlodel* (Generic available)

What this drug does for you:

This drug treats Parkinson's disease. It also stops an unwanted flow of breast milk, either caused by pituitary gland tumors or because a mother doesn't want to breast-feed after pregnancy. Bromocriptine is also used to stimulate regular menstrual cycles and to treat certain fertility problems. Also, this drug treats acromegaly, a condition of middle age causing enlargement of the arms, legs, and head.

Possible side effects of this drug:

- Almost half the people taking this drug experience nausea. Also common are low blood pressure, headache, dizziness, fatigue, stomach cramps, stuffy nose, constipation, diarrhea, drowsiness, and loss of appetite.
- Some people experience pain in the fingers and toes when exposed to cold.
- Less common side effects include difficulty urinating, confusion, and hallucinations.
- Some rare but serious side effects include high blood pressure, seizures, stroke, and heart attack. Report to your doctor severe headaches and blurred vision and have regular blood pressure checks while you're taking this drug.

Special warning:

- Let your doctor know if you have untreated high blood pressure or kidney or liver disease.

Pregnancy and nursing mothers:

Category B. See page 9 for description of categories. Don't take this drug if you want to breast-feed because it prevents milk production.

Possible food and drug interactions:

- This drug, when combined with blood-pressure-lowering drugs, can cause extremely low blood pressure.
- Be sure that you use an alternative form of contraception besides birth control pills because they may decrease the effectiveness of bromocriptine.
- Phenothiazines and butyrophenones may decrease the effectiveness of bromocriptine.

Helpful hints:

- Take with food.
- Have regular liver, kidney, heart, and blood tests while taking this drug.
- You shouldn't drive a car or operate heavy machinery until you are sure the medicine isn't making you drowsy or less than alert.

Levodopa

Brand names: *Dopar, Larodopa*

What this drug does for you:
Levodopa treats the symptoms of Parkinson's disease.

Possible side effects of this drug:
- The most serious side effects of levodopa are rhythmic jerky muscle movements or other muscular abnormalities, irregular heartbeat, low blood pressure when you stand up, heart palpitations followed by very slow heartbeat ("on-off" phenomenon), depression or other mental disorders, and difficulty urinating.
- Other common side effects are loss of appetite, nausea, dry mouth, numbness, dizziness, confusion, nightmares, teeth grinding, and difficulty swallowing. Like many other drugs, levodopa may lower your red blood cell count and cause anemia, or it may lower your white blood cell count and therefore lower your immunity.
- Less common side effects are diarrhea, constipation, hot flashes, flushing, ulcers, intestinal bleeding, fluid retention or swelling, hair loss, hiccups, urinary incontinence, and double vision.

Special warnings:
- This drug should not be used by people with some kinds of glaucoma (consult your doctor), a history of skin cancer, or any undiagnosed skin lesions.
- If you have severe lung or heart disease; an irregular heartbeat; disease of the brain, liver, kidney, or endocrine system; or a history of heart attack, asthma, stomach ulcer, or mental disturbances, talk with your doctor about your condition before you take this drug.

Pregnancy and nursing mothers:
Not known if safe to use in pregnancy. Don't use while nursing.

Possible food and drug interactions:
- Don't take levodopa within two weeks of taking antidepressant drugs called monoamine oxidase (MAO) inhibitors.
- Levodopa can increase the effects of blood-pressure-lowering drugs.
- Vitamin B6 may decrease levels or effects of this drug.

Helpful hints:
- You shouldn't drive a car or operate heavy machinery until you are sure the medicine isn't making you drowsy or less than alert.
- You should have regular liver, blood, heart, and kidney tests while you're taking this drug.
- Since levodopa can cause low blood pressure and dizziness when you stand or sit up, be careful when you change positions.
- Take with food.
- The usual starting dose for adults is 0.5 to 1 g daily. The maximum daily dose is 8 g.

Pergolide

Brand name: *Permax*

What this drug does for you:

Pergolide treats Parkinson's disease in combination with levodopa/carbidopa.

Possible side effects of this drug:

- This drug causes more than half of the people who take it to have abnormal, involuntary muscle movements. Watch yourself for tremors or movements you can't control, and report them immediately to your doctor.
- Many people also have hallucinations, and 10 percent of the people taking the drug have low blood pressure (which causes dizziness) when they stand up.
- Other common side effects are sleepiness, insomnia, nausea, constipation, diarrhea, upset stomach, and stuffy or runny nose.
- Possible but less common side effects are confusion, headache, fluid retention in the hands and feet, weakness, loss of appetite, tremors, difficulty breathing, chest pain, dry mouth, depression, rash, neck pain, heart palpitations, fainting, abnormal dreams, sweating, double vision, frequent urination, back pain, chills, high blood pressure, heart attack, anemia, muscle pain, joint pain, lack of coordination, tingling, abnormal speech, and hiccups.

Special warnings:

- Don't use this drug if you are allergic to ergot derivatives.
- If you have irregular heart rhythms, you should talk with your doctor about your condition before you take this drug. It can cause irregular heartbeats.

Pregnancy and nursing mothers:

Category B. See page 9 for description of categories. Not known if drug is present in mother's milk.

Possible food and drug interaction:

- Effects of this drug may be decreased by phenothiazines, a type of tranquilizer.

Helpful hints:

- An average adult dose is 3 mg a day, taken in divided doses.
- Since this drug causes dizziness when you stand up, make sure you change positions slowly, especially when you first start taking the drug.

Selegiline

Brand name: *Eldepryl*

What this drug does for you:

Selegiline is used along with levodopa and carbidopa to treat Parkinson's disease. It works with levodopa to improve walking ability, speech, and shaking muscles.

Possible side effects of this drug:

- Some of the worst and most common side effects are nausea, hallucinations, confusion, depression, insomnia, uncontrollable muscle movements, irregular heartbeat, agitation, chest pain, and high blood pressure.
- Other possible side effects are swelling ankles, anxiety, burning lips or mouth, constipation, drowsiness, increased sweating, bleeding in the stomach, hair loss, increased shakiness, nervousness, weakness, and weight loss.

Special warnings:

- Call your doctor if you develop a severe headache or any unusual symptoms.

Pregnancy and nursing mothers:

Category C. See page 9 for description of categories. Not known if drug is present in mother's milk.

Possible food and drug interactions:

- Taking selegiline with the pain medicine meperidine (Demerol) may cause high fever, seizures, and coma.
- After taking the antidepressant fluoxetine, you should wait five weeks before you begin taking selegiline. You should wait 14 days after you quit taking selegiline before you begin taking fluoxetine.
- Your doctor may reduce your dosage of levodopa after you begin taking selegiline.

Helpful hints:

- The usual adult dosage is 5 mg taken at breakfast and 5 mg taken at lunch.
- You should never take more than 10 mg of selegiline a day. Taking more than this amount could cause dangerously high blood pressure. Call your doctor if you develop a severe headache — it could be a sign of high blood pressure.

Trihexyphenidyl

Brand name: *Artane*

What this drug does for you:

Trihexyphenidyl is used to treat Parkinson's disease. It is usually combined with levodopa. Trihexyphenidyl is also used to treat stiffness and shaking caused by some medicines.

Possible side effects of this drug:
- Dry mouth, blurred vision, dizziness, nausea, and nervousness are common side effects. These side effects usually go away after you've been taking the drug for a while.
- Other side effects are constipation, confusion, memory loss, hallucinations, mental disturbances, skin rashes, and difficulty urinating.

Special warnings:
- This drug has drying side effects (for instance, it can keep you from sweating properly). You should be very careful in hot weather, and watch yourself for signs of heatstroke.
- People with certain kinds of glaucoma, people with high blood pressure, and people with heart, liver, kidney, or prostate problems should use this drug very carefully.

Pregnancy and nursing mothers:
Not known whether it is safe to use during pregnancy.

Possible food and drug interactions:
- If you also take phenothiazines, haloperidol, tricyclic antidepressants, or other drugs that have drying side effects, make sure you report to your doctor any signs of fever or stomach complaints or any signs that you can't tolerate heat.

Helpful hints:
- You shouldn't drive a car or operate heavy machinery until you are sure the medicine isn't making you drowsy or less than alert.
- If this drug makes you produce extra saliva, you may prefer to take it after meals. If it causes dry mouth, you may want to take it after you eat, unless it causes you to be nauseated.
- Mint candies, chewing gum, and water can help relieve dry mouth.
- The usual daily dose for adults ranges from 5 to 15 mg.

Natural Alternatives

ATTENTION DEFICIT DISORDER

- ◄ Disorganized
- ◄ Emotional difficulties
- ◄ Hyperactive
- ◄ Impulsive
- ◄ Poor planning ability
- ◄ Restless

- ◄ Easily distracted
- ◄ Frequent mood swings
- ◄ Impatient
- ◄ Inattentive
- ◄ Relationship difficulties
- ◄ Short temper

How to succeed in spite of ADD

Pay attention! For many people this simple command may be almost impossible to follow. An estimated 5 percent of American children suffer from attention deficit disorder (ADD). Although most people think that children simply outgrow ADD, 30 to 70 percent of them carry it into adulthood.

Adults with ADD often have career problems. Disorganization can cause poor job performance. Lack of social skills makes relationships with co-workers more difficult. The impulsive nature of the person with ADD may lead him to change jobs frequently.

In order to overcome ADD, you must first identify the problem. Since anxiety and depression cause many of the same symptoms as ADD, you and your doctor will want to rule out those possibilities first.

If you definitely have ADD, there are many strategies for controlling the disorder. The parents of children with ADD must learn to manage the behavior of their children. In the same manner, you can learn to manage your own behavior. Structure your environment. Practice self-control. Easier said than done, right? Here are some suggestions to help get you started on the right track.

Set goals. Think about what you want to accomplish from day to day, and set realistic goals for yourself. Make lists and follow them.

Reward yourself. When you achieve a particular goal, pat yourself on the back. Treat yourself to something special.

Persistence pays off. If you don't accomplish every single goal right away, don't waste time and energy worrying about it. Simply try again.

Take breaks. The inattentiveness caused by ADD can be lessened if you try to structure your day so that you have several short breaks rather than one long lunch hour.

Be active. ADD is often accompanied by hyperactivity. Exercise will work off excess energy, so consider joining an aerobics class or participate in your favorite sport. You'll feel better and probably look better too!

Watch out for sugar. Foods high in carbohydrates may increase inattentiveness and hyperactivity in some people. Making sure you eat some protein whenever you eat carbohydrates may help take the edge off the "sugar high."

Identify allergies. Food allergies and intolerances can sometimes cause or aggravate ADD. The foods that most often cause problems are:

◁ Caffeine
◁ Chocolate
◁ Corn
◁ Eggs
◁ Fish
◁ Food additives such as MSG
◁ Food dyes
◁ Grains (especially wheat)
◁ Milk and milk products
◁ Nuts
◁ Strawberries
◁ Yeast

If you suspect you have food allergies, try eliminating items one at a time from your diet. If you notice an improvement in your ADD symptoms after avoiding a particular food for a few days, you may have uncovered a food allergy.

Take time for therapy. Years of dealing with ADD and its effects can leave you frustrated and tired. Therapy sometimes offers assistance in understanding and coping with your disorder. Short-term psychotherapy, also called "talk therapy," can pinpoint your problems and help you formulate a treatment plan. Long-term psychotherapy can help you maintain stable relationships and control mood swings.

Search out support groups. Sometimes it helps just to know that you're not alone. Others who have experienced the same problems can offer encouragement and support. They also may have helpful suggestions for coping with the disorder.

The frustration experienced by adults with ADD can be devastating. However, you can learn to control the effects of this disorder and overcome its problems. With proper diagnosis and treatment, all that negative frustration can be turned into positive and productive energy.

Sources —
Attention, Please, SPI Press, Atlanta, 1991
C.H.A.D.D. Facts, 499 Northwest 70th Ave., Suite 109, Plantation, Fla. 33317, 1993

EPILEPSY

◀ **Loss of consciousness**   ◀ **Stiffness**
◀ **Tingling sensation**   ◀ **Twitching**
◀ **Uncontrollable jerking**

Stop the shakes

An epileptic seizure can really shake you up, in more ways than one.

Epileptic seizures are caused by electrical malfunctions in the brain. Epilepsy has sort of the same effect as a short circuit in your car, which may cause the headlights to flicker.

There are different types of epileptic seizures. Tonic-clonic, or grand mal, seizures cause you to lose consciousness, become stiff, and jerk uncontrollably. Absence seizures cause you to simply drift into an unconscious state for a few seconds.

While most seizures are not usually dangerous, they can be frightening. Luckily, there are things you can do to control your seizures.

Keep your distance from the television. Video devices such as televisions, computer monitors, and video games have been known to trigger seizures. While video screens don't cause epilepsy, they may provoke seizures in people who are sensitive to the flashing lights and colors they display. The closer you are to the screen, the more sensitive you are. Sit at least six feet away from the television.

Get plenty of sleep and try to control stress. The chances of experiencing a seizure while watching television or playing a video game are made greater by lack of sleep or emotional stress.

Wear sunglasses. People who are sensitive to video screens may also be sensitive to flickering sunlight. Wearing sunglasses or closing one eye may help.

Check the label. Some video games and computer software carry warning labels to people with epilepsy. Also, a program or game which is too complex for your television or computer may lower the frequency of the screen. The screen cannot keep up with images of the program, resulting in a jerky, flickering effect which could bring on a seizure.

Figure out if you have food triggers. Sensitivity to certain foods may increase epileptic seizures. Some people with epilepsy have noticed that foods which contain organic acids (apples, tomatoes, citrus fruits) may cause more frequent attacks.

Also, foods exposed to metal during processing, such as homogenized milk, and food sprayed with metal-containing chemicals like pesticides and fungicides may increase attacks. The time lapse between the food and the seizures is usually about 18 to 24 hours, which may make it harder to recognize the connection.

Can the caffeine. Excessive amounts of caffeine may make epilepsy more difficult to control, so limiting coffee or cola intake may be helpful. A recent study found that many people with severe epilepsy consumed more than 400 milligrams of caffeine a day, enough to cause caffeine intoxication.

Following these suggestions may help you to avoid seizures, and reduce your need for medication.

Sources —
Journal of the Royal Society of Medicine (86,2:110)
The Lancet (344,8930:1102)

NARCOLEPSY

◄ Extreme sleepiness   ◄ Hallucinations
◄ Memory lapses   ◄ Poor sleep at night
◄ Sudden spell of weakness   ◄ Temporary paralysis
◄ Vision problems

Natural ways to keep yourself from nodding off

Two centuries ago, falling asleep in a Puritan church could earn you a rap with a ruler. Today, falling asleep in church might not necessarily mean the sermon is boring. You may have a condition called narcolepsy.

The main symptom of narcolepsy is extreme sleepiness, which is not relieved by sleeping. It occurs most often in boring, nonactive situations. Any type of activity may help relieve the symptoms of extreme sleepiness. Taking a brisk walk outdoors, talking, and even chewing gum can help wake you up.

Another symptom of narcolepsy is cataplexy, a sudden weakness usually brought on by strong emotion such as excitement, laughter, anger, or surprise. Severe attacks can cause paralysis, but normally attacks last less than a minute, and may cause the person to drop things or simply sit down.

The best remedy for narcolepsy is to try and take naps of 15 to 20 minutes at least three times a day. Regular naps may even reduce your need for medication. You may have to change your schedule a bit in order to nab the naps you need, but isn't that better than nodding off just when the sermon is getting good?

Sources —
American Family Physician (42,6:1641)
The New England Journal of Medicine (323,6:389)

PARKINSON'S DISEASE

◀ Arm, hand, or leg tremors   ◀ Shuffling, unbalanced walk
◀ Slowness of movement   ◀ Stiffness
◀ Unblinking, fixed expression   ◀ Weakness

Living with Parkinson's

You've always been an active, outgoing person. And even though you've been diagnosed with Parkinson's, you still have a life to live. With just a few adjustments, you can look forward to living it to the fullest.

Because the main drug used in the treatment of Parkinson's, levodopa (L-dopa), loses its effectiveness over time, you should try to delay the need for medication as long as possible. Your doctor may prescribe other medications in the beginning.

In addition, there are some natural ways you can control the severity of symptoms and improve your quality of life.

Exercise. If you begin an exercise program in the early stages of the disease, you can help prevent or delay some of the stiffness and energy loss. Doctors recommend aerobic exercises, as well as a strengthening program.

Water exercises can be helpful, and fun besides. Because Parkinson's affects a person's balance, certain forms of exercise, such as bicycling, horseback riding, or skiing may be difficult, and even dangerous.

The American Parkinson's Disease Association offers a free booklet of strengthening and flexibility exercises titled *Be Active: A Suggested Exercise Program for People with Parkinson's*. You can call and request the booklet at 1-800-223-2732 or write to them at 60 Bay Street, Suite 401, Staten Island, NY 10301.

Seek support. It can be helpful to meet and talk with other people who are dealing with Parkinson's. Support groups can also help you deal with depression, although you may need professional help as well.

Eat a balanced diet. If you have trouble eating balanced meals on a regular basis, consider taking a multivitamin. Some studies suggest that antioxidant vitamins such as vitamins A, C, and E may help people with Parkinson's. While high doses of these vitamins did not seem to help control the disease, a multivitamin will help ensure that you get the minimum amount your body requires.

Plan for protein. Your protein intake can decrease the effectiveness of L-dopa.

Recent research suggests that you should try to take your medication 45 minutes to an hour before eating.

You may also want to try rationing your protein throughout the day. Experts often recommend the seven-parts-carbohydrate to one-part-protein meal plan.

A company called Elan Pharma offers a line of ready-made products which are formulated according to this seven-to-one ratio. They also have a dietitian available who can answer your questions about meal planning. Their toll-free number is 1-800-473-3663.

Restrict your protein to about 150 grams, the minimum recommended daily allowance. Be sure that you continue to eat the recommended daily allowance of calcium. Most adults require at least 1,000 mg of calcium every day. Watch out for extreme weight loss, which can be a serious problem with Parkinson's. Consulting with a dietitian in your area can be very beneficial.

Bring on the broad beans. Also known as fava beans, broad beans look like large lima beans. Some research suggests that substituting these beans for other protein sources may help control varying responses to L-dopa.

Bulk up your diet with fiber. Since constipation is a common complication of Parkinson's, it will be helpful to add extra fiber and fluids to your diet.

Sign up for speech therapy. The loss of muscle control caused by the disease can affect the way you talk. Therapy can help improve speech patterns, making the disorder less noticeable to others.

Therapy may also help with any swallowing difficulties. One technique that can help with swallowing is to divide your food into small bites.

Even though Parkinson's is a serious and progressive disease, you can improve your situation. Keep a positive attitude, follow your treatment program, and you can control Parkinson's, instead of letting it control you.

Sources —

Nursing Homes and Senior Citizen Care (40,3:33)
Nutrition Research Newsletter (12,4:48; 11,10:115; 11,11:130 and 13,4:48)
Physical Therapy (75,5:363)
The Physician and Sportsmedicine (19,12:85)
The Western Journal of Medicine (161,3:303)

> Please check with your doctor for approval before taking or discontinuing any prescription drug or using a natural healing alternative.

BREATHING PROBLEMS

Prescription Drugs

Natural Alternatives

Prescription Drugs

ASTHMA DRUGS

Albuterol (also known as Salbutamol)
Inhaler, syrup or tablets

Brand names: *Proventil, Ventolin, Volmax* **(Generic available)**

What this drug does for you:
Albuterol is a bronchodilator. It relieves wheezing and the bronchial spasms that accompany asthma, bronchitis, and emphysema by relaxing the bronchial muscles and reducing inflammation. The bronchi are the air passages that lead to the lungs. Albuterol is commonly used to prevent exercise-induced asthma.

Possible side effects of this drug:
- The most common side effects are tremor (shakiness), nervousness, rapid or irregular heartbeat, and a worsening of the asthma symptoms.
- About 3 percent to 6 percent of people taking albuterol get headaches, insomnia, dizziness, high blood pressure, cough, throat irritation, stomachache, and nausea. Headache and a rapid heartbeat may be more common with the extended-release tablets.
- Less common side effects are diarrhea, muscle cramps, heartburn, and weakness.

Special warnings:
- Most importantly, you should never use this drug more frequently than your doctor recommends. The effects of each dose may last from six to eight hours or longer. Extended release tablets last for 12 hours or longer. An overdose can cause a heart attack or sudden death. Talk to your doctor if you aren't getting relief from your asthma symptoms.
- If you have heart disease, an irregular heartbeat, high blood pressure, diabetes, or an overactive thyroid, talk to your doctor about your condition before using this drug. Your doctor should monitor your blood pressure and your heart condition while you are taking albuterol.

Pregnancy and nursing mothers:
Category C. See page 9 for description of categories. Not known if drug is

present in mother's milk.

Possible food and drug interactions:

- Taking other bronchodilators or epinephrine while taking albuterol increases your risk of heart problems such as cardiac arrest. You can use an aerosol inhaler and a tablet or syrup bronchodilator at the same time if you are under the close supervision of your doctor.
- Taking monoamine oxidase (MAO) inhibitors, a type of antidepressant, and tricyclic antidepressants while taking albuterol can raise your blood pressure and cause heart problems.
- Taking beta-blockers (a type of blood pressure drug) while taking albuterol can reduce the effectiveness of both drugs.

Helpful hints:

- For the inhalation aerosol, the effect of the medicine may be decreased if the canister is cold. Shake well before using. Ventolin Nebules Inhalation Solution should be stored in the refrigerator.
- To prevent exercise-induced asthma, the usual adult dosage is two inhalations of the aerosol or one 200-mcg capsule taken with a Rotahaler 15 minutes before exercise.
- For the inhalation aerosol, the usual adult dosage is two inhalations every four to six hours.
- For the inhalation solution, the usual adult dosage is 2.5 mg three to four times daily.
- For the Rotahaler capsules, the usual adult dosage is one 200-mcg capsule every four to six hours.
- For the syrup, the usual adult dosage is 1 to 2 teaspoonfuls three or four times a day.
- For the tablets, the usual adult dosage is 2 to 4 mg three or four times a day.
- The extended-release tablets must be swallowed whole with a liquid. You should not chew or crush the tablet. The usual dosage is 8 mg every 12 hours.
- See page 39 for instructions on how to use your inhaler correctly.

Cromolyn

Brand names: *Gastrocrom, Intal, Nasalcrom* (Generic available)

What this drug does for you:

Cromolyn treats asthma and allergies by preventing the immune cells called "mast cells" from releasing the chemical histamine. Histamine causes allergic reactions and inflammation of the airways.

The aerosol, the inhalation capsules, and the inhalation solution help prevent spasms of the bronchi (the air passages that lead to the lungs) caused by exercise, certain toxins, pollutants, cold air, etc. The nasal solution is used to prevent or treat allergic rhinitis.

The capsule form is commonly used to treat people with mastocytosis. The main sign of mastocytosis is brown, itchy patches on the skin. The capsules help most people with the nausea, vomiting, diarrhea, stomachache, headache, flushing, hives, and itching that accompany the condition.

Possible side effects of this drug:

- The most common side effects of the capsules are headache and diarrhea. The inhaled forms commonly cause coughing, stuffy nose, sneezing, mild wheezing, and nausea. The nasal solution can cause your nose to sting and burn and, rarely, can cause postnasal drip and a bad taste.
- Rarer side effects are itching, muscle pain, stomachache, irritability, and rash.

Special warnings:

- Anyone who has had an allergic reaction to any form of this drug should not use it.
- Rarely, cromolyn may cause a severe allergic reaction.
- People with poor liver or kidney function may need a lower-than-usual dose.
- People allergic to lactose should not take the inhalation capsule form.
- This drug should not be used to treat severe asthma attacks.
- People with coronary artery disease or heart arrhythmias should use inhalers cautiously because of the propellants they contain.

Pregnancy and nursing mothers:

Category B. See page 9 for description of categories. Not known if drug is present in mother's milk.

Possible food and drug interactions:

No significant interactions.

Helpful hints:

- The usual adult dosage for the capsule form is two capsules four times daily — one-half hour before meals and at bedtime. Open the capsules and pour the powder into a half glass of hot water. Stir until completely dissolved, adding cold water while you are stirring. Don't mix with fruit juice, milk, or foods.
- The usual adult dosage for the inhalation capsule form is one capsule inhaled (not swallowed) four times a day at regular intervals. Try rinsing your mouth or taking a drink of water before and after inhaling to prevent coughing and throat irritation.
- The usual adult dosage for the inhalation solution is two metered inhalations four times daily at regular intervals. Don't exceed this dosage.
- The usual adult dosage for the nebulizer solution is one ampule four times a day at regular intervals.
- To prevent bronchospasm caused by exercise, cold air, etc., use the inhaler or nebulizing solution 10 to 15 minutes before exposure to whatever causes your asthma attack.
- The usual adult dosage for the nasal solution form is one spray in each nostril three to four times a day at regular intervals. Clear your nose before spraying. Inhale through your nose while you use the spray.
- You may need to take the drug for several weeks before you notice any

improvement.
- Don't stop taking this drug or reduce the dose without talking to your doctor. Asthma symptoms may get worse.
- You usually begin taking cromolyn in addition to your regular asthma medicine (such as a bronchodilator). You may be able to gradually decrease your other medication under your doctor's supervision.
- See page 39 for instructions on how to use your inhaler correctly.

Dyphylline

Brand names: *Dilor, Lufyllin* **(Generic available)**

What this drug does for you:

Dyphylline is a bronchodilator. It relieves acute asthma and the wheezing and bronchial spasms that accompany bronchitis and emphysema. It works by relaxing the bronchial muscles and the surrounding blood vessels. The bronchi are the air passages that lead to the lungs.

Possible side effects of this drug:

- Possible side effects are nausea, vomiting, headache, irritability, restlessness, insomnia, heart palpitations, or rapid heartbeat.
- Less common side effects are stomach pain, diarrhea, muscle twitching, seizures, flushing, low blood pressure, heart failure, rapid breathing, high blood sugar, and kidney problems.

Special warnings:

- Don't use if you are allergic or hypersensitive to caffeine or any of the other bronchodilators that are "xanthine derivatives."
- Use with caution if you have heart disease, overactive thyroid, high blood pressure, damage to the heart, or stomach ulcer.

Pregnancy and nursing mothers:

Category C. See page 9 for description of categories. Drug is present in mother's milk.

Possible food and drug interactions:

- If you take the gout drug probenecid, your blood levels of dyphylline may increase.
- If you take another bronchodilator (such as theophylline) and ephedrine along with dyphylline, the effects of all three drugs may be increased and your central nervous system may be overstimulated. Some over-the-counter drugs contain theophylline and ephedrine.

Helpful hints:

- The usual adult dosage is 15 mg/kg every six hours.
- Dyphylline may cause less nausea than theophylline, a similar bronchodilator.

Ipratropium

Brand name: *Atrovent*

What this drug does for you:

Ipratropium is a bronchodilator that treats the bronchial spasms associated with emphysema and chronic bronchitis. The bronchi are the air passages that lead to the lungs. Ipratropium is meant for long-term treatment, not for acute episodes of bronchospasm where you need a rapid response.

Ipratropium is different from most other bronchodilators because it is an "anticholinergic." That means it blocks the nerve impulses that cause the bronchial muscles to contract.

Possible side effects of this drug:

- The most common side effects are coughing, dry mouth, and nervousness. You may also experience dizziness, headache, nausea, stomachache, and blurred vision.
- Rare side effects are rapid heartbeat, drowsiness, coordination difficulty, itching, hives, flushing, loss of hair, constipation, tremor, and mouth ulcers.

Special warnings:

- Don't use ipratropium if you are allergic to atropine or its derivatives or if you are allergic to food products such as soybean or lecithin (found in milk, egg yolks, corn, etc.)
- Use ipratropium cautiously if you have some kinds of glaucoma (consult your doctor), bladder neck obstruction, or enlarged prostate.

Pregnancy and nursing mothers:

Category B. See page 9 for description of categories. Not known if drug is present in mother's milk.

Possible food and drug interactions:

No significant interactions.

Helpful hints:

- Avoid accidently spraying ipratropium in your eyes. Your vision may be blurred temporarily.
- Don't skip a dose. You need to use ipratropium consistently to get the full effect.
- People have used this drug with other bronchodilators and asthma drugs without negative effects.
- The usual adult dosage of the inhalation aerosol is two inhalations four times a day. You should not exceed 12 inhalations in 24 hours.
- The usual adult dosage of the inhalation solution is 500 mcg three to four times a day, with doses six to eight hours apart.
- See page 39 for instructions on how to use your inhaler correctly.

How to use your inhaler

The medicine in your inhaler can immediately relax your lung muscles and expand your airways — if you use it correctly. But over half the people who use an inhaler don't know exactly how to use it.

That means most of the medicine ends up in your mouth instead of your lungs. And one recent study revealed that only 4 percent of women with asthma used their inhalers correctly. Women may have more trouble because inhalers are often too large for them. Here's the correct way to use an inhaler:

1) Holding the inhaler upright, shake thoroughly. (Don't forget to remove the cap! One asthma sufferer who woke during the night with shortness of breath forgot to remove the cap and then swallowed it.)
2) Tilt your head back and exhale.
3) Put the mouthpiece in a position that is comfortable for you. Doctors usually suggest one of three positions:
   - Place the inhaler one to two inches away from your mouth.
   - Place the mouthpiece inside your mouth with your lips firmly around it.
   - Use a spacer. Spacers are tubes that connect the inhaler to your mouth. They will hold the medication until you inhale.
4) Start to breathe in slowly just as you press down on the inhaler to release the medicine. This simultaneous action seems to cause the most problems for people using inhalers. Concentrate on the activity and you will soon realize that it's not difficult at all. Remember to breathe in slowly, taking three to five seconds for each breath. You shouldn't see medicine in the air or feel it land on your tongue.
5) In order for the medicine to spread throughout the lungs, hold your breath for 10 seconds.
6) Repeat puffs as directed. You may want to wait one minute between puffs to get the full effect.
7) If you are buying inhaler refills earlier than the date suggested on the label, you may be overusing your inhaler. Consult your doctor because you may need another medication.
8) Finally, don't forget to clean your mouthpiece regularly to avoid buildup. Clean with warm water and soap, and air-dry. Keep the cap on your inhaler when you're not using it so dust and lint will stay out.

Once you start using the inhaler correctly, you will soon realize the medication really does work. It's simple, easy, and provides immediate relief.

Medical Sources —
Medical Tribune (35,24:7)
The Asthma and Allergy Advance (Jan/Feb 1994)

Metaproterenol

Brand names: *Alupent, Metaprel* **(Generic available)**

What this drug does for you:

Metaproterenol is a bronchodilator that works quickly (within five to 30 minutes) to provide temporary relief of the breathing difficulties and wheezing associated with asthma, emphysema, and bronchitis. Some forms of metaproterenol are also used to treat acute asthma attacks in children 6 years and older.

Possible side effects of this drug:

- The most common side effect of metaproterenol is nervousness. A smaller number of the people taking metaproterenol have headaches, dizziness, heart palpitations or an irregular heartbeat, stomachache, tremor (shakiness), throat irritation, nausea, and cough.
- The least common side effects that have been reported are insomnia, fatigue, diarrhea, bad taste, and drowsiness.
- The side effects may be worse for children.
- Very rarely, this drug can cause bronchospasm or a worsening of your asthma. Contact your doctor immediately if this happens.

Special warnings:

- You should use this drug with extreme caution if you have high blood pressure, an irregular heartbeat, heart disease, overactive thyroid, diabetes, or a history of convulsions.

Pregnancy and nursing mothers:

Category C. See page 9 for description of categories. Not known if drug is present in mother's milk.

Possible food and drug interactions:

- Don't use with other bronchodilators.
- Taking monoamine oxidase (MAO) inhibitors, a type of antidepressant, and tricyclic antidepressants while taking metaproterenol can raise your blood pressure and cause heart problems.

Helpful hints:

- The usual adult dose of the inhalation aerosol is two to three inhalations. Don't use more often than every three to four hours. Don't use more than 12 inhalations a day.
- Don't use this drug more frequently than your doctor recommends. An overdose can cause a heart attack or sudden death. Talk to your doctor if you aren't getting relief from your asthma symptoms.
- See page 39 for instructions on how to use your inhaler correctly.

Pirbuterol

Brand names: *Maxair Autohaler, Maxair Inhaler*

What this drug does for you:
Pirbuterol is a bronchodilator. It prevents and reverses bronchospasm caused by asthma by relaxing the bronchial muscles and reducing inflammation. The bronchi are the air passages that lead to the lungs. Pirbuterol can be used along with theophylline and/or steroid therapy.

Possible side effects of this drug:
- The most common side effects of pirbuterol are nervousness, tremors (shakiness), headache, dizziness, heart palpitations or a rapid heartbeat, coughing, and nausea.
- Rare side effects are depression, anxiety, insomnia, weakness, fainting, low blood pressure, chest pain, dry mouth, stomach pain, diarrhea, smell and taste changes, rash, hair loss, bruising, weight gain, and flushing.

Special warnings:
- People with a history of seizures, diabetes, overactive thyroid, high blood pres-sure, irregular heartbeat, or heart disease should use this drug with caution.
- Pirbuterol can affect your blood pressure. You should have it tested regularly while taking the drug.

Pregnancy and nursing mothers:
Category C. See page 9 for description of categories. Not known if drug is present in mother's milk.

Possible food and drug interactions:
- Don't use with other beta adrenergic aerosol bronchodilators.
- Taking monoamine oxidase (MAO) inhibitors, a type of antidepressant, and tricyclic antidepressants while taking pirbuterol can raise your blood pressure and cause heart problems.

Helpful hints:
- Don't take more medicine than you are prescribed or stop taking your medicine without consulting your doctor. Call your doctor if your asthma symptoms get worse.
- The usual adult dose is two inhalations every four to six hours. You should not take more than 12 inhalations in one day.
- See page 39 for instructions on how to use your inhaler correctly.

Terbutaline

Brand names: *Brethaire, Brethine, Bricanyl*

What this drug does for you:
Terbutaline is a bronchodilator that works within five to 30 minutes to relieve wheezing and the bronchial spasms that accompany asthma, bronchitis, and emphysema. It relaxes the bronchial muscles and reduces inflamma-

tion. The bronchi are the air passages that lead to the lungs.

Possible side effects of this drug:

- Common side effects are a rapid or irregular heartbeat, headache, tremors (shakiness), nervousness, drowsiness, and dizziness. Other possible side effects are nausea, stomachache, chest pain, sweating, flushing, insomnia, and dry mouth and throat. Most of these side effects are temporary and will go away after you've been taking terbutaline for a while.
- There have been rare reports of seizures in people taking this drug.

Special warning:

- If you have heart disease, an irregular heartbeat, low potassium levels, high blood pressure, diabetes, or an overactive thyroid, talk to your doctor about your condition before using this drug. Your doctor should monitor your blood pressure and your heart condition while you are taking terbutaline.

Pregnancy and nursing mothers:

Category B. See page 9 for description of categories. Drug is present in mother's milk.

Possible food and drug interactions:

- Taking other bronchodilators or epinephrine while taking terbutaline increases your risk of heart problems such as cardiac arrest. You can use an aerosol inhaler and a tablet or syrup bronchodilator at the same time if you are under the close supervision of your doctor.
- Taking monoamine oxidase (MAO) inhibitors, a type of antidepressant, and tricyclic antidepressants while taking terbutaline can raise your blood pressure and cause heart problems.
- Taking beta-blockers (a type of blood pressure drug) while taking terbutaline can reduce the effectiveness of both drugs.

Helpful hints:

- Don't take more medicine than you are prescribed or stop taking your medicine without consulting your doctor. Call your doctor if your asthma symptoms get worse.
- The usual adult dose of the inhalation aerosol is two inhalations separated by one minute every four to six hours.
- The usual adult dose of the tablets is 5 mg three times a day, approximately every six hours.
- After you've taken terbutaline for a while, you may develop a tolerance to it. In other words, each dose may not relieve your symptoms for as long as it once did.
- The usual adult dose of the injection is 0.25 mg in the side of the deltoid muscle, which covers the shoulder and upper arm. If your symptoms don't improve in 15 to 30 minutes, you can inject another 0.25 mg dose.
- See page 39 for instructions on how to use your inhaler correctly.

Theophylline

Brand names: *Aerolate, Aerolate Jr. T.D., Aerolate SR & JR, Elixophyllin, Elixophyllin SR, Quibron-T, Quibron-T/SR, Respbid, Slo-bid, Slo-Phyllin, Theo-24, Theo-Dur, Theo-X, Theoclear, Theolair, Theolair SR, T-PHYL, Uniphyl*

What this drug does for you:

Theophylline is a bronchodilator. It relieves acute asthma and the wheezing and bronchial spasms that accompany bronchitis and emphysema. The bronchi are the air passages that lead to the lungs. Theophylline works by relaxing the bronchial muscles and the surrounding blood vessels, expanding your lung capacity and improving lung circulation.

Possible side effects of this drug:

- This drug may cause nausea, diarrhea, stomach pain, vomiting blood, palpitations or a rapid heartbeat, low blood pressure, respiratory problems, flushing, high blood sugar levels, hair loss, rash, headache, insomnia, irritability, restlessness, convulsions, and muscle twitching.

Special warnings:

- This drug should not be taken by people with stomach ulcers or a seizure disorder, unless it is being controlled by a seizure drug.
- Don't use if you are allergic or hypersensitive to caffeine or any of the other bronchodilators that are "xanthine derivatives."
- Use this drug cautiously if you have high blood pressure.
- Theophylline can accumulate to toxic levels if you have poor liver function or heart failure, or if you are over 55 with lung disease, or if you are taking other bronchodilators or ephedrine. Toxicity can cause serious side effects, even death, without warning. Contact your doctor immediately if you experience nausea, restlessness, irregular heartbeat, or convulsions.

Pregnancy and nursing mothers:

Category C. See page 9 for description of categories. Drug is present in mother's milk.

Possible food and drug interactions:

- Theophylline may decrease blood levels of the seizure drug phenytoin and the antipsychotic drug lithium.
- The ulcer drug cimetidine, birth control pills, the beta-blocker propanolol, the gout drug allopurinol, the antibiotics erythromycin and troleandomycin, and the antibacterial drug ciprofloxacin may increase blood levels of theophylline.
- The tuberculosis drug rifampin and the seizure drug phenytoin may decrease blood levels of theophylline.
- If you take another bronchodilator or ephedrine along with theophylline, the effects of both drugs may be increased.

Helpful hints:
- Don't crush, dissolve, or chew tablets.
- Don't take the tablets more often than your doctor prescribes.
- Taking theophylline after a high-fat meal may slightly slow down the rate your body absorbs the drug. However, unless your doctor tells you otherwise, you can take the drug without regard to when you eat.
- Take your medicine at the same time every day.
- If you are taking a tablet once a day, take the whole tablet. Don't split it.

ANTIHISTAMINES

Astemizole

Brand name: *Hismanal*

What this drug does for you:
Astemizole is a long-lasting, nonsedating antihistamine meant to relieve allergy symptoms such as sneezing, runny nose, itching, rashes, hives, swelling, and difficulty breathing.

Possible side effects of this drug:
- The most common side effects are fatigue, increased appetite and weight gain, nervousness, dizziness, and dry mouth. Astemizole doesn't have the sedating effect that many of the older antihistamines have.
- Rare heart rhythm disturbances are the most serious risk of taking astemizole. If you feel dizzy or faint while taking astemizole, you should immediately contact your doctor. It could be a warning sign of severe heart problems.

Special warnings:
- This drug should not be used by people with liver disease, and probably shouldn't be used by people with kidney disease.
- You shouldn't use astemizole if you have a lower respiratory disease, such as asthma, bronchitis, or pneumonia. Astemizole can dry out and thicken the mucus in your airways, making it more difficult to remove.

Pregnancy and nursing mothers:
Category C. See page 9 for description of categories. Not known if drug is present in mother's milk.

Possible food and drug interactions:
- You should not use astemizole while using the antibiotic erythromycin or the similar antibiotics troleandomycin, azithromycin, and clarithromycin.
- Don't use astemizole while taking the antifungals ketoconazole or itraconazole. The drug interaction could cause serious heart problems. Other similar antifungals you may want to avoid using while you are taking astemizole are fluconazole, metronidazole, and miconazole.
- Using astemizole witn certain drugs may put you at a greater risk for

heart problems. These drugs are probucol, certain drugs for irregular heart rhythms, certain tricyclic antidepressants, certain phenothiazines, certain calcium channel blockers such as bepridil, and terfenadine.

Helpful hints:
- You will not get the full effect of astemizole if you take it with a meal because you won't absorb it all. Take the medicine on an empty stomach, at least two hours after or one hour before a meal.
- Astemizole will not relieve your symptoms immediately. Some people, trying to speed up the action of the drug, have taken extra medicine and have had trouble with side effects. You shouldn't take more than the recommended dose, which is one tablet (10 mg) a day.

Clemastine

Brand name: *Tavist* **(Generic available)**

What this drug does for you:
This 12-hour antihistamine relieves allergy symptoms such as sneezing, runny nose, tearing eyes, itching, rashes, hives, swelling, and difficulty breathing.

Possible side effects of this drug:
- Clemastine is a sedating antihistamine. The most common side effects are sleepiness and dry mouth. Also common are dizziness, lack of coordination, stomachache, and a thickening of the mucus in your airways.
- If you are over 60, you're more likely to feel dizzy and sedated and have low blood pressure while taking clemastine.
- Rare side effects common to most antihistamines are fatigue, confusion, restlessness, nervousness, tremor (shakiness), irritability, insomnia, euphoria, tingling, blurred or double vision, pain or ringing in the ears, hysteria, nerve inflammation, convulsions, loss of appetite, nausea, vomiting, diarrhea, constipation, tightness of the chest, wheezing, stuffy nose, low blood pressure, headache, palpitations, rapid heartbeat, anemia and various blood disorders, urinary problems, menstrual cycle problems, hives, drug rash, allergic shock reaction, sensitivity to light, and sweating.

Special warnings:
- This drug should not be used by people with some kinds of glaucoma, bladder neck obstruction, obstruction of the pylorus (opening from the stomach to the intestine), stomach ulcer, or an enlarged prostate.
- You shouldn't use clemastine if you have a lower respiratory disease, such as asthma, bronchitis, or pneumonia. Clemastine can dry out and thicken the mucus in your airways, making it more difficult to remove.
- You should use clemastine cautiously if you have increased pressure in the eye, an overactive thyroid, heart disease, or high blood pressure.

Pregnancy and nursing mothers:

Category B. See page 9 for description of categories. Don't use while breast-feeding. Babies, especially newborn and premature infants, have a higher risk of severe reactions to clemastine.

Possible food and drug interactions:

- Don't take clemastine if you are taking antidepressant drugs called monoamine oxidase (MAO) inhibitors. The effects of both drugs are increased and can result in very low blood pressure and other serious reactions.
- While taking clemastine, avoid alcohol and other depressants such as sleeping pills and tranquilizers.

Helpful hints:

- This drug may make you feel sleepy and sedated, so drive cautiously. Don't try to mow your lawn or operate machinery until you figure out how the medicine affects you.
- The usual adult starting dose of the syrup is 2 teaspoonfuls of clemastine twice daily. You shouldn't take more than 12 teaspoonfuls a day.
- The maximum recommended dosage of the 2.68 mg tablets is one tablet three times daily.

Cyproheptadine

Brand name: *Periactin*

What this drug does for you:

This antihistamine relieves symptoms of food allergies, hay fever, allergy to cold temperatures, and other allergies. It helps relieve sneezing, runny nose, itching, rashes, hives, swelling, and difficulty breathing. Cyproheptadine can be used to treat severe allergic reactions in addition to epinephrine.

Possible side effects of this drug:

- Cyproheptadine is a sedating antihistamine. The most common side effects are sleepiness and dry mouth. The sleepiness may go away after you've been taking the drug for a while. Also common are dizziness, lack of coordination, stomachache, and a thickening of the mucus in your airways.
- If you are over 60, you're more likely to feel dizzy and sedated and have low blood pressure while taking cyproheptadine.
- Rare side effects common to most antihistamines are fatigue, confusion, restlessness, nervousness, tremor (shakiness), irritability, insomnia, euphoria, tingling, blurred or double vision, pain or ringing in the ears, hysteria, nerve inflammation, convulsions, loss of appetite, nausea, vomiting, diarrhea, constipation, tightness of the chest, wheezing, stuffy nose, low blood pressure, headache, palpitations, rapid heartbeat, anemia and various blood disorders, urinary problems, menstrual cycle problems, hives, drug rash, allergic shock reaction, sensitivity to light, and sweating.

Special warnings:

- This drug should not be used by people with some kinds of glaucoma, bladder neck obstruction, obstruction of the pylorus (opening from the stomach to the intestine), stomach ulcer, or an enlarged prostate.
- You shouldn't use cyproheptadine if you have a lower respiratory disease, such as asthma, bronchitis, or pneumonia. Cyproheptadine can dry out and thicken the mucus in your airways, making it more difficult to remove.
- You should use cyproheptadine cautiously if you have increased pressure in the eye, an overactive thyroid, heart disease, or high blood pressure.

Pregnancy and nursing mothers:

Category B. See page 9 for description of categories. Don't use while breast-feeding. Babies, especially newborn and premature infants, have a higher risk of severe reactions to cyproheptadine.

Possible food and drug interactions:

- Don't take cyproheptadine if you are taking antidepressant drugs called monoamine oxidase (MAO) inhibitors. The effects of both drugs are increased and can result in very low blood pressure and other serious reactions.
- While taking cyproheptadine, avoid alcohol and other depressants such as sleeping pills and tranquilizers.

Helpful hints:

- This drug may make you feel sleepy and sedated, so drive cautiously. Don't try to mow your lawn or operate machinery until you figure out how the medicine affects you.
- Most people need 12 to 16 mg of cyproheptadine a day to relieve their allergy symptoms.

Diphenhydramine

Brand name: *Benadryl* (Generic available)

What this drug does for you:

This sedating antihistamine relieves symptoms of food allergies, hay fever, and other allergies. It helps relieve sneezing, runny nose, itching, rashes, hives, swelling, and difficulty breathing. Diphenhydramine can be used to treat severe allergic reactions in addition to epinephrine.

This drug also treats motion sickness and mild cases of parkinsonism.

Possible side effects of this drug:

- Diphenhydramine is a sedating antihistamine. The most common side effects are sleepiness and dry mouth. The sleepiness may go away after you've been taking the drug for a while. Also common are dizziness, lack of coordination, stomachache, and a thickening of the mucus in your airways.
- If you are over 60, you're more likely to feel dizzy and sedated and have

low blood pressure while taking diphenhydramine.
- Rare side effects common to most antihistamines are fatigue, confusion, restlessness, nervousness, tremor (shakiness), irritability, insomnia, euphoria, tingling, blurred or double vision, pain or ringing in the ears, hysteria, nerve inflammation, convulsions, loss of appetite, nausea, vomiting, diarrhea, constipation, tightness of the chest, wheezing, stuffy nose, low blood pressure, headache, palpitations, rapid heartbeat, anemia and various blood disorders, urinary problems, menstrual cycle problems, hives, drug rash, allergic shock reaction, sensitivity to light, and sweating.

Special warnings:
- This drug should not be used by people with some kinds of glaucoma, bladder neck obstruction, obstruction of the pylorus (opening from the stomach to the intestine), stomach ulcer, or an enlarged prostate.
- You shouldn't use diphenhydramine if you have a lower respiratory disease, such as asthma, bronchitis, or pneumonia. Diphenhydramine can dry out and thicken the mucus in your airways, making it more difficult to remove.
- You should use diphenhydramine cautiously if you have increased pressure in the eye, an overactive thyroid, heart disease, or high blood pressure.

Pregnancy and nursing mothers:
Category B. See page 9 for description of categories. Don't use while breast-feeding. Babies, especially newborn and premature infants, have a higher risk of severe reactions to diphenhydramine.

Possible food and drug interactions:
- Don't take diphenhydramine if you are taking antidepressant drugs called monoamine oxidase (MAO) inhibitors. The effects of both drugs are increased and can result in very low blood pressure and other serious reactions.
- While taking diphenhydramine, avoid alcohol and other depressants such as sleeping pills and tranquilizers.

Helpful hints:
- This drug may make you feel sleepy and sedated, so drive cautiously. Don't try to mow your lawn or operate machinery until you figure out how the medicine affects you.
- To ease motion sickness, take 30 minutes before traveling. While traveling, take the medicine before meals and when you go to bed.
- Diphenhydramine tablets reach their maximum effectiveness about one hour after you take them. They continue to work for four to six hours after you take the medicine.
- The usual adult dosage of the tablets is 25 to 50 mg three or four times daily.

Loratadine

Brand name: *Claritin*

What this drug does for you:

Loratadine is a long-acting, nonsedating antihistamine used to relieve seasonal allergy symptoms such as sneezing, runny nose, itching, rashes, hives, swelling, and difficulty breathing.

Possible side effects of this drug:

- Headache, sleepiness, fatigue, and dry mouth were the only side effects reported by more than 2 percent of the people taking the drug when it was tested.

Special warning:

- You may need to take the tablets every other day if you have cirrhosis or another liver disease.

Pregnancy and nursing mothers:

Category B. See page 9 for description of categories. Drug is present in mother's milk.

Possible food and drug interaction:

- The antifungal drug ketoconazole may increase the levels of loratadine in your blood.

Helpful hints:

- Take this drug on an empty stomach — at least two hours after or one hour before a meal. Food makes your body absorb the drug more slowly.
- This drug begins working within one to three hours and reaches maximum effectiveness at eight to 12 hours. Loratadine relieves symptoms for over 24 hours.
- The usual adult dosage is one 10 mg tablet once a day.

Promethazine

Brand names: *Phenergan, Prometh Syrup Plain, Prometh VC Plain*
(Generic available)

What this drug does for you:

Promethazine is a sedating antihistamine that relieves symptoms of food allergies, hay fever, and other allergies. It helps relieve sneezing, runny nose, itching, rashes, hives, swelling, and difficulty breathing. Promethazine can be used to treat severe allergic reactions in addition to epinephrine. This drug also treats motion sickness and prevents or controls nausea and vomiting.

Promethazine is also used as a sedative before or after some surgeries, and given along with some pain relievers after surgery.

Possible side effects of this drug:

- Promethazine can cause sleepiness, changes in blood pressure levels, rash, and nausea.

- It occasionally causes blurred vision, dry mouth, and dizziness.
- Rare side effects are confusion, disorientation, sensitivity to light, jaundice, and blood disorders.

Special warnings:

- You shouldn't use promethazine if you have a lower respiratory disease, such as asthma, bronchitis or pneumonia. Promethazine can dry out and thicken the mucus in your airways, making it more difficult to remove.
- You shouldn't use promethazine if you are allergic to any phenothiazine.
- You shouldn't use promethazine if you have sleep apnea.
- This drug should not be used by people with some kinds of glaucoma, bladder neck obstruction, obstruction of the pylorus (opening from the stomach to the intestine), stomach ulcer, or an enlarged prostate.
- People with seizure disorders, poor liver function, or heart disease should use promethazine cautiously.

Pregnancy and nursing mothers:

Category C. See page 9 for description of categories. Not known if drug is present in mother's milk.

Possible food and drug interactions:

- While taking promethazine, avoid alcohol and other depressants such as sleeping pills, tranquilizers, and tricyclic antidepressants. Doctors will usually reduce your dose of barbiturates or analgesic depressants such as morphine by one-half if you are taking promethazine.

Helpful hints:

- This drug may make you feel sleepy and sedated, so drive cautiously. Don't try to mow your lawn or operate machinery until you figure out how the medicine affects you.
- This drug may affect pregnancy test results and may increase blood sugar levels.
- Call your doctor if you experience any involuntary muscle movements or abnormal sensitivity to sunlight.
- The usual adult dosage for allergy is 25 mg taken before you go to bed. For motion sickness, the average adult dose is 25 mg twice a day — when you wake up and when you go to bed. You should take the first dose a half-hour to an hour before you travel. For nausea, the average dose is 25 mg.

Terfenadine

Brand name: *Seldane*

What this drug does for you:

Terfenadine is a long-lasting, nonsedating antihistamine meant to relieve hay fever or seasonal allergy symptoms. It relieves sneezing, runny nose, itching of the nose and throat, and itchy, watery eyes.

Possible side effects of this drug:

- The most common side effects are headache and upset stomach. Terfen-

adine doesn't have the sedating effect that many of the older antihistamines have.

- Other possible side effects are drowsiness, fatigue, dizziness, nervousness, weakness, increased appetite, dry mouth, cough, rash, and itching.
- Rare heart rhythm disturbances are the most serious risk of taking terfenadine. If you feel dizzy or faint or have any unusual heartbeats while
taking terfenadine, you should immediately contact your doctor. It could
be a warning sign of severe heart problems.

Special warning:

- People with liver disease, kidney disease, or heart disease should talk to
their doctors before using terfenadine.

Pregnancy and nursing mothers:

Category C. See page 9 for description of categories. You should not use terfenadine while you are nursing.

Possible food and drug interactions:

- You should not use terfenadine while using the antibiotic erythromycin
or the similar antibiotics troleandomycin, azithromycin, and clarithromycin.
- Don't use terfenadine while taking the antifungals ketoconazole or itraconazole. The drug interaction could cause serious heart problems.
Other similar antifungals you may want to avoid using while you are
taking terfenadine are fluconazole, metronidazole, and miconazole.
- Using terfenadine with certain drugs may put you at a greater risk for
heart problems. These drugs are probucol, certain drugs for irregular
heart rhythms, certain tricyclic antidepressants, certain phenothiazines, certain calcium channel blockers such as bepridil, and astemizole.

Helpful hint:

- Don't take more than one tablet (60 mg) every 12 hours. Taking more
medicine will increase your risk of serious heart problems.

Trimeprazine

Brand name: *Temaril*

What this drug does for you:

This antihistamine mainly relieves itching. The itching can be caused by a
variety of conditions, including hives, allergies, and poison ivy.

Possible side effects of this drug:

- The most common side effects of trimeprazine are sleepiness, dizziness
when you stand up, thickening of mucus, and dry mouth.
- Less common side effects are rash, hives, nausea, stomachache, constipation, blurred vision, heart palpitations or irregular rhythms, urinary
problems, ringing in the ears, headache, and sensitivity to light.
- People over 60 are more prone to certain side effects — low blood pressure, fainting, and sleepiness.

- Staying on a high dose of this drug for a long time may cause vision problems and coloring of the skin.

Special warnings:

- If you have glaucoma, heart disease, poor liver function, bladder neck obstruction, asthma, obstruction of the pylorus (opening from the stomach to the intestine), a stomach ulcer, or an enlarged prostate, talk with your doctor about your condition before taking this drug.
- This drug should be given very cautiously to children with a family history of sudden infant death syndrome (SIDS) or sleep apnea.
- People who have had breast cancer probably should avoid trimeprazine. There is some possibility that the drug will promote the growth of already-present breast cancer.

Pregnancy and nursing mothers:

You should not use this drug if you are pregnant. You should not use this drug if you are nursing.

Possible food and drug interactions:

- Don't use trimeprazine if you are taking antidepressants called monoamine oxidase (MAO) inhibitors or thiazide diuretics. The combination can result in very low blood pressure and other serious reactions.
- While taking trimeprazine, avoid alcohol and other depressants such as sedatives, tranquilizers, and sleeping pills. Doctors will usually reduce your dose of barbiturates or analgesic depressants such as morphine by one-half if you are taking trimeprazine.
- Other drugs that may increase the effects of trimeprazine are birth control pills, progesterone, or the blood pressure drug reserpine.

Helpful hints:

- This drug may make you feel sleepy and sedated, so drive cautiously. Don't try to mow your lawn or operate machinery until you figure out how the medicine affects you.
- The usual adult dosage of the tablets and syrup is 2.5 mg four times daily. The usual adult dosage of the extended-release capsules is one capsule every 12 hours.

Tripelennamine

Brand names: *PBZ, PBZ-SR*

What this drug does for you:

This sedating antihistamine relieves symptoms of food allergies, hay fever, and other allergies. It helps relieve sneezing, runny nose, itching, rashes, hives, swelling, and difficulty breathing. Tripelennamine can be used to treat severe allergic reactions in addition to epinephrine.

Possible side effects of this drug:

- Tripelennamine is a sedating antihistamine. The most common side effects are sleepiness and dry mouth. The sleepiness may go away after you've been taking the drug for a while. Also common are dizziness, lack of coordination, stomachache, and a thickening of the mucus in your airways.

- If you are over 60, you're more likely to feel dizzy and sedated and have low blood pressure while taking tripelennamine.
- Rare side effects common to most antihistamines are fatigue, confusion, restlessness, nervousness, tremor (shakiness), irritability, insomnia, euphoria, tingling, blurred or double vision, pain or ringing in the ears, hysteria, nerve inflammation, convulsions, loss of appetite, nausea, vomiting, diarrhea, constipation, tightness of the chest, wheezing, stuffy nose, low blood pressure, headache, palpitations, rapid heartbeat, anemia and various blood disorders, urinary problems, menstrual cycle problems, hives, drug rash, allergic shock reaction, sensitivity to light, and sweating.

Special warnings:

- This drug should not be used by people with some kinds of glaucoma, bladder neck obstruction, obstruction of the pylorus (opening from the stomach to the intestine), stomach ulcer, or an enlarged prostate.
- You shouldn't use tripelennamine if you have a lower respiratory disease, such as asthma, bronchitis, or pneumonia. Tripelennamine can dry out and thicken the mucus in your airways, making it more difficult to remove.
- You should use tripelennamine cautiously if you have increased pressure in the eye, an overactive thyroid, heart disease, or high blood pressure.

Pregnancy and nursing mothers:

You shouldn't use this drug while you're pregnant because it may not be safe. Don't use this drug while breast-feeding. Babies, especially newborn and premature infants, have a higher risk of severe reactions to tripelennamine.

Possible food and drug interactions:

- Don't take tripelennamine if you are taking antidepressant drugs called monoamine oxidase (MAO) inhibitors. The effects of both drugs are increased and can result in very low blood pressure and other serious reactions.
- While taking tripelennamine, avoid alcohol and other depressants such as sleeping pills and tranquilizers.

Helpful hints:

- This drug may make you feel sleepy and sedated, so drive cautiously. Don't try to mow your lawn or operate machinery until you figure out how the medicine affects you.
- The usual adult dose is 25 to 50 mg every four to six hours. You shouldn't take more than 600 mg a day.
- The usual dose of the extended-release tablets is one 100-mg tablet in the morning and one in the evening. The extended-release tablets must be swallowed whole — never crushed or chewed.

ANTIHISTAMINE AND DECONGESTANT COMBINATIONS

Azatadine with Pseudoephedrine

Brand name: *Trinalin*

What this drug does for you:

This long-acting drug combines an antihistamine and decongestant to relieve congestion in the nose, sinuses, ears, and chest. You can take this drug along with pain relievers or antibiotics if you need them.

Possible side effects of this drug:

- The most common side effects of drugs containing antihistamines are sleepiness and dry mouth. The sleepiness may go away after you've been taking the drug for a while. Also common are dizziness, lack of coordination, stomachache, and a thickening of the mucus in your airways.
- Rare side effects common to most drugs that contain antihistamines are fatigue, confusion, restlessness, nervousness, tremor (shakiness), irritability, insomnia, euphoria, tingling, blurred or double vision, pain or ringing in the ears, hysteria, nerve inflammation, convulsions, loss of appetite, nausea, vomiting, diarrhea, constipation, tightness of the chest, wheezing, stuffy nose, low blood pressure, headache, palpitations, rapid heartbeat, anemia and various blood disorders, urinary problems, menstrual cycle problems, hives, drug rash, allergic shock reaction, sensitivity to light, and sweating.

Special warnings:

- This drug should not be used by people with some kinds of glaucoma, urinary retention, bladder neck obstruction, obstruction of the pylorus (opening from the stomach to the intestine), diabetes, stomach ulcer, an enlarged prostate, severe high blood pressure, severe heart disease, and an overactive thyroid.
- If you have diabetes, asthma, or pressure in the eye, talk to your doctor before taking this drug.
- You shouldn't use this drug to treat a lower respiratory disease, such as asthma, bronchitis, or pneumonia.
- Side effects of both antihistamines and decongestants can be worse for people over 60. Older people may want to test their reaction to a short-acting decongestant before trying the long-acting varieties.

Pregnancy and nursing mothers:

Category C. See page 9 for description of categories. Not known if drug is present in mother's milk.

Possible food and drug interactions:

- Don't take this drug if you are taking antidepressant drugs called monoamine oxidase (MAO) inhibitors or tricyclic antidepressants, or if you have stopped taking MAO inhibitors in the last 10 days. The combination can result in very high blood pressure and other serious reactions.

- If you are taking digitalis or oral anticoagulants, you should let your doctor know before you begin taking this drug.
- While taking this drug, avoid alcohol and other depressants, such as sleeping pills and tranquilizers.
- Pseudoephedrine can reduce the effectiveness of beta blockers and other high blood pressure drugs, including methyldopa, mecamylamine, reserpine, and veratrum alkaloids.
- Antacids increase how quickly pseudoephedrine is absorbed.
- Kaolin decreases how quickly pseudoephedrine is absorbed.

Helpful hints:
- This drug may make you feel sleepy and sedated, so drive cautiously. Don't try to mow your lawn or operate machinery until you figure out how the medicine affects you.
- The usual adult dosage is one tablet twice a day.

Brompheniramine with Pseudoephedrine

Brand names: *Bromfed, Bromfed-PD, Dallergy-JR, Lodrane, Lodrane LD, Touro A&H, Ultrabrom, Ultrabrom PD*

What this drug does for you:
This drug combines an antihistamine and decongestant to relieve congestion in the nose, sinuses, ears, and chest.

Possible side effects of this drug:
- This drug does have sleepiness as a side effect, but it doesn't cause sleepiness as often as some of the other antihistamine-containing drugs.
- Other possible side effects are nausea, giddiness, dry mouth, blurred vision, heart palpitations, flushing, irritability, and excitement.

Special warnings:
- This drug should not be used by people with some kinds of glaucoma, urinary retention, bladder neck obstruction, obstruction of the pylorus (opening from the stomach to the intestine), diabetes, stomach ulcer, an enlarged prostate, severe high blood pressure, severe heart disease, and an overactive thyroid.
- If you have diabetes, asthma, or pressure in the eye, talk to your doctor before taking this drug.
- You shouldn't use this drug to treat a lower respiratory disease, such as asthma, bronchitis, or pneumonia.

Pregnancy and nursing mothers:
Don't use this drug while you're pregnant because it may not be safe.

Possible food and drug interactions:
- Don't take this drug if you are taking antidepressant drugs called monoamine oxidase (MAO) inhibitors or tricyclic antidepressants, or if you have stopped taking MAO inhibitors in the last 10 days. The combination can result in very high blood pressure and other serious reactions.

- If you are taking digitalis or oral anticoagulants, you should let your doctor know before you begin taking this drug.
- While taking this drug, avoid alcohol and other depressants, such as sleeping pills and tranquilizers.
- Pseudoephedrine can reduce the effectiveness of beta blockers and other high blood pressure drugs, including methyldopa, mecamylamine, reserpine, and veratrum alkaloids.
- Antacids increase how quickly pseudoephedrine is absorbed.
- Kaolin decreases how quickly pseudoephedrine is absorbed.

Helpful hints:
- This drug may make you feel sleepy and sedated, so drive cautiously. Don't try to mow your lawn or operate machinery until you figure out how the medicine affects you.

Brompheniramine with Phenylpropanolamine and Codeine

Brand names: *Dimetane-DC, Poly-Histine CS*

What this drug does for you:
This combination of antihistamine, nasal decongestant, and opiate pain reliever works to relieve coughing and other symptoms of allergies and the common cold. It relieves congestion in the nose, sinuses, ears, and chest.

Possible side effects of this drug:
- The most common side effects of drugs containing antihistamines are sleepiness and dry mouth. The sleepiness may go away after you've been taking the drug for a while. Also common are dizziness, lack of coordination, stomachache, and a thickening of the mucus in your airways.
- Codeine commonly causes constipation.
- Rare side effects common to most drugs that contain antihistamines are fatigue, confusion, restlessness, nervousness, tremor (shakiness), irritability, insomnia, euphoria, tingling, blurred or double vision, pain or ringing in the ears, hysteria, nerve inflammation, convulsions, loss of appetite, nausea, vomiting, diarrhea, tightness of the chest, wheezing, stuffy nose, low blood pressure, headache, palpitations, rapid heartbeat, anemia and various blood disorders, urinary problems, menstrual cycle problems, hives, drug rash, allergic shock reaction, sensitivity to light, and sweating.

Special warnings:
- This drug should not be used by people with some kinds of glaucoma, urinary retention, bladder neck obstruction, obstruction of the pylorus (opening from the stomach to the intestine), diabetes, stomach ulcer, an enlarged prostate, severe high blood pressure, severe heart disease, and an overactive thyroid.
- If you have diabetes, asthma, or pressure in the eye, talk to your doctor before taking this drug.
- You shouldn't use this drug to treat a lower respiratory disease, such as asthma, bronchitis, or pneumonia.

- You can become addicted to codeine if you use this drug for a long time.

Pregnancy and nursing mothers:
Category C. See page 9 for description of categories. Don't use this drug if you are nursing. Antihistamines and codeine can be dangerous to babies.

Possible food and drug interactions:
- Don't take this drug if you are taking antidepressant drugs called monoamine oxidase (MAO) inhibitors or tricyclic antidepressants, or if you have stopped taking MAO inhibitors in the last 10 days. The combination can result in very high blood pressure and other serious reactions.
- If you are taking digitalis or oral anticoagulants, you should let your doctor know before you begin taking this drug.
- While taking this drug, avoid alcohol and other depressants, such as sleeping pills and tranquilizers.
- Phenylpropanolamine can reduce the effectiveness of beta blockers and other high blood pressure drugs, including methyldopa, mecamylamine, reserpine, and veratrum alkaloids.

Helpful hints:
- This drug may make you feel sleepy and sedated, so drive cautiously. Don't try to mow your lawn or operate machinery until you figure out how the medicine affects you.
- The usual adult dosage is 2 teaspoonfuls every four hours.

Carbinoxamine with Pseudoephedrine

Brand name: *Rondec*

What this drug does for you:
This drug combines an antihistamine and decongestant to relieve a stuffy nose caused by allergies or a cold.

Possible side effects of this drug:
- The most common side effects of drugs containing antihistamines are sleepiness and dry mouth. The sleepiness may go away after you've been taking the drug for a while. Also common are dizziness, lack of coordination, stomachache, and a thickening of the mucus in your airways. Rarely, you may experience double vision, nausea, loss of appetite, and heartburn.
- Decongestants such as pseudoephedrine can make you feel shaky and nervous and can cause a rapid heartbeat and insomnia.
- Rare and more dangerous side effects are convulsions, an irregular heartbeat, difficulty breathing or urinating, high blood pressure, and hallucinations.

Special warnings:
- This drug should not be used by people with some kinds of glaucoma, urinary retention, stomach ulcer, severe high blood pressure, and severe heart disease. You shouldn't use this drug during an asthma attack.

- If you have diabetes, asthma, an enlarged prostate, an overactive thyroid, mild high blood pressure, mild heart disease, or pressure in the eye, talk to your doctor about your condition before taking this drug.
- Anyone over 60 should use this drug cautiously.

Pregnancy and nursing mothers:
Category C. See page 9 for description of categories. Use this drug cautiously if you are nursing.

Possible food and drug interactions:
- Don't take this drug if you are taking antidepressant drugs called monoamine oxidase (MAO) inhibitors or tricyclic antidepressants, or if you have stopped taking MAO inhibitors in the last 10 days. The combination can result in very high blood pressure and other serious reactions.
- While taking this drug, avoid alcohol and other depressants, such as sleeping pills and tranquilizers.
- Pseudoephedrine can reduce the effectiveness of beta blockers and other high blood pressure drugs, including methyldopa, mecamylamine, reserpine, and veratrum alkaloids.
- Antacids increase how quickly pseudoephedrine is absorbed.
- Kaolin decreases how quickly pseudoephedrine is absorbed.

Helpful hints:
- This drug may make you feel sleepy and sedated, so drive cautiously. Don't try to mow your lawn or operate machinery until you figure out how the medicine affects you.
- The usual adult dosage is 1 teaspoonful of the syrup or 1 tablet four times a day. The timed-release tablets last for 12 hours.

Terfenadine and Pseudoephedrine

Brand name: *Seldane-D*

What this drug does for you:
This long-lasting drug combines an antihistamine and a decongestant to relieve hay fever or seasonal allergy symptoms. It relieves sneezing, itching of the nose and throat, watery eyes, and a stuffy nose.

Possible side effects of this drug:
- The most common side effects are difficulty falling asleep, nervousness, dry mouth, headaches, and stomach problems.
- Rare heart rhythm disturbances are the most serious risk of taking terfenadine. If you feel dizzy or faint or have any unusual heartbeats while taking terfenadine, you should immediately contact your doctor. It could be a warning sign of severe heart problems.

Special warnings:
- People with liver disease, kidney disease, or heart disease should talk to their doctors about their condition before using terfenadine.
- People with high blood pressure, diabetes, heart disease, increased pres-

sure in the eye, an overactive thyroid, or an enlarged prostate should talk to their doctors about their condition before taking any drug containing pseudoephedrine.

Pregnancy and nursing mothers:
Category C. See page 9 for description of categories. You should not use this drug while you are nursing.

Possible food and drug interactions:
- You should not use terfenadine while using the antibiotic erythromycin or the similar antibiotics troleandomycin, azithromycin, and clarithromycin.
- Don't use terfenadine while taking the antifungals ketoconazole or itraconazole. The drug interaction could cause serious heart problems. Other similar antifungals you may want to avoid using while you are taking terfenadine are fluconazole, metronidazole, and miconazole.
- Using terfenadine with certain drugs may put you at a greater risk for heart problems. These drugs are probucol, certain drugs for irregular heart rhythms, certain tricyclic antidepressants, certain phenothiazines, certain calcium channel blockers such as bepridil, and astemizole.
- Don't take drugs containing pseudoephedrine if you are taking antidepressant drugs called monoamine oxidase (MAO) inhibitors, or if you have stopped taking MAO inhibitors in the last 10 days. The combination can result in very high blood pressure and other serious reactions.
- Pseudoephedrine can reduce the effectiveness of beta blockers and other high blood pressure drugs, including methyldopa, mecamylamine, reserpine, and veratrum alkaloids.

Helpful hints:
- Don't take more than one tablet every 12 hours. Taking more medicine will increase your risk of serious heart problems.
- Make sure you swallow the tablet whole — don't chew or crush it.

CORTISONE-LIKE DRUGS

Beclomethasone Dipropionate

Brand names: *Beclovent, Beconase, Beconase AQ, Vancenase, Vancenase AQ, Vanceril*

What this drug does for you:
Beclomethasone dipropionate is an anti-inflammatory steroid. The forms that you inhale through your mouth are used to treat and control asthma.

The forms that you inhale through or spray into your nose are used to treat congested, swollen nasal passages, often caused by allergies. They also treat nasal polyps (tumors in your nose).

These steroids are a man-made copy of the natural hormones produced by the adrenal glands. One function of the natural hormones is reducing inflammation.

Inhaled steroids don't have the sometimes serious side effects associated with steroid pills or shots.

Possible side effects of this drug:

- The inhaled forms can cause hoarseness, dry mouth, and yeast infections in the mouth and throat (oral thrush).
- The nasal forms may irritate the inside of your nose or cause you to sneeze.
- You could have a rare allergic reaction to the drug, which may include rash, hives, swelling, and difficulty breathing.
- Inhaled steroids are very safe compared with steroid pills or shots, but if you use them more often than your doctor recommends, you may suffer some serious side effects: cataracts, osteoporosis, weight gain, high blood pressure, increased blood sugar, easy bruising, slowed growth (in children), muscle weakness, acne, low resistance to infection, water retention, and mood changes. Your adrenal glands may also quit producing natural steroids.

Special warnings:

- You should not use beclomethasone dipropionate if you can get relief from your asthma through bronchodilators and other nonsteroid drugs.
- This drug is not meant to treat nonasthmatic bronchitis.
- This drug won't stop a severe asthma attack.
- If you are switching to beclomethasone from steroid pills or shots, make sure you get off the other drug slowly. People have died after switching quickly from steroid pills to inhaled steroids. You should report to your doctor any signs of corticosteroid withdrawal, including fatigue, weakness, painful joints or muscles, low blood pressure when you stand up, and difficulty breathing.
- If you were taking steroid pills and you are now taking beclomethasone, you may need to get back on the former drug during a severe asthma attack or during times of stress: surgery, infection, or an injury. It can take your body several months to begin producing enough steroid hormones on its own after you have been taking steroid pills. In case of an emergency, you should carry a card that says you have used cortisone-related drugs in the past year.
- Take extra care to avoid exposure to people with chicken pox or measles because corticosteroid drugs can weaken your immune system. If you are exposed, let your doctor know right away.

Pregnancy and nursing mothers:

Category C. See page 9 for description of categories. Not known if drug is present in mother's milk.

Possible food and drug interactions:

No significant interactions.

Helpful hints:

- See page 39 for instructions on how to use your inhaler correctly.
- Beclomethasone may begin relieving your stuffy nose or your asthma

after three days or less, but it may take as long as two or three weeks. If you don't experience relief eventually, your doctor will probably decide to take you off the drug.

- Since beclomethasone probably won't relieve your stuffy nose right away, you may need to also take an antihistamine tablet or a decongestant nasal spray for a few days.
- You can avoid fungal infections in your mouth and throat by rinsing your mouth and gargling with warm water after using your inhaler. Don't swallow the water.
- You should do your best to take your medicine at regular time intervals.

Flunisolide

Brand names: *AeroBid, Nasalide*

What this drug does for you:

Flunisolide is an anti-inflammatory steroid. The forms that you inhale through your mouth are used to treat and control asthma.

The forms that you inhale through or spray into your nose are used to treat congested, swollen nasal passages, often caused by allergies. They also treat nasal polyps (tumors in your nose). These steroids are a man-made copy of the natural hormones produced by the adrenal glands. One function of the natural hormones is reducing inflammation.

Inhaled steroids don't have the sometimes serious side effects associated with steroid pills or shots.

Possible side effects of this drug:

- The inhaled forms can cause hoarseness, dry mouth, and yeast infections in the mouth and throat (oral thrush).
- The nasal forms may irritate the inside of your nose, cause you to sneeze, cause your eyes to water, or cause a fungal infection in your nose.
- Other side effects are nausea, vomiting, and headache. You could have a rare allergic reaction to the drug, which may include rash, hives, swelling, and difficulty breathing.
- Inhaled steroids are very safe compared with steroid pills or shots, but if you use them more often than your doctor recommends, you may suffer some serious side effects: cataracts, osteoporosis, weight gain, high blood pressure, increased blood sugar, easy bruising, slowed growth (in children), muscle weakness, acne, low resistance to infection, water retention, and mood changes. Your adrenal glands may also quit producing natural steroids.

Flunisolide may be more likely to cause these side effects than the other inhaled steroids. It is one of the more potent inhaled steroids, and your body may absorb more of it. You and your doctor should watch for any problems.

Special warnings:

- You should not use flunisolide if you can get relief from your asthma through bronchodilators and other nonsteroid drugs.

- This drug is not meant to treat nonasthmatic bronchitis.
- This drug won't stop a severe asthma attack. If you do have an asthma attack and you don't get relief from a bronchodilator, you should contact your doctor immediately. You may need steroid pills or shots.
- If you are switching to flunisolide from steroid pills or shots, make sure you get off the other drug slowly. People have died after switching quickly from steroid pills to inhaled steroids. You should report to your doctor any signs of corticosteroid withdrawal, including fatigue, weakness, painful joints or muscles, low blood pressure when you stand up, and difficulty breathing.
- If you were taking steroid pills and you are now taking flunisolide, you may need to get back on the former drug during a severe asthma attack or during times of stress: surgery, infection, or an injury. It can take your body several months to begin producing enough steroid hormones on its own after you have been taking steroid pills. In case of an emergency, you should carry a card that says you have used cortisone-related drugs in the past year.
- Take extra care to avoid exposure to people with chicken pox or measles because corticosteroid drugs can weaken your immune system. If you are exposed, let your doctor know right away.
- People with tuberculosis, herpes simplex of the eye, or an untreated infection (fungal, viral, or bacterial) shouldn't use flunisolide.

Pregnancy and nursing mothers:

Category C. See page 9 for description of categories. Not known if drug is present in mother's milk.

Possible food and drug interactions:

No significant interactions.

Helpful hints:

- See page 39 for instructions on how to use your inhaler correctly.
- Flunisolide may begin relieving your stuffy nose or your asthma after three days or less, but it may take as long as two or three weeks. If you don't experience relief eventually, your doctor will probably decide to take you off the drug.
- You can avoid fungal infections in your mouth and throat by rinsing your mouth and gargling with warm water after using your inhaler. Don't swallow the water.
- You should do your best to take your medicine at regular time intervals.
- For people with asthma, if you use a bronchodilator, you should use it several minutes before the flunisolide. This will help you get the full effect of your medicine.
- The usual adult dose of the inhaled form is two inhalations in the morning and two inhalations in the evening.
- Since the nasal form of flunisolide probably won't relieve your stuffy nose right away, you may need to also take an antihistamine tablet or a decongestant nasal spray for a few days. Use the decongestant a few minutes before the flunisolide to help you get the full effect of your med-

icine. Also, blow your nose before using the flunisolide.

Triamcinolone Acetonide

Brand names: *Aristocort A, Azmacort, Nasacort, Tac-3* **(Generic available)**

What this drug does for you:

Triamcinolone is an anti-inflammatory steroid. The forms that you inhale through your mouth are used to treat and control asthma.

The forms that you inhale through or spray into your nose are used to treat congested, swollen nasal passages, often caused by allergies. They also treat nasal polyps (tumors in your nose).

The creams and ointments are used to relieve itchy, inflamed skin.

These steroids are a man-made copy of the natural hormones produced by the adrenal glands. One function of the natural hormones is reducing inflammation.

Inhaled steroids don't have the sometimes serious side effects associated with steroid pills or shots.

Possible side effects of this drug:

- The inhaled forms can cause hoarseness, dry mouth, and yeast infections in the mouth and throat (oral thrush). You may also wheeze, cough, and have some swelling in your face.
- The nasal forms may irritate the inside of your nose; cause sneezing, watery eyes or headache; or cause a fungal infection in your nose.
- The cream or ointment forms may cause burning, itching, and dryness. They rarely cause more serious skin reactions, but you should report any reaction to your doctor.
- Inhaled, sprayed, or cream steroids are very safe compared with steroid pills or shots, but if you use them more often than your doctor recommends, you may suffer some serious side effects: cataracts, osteoporosis, weight gain, high blood pressure, increased blood sugar, easy bruising, slowed growth (in children), muscle weakness, acne, low resistance to infection, water retention, and mood changes. Your adrenal glands may also quit producing natural steroids.

Special warnings:

- You should not use triamcinolone if you can get relief from your asthma through bronchodilators and other nonsteroid drugs.
- This drug is not meant to treat nonasthmatic bronchitis.
- This drug won't stop a severe asthma attack. If you do have an asthma attack and you don't get relief from a bronchodilator, you should contact your doctor immediately. You may need steroid pills or shots.
- If you are switching to triamcinolone from steroid pills or shots, make sure you get off the other drug slowly. People have died after switching quickly from steroid pills to inhaled steroids. You should report to your doctor any signs of corticosteroid withdrawal, including fatigue, weakness, painful joints or muscles, low blood pressure when you stand up, and difficulty breathing.

- If you were taking steroid pills and you are now taking triamcinolone, you may need to get back on the former drug during a severe asthma attack or during times of stress: surgery, infection, or an injury. It can take your body several months to begin producing enough steroid hormones on its own after you have been taking steroid pills. In case of an emergency, you should carry a card that says you have used cortisone-related drugs in the past year.
- Take extra care to avoid exposure to people with chicken pox or measles because corticosteroid drugs can weaken your immune system. If you are exposed, let your doctor know right away.
- People with tuberculosis, herpes simplex of the eye, or an untreated infection (fungal, viral, or bacterial) shouldn't use triamcinolone.

Pregnancy and nursing mothers:

Category C. See page 9 for description of categories. Not known if drug is present in mother's milk.

Possible food and drug interactions:

No significant interactions.

Helpful hints:

- If you are using the steroid creams or ointments, don't put a bandage or cover over the medicine unless your doctor tells you to use a bandage. Parents shouldn't put a tight-fitting diaper or plastic pants on a child if the medicine is being used in the diaper area. Covering up the medicine may make you or your child absorb more of it than you should.
- See page 39 for instructions on how to use your inhaler correctly.
- Triamcinolone may begin relieving your stuffy nose or your asthma after four to seven days, but it may take as long as two or three weeks. If you don't experience relief eventually, your doctor will probably decide to take you off the drug.
- You can avoid fungal infections in your mouth and throat by rinsing your mouth and gargling with warm water after using your inhaler. Don't swallow the water.
- You should do your best to take your medicine at regular time intervals.
- For people with asthma, if you use a bronchodilator, you should use it several minutes before the triamcinolone. This will help you get the full effect of your medicine.
- The usual adult dose of the inhaled form is two inhalations three or four times a day.
- The usual adult dose of the nasal spray is two sprays in each nostril once a day.
- The usual adult dose of the cream and ointment is a thin film applied three or four times a day.
- Since the nasal form of triamcinolone probably won't relieve your stuffy nose right away, you may need to also take an antihistamine tablet or a decongestant nasal spray for a few days. Use the decongestant a few minutes before the triamcinolone to help you get the full effect of your medicine. Also, blow your nose before using the triamcinolone.

COUGH SUPPRESSANTS/EXPECTORANTS

Benzonatate

Brand name: *Tessalon* **(Generic available)**

What this drug does for you:
This non-narcotic relieves coughing by deadening the nerves in the airways and reducing the cough reflex. It begins to act within 15 to 20 minutes and lasts for three to eight hours.

Possible side effects of this drug:
- This drug may cause sleepiness, headache, dizziness, confusion, hallucinations, constipation, nausea, upset stomach, itching, skin eruptions, nasal congestion, chills, burning eyes, and numbness in the chest.

Special warnings:
- Don't chew or suck the soft capsules. This can completely deaden the nerves in your mouth and throat, possibly leading to difficulty breathing, choking, a spasm of the airways, or cardiovascular collapse.
- Don't use if allergic to any related anesthetics (ester-type local anesthetics).

Pregnancy and nursing mothers:
Category C. See page 9 for description of categories. Not known if drug is present in mother's milk.

Possible food and drug interactions:
- No specific interactions, but benzonatate may cause bizarre behavior or hallucinations when combined with some other prescribed drugs. Make sure you tell your doctor what other prescriptions you are taking.

Helpful hint:
- The usual adult dosage is one 100 mg capsule taken three times a day. You can take up to six capsules a day. An overdose can be fatal.

Guaifenesin

Brand names: *Humibid LA, Humibid Sprinkle, Liquibid, Organidin NR, Phencen, Pneumomist, Touro EX* **(Generic available)**

What this drug does for you:
Guaifenesin is an expectorant which loosens phlegm and thins the secretions in the air passages. This helps make your coughing more productive and less frequent. Guaifenesin relieves coughing and chest congestion associated with respiratory tract infections, sinusitis, bronchitis, and asthma.

Possible side effects of this drug:
- Guaifenesin should not cause any serious side effects, but you may experience nausea and vomiting.
- Very rare side effects are headaches, rash, hives, and dizziness.

Pregnancy and nursing mothers:

Category C. See page 9 for description of categories. Not known if drug is present in mother's milk.

Helpful hints:

- For people who don't like swallowing pills, the contents of the Sprinkle capsules may be sprinkled on a small amount of soft food just before you eat it. Liquid forms are also available.

DECONGESTANTS AND EXPECTORANTS

Phenylephrine, Phenylpropanolamine, and Guaifenesin

Brand name: *Entex*

What this drug does for you:

This drug combines two decongestants and an expectorant and is used when you have a cold, bronchitis, or sinusitis. It relieves a congested nose and thick mucus in the chest.

Possible side effects of this drug:

- Common side effects are nervousness, insomnia, restlessness, headache, nausea, and stomachache.
- This drug may make urinating more difficult if you have an enlarged prostate.

Special warnings:

- You should not use this drug if you have very high blood pressure.
- If you have mild high blood pressure, diabetes, heart or blood vessel disease, increased pressure in the eye, an overactive thyroid, or an enlarged prostate, you should talk to your doctor about your condition before taking this drug.

Pregnancy and nursing mothers:

Category C. See page 9 for description of categories. Not known if drug is present in mother's milk.

Possible food and drug interactions:

- You should not use this drug if you are taking monoamine oxidase (MAO) inhibitors, an antidepressant.
- You shouldn't take this drug if you are taking other drugs that stimulate the sympathetic nervous system, such as epinephrine or other decongestants.

Helpful hint:

- The usual adult dose is 2 teaspoonfuls four times a day (every six hours).

Natural Alternatives

ALLERGIES

- Coughing
- Headache
- Itching
- Shortness of breath
- Sneezing
- Stuffy or runny nose
- Vomiting

- Diarrhea
- Hives
- Red, watery, itchy eyes
- Skin rash
- Stomach cramps
- Swollen lips
- Wheezing

Home remedies fight off airborne allergens

"If you're happy and you know it, then your face will surely show it. If you're happy and you know it, clap your hands."

If you've got allergies, you know it, and your face will surely show it (red eyes, runny nose), but unlike the popular children's song suggests, you probably won't feel like clapping your hands.

An allergic reaction means your body activates your immune system to fight off a substance it identifies as foreign and dangerous. Your immune system produces antibodies to halt the "invasion." The resulting chemical release can cause skin reactions, breathing problems, and digestive difficulties.

Each day, you inhale enough air to fill a standard-sized bedroom. Since even one-tenth of that amount can contain hundreds of pollen grains and tens of thousands of mold spores, among other things, it's not surprising that the most common allergies come from substances you inhale.

Hay fever (also called allergic rhinitis) is a common allergic reaction, usually inherited, that causes the lining of your nose and sinuses to swell. The result is an itchy or runny nose, sneezing, sore throat, stuffy head, and even a decreased attention span. Though pollen from blooming plants makes spring the most likely time to have hay fever, other allergens like mold, dust mites, and pet dander can cause hay fever at any time of the year.

Many medications are available to treat hay fever, but side effects like drowsiness can make the cure worse than the disease. By evaluating your home and workplace, and adjusting your lifestyle a little, you can eliminate many of the things that cause your hay fever.

Remove as much house dust as possible. Dust mites love dust. And they thrive wherever dust decides to land, on furniture, bedding, toys, carpet, and clothes. You can kill dust mites by regularly washing clothes, bedding, and curtains in hot water (at least 130 degrees F). Use washable synthetic materials instead of feather or down pillows, and put dustproof covers on your pillows, mattresses, and box springs. Consider a dehumidifier if you live in a humid climate. Dust mites are most common in humid areas, but they can't survive if the humidity is below 50 percent.

Try this quick freezer trick to keep those bothersome bugs out of children's stuffed toys and small pillows: Place the item in a plastic bag in the freezer for several hours to kill the resident dust mites. Remove from the freezer and wash, shake, or vacuum to remove the debris.

The latest research from Australia suggests that sunlight may be an important key to fighting dust mites. Researchers there found that leaving mite-infested rugs outdoors for four hours on a hot, sunny day killed 100 percent of the mites and their eggs. This approach would probably work well for bedding, pillows, and upholstered furniture.

Try tannic acid and acaricides for rugs and carpets. Researchers at the University of Virginia in Charlottesville found that the product Allersearch ADS reduced dust mites in carpet by up to 92 percent. This natural product contains tannic acid. It does not actually remove dust mites; it just makes the enzyme coating found on mites' feces inactive. This means dust mite droppings will no longer trigger an allergic or asthmatic reaction in people who are susceptible.

The tannic acid product is also effective in neutralizing the allergen in pet dander. For more information on Allersearch ADS, call 1-800-422-DUST (3878).

Acaricides, chemicals which kill the dust mites themselves, are also available. They must be applied regularly, and they won't remove the dust mite droppings that are already in your house. You'll need to clean and vacuum to do that.

Vacuum your house twice a week. Even better, have someone who doesn't suffer from hay fever vacuum for you. Stirring up dust as the vacuum rolls along could make your hay fever worse, but it's necessary to help eliminate dust, dust mites, and pet dander. It's wise to throw away the vacuum bag immediately after each vacuuming.

Some people swear by the special "anti-allergic" vacuum cleaners, but studies show that these vacuum cleaners don't work any better than regular vacuums. You should at least consider the small expense of a special bag for your vacuum. Certain vacuum cleaner bags and filters do a better job of trapping microscopic particles than others.

If you have serious allergies to dust, you may have to remove your carpet. Even a professional cleaning only works for a short while. Dust mites can't live on dry, polished wood floors.

Wear a mask when you work in the yard, especially while cutting your grass. Blocking pollen and dust from your airways can provide significant relief, particularly during the growing season. Sunglasses can help protect your eyes from pollen too.

Not everyone is allergic to the same pollen, and different geographic areas have different "pollen seasons," so it's impossible to say when you should be wary of the outdoors. Note which time of year seems to produce the worst hay fever symptoms for you, and be extra careful at that time.

Pollen is usually worst in the early evening, when it's settling back to the ground. The best time for allergy sufferers to go outside on hot, dry days is midmorning.

Wash your hair and clothes. Your hair, especially if it's long, acts as a pollen net. Washing it before you go to bed should help you rest easier.

If you or your children have been outside for a while, especially working or playing in the yard, change clothes, and put the work or play clothes in the laundry hamper. Better yet, wash them right away. Your clothes can bring outdoor dust and pollen into the house.

Use air conditioning. If pollen causes your hay fever, opening your windows to let in fresh air is the worst thing you can do. Air conditioning can keep the pollen out while helping you keep your cool.

Use the air conditioner in your car as well. It may be fun to drive with the windows open or the top down, but that just blows pollen up your nose at the speed you are driving.

Air conditioning also keeps the humidity down in your house. By holding down the moisture, you prevent mold from growing. Mold spores can cause severe hay fever in some people. Studies show that central air conditioning is better at preventing mold than window units, but a window unit is better than no air conditioning at all.

Be sure to clean or change your air conditioner filter regularly.

Injected allergens — when the bee stings

If you are severely allergic to certain insect bites, don't take unnecessary risks. It might be better to skip the family picnic, or at least relocate it to a safer, screened-in area, than to expose yourself to the possibility of a bite. If you are stung, however, follow this course of action:

Remove the stinger immediately. A honeybee stinger left in the skin continues to release venom. Most other common insects take their stingers with them. To remove a honeybee stinger, use a flat, thin object such as a driver's license to gently flick the stinger out of the skin. If you try to pull the stinger out, you will just release more venom into your wound.

Wash wound thoroughly with soap and water. Then to neutralize the venom, make a paste of unseasoned meat tenderizer and water and apply it to your sting site.

Apply an ice pack. Ice helps to relieve the itching, swelling, and pain and slows down the absorption of the venom. Don't apply ice directly to the skin, or you may make matters worse by giving yourself frostbite. Use an ice pack or place a few ice cubes in a plastic bag, then wrap the plastic bag in a clean towel and apply to your injury.

Seek first aid. If you know that you are allergic to an insect sting and have an emergency epinephrine kit, use it, then seek medical help. If you don't know of an allergy, but begin to feel agitated, dizzy, nauseated, have difficulty breathing, start vomiting, or develop cramps, hives, or a rapid heartbeat, get to an emergency room immediately.

Sources —
Emergency Medicine (27,2:79)
Before You Call the Doctor, Random House, New York, 1992

Don't let furry pets inside. You may love Fluffy very much, but she could be the reason you always feel sick. Pet dander, or dead skin cells, ranks with dust mites as a primary cause of hay fever. It can also cause asthma and eczema in some allergic people.

Other allergy triggers from animals are saliva (which cats deposit on their fur while grooming), dog urine, and fleas. That's why you can be allergic to some pets but not others — it may be the fleas that make you sneeze, not the pet.

Your pet's hair and dead skin cells are blown through your house by your heating and cooling systems. For some people who are extremely sensitive to pet dander, even keeping the animal outside may not be enough to prevent hay fever. Consider keeping a pet that doesn't cause allergies. Fish, turtles, frogs, snakes, and sand crabs are ideal for hay fever sufferers. If you absolutely can't part with Fluffy, bathe her every week. If possible, get someone who isn't allergic to do it for you. Keep your pet out of your bedroom at all times.

You should also place specially made filters over forced-air heating and cooling vents to keep the dander down. In the winter, you can close the air ducts in the allergic person's room and use an electric heater instead.

What about an electronic filter? Electrostatic desktop filters don't seem to be very effective in controlling allergens. High-Efficiency Particulate-Air (HEPA) filters are effective for long periods of time, but they are very expensive. They can remove pet dander from the air, but even they won't be effective unless you can keep down the amount of dander elsewhere. Try other less expensive measures before you invest in a HEPA filter.

Check your house for mold. Dark, damp areas such as basements are prime spots for mold growth. A dehumidifier in damp parts of the house should help.

Also check sinks, shower and toilet areas, refrigerators, and washing machines. Try to keep these areas squeaky clean. Even the air conditioner, which can be so helpful in preventing mold, can be an area of concern if it does not drain properly. Wipe moldy surfaces with a solution of bleach and water.

House plants can also harbor mold, especially those in wicker baskets. You can purchase mold retardants from your local nursery for use in the home.

Check your yard for mold as well. Compost piles, poorly landscaped or heavily shaded areas, along with areas that don't drain well, are susceptible to mold. Again, check with your local nursery for mold retardants. Rake the leaves in your yard regularly. Fallen leaves provide a perfect environment for molds and mildews to grow.

Steer clear of smoke. People with allergies should not smoke and should ask smokers not to smoke around them. Avoiding smoke not only helps your allergies, but it also helps prevent other respiratory problems like lung cancer and emphysema. Don't allow smoking inside the house. Even a few puffs of smoke can linger on furniture and in carpet for months, causing irritation and allergic reactions.

Use pump or roll-on products instead of aerosols. Breathing in the spray of aerosols irritates upper and lower airways.

Stay away from strong odors. Perfumes, scented soaps and tissues, paints, and insecticides all contain chemicals which can trigger allergic reactions.

Take a beach vacation. One of the best vacation spots for allergy sufferers is the seashore. Sea breezes keep pollen inland and away from the beach.

Clear out the cockroaches. Like dust mites, cockroaches thrive in warm, humid climates. They, too, can cause an allergic reaction, especially in people with allergic asthma. You can use a professional pest control service to eliminate the roaches, but it is also very important to remove the bug debris, which actually causes the allergy.

Don't move; improve. Sound advice for many homeowners also applies to people who suffer from severe allergies. People who move to what they believe is a better climate for their allergies often find that any improvement in their condition is short-lived, as new allergies replace old ones. Working hard to control the allergens in your present environment often works much better than moving.

Vitamins and herbs that offer allergy relief

Get enough vitamin C. Dr. Robert Cathcart, who has treated over 1,000 patients for allergies, recommends massive doses of vitamin C. He has even treated himself for hay fever with great success.

How to stop an allergic emergency

In worst cases, an allergic reaction may trigger anaphylactic shock. Without immediate treatment, breathing becomes extremely difficult, blood pressure drops, the mouth and throat swell, and the victim has a feeling of impending disaster and may lose consciousness. Anaphylaxis can be fatal.

This type of reaction often occurs within 15 minutes of coming in contact with the allergen. Symptoms can last for several hours. The quicker anaphylaxis is treated, the greater the chance of survival. Anyone with symptoms of anaphylaxis should go to a hospital emergency room, even if symptoms seem to subside on their own.

Treatment of anaphylaxis requires an injection of epinephrine, a synthetic version of the natural hormone adrenaline. If you have ever experienced a severe allergic reaction, you should carry an emergency dose of epinephrine with you at all times. Also carry a tag or identification card that includes your medical history and allergies.

Your doctor can write you a prescription for epinephrine if you need one. Ask your doctor or pharmacist to instruct you in its proper use. The quantity of epinephrine these syringes contain could cause serious complications if accidentally injected into a vein. Epinephrine is now available in easy-to-use "pen" form, which can be injected quickly right through your clothing.

Source —

Food Allergies, FDA Consumer Reprint, Publication No. (FDA) 94-2279, Department of Health and Human Services, Food and Drug Administration, HFI-40, Rockville, Md. 20857

Dr. Mary Eades, a physician from Little Rock, Arkansas, recommends beginning with a dosage of 500 mg per day and working up to 4 grams (about a teaspoon) per day over a period of a week or two. She finds it is easier to use powdered vitamin C and mix it into a citrus-flavored carbonated beverage.

If you have high blood pressure or kidney problems, make sure that the form of vitamin C you use does not contain sodium ascorbate, a form of salt.

Make sure you get enough calcium and magnesium. Any deficiency in these minerals can make allergic/asthmatic symptoms worse. The recommended daily allowance (RDA) for magnesium is 300 mg for women and 350 mg for men. Both men and women need at least 800 mg of calcium per day. Doctors often recommend 1,000 mg of calcium a day for women and 1,500 mg for postmenopausal women and older men.

Consider quercetin. Quercetin is a bioflavonoid (a substance which helps make vitamin C more effective). Try a daily dose of 1 to 2 grams of bioflavonoid complex, which contains quercetin. A 500-mg tablet three times a day for no longer than three weeks should be sufficient.

Add some spice to your life. Everyday spices may help suppress allergy symptoms. Try adding more garlic, ginger, black pepper, and onion to your food. Cayenne pepper can be especially effective as a natural treatment for allergies.

Always be sure to discuss any use of supplements with your doctor.

Defending yourself from food allergies

If you have a food allergy, you probably won't have a reaction to the food the first time you eat it. After the first exposure, your body classifies a particular food as foreign and will be prepared to attack quickly at the next encounter. The second time you eat the offending food, your body may respond in a number of ways, including:

◁ swollen lips
◁ stomach cramps, vomiting, or diarrhea
◁ skin reactions, including hives or rash
◁ wheezing or breathing difficulties
◁ migraine headache
◁ fluid buildup behind the ear drum (this reaction is usually seen only in children)

If you suspect you have a food allergy, keep a food diary. Write down everything you eat or drink for a two-week period. Note any symptoms and how long it took for them to develop. Even though you may think you are reacting to certain foods, only a doctor who has specialized training in allergy and immunology can correctly identify a food allergy. Incorrectly labeling a reaction to food as a food allergy can make you avoid the food unnecessarily, which can cause nutritional deficiencies.

If you are diagnosed with a food allergy, you will need to completely avoid the offending food. It's critical that allergy sufferers take these precautions:

◁ Read labels carefully. If you are allergic to milk, check labels for words such as casein, whey, or lactose that indicate the presence of milk products. If you are allergic to eggs, check labels for words such as albumin.

Soy in products is sometimes identified as hydrogenated vegetable protein.

◁ Watch out for additives. Some people don't respond well to various preservatives and additives used in food preparation. The artificial sweetener aspartame, the flavor enhancer monosodium glutamate (MSG), the food dye FD&C Yellow No. 5 (listed as tartrazine on medicine labels), and the sulfur-based preservatives called sulfites cause adverse reactions in certain people.

◁ Consult restaurant staff concerning menu ingredients when you eat out. Even food cooked in the same pan as an allergen can cause a reaction.

◁ Warn school employees if your child is allergic.

◁ Instruct children and their friends and caregivers about the type and seriousness of the allergy.

◁ Keep epinephrine on hand and know how to administer it.

◁ Have children retested. Many children outgrow their food allergies by the age of 3. In some instances, the allergy-causing foods may be reintroduced into the diet.

A combination of factors may trigger an allergy. Just like it takes two to tango, sometimes it takes two or more triggers to stimulate an allergic response. In the last few years, researchers have found that certain people can develop life-threatening allergic reactions when they eat a certain food, then exercise strenuously. Separately, neither the food nor the exercise causes any problems.

Natural help for hives and rashes

Some people are allergic to certain substances in cosmetics, hair-care products, cleaning products, plants, clothing, shoes, and costume jewelry. You may not have a reaction until you have been exposed to a substance several times. To treat allergic skin reactions naturally, try the following:

Find the cause. If you experience welts, blisters, or other rashes, including dry, itchy skin, try to figure out what has caused the problem, and do everything you can to avoid that substance.

Help your hives. A warm (not hot) shower may help relieve the itching of hives. Treat blisters with cold compresses soaked with water or saline solution. The compresses help dry the blisters and promote healing.

Limit contact with soaps, solvents, and detergents. Wear rubber gloves for washing dishes and specially made heavy-duty gloves when you work with strong chemicals. If you find that the residual laundry detergent left on clothes after washing irritates your skin, run each load of clothes through the rinse cycle one extra time.

Go natural. All-cotton clothing and bedding are less irritating to allergy-prone skin than synthetic or wool fibers.

Monitor your medicines. Aspirin, NSAIDs, or alcohol may make you more prone to react to an allergen by getting hives. People with thyroid problems may also be more prone to hives.

Other factors which may set the stage for hives are heat and humidity, tight clothing, rigorous exercise (especially after eating), exposure to sunlight, and exposure to cold, fever, and anxiety.

Stay calm. The emotional stress of having a skin rash can make the condition worse. Try stress management techniques to keep calm and maintain a positive outlook.

Soothe skin with the "soak-grease" method. To treat an allergic reaction that results in dry, itchy skin, try showering and bathing with a very gentle, nonperfumed soap. While skin is still damp, apply petroleum jelly, oil, or nonperfumed skin cream to seal in moisture. Do this once or twice a day until the condition improves.

Beware of latex products. If you're allergic to bananas, chestnuts, avocados, celery, cherries, figs, nectarines, papaya, passion fruit, or peaches, you may be allergic to products containing latex. Recently, researchers confirmed a link between allergies to certain foods and allergies to latex products.

If you think you have a latex allergy, let your doctor know, especially before he performs any procedure that might expose you to latex, such as using latex surgical gloves or latex bandages.

For more skin self-help, see the *Skin Conditions* chapter.

Sources —

Advance Plus, The Asthma and Allergy Foundation of America, 1125 Fifteenth St. N.W., Suite 502, Washington, D.C. 20005

Alternative Medicine, The Definitive Guide, Future Medicine Publishing, Puyallup, Wash., 1993

American Family Physician (49,6:1411 and 48,5:773)

Annals of Allergy (70,1:31)

Cutis (52,2:70)

Food Allergies, FDA Consumer Reprint, Publication No. (FDA) 94-2279, Department of Health and Human Services, Food and Drug Administration, HFI-40, Rockville, Md. 20857

Journal of the American Medical Association (268,20:2807,2830)

Journal Watch (14,12:93)

Medical Tribune (33,6:112 and 36,7:18)

Medical Tribune for the Family Physician (35,7:24 and 35,18:22)

New England Journal of Medicine (332,26:1769)

Physician Assistant (117,5:52)

Science News (145,2:28 and 146,15:231)

The Allergy Book, Atlanta Allergy Clinic, P.A., Suite 200, 1965 N. Park Place, N.W., Atlanta, Ga. 30339

The Asthma and Allergy Advance (Nov./Dec. 1993)

The Doctor's Complete Guide to Vitamins and Minerals, Dell Publishing, N.Y., 1994

The Journal of Allergy and Clinical Immunology (81,3:495)

U.S. Pharmacist (20,7:37)

Understanding Allergy, National Jewish Center for Immunology and Respiratory Medicine, 1400 Jackson Street, Denver, Colo. 80206, 1993

ASTHMA

◄ Anxiety   ◄ Chest pain
◄ Coughing   ◄ Gasping
◄ Shortness of breath   ◄ Wheezing

Natural strategies for dealing with asthma

You feel like you're choking, but you know you're not. You feel like you've had the breath knocked out of you, but you know you haven't. You sound like the little locomotive that couldn't, but you know you can — if only you could get a deep breath.

When asthma strikes, your airways narrow as lung muscles contract, the airway walls swell, and thick mucus is produced. Along with the painful attempt to catch your breath comes a wheezing cough that may last for days or weeks.

Don't let asthma run your life anymore. Here's how to take control.

Keep your house clean. Allergic reactions trigger most asthma attacks. Allergy triggers, or allergens, include pollen, dust, mold, animal hair, and feathers. Clean your house regularly to keep dust and mold to a minimum. See the allergy section of this chapter for more house-cleaning and allergen-avoiding tips.

But watch out for cleaning-product fumes! While cleaning your house is a must for eliminating allergens, be aware that certain house-cleaning products contain chemical fumes that may bring on an asthma attack. Be especially careful when you buy and use new chemical cleaners.

Use caution in the great outdoors. Asthma triggers not only exist inside the house, they are outside as well. Air pollution and smog are terrible for asthma sufferers. Always carry your medication with you when you plan a long day outdoors. Stay indoors as much as possible when pollen and pollution are at their peak.

Avoid cigarette smoke like the plague. If your friends smoke, ask them politely to take their habit elsewhere. If you smoke, the best and only advice is to quit immediately. One cigarette can hinder your breathing and cause mucus to build up in your lungs. Always ask for nonsmoking sections in restaurants and on airplanes.

Stay away from sick people. Viral infections tend to provoke asthma attacks. Avoid unnecessary exposure to people and situations where you might catch a virus.

Don't read fashion and other popular magazines that contain scented advertisement cards. Doctors say that as many as 20 percent of asthmatics could suffer an attack caused by perfume advertising inserts. You should also try to stay away from perfume counters in department stores, as well as scented air fresheners.

Figure out your food triggers and avoid them. Studies show that certain foods can bring on asthma attacks. In particular, seafood, eggs, and some dairy products like milk have been linked to asthma flare-ups.

Search out sulfites. Eating foods with sulfites (food preservatives) and artificial coloring products can also trigger asthma. Manufacturers add sulfites to foods such as dried fruits and dehydrated potatoes to prevent discoloration. Some foods that tend to have high sulfite levels are dried apricots, dried peaches, instant mashed potatoes, imported peppers, shrimp, and hominy. Wine is also high in sulfites; just one glass can cause sensitive people to become short of breath.

If you think you may be sensitive to sulfites, check labels for sodium sulfite, sulfur dioxide, or sodium or potassium bisulfite or metabisulfite.

Be wary of benzoates. The benzoate preservatives can trigger asthmatic reactions in some people. Check labels for benzoic acid, sodium benzoate, butylated hydroxyanisole (BHA), butylated hydroxytoluene (BHT). You'll find benzoates in bread, chocolate, fat, instant drink powders, jam, margarine, mayonnaise, milk powder, oil, potato powder, and soft drinks.

Load up on cereals, dairy products, nuts, and green vegetables. These foods contain magnesium — a mineral that can do wonders for your lungs. Eating magnesium-rich foods can prevent wheezing and reduce your chances of suffering an asthma attack. Eat more fresh food and avoid eating too many processed foods. Processed food tends to be very low in magnesium.

Enjoy your morning cup of coffee. Caffeine has been found to reduce asthma attacks by widening the blood vessels in the lungs. During an asthma attack, caffeine can be particularly helpful as an emergency backup if you've forgotten your inhaler. Don't overdose on caffeine, but a can or two of cola or two cups of coffee can help. Now your morning coffee can serve the dual purpose of fighting asthma and giving you a jump-start on the day.

Chase away headaches with acetaminophen, not aspirin. Many people with asthma are sensitive to aspirin. Because aspirin is one of the most widely used drugs in the world, it is important for everyone with asthma to be tested for aspirin sensitivity. Doctors strongly recommend using acetaminophen in place of aspirin. Always ask your pharmacist about the possible aspirin content of any prescription or nonprescription medicine you take.

Take a cold-water bath. Cold-water baths, though they may not be comfortable, seem to ease asthma symptoms. Studies show remarkable improvements in wheezing and breathing after bathing in cold water for one minute or taking a 30-second cold shower every day. So if you can stand the chill, a cold shower a day can help keep the asthma attacks away.

Be careful with winter fires. Burning wood gives off tiny particles that can get into your lungs and cause shortness of breath. To enjoy your fireplace in good health, take these precautions: Don't sit close to the fireplace; don't use chemicals, such as kerosene, to light the fire; and keep the chimney clean to prevent fumes. Be sure to air the room out after the fire, and dust and vacuum as soon as possible.

Take vitamin C to protect your body from toxins. Cigarette smoke and other pollutants can be deadly for people with asthma. Vitamin C, the most important fighter of free radicals in the lungs, helps protect your body from environmental pollutants. Make sure your diet is high in vitamin C. The recommended daily allowance is 60 mg, but most multivitamins contain much more than that.

Monitor your breathing with a peak flow meter. Some people with asthma can't tell when they're not getting enough oxygen until it's too late. If you have trouble knowing when you are breathless, you need to use a peak flow meter every day. Peak flow meters measure how fast you blow air out of your lungs. They are portable and can alert you to the early signals of an asthma attack.

Although these suggestions and the tips that follow may require some extra work on your part, the time and effort are definitely worth it. Asthma does not have to control your life. Instead of living with the chest pains, wheezing and coughing, fight asthma and win!

Prevent nighttime asthma attacks

Most people's asthma gets worse at night. Here are some strategies for more restful nights:

Wash 'em out. Use saline nasal washes to rinse out your sinuses and keep allergens out of your breathing passages.

Aid your digestion. The way your body digests food can have an effect on your asthma. Heartburn can make asthma worse, especially at night. If heartburn is a problem for you, avoid food and drink for several hours before you go to bed. Put 4-inch blocks under the head of your bed to keep your head above the level of your stomach and to keep stomach acid in its place. Antacids can also help, but long-term use may do more harm than good.

Breathe easier. If you have sleep apnea (you stop breathing for short periods during the night), talk to your doctor about a device that applies "continuous positive airway pressure." This is a mask and pump you can use that will help control your apnea as well as your nighttime asthma.

Be cautious at night. Allergens affect you more at night than during the day because your body is more vulnerable during sleep. So watch out for anything in your bedroom (pets, pollen, dust, etc.) that might cause you to lose sleep to asthma.

Check your daytime activities. About half of the people with asthma have a delayed response to breathing in allergens during the day, so that the reaction occurs at night. If you cannot find a substance in your nighttime environment that seems to be causing your problem, check the substances that you are exposed to at work or at home during the day. Do your symptoms lessen during holidays away from your job? You may need to stay away from some substance in your work environment.

If you have questions about asthma, you can call the Lung Line at 1-800-222-LUNG. Specially trained nurses at the National Jewish Center for Immunology and Respiratory Medicine will answer your questions.

Steps to easier exercising with asthma

Asthma may make exercise extra challenging, but it definitely doesn't make it impossible. Many people with asthma avoid exercise because they fear an attack. Exercise-induced asthma is extremely common, but it can be prevented and controlled. Follow these suggestions, and you'll be able to enjoy a fun, daily exercise program.

Choose an asthma-friendly exercise. Some activities are going to be easier on your lungs than others. Most experts believe exercise-induced asthma occurs when your lungs lose heat and water. There are three reasons for this: long periods of hard breathing, breathing in allergens, and breathing in cold air.

Therefore, sports such as running and bicycling, especially during the winter, will increase your chances of an exercise-induced attack. Long-lasting endurance sports, such as baseball and downhill skiing, are less likely to trigger asthma than a high-intensity sport like basketball or soccer.

Water sports cause the least problems because the moist, warm air prevents the airways from cooling. Walking and weight training rarely trigger asthma.

Choose the proper environment. Try to exercise in warm, humid, unpolluted environments. Early morning is the least-polluted time of day in an urban area.

On cold days, wear a face mask or scarf over your nose and mouth. This will make the air you breathe warmer and more humid. Foam nylon masks will help warm the air before it enters your lungs.

Use an inhaler five minutes to an hour before vigorous exercise. Always carry your inhaler in case you need it during exercise as well.

Always warm up thoroughly before starting vigorous exercise. Follow up with a long cool down after exercise. This is an excellent way to gradually increase your physical strength and lung capacity without triggering an asthma attack.

Avoid eating certain foods up to two hours before exercise. Shrimp, celery, peanuts, egg whites, almonds, and bananas are some of the foods that can trigger exercise-induced attacks. Eating these foods before exercise can actually cause breathlessness, a drop in blood pressure, and extreme weakness.

Breathe through your nose. This will warm and moisten the air in your nasal passages. Asthma and Exercise by Nancy Hogstead and Gerald Couzens and The Breath Approach to Whole Life Fitness by Ian Jackson outline other useful breathing techniques that will reduce your chances of asthma during exercise.

Keep a positive attitude and believe in yourself. Don't give up exercise altogether if you have a bad experience. One negative experience does not even compare to all of the positive benefits of exercise.

Sources —
American Family Physician (48,5:865)
American Journal of Medicine (85S,18:6)
American Review of Respiratory Diseases (147:525 and 142:1153)
Asthma Facts, Whitehall Laboratories, No. 5 Giralda Farms, Madison, N.J. 07940, 1992
Asthma: What Every Parent Should Know, American Lung Association and Fisons Corp., P.O. Box 1766, Rochester, N.Y. 14603, 1992
British Medical Journal (306,6881:854; 307,6913:1159 and 308,6922:200)
Drug Therapy (23,4:29 and 24,6:20)
Emergency Medicine (26,2:40)
FDA Consumer (28,1:30)
Food Safety Notebook (4,2:18)
LungLine Letter (8,2:3 and 7,5:4)
Medical Tribune for the Internist and Cardiologist (34,23:7; 35,7:12 and 35,16:19)
More Than Snuffles: Childhood Asthma, FDA Consumer Reprint, Publication No. (FDA) 91-3181, Dept. of Health and Human Services, Food and Drug Administration, Rockville, Md. 20857, 1991
One Minute Asthma, Pedipress Inc., Amherst, Mass. 01002, 1992
Postgraduate Medicine (95,8:185 and 97,6:83)
The American Journal of Clinical Nutrition (61,3S:625S)
The Journal of the American Medical Association (268,20:2807)
The Lancet (344,8919:357)
The PDR Family Guide to Nutrition and Health, Medical Economics, Montvale, N.J., 1995
The Physician and Sportsmedicine (21,10:7 and 22,9:15)
Western Journal of Medicine (163,1:49)
What Everyone Needs To Know About Exercise-Induced Asthma, UCLA School of Medicine, Los Angeles, Calif. 90024, 1993

CHRONIC OBSTRUCTIVE PULMONARY DISEASE (CHRONIC BRONCHITIS AND EMPHYSEMA)

◄ Constant feeling of breathlessness
◄ Fatigue
◄ Persistent, wrenching cough

12 steps to easier breathing

If you have chronic obstructive pulmonary disease (COPD), you may think that breathing easy is like making the impossible dream come true.

COPD refers to chronic bronchitis and emphysema. These conditions may exist separately, but usually they're found together. A cough that won't go away, caused by too much mucus in the lungs, is the main sign of chronic bronchitis.

Emphysema involves damage to lung tissue and the inability to catch your breath. Cigarette smoking is the major cause of COPD. If you have either chronic bronchitis or emphysema, or both, you need to be under a doctor's care.

While breathing may never be the effortless endeavor that it once was, there are ways you can make it easier. Here's how:

Don't smoke! And don't spend time around others who are smoking. It could irritate your lungs further.

Avoid allergens. Dust and pollen will irritate your lungs too.

Don't catch colds. Washing your hands frequently is the best defense.

Plan to get a flu vaccination each year. Seek treatment from your doctor immediately if you do catch an infection.

Exercise regularly. If you are able to exercise, it will strengthen your muscle tone and endurance. It will also help reduce breathlessness, lead to greater independence, and enable you to participate in a wider range of activities. Walking, using a treadmill, stair climbing, and riding a stationary bike are good activities to increase your strength.

Follow a healthy diet. Between 30 and 50 percent of people with COPD suffer from some degree of malnutrition. This causes further complications and weakens the body more, especially if you are underweight. A healthy, balanced diet with added calories and protein can increase your health and even slow the progress of the disease.

Drink plenty of liquids. Drinking six to eight glasses of liquids a day will help thin mucus that must be coughed up from your lungs.

Blow up a balloon. A study was conducted with 28 volunteers who blew up balloons 40 times a day for eight weeks. At the end of the eight weeks, the volunteers had a huge decrease in their symptoms of breathlessness. They also felt a greater ability to walk around without losing their breath. Blowing up balloons is an easy and inexpensive way to decrease your breathlessness.

Learn to breathe and cough properly. Your doctor or physical therapist can show you techniques to improve your breathing and coughing to make them more productive.

Enroll in a class. A pulmonary rehabilitation class can help you and your family deal with the physical and emotional aspects of COPD.

Consider oxygen therapy. Portable oxygen tanks are available now and are a convenient way to ease your breathing. It's important to take care of yourself and follow your doctor's advice. With courage and a positive attitude, you can manage your COPD and have a healthier, better quality life.

Diet remedies ease COPD

Along with your medicines and other therapies, here are some healthy and comforting natural remedies.

Eat more whole foods. A diet rich in whole, unprocessed foods is more nutritious and healthier for you in general. Raw grapes are a good food to add to your diet, as well as fresh grape, orange, lemon, and black currant juices. Carrots, celery, spinach, and watercress are high in vitamins and provide good nutrition in either whole or juice form.

Enjoy hot, spicy foods. Chili peppers, horseradish, mustard, cayenne pepper, garlic, and onion will help open your air passages and bring relief.

Get enough vitamins and minerals. Be sure to get at least the recommended daily allowance to maintain your health. Vitamins A, C, and E are especially important.

Dine on healthy fish. There is evidence that eating 2 1/2 servings of fish a week may help prevent COPD in some people who smoke. (Of course, not smoking is the best prevention.)

The omega-3 fatty acids contained in fish seem to interfere with smoking's inflammation of the lungs. Fish is a healthy protein to add to your diet even if you already have COPD.

Sources —
Alternative Medicine: The Definitive Guide, Future Medicine Publishing, Puyallup, Wash., 1993
British Medical Journal (304,6843:1642)
Consultant (31,2:75)
Geriatrics (48,1:59)
Med Facts: Chronic Bronchitis, National Jewish Center for Immunology and Respiratory Medicine, 1400 Jackson Street, Denver, Colo. 80206,1987
Med Facts: Management of COPD, National Jewish Center for Immunology and Respiratory Medicine, 1400 Jackson Street, Denver, Colo. 80206,1993
Taber's Cyclopedic Medical Dictionary, F.A. Davis Company, Philadelphia, Pa., 1989
The Merck Manual, 16th edition, Merck Research Laboratories, Rahway, N.J., 1992

COLDS

◀ Coughing
◀ Nose or chest congestion
◀ Sneezing
◀ Watery eyes
◀ Mild fatigue
◀ Runny nose
◀ Sore throat

Seven ways to comfort the common cold

You may be the cleanest and most cautious person in the world, but you will probably still catch a cold or two each year. Colds are caused by viruses. They are highly contagious and easily spread from person to person through coughs, sneezes, handshakes, and touching surfaces contaminated by other people's germs.

Unlike bacterial infections that can be cured with antibiotics, cold viruses have no cure except time. They must run their course, and usually go away in about seven to 10 days. Here's what you can do until the time passes.

Gargle with warm, salty water. Your sore throat will thank you for this time-tested remedy.

Breathe hot, moist air. A vaporizer or similar device for inhaling hot, moist air may help you breathe easier if your chest is tight. Hot showers can also help your airways open.

Drink lots of fluids. Most people don't drink enough fluids when they are healthy, but your body is strong enough to manage. When you are sick, however, it's very important to drink so that your body has the strength to fight the illness. Drinking eight to 10 glasses of liquid each day is a good guideline. Hot drinks are better than cold.

Use the color of your urine as an indicator. If your urine is dark yellow, you need to drink more. If your urine is clear, you are drinking enough.

Get plenty of rest. If you feel tired, your body is trying to tell you something. Take a nap or a day off work. Your body will appreciate it, and your co-workers will thank you for not spreading your cold throughout the office.

Use disposable tissues instead of handkerchiefs. Cold germs can live for hours in your handkerchief. Wash your hands after disposing of soiled tissues.

Wash out your nostrils. This will help prevent stuffy sinuses from becoming infected. Take a syringe and fill it with warm water, then gently inject the water into one nostril. The water (and mucus) will drain out through your mouth into the sink. Repeat a few times for each nostril until the drainage is clean. It sounds kind of unpleasant, but it really will help clear your sinuses.

Take your vitamin C. Studies show that vitamin C can help prevent colds. Citrus juices like orange and grapefruit are excellent sources of vitamin C. You could also take vitamin supplements. Even if vitamin C doesn't keep the cold away, researchers say it can make the cold less severe and make it go away faster.

No matter where you live or what you do, it seems that colds are part of life in a crowded world. If you get a cold, don't be distressed or embarrassed. Do everything you can to avoid giving it to someone else, and follow our advice to make it more bearable for yourself. And remember, this too shall pass!

Herbal remedies for the common cold

Herbs can help relieve some of your cold symptoms. With the safe, natural remedies listed here, you won't have to worry as much about drug side effects. If you plan to use herbs, be sure to let your doctor know. Herbs may interfere with or intensify the effects of other medicines you take.

Hyssop

Drink hyssop tea for relief of coughs, hoarseness, fever, and sore throats. It is especially effective as an expectorant, helping you get rid of fluid in your chest. The taste is bitter, so many people add honey to tea made from hyssop leaves.

Horehound

You've probably heard of horehound lozenges to relieve sore throats and coughs. Lozenges containing horehound may be available at your pharmacy, natural health food store, or herbal remedy store. Horehound is such an effective remedy that German health officials approved it as a drug to fight colds.

Echinacea

Echinacea works by stimulating your body's defenses against germs. It doesn't relieve symptoms of a cold, but it may keep the cold from becoming severe or lasting a long time, especially if you take the herb in the early stages of your cold. You can find echinacea in a liquid or tablet form in stores that sell herbal remedies. If you choose the liquid, take 10 to 25 drops per day. If you choose tablets, take one or two a day.

Chamomile

Chamomile clears clogged sinuses and stuffy noses. Place a handful of chamomile flower heads into a bowl and pour boiling water over them. Place a towel over your head, lean over the bowl, and inhale the steam.

Chamomile also soothes minor irritations of the mouth, gums, and throat. To relieve discomfort, gargle with a cup of hot chamomile tea every hour. To prepare chamomile tea, pour boiling water over 1 heaping tablespoon of chamomile flower heads. Cover and let steep for 10 to 15 minutes. Strain. You may find the tea more enjoyable if you add a spoonful of honey or sugar.

Horseradish

For quick and natural sinus relief, grate some fresh horseradish. A few whiffs and your sinuses will open right up. You can also grate horseradish into a mixture of honey and water and gargle with it to relieve hoarseness.

Betony

You can buy betony in health food stores as dried leaves or a liquid extract. To soothe a sore throat or mouth, place 2 heaping teaspoons of dried betony or 8 to 12 drops of betony extract into a cup and add boiling water. If you use the dried herb to prepare your tea, you must strain it before drinking. You can either drink the tea or let it cool and use as a gargle. Don't drink more than three cups of betony tea a day because it might irritate your stomach.

For more self-help solutions for colds, flu, and other respiratory disorders, see the **Infections** chapter.

Sources —
American Family Physician (48,7:1302)
Herbal Medicine, Beaconsfield Publishers, Beaconsfield, England, 1988
HerbalGram (30:45)
Herbs of Choice: The Therapeutic Use of Phytomedicinals, The Haworth Press, Binghamton, N.Y., 1994
Herbs, Reader's Digest, Pleasantville, N.Y., 1990
Journal of Pediatrics (122,5:799)
Journal Watch (12,1:5)
Medical World News (34,3:31)
Miracle Medicine Herbs, Parker Publishing, West Nyack, N.Y., 1991
Nutrition Research Newsletter (12,3:29 and 12,11/12,121)
Parent's Guide to Coldproofing Your Home, Dixie Child Care Challenge, James River Corporation, 1993
Postgraduate Medicine (91,5:281 and 91,6:55)
The Honest Herbal, The Haworth Press, Binghamton, N.Y., 1993
The Journal of the American Medical Association (269,17:2258 and 271,14:1109)
The Lancet (338,8765:522)
The Lawrence Review of Natural Products, Facts and Comparisons, St. Louis, Mo., 1991
U.S. Pharmacist (18,101:35)

COUGHS

◀ Deep, wrenching cough
◀ Sputum-producing cough
◀ Tickling or hacking dry cough

How to quit coughing

You've snuggled cozily into your chair in the concert hall, enjoying the quiet, lyrical violin solo, when suddenly you are struck by a fit of coughing. As the dry, hacking cough continues, you feel suddenly as if you are "center stage," and the embarrassment follows you all the way from your seat to the water fountain in the lobby.

From a dry tickle at the back of your throat to a never-ending hacking to a gut-wrenching, sputum-producing heave — coughing is one miserable symptom that seems to accompany a variety of health problems. Colds, flu, heartburn, and even some drugs such as ACE inhibitors cause coughing. Allergies and the accompanying sinus drainage can also cause coughs.

Coughing can lead to serious health problems like urinary incontinence and rectal and vaginal muscle strain. But even without additional problems, coughing is irritating enough in itself to warrant some cures. Here are some ways to relieve your discomfort when coughing strikes.

Drink warm liquids and plain water. Warm liquids and water are the best ways to loosen mucus in your lungs so that it's easier to cough up. If your cough accompanies other cold and flu symptoms, try to drink at least eight to 10 glasses of liquids a day. Liquids will keep a fever down, soothe a sore throat, and help your body flush out germs.

Try the ice trick. Suppress your cough by keeping an ice cube in your mouth until it melts. (Be careful not to swallow the ice cube.)

Put down that cigarette. Have you ever met a smoker who didn't have a chronic cough? Even if you don't smoke, if you work or live with people who do, passive smoke could be the culprit responsible for your cough. Find a way to free yourself from smoky environments, or you could be coughing and wheezing forever.

Eat a banana. Heartburn is the culprit for about one in every 10 chronic coughers, and researchers have found that bananas are a great natural solution for heartburn. Banana powder, a dried, ground-up form of the fruit, also works well. Other heartburn remedies include raising the head of your bed, avoiding food and drink before bedtime, losing weight, and eating more slowly.

Get that chicken soup comfort. If you are coughing up phlegm, you need to let nature take its course and even help it along. Warm soup will help speed up the process of coughing up the phlegm and mucus caught in your lungs. When your body coughs productively, it can clean out unwanted substances in your lungs.

Take a hot shower or a steamy bath. Use a humidifier or sit in a steamy room to help loosen the mucus in your lungs.

Take the right kind of cough medicine. If you are coughing up phlegm, you need to take an expectorant that will help you cough. If you have a dry cough that doesn't bring up any mucus, you can use a cough suppressant. Suppressants are also called antitussives, and they come in both liquid form and lozenge form.

Herbal cough remedies

These herbs may help your cough. If you plan to use herbs, be sure to let your doctor know. Herbs may interfere with or intensify the effects of other medicines you take.

Hyssop and chamomile teas will soothe your throat and relieve a cough.

Horehound works well too. You can usually find horehound lozenges at health-food stores.

Marshmallow-root tea soothes sore throats. Put 1 to 2 teaspoonfuls in about 1/2 cup of water.

Mullein flowers are good for throat irritations and cough. Use 3 to 4 teaspoonfuls to prepare about 1/2 cup of tea. You may drink this concoction several times daily.

Plantain leaves, fresh or dried, are a cough suppressant. Add 3 to 4 teaspoonfuls of the herb to about 1/2 cup of boiling water.

Slippery elm lozenges release mucilage (a slippery vegetable substance) to soothe the throat.

Sources —
British Medical Journal (298,6683:1280)
Health Letter (6,2:1)
Herbs of Choice: The Therapeutic Use of Phytomedicinals by Varro E. Tyler, Ph.D., ScD, Haworth Press, Binghamton, N.Y., 1994
The Lancet (336,8710:282)

CANCER

Prescription Drugs ℞

Chlorambucil

Brand name: *Leukeran*

What this drug does for you:
This drug treats various types of cancer.

Possible side effects of this drug:
- You may experience nausea, vomiting, diarrhea, mouth ulcers, skin rash, lung problems, liver problems, drug fever, nerve problems, pneumonia, and inflammation of the bladder.
- Rare side effects include tremors, muscle twitching, confusion, agitation, lack of coordination, loss of muscle tone or reflexes, seizures, and hallucinations.

Special warnings:
- This drug should only be taken by people with certain kinds of cancer.
- People taking chlorambucil should have their blood checked weekly.
- Chlorambucil causes chromosome damage and may cause permanent sterility.
- Do not have any live virus vaccines while taking this drug.

Pregnancy and nursing mothers:
Category D. See page 9 for description of categories. Not known if drug is present in mother's milk.

Possible food and drug interactions:
- Taking anticoagulants or aspirin with this drug may increase the chance of unusual bleeding or bruising.
- Use with extreme caution when you are taking any drugs that have a risk of seizure.

Helpful hints:
- Eat small, frequent meals to help prevent nausea and vomiting.
- Drink seven to 12 glasses of water or other clear liquids every day.

Cyclophosphamide

Brand name: *Cytoxan* **(Generic available)**

What this drug does for you:

This drug treats various types of cancer.

Possible side effects of this drug:

- Common side effects include loss of appetite, nausea, and vomiting.
- Less common side effects include abdominal pain, diarrhea, rash, changes in skin color, temporary hair loss, mouth sores, and infertility.
- Even though it is very rare, cyclophosphamide can lower the number of blood cells you have. If you don't have enough white blood cells, your immunity is down, and you can get a fever, sore throat or pneumonia. If you are lacking red blood cells, you can become anemic, and that makes you tired and weak. Not having enough blood platelets makes you bruise easily and keeps your blood from clotting properly when you're injured. Be on the lookout for any of these symptoms of bone marrow depression.

Special warnings:

- Cyclophosphamide may cause new cancerous growths, sometimes several years after treatment has stopped.
- Cyclophosphamide can also cause liver and kidney damage. You should have regular liver and kidney tests while you're taking this drug.
- Dose may need to be reduced in people who have had one or both adrenal glands removed.
- May cause sterility in men and women.

Pregnancy and nursing mothers:

Category D. See page 9 for description of categories. Drug is present in mother's milk.

Possible food and drug interaction:

- Cyclophosphamide may change the effects of phenobarbital and the anticancer drug doxorubicin hydrochloride.

Helpful hint:

- Take cyclophosphamide on an empty stomach. If stomach upset occurs, you may take it with food.

Flutamide

Brand name: *Eulexin*

What this drug does for you:

This drug treats cancer of the prostate that has spread to other parts of the body.

Possible side effects of this drug:

- Side effects include vomiting, nausea, diarrhea, hot flashes, impotence, enlargement of breasts in men, decreased sex drive, anemia, low white

blood cell count (lowered immunity), depression, nervousness, anxiety, confusion, loss of appetite, fluid retention, and high blood pressure.
- Rare side effects include hepatitis and jaundice.

Special warnings:
- Do not stop treatment without consulting your doctor.
- Periodic liver function tests should be performed.

Pregnancy and nursing mothers:
Drug not used in women.

Mercaptopurine

Brand name: *Purinethol*

What this drug does for you:
This drug is used to induce and maintain remission in leukemia.

Possible side effects of this drug:
- Side effects include increased skin pigmentation, nausea, vomiting, stomach ulcers, and increased levels of uric acid in the blood.
- Mercaptopurine can suppress your bone marrow, which makes your blood cells, and therefore lower the number of blood cells you have. If you don't have enough white blood cells, your immunity is down, and you can get a fever, sore throat or pneumonia. If you are lacking red blood cells, you can become anemic, and that makes you tired and weak. Not having enough blood platelets makes you bruise easily and keeps your blood from clotting properly when you're injured.
- Drug fever is a rare side effect.
- Call your doctor if you experience anemia, bleeding, infection, nausea, vomiting, jaundice, fever, or sore throat.

Special warnings:
- Do not used if you have previously been resistant to the leukemia drug thioguanine.
- Blood counts should be done weekly throughout treatment.
- Liver functions should be checked weekly when treatment is started.

Pregnancy and nursing mothers:
Category D. See page 9 for description of categories. Discuss any plans for pregnancy with your doctor before taking this drug. Not known if drug is present in mother's milk.

Possible food and drug interactions:
- The drug allopurinol increases the effects of this drug. You may need a smaller dose of mercaptopurine if you are taking allopurinol.
- Using the antibacterial combination drug trimethoprim-sulfamethoxazole and mercaptopurine together may increase suppression of bone marrow.

Helpful hint:
- Drink plenty of fluids while taking this drug.

Methotrexate

Brand name: *Rheumatrex* (Generic available)

What this drug does for you:

This drug treats various cancers including certain types of breast and lung cancers, certain skin cancers of the head and neck, non-Hodgkin's lymphomas, and leukemia. It is also used to treat severe psoriasis that does not respond to other treatments. Lower doses are used to treat severe rheumatoid arthritis.

Possible side effects of this drug:

- Side effects include upset stomach, inflammation of the mouth, fever, chills, dizziness, suppressed immune system, sore throat, diarrhea, headache, loss of appetite, bleeding ulcers, blurred vision, difficulty speaking, rash, itching, hives, hair loss, sensitivity to light, acne, kidney failure, menstrual abnormalities, pneumonia, abortion, and birth defects.
- Rare side effects include eye pain, ringing in the ears, impotence, muscle pain, diabetes, and sudden death.

Special warnings:

- Methotrexate can be extremely toxic. Symptoms include back pain, fever, headache, confusion, lack of coordination, and, sometimes, convulsions.
- This drug should not be used to treat rheumatoid arthritis in people with blood disorders, alcoholism, or chronic liver disease. Routine blood counts, liver and kidney functions, and a chest X-ray should be performed before treatment begins.
- People with infections or whose immune systems are weak, as well as people with poor liver or kidney functions, should take this drug with extreme caution.

Pregnancy and nursing mothers:

Category X. See page 9 for description of categories. Pregnancy should be avoided if either partner is taking this drug. Do not use for psoriasis or rheumatoid arthritis during pregnancy. Drug is present in mother's milk.

Possible food and drug interactions:

- Avoid taking this drug with nonsteroidal anti-inflammatory drugs (NSAIDs). The combination may cause severe intestinal problems and bone marrow toxicity, which may be fatal.
- Levels or effects may be increased by the gout drug probenecid, the seizure drug phenytoin, aspirin, the NSAID phenylbutazone, and the sulfonamide antibiotics.

Tamoxifen

Brand name: *Nolvadex*

What this drug does for you:

This drug is used to treat some forms of breast cancer.

Possible side effects of this drug:

- Common side effects include nausea, hot flashes, vomiting, diarrhea, menstrual cycle disturbances, vaginal discharge or bleeding, eye or vision disorders, mental depression, high calcium levels, ovarian cysts, liver disorders, fatigue, bone pain, rash, phlebitis, cough, and loss of appetite.
- Less common side effects include hair loss, dizziness, vaginal itching, headache, fluid retention or swelling of the hands or feet, and an abnormal sense of taste.

Special warnings:

- This drug may cause eye problems, uterine abnormalities, and liver disorders.
- People with blood disorders should take this drug with extreme caution. Blood counts should be done regularly during treatment. Notify your doctor if menstrual disorders or abnormal bleeding occurs.

Pregnancy and nursing mothers:

Category D. See page 9 for description of categories. Do not take during pregnancy as it may cause spontaneous abortions or birth defects. Use effective contraception other than birth control pills throughout treatment. If you do become pregnant, inform your doctor immediately. Not known if drug is present in mother's milk.

Possible food and drug interactions:

- This drug may increase the effects of anticoagulants.
- The effects of this drug may be increased by the antiparkinson drug bromocriptine.

Natural Alternatives

CANCER

- ◀ Bleeding or itchy mole
- ◀ Change in bowel or bladder habits that lasts more than a week
- ◀ Difficulty swallowing
- ◀ Lump or change in breast shape
- ◀ Rapid, unexpected weight loss
- ◀ Severe, recurrent headaches
- ◀ Blood in urine
- ◀ Change in testes size
- ◀ Coughing up blood
- ◀ Frequent stomach cramps
- ◀ Nagging cough or persistent hoarseness
- ◀ Scab, sore, or ulcer that hasn't healed after three weeks

Battle plan for winning the war against cancer

It's a frightening experience to hear your doctor say, "You have cancer." However, it's no longer a death sentence, as it often was years ago. Today, with new treatments and greater knowledge, it's a whole new ballgame. Along with your medical treatments, here are some self-help strategies that can give you a better crack at recovery.

Remember to work directly with your doctor and never substitute any of the following suggestions for his treatment plan. Get his approval for any natural remedies you want to use in addition to your cancer treatment.

Practice positive thinking. You may be tired of hearing this sermon, but study after study proves that attitude affects health. If you have cancer, your attitude has a big influence on your condition.

In a study at UCLA, researchers found that people with cancer live longer when they are relaxed and optimistic about their chances of survival. A six-week program of relaxation techniques, coping strategies, and cancer education resulted in a higher percentage of long-term survival for a group of people with deadly skin cancer. Another group the same age, sex, and with the same seriousness of cancer didn't receive counseling, and their survival rate was one-fifth lower.

Join a group. Doctors at universities in New York and California found that people with cancer live longer, happier lives when they join support groups. This proved true for groups of women with breast cancer, as well as for groups of men with prostate cancer. Talking with others who have the same disease, and lending each other psychological and emotional support, restores self-esteem and confidence and reduces depression in people with cancer.

Soak up some sunshine. If you have prostate cancer, spend some time in the sun. Sunlight helps your body produce vitamin D, and vitamin D seems to slow prostate tumor growth. Studies show that men with prostate cancer often have low levels of vitamin D in their bodies.

Shed excess pounds. Obese men have up to 44 percent more deaths from cancer than men at their normal weights.

Beating cancer: The right foods pack a powerful punch

If you have cancer, you should do everything you can to nourish your body for its fight against the disease. Here are some ways you can make your diet healthier.

Live low-fat. Your latest defense against skin cancer seems to be the cure-all for everything that ails people these days — a low-fat diet. Researchers at the Baylor College of Medicine in Houston found that people who eat low-fat diets develop fewer solar keratoses, those scaly, reddish patches on the skin that often precede skin cancer.

Researchers followed a group of people who previously had skin cancer. Over a two-year period, the people following their usual diets had an average of 10 precancerous skin growths, while the people following low-fat diets averaged only three.

Researchers at Memorial Sloan-Kettering Cancer Center in New York have also found that a low-fat diet seems to slow the growth of prostate cancer. Human prostate tumors injected into mice grew only half as fast in mice who ate diets with 21 percent fat as compared to those who ate 40 percent fat. Most days, try to eat only 15 percent of your daily calories in fat. Some dietary fats are more dangerous than others. The most harmful fats are contained in meats, eggs, cheese, cream, hydrogenated vegetable oils, butter, mayonnaise, salad dressings, and many baked goods.

Poultry fat, on the other hand, has not been linked to prostate cancer. And Omega-3 fatty acids from fish oils seem to suppress tumor growth.

Recent findings on linoleic acid, a fatty substance previously thought to benefit people with breast cancer, show that this natural substance found in nuts, corn oil, and most margarines may increase the risk that a breast cancer will produce additional small tumors throughout the body.

Fill up on fiber. Enjoy whole-grain breads and at least five servings of fruits and vegetables every day.

High-fiber vegetables include broccoli, cabbage, brussels sprouts, and legumes such as dried beans, lentils, peas, and lima beans. Eat fresh vegetables raw, steamed, or microwaved.

Fresh and dried fruits, such as raisins and dates, are good sources of fiber. For maximum benefit, leave the skins on fresh fruits.

Limit meat. In countries where people eat a lot of meat and fats, there are many more cases of prostate cancer than in other countries. In a Harvard University study, men who ate beef, lamb, and pork nearly every day suffered from the worst complications of prostate cancer 2 1/2 times more often than men who ate meat as little as once a month. A low-fat, high-fiber diet reduces the risk that microscopic prostate cancers will spread and become life-threatening.

Feast on seafood, lean meats, and rich grain products to ensure that you are eating enough selenium. Selenium is a powerful anti-cancer mineral. One of the best sources of selenium is Brazil nuts. You may want to eat three to six Brazil nuts a day to increase your body's selenium content. Keep in mind that Brazil nuts are high in fat and plan the rest of your fat intake accordingly.

Large amounts of selenium are toxic. Don't overdo it on the nuts, especially if you are taking a multivitamin that contains selenium.

And don't forget your antioxidants. Vitamins A, C, E, and beta carotene are all important antioxidant sources. Antioxidants sweep up unstable oxygen molecules, called free radicals, that promote cancer. Antioxidants can be harmful if taken in very high doses, so get them by eating a variety of fresh foods.

Good sources of vitamin A are deep-green and yellow vegetables and fruits, including broccoli, winter squash, apricots, peaches, and cantaloupe.

Citrus fruits, including oranges, grapefruit, berries, and melons, are rich in vitamin C. Vegetable sources include cabbage and cauliflower. Sources rich in both vitamins A and C are brussels sprouts, leafy greens, spinach, tomatoes, sweet green and red peppers, and sweet potatoes.

Whole-grain cereals and dark-green vegetables contain vitamin E, as do wheat germ and nuts.

Savor the stomach-friendly spice. In recent studies, turmeric, the spice that gives curry powder its yellow tint, was shown to stop the growth of certain types of stomach and skin tumors caused by common chemicals found in smog. An ingredient in turmeric, called curcumin, is the compound that suppressed the tumors, scientists say.

In fighting cancer, turmeric appears to act in the same way as antioxidant vitamins. The curcumin soaks up damaging free radicals. It seems that the curcumin in turmeric works even faster than antioxidant vitamins in attacking free radicals.

Season with soy. In a recent study at the University of Wisconsin, scientists found that soy sauce acted as an antioxidant, preventing the growth of cancer. Several components of soy sauce reduced the number of stomach tumors in rats by 66 percent.

In a recent Japanese study, scientists showed that miso, a type of fermented soy paste used as a seasoning or pickling ingredient in Asian cuisine, is a free-radical-fighting antioxidant. Large population studies have shown that eating miso soup is associated with a lower death rate from stomach cancer.

For more information on dealing with nutritional problems specific to certain cancers, call the American Institute of Cancer Research at 1-800-843-8114 or write to them at 1759 R Street, N.W., Washington, D.C. 20069. Request their booklet entitled Nutrition of the Cancer Patient.

In coping with cancer, don't feel that you are alone. Talk to others who have it so that you can give and receive emotional support. And be sure to meet your nutritional needs as well. Along with good medical treatment, taking care of yourself is the way to take cancer out of the game.

Sources —
American Family Physician (47,5:1253)
American Journal of Cardiology (71,4:263)
Cancer Weekly (Nov. 2, 1992)
Diet, Nutrition, and Prostate Cancer, American Institute for Cancer Research, 1759 R Street, N.W., Washington, D.C. 20069, 1991
Food Safety Notebook (4,2:23)
Journal of the American College of Nutrition (12,2:203)
Journal of the National Cancer Institute (87,19:1456)
Medical Tribune (34,3:13)
Medical Tribune for the Family Physician (35,7:12, 10:3, 15:8 and 18:19)
Medical Tribune for the Internist and Cardiologist (34,22:8)
Nutrition and Cancer (22,1:1)
Nutrition Research Newsletter (12,3:28 and 12,11/12:117)
Pharmacy Times (59,12:29)
Science News (146,26/27:421)
The American Journal of Clinical Nutrition (60,3:333)
The American Medical Association Encyclopedia of Medicine, Random House, New York, 1989
The Atlanta Journal / Constitution (Sept. 22, 1993, B4)
The Johns Hopkins White Papers, 1994: Prostate Disorders, The Johns Hopkins Medical Institutions, Baltimore, Md.
The Lancet (2,8668:888)
The New England Journal of Medicine (330,18:1272)
What You Need to Know About Cancer, National Cancer Institute, NIH Publication No. 90-1566, 9000 Rockville Pike, Bethesda, Md., 20892, 1989

DIABETES

Prescription Drugs

Chlorpropamide

Brand name: *Diabinese* **(Generic available)**

What this drug does for you:
This drug is used to treat noninsulin dependent (type II) diabetes by encouraging your pancreas to secrete more insulin.

Possible side effects of this drug:
- The most common side effects are nausea, diarrhea, and constipation.
- Side effects that are common but usually temporary are dizziness, drowsiness, headache, and allergic skin reactions such as itching or hives. This drug may make your skin sensitive to light.
- Jaundice (yellow skin and eyes, dark urine) is a rare side effect.

Special warnings:
- Don't take chlorpropamide if you have ever had an allergic reaction to it.
- Your doctor should not prescribe this drug to you if you have diabetic ketoacidosis.
- Be sure to let your doctor know if you have liver or kidney disease or are at high risk of heart attack.
- Check your blood and urine periodically for abnormal sugar levels while taking this drug.

Pregnancy and nursing mothers
Category C. See page 9 for description of categories. Drug is present in mother's milk.

Possible food and drug interactions:
- Avoid alcohol while you are taking this drug.
- Chlorpropamide is more likely to cause a drop in blood sugar if you are also taking nonsteroidal anti-inflammatories (NSAIDs), some antibiotics, the gout drug probenecid, or some high blood pressure drugs.
- Loss of control of blood sugar may be caused by some high blood pressure drugs, corticosteroids, thyroid drugs, estrogen, birth control pills, seizure drugs, niacin (vitamin B3), and the tuberculosis drug isoniazid.

Helpful hints:
- Wear identification that states you are diabetic.
- This drug may make your skin extra-sensitive to sunlight, so protect

your skin if you'll be outdoors in sunny weather.

- Losing weight and exercising are the most effective and safest ways to control diabetes. You should only use chlorpropamide as an addition to a healthy lifestyle.
- Since this drug can cause low blood sugar, especially when you haven't eaten enough, when you've exercised, or when you've consumed alcohol, learn to recognize the signs of hypoglycemia and know how to treat it.
- This drug can lose its effectiveness when you've taken it for a long period of time.
- Tell your doctor about any stressful events you experience, such as surgery, trauma, infection, or fever. You may need insulin or some other special treatment.

Glipizide

Brand name: *Glucotrol* **(Generic available)**

What this drug does for you:
This drug is used to treat noninsulin dependent (type II) diabetes by lowering blood sugar. Glipizide encourages the pancreas to release insulin after a meal.

Possible side effects of this drug:
- The most common side effects are nausea, diarrhea, and constipation.
- Side effects that are common but usually temporary are dizziness, drowsiness, headache, and allergic skin reactions such as itching or hives. This drug may make your skin sensitive to light.
- Jaundice is a rare side effect.

Special warnings:
- Don't use this drug if you have diabetes complicated by ketoacidosis.
- If you have liver or kidney problems or congestive heart failure, you should use this drug with caution.
- Check your blood and urine periodically for abnormal sugar levels while taking this drug.

Pregnancy and nursing mothers:
Category C. See page 9 for description of categories. Avoid using this drug while you are pregnant if possible. However, if you must take this drug, ask your doctor if you can stop taking it at least a month before your due date because of the risk of severe hypoglycemia in the baby. Not known if drug is present in mother's milk.

Possible food and drug interactions:
- Glipizide is more likely to cause low blood sugar if you are also taking antidepressant drugs called monoamine oxidase (MAO) inhibitors, blood pressure drugs called beta-blockers, anticoagulants, sulfonamides, the gout drug probenecid, nonsteroidal anti-inflammatory drugs (NSAIDs), the antifungal miconazole, or the antibiotic chloramphenicol.
- Glipizide may cause high blood sugar if you take it with calcium chan-

nel blockers, diuretics, the seizure drug phenytoin, corticosteroids, sympathomimetics, estrogen, or the tuberculosis drug isoniazid.

Helpful hints:
- Wear identification that states you are diabetic.
- Take this drug 30 minutes before eating a meal.
- Losing weight and exercising are the most effective and safest ways to control diabetes. You should only use glipizide as an addition to a healthy lifestyle.
- Since this drug can cause low blood sugar, especially when you haven't eaten enough, when you've exercised, or when you've consumed alcohol, learn to recognize the signs of hypoglycemia and know how to treat it.
- This drug can lose its effectiveness when you've taken it for a long period of time.
- Tell your doctor about any stressful events you experience, such as surgery, trauma, infection, or fever. You may need insulin or some other special treatment.

Glyburide

Brand names: *DiaBeta, Glynase PresTab, Micronase*

What this drug does for you:
This drug is used to treat noninsulin dependent (type II) diabetes by encouraging the pancreas to release insulin. Glyburide also has some diuretic effect (it helps your kidneys get rid of water).

Possible side effects of this drug:
- The most common side effects are nausea and heartburn.
- Allergic skin reactions such as itching or hives can be a common and temporary side effect. This drug may make your skin sensitive to light.
- Blurred vision, muscle pain, jaundice, and hepatitis are rare side effects.

Special warnings:
- Don't use this drug if you have diabetes complicated by ketoacidosis.
- If you have liver or kidney problems or congestive heart failure, you should use this drug with caution.
- This drug shouldn't be used as the only therapy for type I diabetes.
- Check your blood and urine periodically for abnormal sugar levels while taking this drug.

Pregnancy and nursing mothers:
Category C. See page 9 for description of categories. Avoid taking this drug while you're pregnant if possible. However, if you must take this drug, ask your doctor if you can stop taking it at least two weeks before your due date because of the risk of severe hypoglycemia in the baby. Not known if drug is present in mother's milk.

Possible food and drug interactions:
- Glyburide is more likely to cause low blood sugar if you are also taking antidepressant drugs called monoamine oxidase (MAO) inhibitors, blood

pressure drugs called beta-blockers, anticoagulants, sulfonamides, the gout drug probenecid, nonsteroidal anti-inflammatory drugs (NSAIDs), the antifungal miconazole, the antibiotic chloramphenicol, or the fluoro-quinolone antibiotics.

- Glyburide may cause high blood sugar if you take it with calcium channel blockers, diuretics, the seizure drug phenytoin, corticosteroids, nicotinic acid, sympathomimetics, estrogen, or the tuberculosis drug isoniazid.

Helpful hints:
- Wear identification that states you are diabetic.
- Losing weight and exercising are the most effective and safest ways to control diabetes. You should only use glyburide as an addition to a healthy lifestyle.
- Since this drug can cause low blood sugar, especially when you haven't eaten enough, when you've exercised, or when you've consumed alcohol, learn to recognize the signs of hypoglycemia and know how to treat it.
- This drug can lose its effectiveness when you've taken it for a long period of time.
- Tell your doctor about any stressful events you experience, such as surgery, trauma, infection, or fever. You may need insulin or some other special treatment.

Insulin, Human NPH and Human Regular Mixture

Brand names: *Humulin N, Novolin N* **(Generic available)**
Humulin 50/50, Humulin 70/30, Novolin 70/30

What this drug does for you:
This drug is used to treat diabetes when oral medications and changes in diet are not effective. Insulin will help keep your blood sugar at a normal level.

Possible side effects of this drug:
- Side effects from insulin are rare, but you may have an allergic reaction to it or low blood sugar.
- The symptoms of an allergic reaction include swelling, itching or redness at the site of the injection, and more serious symptoms such as shortness of breath, wheezing, low blood pressure, fast pulse, perspiration, and rash over the entire body.
- Symptoms of low blood sugar include sweating, dizziness, fatigue, blurred vision, headache, hunger, nausea, irritability, anxiety, palpitation, and an inability to concentrate. Signs of severe low blood sugar include seizures, disorientation, and unconsciousness.

Special warnings:
- If you are traveling across more than two time zones, your insulin schedule will need to be adjusted.
- Nausea and vomiting, as well as any illness, may cause your insulin needs to change. Test your blood and urine frequently if you are sick, and

call your doctor for advice.

Pregnancy and nursing mothers:

Managing diabetes during pregnancy is difficult. Talk with your doctor if you are planning to have a baby, or if you are pregnant or nursing a baby.

Possible food and drug interactions:

- Oral contraceptives, corticosteroids, or thyroid replacement therapy may increase your insulin requirements.
- Aspirin, sulfa antibiotics, oral hypoglycemics, and certain antidepressants may decrease your insulin requirements.

Helpful hints:

- Insulin should be stored in your refrigerator. If this is not possible, store it in a cool place (below 86 degrees Fahrenheit) away from heat and light.
- Wear identification that states you are diabetic. If you have been diagnosed as Type I, it should also state that you are insulin dependent.
- Since this drug can cause low blood sugar, especially when you haven't eaten enough, when you've exercised, or when you've consumed alcohol, learn to recognize the signs of hypoglycemia and know how to treat it.
- Tell your doctor about any stressful events you experience, such as surgery, trauma, infection, or fever. Your insulin schedule may need to be adjusted.

Tolazamide

Brand name: *None available* **(Generic available)**

What this drug does for you:

People with noninsulin dependent (type II) diabetes use this drug to lower their blood sugar levels when they can't control their blood sugar by diet alone.

Possible side effects of this drug:

- This drug may cause nausea, heartburn, feelings of fullness, itching, hives, skin eruptions, sensitivity to sunlight, weakness, fatigue, dizziness, numbness or tingling sensations, headache, and ringing in the ears.
- Jaundice is a rare side effect.
- Even though it is rare, tolazamide can lower the number of blood cells you have. If you don't have enough white blood cells, your immunity is down, and you can get a fever, sore throat, or pneumonia. If you are lacking red blood cells, you can become anemic, and that makes you tired and weak. Not having enough blood platelets makes you bruise easily and keeps your blood from clotting properly when you're injured. Be on the lookout for any of these symptoms of bone marrow depression.

Special warnings:

- Don't use this drug if you have diabetes complicated by ketoacidosis.
- If you have liver or kidney problems or congestive heart failure, you

should use this drug with caution.
- This drug shouldn't be used as the only therapy for type I diabetes.
- Check your blood and urine periodically for abnormal sugar levels while taking this drug.

Pregnancy and nursing mothers:
Category C. See page 9 for description of categories. Not known if drug is present in mother's milk.

Possible food and drug interactions:
- Tolazamide is more likely to cause low blood sugar if you are also taking aspirin, beta-blockers, the antibiotic chloramphenicol, anticoagulants, monoamine oxidase (MAO) inhibitors, the antifungal drug miconazole, nonsteroidal anti-inflammatory drugs (NSAIDs), or the gout drug probenecid.
- You increase your risk of high blood sugar if you take this drug along with birth control pills, corticosteroids, diuretics, estrogen, the tuberculosis drug isoniazid, phenothiazine tranquilizers, thyroid drugs, or the seizure drug phenytoin.

Helpful hints:
- Losing weight and exercising are the most effective and safest ways to control diabetes. You should only use tolazamide as an addition to a healthy lifestyle.
- Since this drug can cause low blood sugar, especially when you haven't eaten enough, when you've exercised, or when you've consumed alcohol, learn to recognize the signs of hypoglycemia and know how to treat it.
- This drug can lose its effectiveness when you've taken it for a long period of time.
- Tell your doctor about any stressful events you experience, such as surgery, trauma, infection, or fever. You may need insulin or some other special treatment.

Tolbutamide

Brand name: *None available* **(Generic available)**

What this drug does for you:
People with noninsulin dependent (type II) diabetes use this drug to lower their blood sugar levels when they can't control their blood sugar by diet alone.

Possible side effects of this drug:
- This drug may cause nausea, heartburn, feelings of fullness, itching, hives, skin eruptions, sensitivity to sunlight, weakness, fatigue, dizziness, numbness or tingling sensations, headache, and ringing in the ears.
- Jaundice is a rare side effect.
- Even though it is rare, tolbutamide can lower the number of blood cells you have. If you don't have enough white blood cells, your immunity is

down, and you can get a fever, sore throat, or pneumonia. If you are lacking red blood cells, you can become anemic, and that makes you tired and weak. Not having enough blood platelets makes you bruise easily and keeps your blood from clotting properly when you're injured. Be on the lookout for any of these symptoms of bone marrow depression.

Special warnings:
- Don't use this drug if you have diabetes complicated by ketoacidosis.
- If you have liver or kidney problems or congestive heart failure, you should use this drug with caution.
- This drug shouldn't be used as the only therapy for type I diabetes.
- Check your blood and urine periodically for abnormal sugar levels while taking this drug.

Pregnancy and nursing mothers:
Category C. See page 9 for description of categories. Not known if drug is present in mother's milk.

Possible food and drug interactions:
- Tolbutamide is more likely to cause low blood sugar if you are also taking aspirin, beta-blockers, the antibiotic chloramphenicol, anticoagulants, monoamine oxidase (MAO) inhibitors, the antifungal drug miconazole, nonsteroidal anti-inflammatory drugs (NSAIDs), or the gout drug probenecid.
- You increase your risk of high blood sugar if you take this drug along with birth control pills, corticosteroids, diuretics, estrogen, the tuberculosis drug isoniazid, phenothiazine tranquilizers, thyroid drugs, or the seizure drug phenytoin.

Helpful hints:
- Losing weight and exercising are the most effective and safest ways to control diabetes. You should only use tolbutamide as an addition to a healthy lifestyle.
- Since this drug can cause low blood sugar, especially when you haven't eaten enough, when you've exercised, or when you've consumed alcohol, learn to recognize the signs of hypoglycemia and know how to treat it.
- This drug can lose its effectiveness when you've taken it for a long period of time.
- Tell your doctor about any stressful events you experience, such as surgery, trauma, infection, or fever. You may need insulin or some other special treatment.

Natural Alternatives

DIABETES

◀ Blurred vision
◀ Fatigue
◀ Itchiness
◀ Slow healing of cuts and bruises
◀ Weakness
◀ Weight loss

◀ Excessive thirst and hunger
◀ Frequent urination, especially at night
◀ Tingling or numbness in the hands and feet

Sweet news for diabetics

"Roses are red, violets are blue, sugar is sweet and so are you." Having a sweet disposition is good, but having too much sugar in your body isn't.

When you have diabetes, your pancreas may not produce any insulin, the hormone that helps your cells take in sugar for nourishment. That's called Type I diabetes.

When your pancreas doesn't produce enough insulin or your cells don't respond properly to it, it's called Type II diabetes. For both types, the result is the same: too much sugar circulates in your bloodstream.

Diet and exercise are the most important aspects of controlling your diabetes, even if you have to take insulin. Deciding what to eat can be a problem for everyone, and it's worse if you have diabetes. Doctors used to recommend a standard, very strict diet to every diabetic. Now, researchers have learned so much about the effects of carbohydrates, proteins, and fats that the American Diabetes Association has revised its guidelines.

The new guidelines let you create an individual diet, using advice from a registered dietician. Your ideal diet will depend on what type of diabetes you have, your lifestyle, and your health profile. Here are some healthy tips to use along with your own specific diet:

Satisfy your sweet tooth sometimes. Experts used to believe that simple carbohydrates like sugar entered the blood more quickly than the complex carbohydrates you find in breads and vegetables. But the thought now is that moderate amounts of sugar are no more damaging for diabetics than other carbohydrates. You just have to remember that carbohydrates can make up no more than 55 to 60 percent of your total calorie intake.

So satisfy your sweet tooth every now and then, but be sure to adjust your diet accordingly. Cut back on calories from starches by a corresponding amount and watch your fat intake, since many sweets contain large amounts of fat.

You can eat some fat. But you must keep track of the kind of fat you're eating. Stay away from saturated fats, which are found in animal products and in coconut, palm, and palm-kernel oils. Instead, choose one of the two types of unsaturated fat: polyunsaturated fat, found in corn, safflower, sunflower, and soybean oils; and monounsaturated fat, now thought to be the healthier of the two, found in olive and canola oils and in some deep-water fish. Whether you're diabetic or not, you should get no more than 30 percent of your daily calories from fat.

Fill up on fiber. Researchers say fiber helps you regulate your blood sugar, and possibly decreases your need for insulin. Add to your diet at least five servings of fruits and vegetables a day. (Be sure to stay within your diet guidelines.)

Apples, berries, figs, oranges, pears, prunes, broccoli, brussels sprouts, carrots, cauliflower, lettuce, and potatoes are good sources of fiber, as are whole-grain breads and cereals. When you increase the fiber in your diet, drink at least six glasses of water a day to avoid constipation. It's also a good idea to increase your fiber intake gradually to avoid cramping or bloating.

Load up on legumes. Legumes come in all shapes and sizes, including black beans, kidney beans, lima beans, navy beans, pinto beans, red beans, soybeans, chick-peas, black-eyed peas, and many more. Beans are a boon to diabetics because they help lower the need for insulin.

Eat four to six small meals instead of three large ones. Participants in a recent study lowered their blood sugar levels and insulin requirements by grazing instead of eating three square meals a day. This doesn't mean you should eat more. Just eat smaller quantities more frequently.

If you're taking insulin, remember that you must eat at regular times, according to the time and amount of your injection. Plan your snacks to keep your blood-sugar level up between meals.

Four nutrients that boost blood sugar control

New research suggests that these common vitamin and mineral supplements may be a big help to diabetics trying to control their blood sugar. Make sure you tell your doctor about your supplement plans so he can watch out for any side effects. Unless you have kidney problems, supplementing your diet with magnesium, chromium, vitamin C, and vitamin E could help you get control of your diabetes.

Magnesium

Daily magnesium supplements may help people with diabetes handle their extra blood sugar better. Magnesium helps insulin work more effectively, so make sure that you get enough magnesium in your diet.

Foods high in magnesium are bran cereal, cashews, peanuts, soybeans, whole wheat, chocolate, rice, dried fruits, and shrimp. Many of these foods are high in calories and sugar, so you may want to take a magnesium supplement. Researchers suggest 20 to 130 mg of magnesium chloride a day. Talk with your doctor or dietician to determine the best amount for you.

Chromium

Chromium acts as insulin's overseer: It makes sure that insulin does a good job moving excess sugar from the bloodstream to the cells. Chromium has to work hard after you eat a lot of simple sugar.

If you're already getting enough chromium in your diet, supplements won't help. But if you have a chromium deficiency, supplements will decrease, and possibly eliminate, your resistance to insulin. For adults, the recommended daily allowance for chromium is .05 to .20 mg.

Vitamin C

New studies offer good news for fans of vitamin C. Large supplements of vitamin C (one study used 1,000 mg a day) may help you sidestep many complications of diabetes. Some studies had successful results with only 100 mg of vitamin C a day.

If your blood sugar level stays out of control for too long, the proteins in your body could bind to the sugar in your bloodstream. This process can cause all sorts of problems with blood vessels and circulation. Further studies are needed, but researchers presently believe that vitamin C puts a stop to this process.

A word of caution for those of you who test your blood sugar with urine tests: Large doses of vitamin C can distort urinary glucose test results. So if you do take vitamin C supplements, use blood tests instead.

Vitamin E

Researchers report that vitamin E may make cell walls more physically fit. This helps insulin move sugar around more easily. One study found that non-insulin dependent diabetics who used large doses of vitamin E improved their insulin action.

Also, like vitamin C, vitamin E supplements may reduce your risk of cataracts by preventing protein and sugar binding. Because it's an antioxidant, it may also help prevent clogged arteries.

Good food sources of vitamin E are vegetable oils, green vegetables, wholegrain cereals, and wheat germ. Many vitamin E sources are high in fat (oils, nuts, and olives, for instance) so eating large amounts of vitamin E is difficult. Some studies recommend supplements of 800 mg a day, but if you want to take more than 400 mg, be sure to check with your doctor first. Vitamin E could cause side effects.

Tips for healthy workouts

The more you exercise, the more control you have over your blood sugar. Even people with Type I diabetes may need less insulin if they exercise regularly. Exercise also lowers your risk of complications like eye disease, heart and circulatory disease, and neuropathy.

Ideally, you should exercise between three and five times a week for 30 minutes at a time. Aim for a heart rate of around 100 to 160 beats per minute. Pushing yourself over this rate increases your risk of fatigue, injury, and hypoglycemia. Here are some other guidelines for exercising safely:

Ease into it. Begin with light exercise for a few minutes each day. Slowly increase how hard and how long you work out.

Warm up and cool down. Before and after exercise, spend five to 10 minutes stretching and doing light exercises such as sit-ups and shoulder shrugs.

Don't dehydrate. Drink three or four cups of water before exercise, 1/2 cup every 15 minutes during exercise, and enough afterward to regain any pounds you sweat away.

Be light on your feet. Choose activities that are easy on your feet, like walking, swimming, or cross-country skiing. Wear comfortable shoes and socks during exercise and inspect your feet afterwards. Check your feet for blisters and cuts. Apply an antiseptic to any problem areas. See a doctor if your injuries aren't looking better after a few days.

Don't exercise on an empty stomach. Three hours before your workout, eat a high-carbohydrate, low-fat meal. Snack on fruit juice or low-fat crackers 30 minutes to an hour before you exercise. Always eat something two or three hours after you exercise.

Head off hypoglycemia. Avoid alcohol and beta blocker drugs around the time of exercise. Both promote hypoglycemia.

Exercise with a buddy who knows the signs of hypoglycemia. Keep hard candy, glucose tablets or fruit juice, and diabetic identification with you while you exercise.

To prevent nighttime hypoglycemia, exercise earlier in the day and reduce your evening insulin dose after you are through exercising. You may need extra carbohydrates before you go to sleep.

Know your numbers. Log your blood sugar level, insulin dosage (if you use it), diet, and exercise for a few months. Learn how changes in your exercise affect your blood sugar, and adjust your diet and insulin dosage accordingly.

Check your blood-sugar level before exercising. If it's less than 100 mg/dl, eat a slice of bread or piece of fruit and check it again. Don't exercise if your blood-sugar level is less than 60 mg/dl.

Follow two tips for insulin shots. Inject your insulin at least an hour before you start exercising, and try to keep the injection away from active muscle groups.

Don't forget your feet

Adults with diabetes frequently develop ulcer-type sores on their feet. If not cared for properly, foot ulcers can become quite serious.

The only sure methods for preventing foot problems are constant vigilance, careful hygiene, and frequent foot checkups by your doctor or podiatrist. You must care for even the most minor injury to your feet to ensure rapid and complete healing. Here are some foot care tips:

Pass on that barefoot stroll. As a diabetic, you should never walk barefoot or in sandals. Shoes protect your feet from injury.

Wear the shoe that fits. Shoes must be fitted carefully by a professional familiar with your special needs as a diabetic. A good fit is extremely important since nerve damage can prevent you from noticing a badly-fitting shoe.

Shoes should be sturdy with ample toe room, good support, and should have soft leather uppers. Running or walking shoes are generally a good choice, but you may require specially designed orthopedic shoes. Break in new shoes gradually to prevent blisters by wearing them for short periods of time.

Treat your feet well. Keep your feet clean and dry at all times. Daily foot care should include careful inspection, washing in lukewarm water, and the use of moisturizing lotion. Your feet should never be exposed to extreme temperatures such as hot water soaks, heating pads, or very cold outdoor weather. Nails should be trimmed straight across, not rounded. Corns or calluses should only be removed by your doctor or podiatrist.

Follow a diet fit for your feet. Diabetic foot problems can also be prevented by controlling the underlying causes. Tight control of your blood sugar levels can reduce damage to your nerves and circulatory system.

Other tips for living with diabetes

A person with diabetes has special health needs and is sometimes confronted with unusual situations. Here are some ways of dealing with them:

Try capsaicin cream for diabetic neuropathy. Capsaicin, the active ingredient in hot chili peppers, has been found to help relieve the severe burning sensation in the ankles and feet that many diabetic people experience. It is now available in over-the-counter ointment form.

Take food along for the ride. Diabetics should never drive a car when they've missed a meal or a regular snack. Carry food with you in case you start getting shaky.

Control stress. Any stress, whether it's from a physical illness or mental overload, can affect how your body handles glucose. You should be especially careful about controlling your blood sugar during trying times.

Test regularly. If you have diabetes, know what your blood sugar level should be, and test it whenever you feel any of the symptoms of hypoglycemia. If your blood sugar level is low, eat a piece of hard candy.

Once you've raised your blood sugar, wait 15 to 20 minutes and test again.

Inject glucagon, not insulin. If you pass out, you'll need immediate treatment in a hospital or an injection of glucagon. Glucagon raises blood sugar and is injected like insulin.

Tell people around you how and when to inject it. People should never give you insulin when you are unconscious.

Tell others to keep their hands to themselves. Naturally, if you're unconscious, people will want to help you. Warn friends and family not to put their hands in your mouth or try to give you food or fluids.

Call for emergency help. Make sure that children know how and when to dial 911.

Use caution with over-the-counter drugs. Many over-the-counter medications can influence the amount of sugar in the blood and could cause problems for diabetics who need to control their blood sugar levels. Some of the most popular over-the-counter medications contain sugar or alcohol.

Researchers warn that an illness by itself makes it harder to control blood sugar levels. Adding an over-the-counter medication that affects blood sugar might make control much more difficult. Check with your doctor for over-the-counter products that are safe for you.

Watch out for other health problems. Your risk of heart disease, kidney disease, tooth and gum problems, eye disease, and nerve damage are greater if you have diabetes. It's very important to have regular checkups with your doctor to look out for these problems.

Your main goal as a diabetic is to stay healthy by controlling your blood sugar level. You will need to eat a carefully balanced diet, watch your weight, exercise, and test your blood sugar regularly. You may have to take insulin, too.

All this will take some effort and determination, but even small changes can make a big difference in feeling healthy. And if you feel good, you'll have that sweet disposition.

Sources —

American Family Physician (47,1:216 and 51,2:419)
Arteriosclerosis and Thrombosis (14,9:1425)
Cardiac Alert (16,10:3)
Complete Guide to Vitamins, Minerals & Supplements, Fisher Books, Tucson, Ariz., 1988
Diabetes. Take the test. Know the score., American Diabetes Association, 1660 Duke Street, Alexandria, Va. 22314
Geriatrics (50,2:48)
Hamilton and Whitney's Nutrition Concepts and Controversies, 6th ed., West Publishing, New York, 1994
Journal of Gerontology (48,3:M84)
Journal of the American College of Nutrition (13,4:344)
Journal of the American Dietetic Association (94,5:504; 94,7:752 and 94,11:1259)
Journal of the American Geriatrics Society (42,12:1235)
Medical Tribune for the Internist and Cardiologist (36,7:18)
NCRR Reporter (17,4:10)
Nutrition Research Newsletter (11,10:113)
Nutrition Today (29,1:6)
Postgraduate Medicine (1994,96:177)
The American Journal of Clinical Nutrition (55,2:461; 55,6:1161; 57,5;650 and 61,2:334))
The Diabetes Educator (18,5:420)
The Journal of Nutrition (123,4:626)
The Journal of the American Medical Association (271,18:1421)
The New England Journal of Medicine (329,14:977)
The Physician and Sportsmedicine (23,3:41)
U.S. Pharmacist (18,1:65)
What is Hypoglycemia?, American Diabetes Association, 1660 Duke Street, Alexandria, Va. 22314

GASTROINTESTINAL DISORDERS

Prescription Drugs

Natural Alternatives

Prescription Drugs ℞

DRUGS FOR DIARRHEA

Diphenoxylate HCL with Atropine

Brand name: *Lomotil* **(Generic available)**

What this drug does for you:

Diphenoxylate and atropine is a combination medicine that relieves diarrhea by slowing down the movements of the intestines.

Possible side effects of this drug:

- This drug may cause tiredness, confusion, dizziness, numbness of fingers or toes, drowsiness, restlessness, itching, swelling, rash, headache, stomach pain, and nausea.
- Other common side effects are fever, rapid heartbeat, difficulty urinating, flushing, and dry skin and mouth.

Special warnings:

- People with some types of jaundice or some types of colitis (consult your doctor) should not use this drug.
- You must not take more than the recommended dose. Use with extreme caution in children. Children are very susceptible to overdose. This drug should not be given to children under 2 years of age.
- If you have liver or kidney problems, talk to your doctor about your condition before taking this drug.

Pregnancy and nursing mothers:

Category C. See page 9 for description of categories. Drug may be present in mother's milk.

Possible food and drug interactions:

- Don't use this drug at the same time as antidepressant drugs called monoamine oxidase (MAO) inhibitors. The combination can cause dangerously high blood pressure.
- If you take this drug along with a drug that depresses your nervous

system, such as tranquilizers, alcohol, antihistamines, or muscle relaxers, the combination may dangerously depress your nervous system.

Helpful hints:

- When you have diarrhea, you are losing water along with minerals such as salt and potassium. This drug can put you at greater risk for dehydration. Make sure you drink extra fluids and eat a balanced diet.
- You shouldn't drive a car or operate heavy machinery until you are sure the medicine isn't making you drowsy or less than alert.
- The usual starting dosage for adults is 20 mg per day (two tablets four times daily or two teaspoonfuls of liquid four times daily).

Loperamide

Brand name: *Imodium* **(Generic available)**

What this drug does for you:

Loperamide relieves diarrhea, including traveler's diarrhea, by slowing down the movements of the intestines.

Possible side effects of this drug:

- Possible side effects include nausea, vomiting, constipation, stomach pain or bloating, dry mouth, tiredness, drowsiness, dizziness, and allergic reactions including skin rash.

Special warnings:

- Don't take loperamide if you have bloody diarrhea or a fever over 101 degrees Fahrenheit. Contact your doctor immediately if you develop a fever or severe stomach pain.
- If you are taking antibiotics or have poor liver function, talk with your doctor before taking loperamide.

Pregnancy and nursing mothers:

Category B. See page 9 for description of categories. Not known if drug is present in mother's milk.

Helpful hints:

- When you have diarrhea, you are losing water along with minerals such as salt and potassium. This drug can put you at greater risk for dehydration. Make sure you drink extra fluids and eat a balanced diet.
- You shouldn't drive a car or operate heavy machinery until you are sure the medicine isn't making you drowsy or less than alert.
- The usual adult dosage for adults is 4 teaspoonfuls or 2 caplets after your first loose bowel movement, then two teaspoonfuls or one caplet after any following bowel movements. Unless your doctor tells you to, you shouldn't take more than 8 teaspoonfuls or 4 caplets in a 24-hour period.
- Don't use this drug for more than two days unless your doctor has told you to do so. Tell your doctor if diarrhea has not improved within 48 hours.

DRUGS FOR NAUSEA, MOTION SICKNESS, AND HEARTBURN

Cisapride

Brand name: *Propulsid*

What this drug does for you:
This drug relieves nighttime heartburn by increasing the contractions of the stomach and the intestines. It helps keep stomach acid out of the esophagus and helps food move through the stomach more quickly.

Possible side effects of this drug:
- Cisapride may cause headache, diarrhea, stomach pain, constipation, gas, stuffy nose, fever, frequent urination, insomnia, anxiety, nervousness, and abnormal vision. It may also make you more prone to infections — urinary infections, viral infections, and respiratory tract infections (such as a common cold).

Special warning:
- People with bleeding in the stomach or some kind of intestinal blockage should not take cisapride. More movement in the intestines could be harmful for these people.

Pregnancy and nursing mothers:
Category C. See page 9 for a description of the categories. Cisapride is present in mother's milk.

Possible food and drug interactions:
- Cisapride doesn't cause sleepiness when you take it by itself, but if you take it along with a drug that depresses your nervous system, such as tranquilizers, alcohol, antihistamines, or muscle relaxers, the combination may make you even more sleepy and sedated.
- Cisapride can make anticoagulants such as warfarin less effective.
- The ulcer drug cimetidine can increase the levels of cisapride.

Helpful hints:
- Cisapride begins working in 30 minutes to one hour.
- The usual starting dosage for adults is 10 mg four times a day — 15 minutes before meals and at bedtime.

Meclizine

Brand names: *Antivert, Bonine* **(Generic available)**

What this drug does for you:
Meclizine is an antihistamine which controls the nausea, vomiting, and dizziness associated with motion sickness.

Possible side effects of this drug:
- This drug may cause dry mouth or drowsiness.

- Blurred vision is a rare side effect.

Special warning:
- People with glaucoma, emphysema, asthma, chronic bronchitis, or an enlarged prostate should use this drug cautiously.

Pregnancy and nursing mothers:
Category B. See page 9 for a description of the categories. Not known if drug is safe to use while nursing.

Possible food and drug interaction:
- If you take meclizine along with a drug that depresses your nervous system, such as tranquilizers, alcohol, antihistamines, or muscle relaxers, the combination may dangerously depress your nervous system.

Helpful hints:
- You shouldn't drive a car or operate heavy machinery until you are sure the medicine isn't making you drowsy or less than alert.
- For motion sickness, the usual adult dose is 25 to 50 mg one hour before traveling. You may repeat the dose every 24 hours for the rest of the journey.

Metoclopramide

Brand name: *Reglan* (Generic available)

What this drug does for you:
Metoclopramide increases the contractions of the stomach and intestines. It is used to treat severe heartburn (stomach acid washing back up into the esophagus), nausea and vomiting after surgery or cancer chemotherapy, and a condition called diabetic gastroparesis (delayed emptying of the stomach). People with diabetic gastroparesis experience nausea, vomiting, heartburn, loss of appetite, or continued feelings of fullness after meals.

Possible side effects of this drug:
- About one out of every 10 people taking metoclopramide experience restlessness, drowsiness, and tiredness.
- Less common side effects are dizziness, headache, depression, insomnia, confusion, anxiety, hallucinations, seizures, irregular menstrual periods, impotence, breast development in men, fluid retention, diarrhea and other bowel disorders, high or low blood pressure, slow or rapid heartbeat, frequent urination, incontinence, flushing, and visual problems. If you are allergic to the drug, you may develop a rash, hives or wheezing.
- A rare side effect of metoclopramide is tardive dyskinesia, a disorder where certain muscles or muscle groups move slowly and uncontrollably. This side effect is dangerous because it may not go away when you quit taking the drug. Lip smacking, puffing of cheeks, or any uncontrolled movement is a sign of tardive dyskinesia.
- This drug can also cause other nerve or muscle disorders such as foot tapping and other restless movements or difficulty talking or breathing because of spasms of the larynx. The longer you take the drug and the

higher the dose, the more likely these side effects are. Let your doctor know immediately if you experience any unusual movements, trembling, or spasms.

Special warnings:

- People with bleeding in the stomach or some kind of intestinal blockage should not take metoclopramide. More movement in the intestines could be harmful for these people.
- People with pheochromocytoma (tumor of the adrenal system) should not use metoclopramide because it can cause severe high blood pressure.
- People with epilepsy or people taking drugs that can cause nerve and muscle disorders (such as tardive dyskinesia) shouldn't take this drug. Metoclopramide increases your risk of seizures and nerve disorders.
- Metoclopramide may cause mental depression. People with a history of depression should take this drug very cautiously.
- People with Parkinson's disease or high blood pressure should take this drug with caution.

Pregnancy and nursing mothers:

Category B. See page 9 for description of categories. Drug is present in mother's milk.

Possible food and drug interactions:

- If you take metoclopramide along with a drug that depresses your nervous system, such as tranquilizers, alcohol, antihistamines, or muscle relaxers, the combination may dangerously depress your nervous system.
- People taking antidepressant drugs called monoamine oxidase (MAO) inhibitors should take metoclopramide very cautiously.
- Metoclopramide may increase levels or effects of the analgesic acetaminophen, the antibiotic tetracycline, and the antiparkinson drug levodopa.
- Metoclopramide may decrease levels of the heart drug digoxin.
- Effects of metoclopramide may be reduced by narcotic analgesics and anticholinergics.

Helpful hints:

- You shouldn't drive a car or operate heavy machinery until you are sure the medicine isn't making you drowsy or less than alert.
- The usual adult dosage for heartburn is 10 to 15 mg up to four times a day — 30 minutes before meals and at bedtime.

Prochlorperazine

Brand name: *Compazine*

What this drug does for you:

Like many of the drugs used to treat anxiety, prochlorperazine is a phenothiazine. It is usually used to relieve severe nausea and vomiting, but it is occasionally used as a tranquilizer to treat anxiety and mental disorders.

Possible side effects of this drug:

- All phenothiazines commonly cause sleepiness, dry mouth, urine retention, confusion, and low blood pressure.

- Some of the less common side effects of prochlorperazine are restlessness, excitement, bizarre dreams, nausea, loss of appetite, sweating, headache, constipation, frequent urination, blurred vision, rapid heartbeat, nasal congestion, swelling, enlargement of breasts in men, impotence, increased sex drive in women, and skin disorders including a sensitivity to light.
- This drug may cause liver problems. If you develop a fever with flu-like symptoms, let your doctor know immediately.
- With any phenothiazine you take, you risk nerve problems as a rare side effect. These problems include tardive dyskinesia (out-of-control movements of the lips, tongue, fingers, toes, or other muscle groups), drug-induced parkinsonism (difficulty speaking or swallowing, loss of balance, muscle spasms, stiff arms or legs, trembling, and shaking), restless leg syndrome, and weak or tired muscles. Very rarely, these problems remain even after you quit taking the drug. Catching the nerve disorders quickly is important, so be sure to let your doctor know immediately if you notice any of these symptoms.
- Even though it is very rare, prochlorperazine can lower the number of blood cells you have. If you don't have enough white blood cells, your immunity is down, and you can get a fever, sore throat, or pneumonia. If you are lacking red blood cells, you can become anemic, and that makes you tired and weak. Not having enough blood platelets makes you bruise easily and keeps your blood from clotting properly when you're injured. Be on the lookout for any of these symptoms.

Special warnings:
- This drug can cause very low blood pressure, so you should take it with caution if you have a history of heart disease.
- Use prochlorperazine with caution if you have a history of epilepsy or glaucoma. This drug may increase the risk of seizures.
- Use prochlorperazine with caution if you have glaucoma.
- This drug can make you become overheated if you are exposed to hot weather.

Pregnancy and nursing mothers:
Not known if safe to use while pregnant. Drug is present in mother's milk.

Possible food and drug interactions:
- If you take prochlorperazine along with a drug that depresses your nervous system, such as other tranquilizers, alcohol, antihistamines, or muscle relaxers, the combination may dangerously depress your nervous system.
- This drug may decrease the effectiveness of anticoagulants and blood-pressure-lowering medicines.
- If you take prochlorperazine with a diuretic, you may experience dizziness and very low blood pressure when you stand up or exercise.

Helpful hints:
- Because of the side effects of prochlorperazine, other drugs are usually

tried first to treat anxiety. When used for nonpsychotic anxiety, your doctor shouldn't prescribe doses higher than 20 mg a day or for longer than 12 weeks.

- As with any drug that affects your central nervous system, you shouldn't drive a car or operate heavy machinery until you are sure the medicine isn't making you drowsy or less than alert.
- This drug can cause low blood pressure and dizziness when you stand up. You may want to remain lying down for a while after you take a dose.

Scopolamine

Brand name: *Transderm Scop*

What this drug does for you:
This circular, flat patch is placed behind the ear several hours before you travel to prevent nausea and vomiting due to motion sickness. It works for up to three days by reducing the activity of the nerve fibers in your ear that help you keep your balance.

Possible side effects of this drug:
- Most people who use a scopolamine patch will experience dry mouth. Many people will also feel drowsy. You may have temporary blurred vision and dilated pupils, especially if you get the medicine in your eyes.
- Rare side effects are memory loss, dizziness, restlessness, hallucinations, confusion, difficulty urinating, and skin rashes or redness. If you have any of these side effects, remove the patch and call your doctor.

Special warnings:
- People with glaucoma should not use scopolamine.
- People with stomach, intestinal, or bladder obstruction, poor liver or kidney functions, or problems with metabolism should use this drug cautiously.

Pregnancy and nursing mothers:
Category C. See page 9 for description of categories. Not known if drug is present in mother's milk.

Possible food and drug interaction:
- If you take scopolamine along with alcohol or a drug that depresses your nervous system, such as tranquilizers, antihistamines, or muscle relaxers, the combination may dangerously depress your nervous system.

Helpful hints:
- This drug can cause your pupils to dilate and cause blurred vision if it comes in contact with your eyes. Wash your hands with soap and water after you handle the patch to avoid getting the medicine in your eyes. If the drug does get in your eye, remove the patch and call your doctor if your eyes feel itchy, red, dry, or painful.
- This drug can cause drowsiness and confusion, so you should be very cautious about driving a car or operating heavy machinery.
- You may have withdrawal symptoms when you remove the patch, including

nausea, vomiting, headache, and dizziness.
- When you throw the patch away, fold it in half with the sticky side together to avoid accidental contact with children or pets.

Trimethobenzamide

Brand name: *Tigan*

What this drug does for you:

This drug controls nausea and vomiting. It comes in capsules, suppositories, and injection form.

Possible side effects of this drug:

- This drug may cause Parkinson-like symptoms, drowsiness, blood disorders, convulsions, diarrhea, jaundice, allergic skin reactions, dizziness, blurred vision, disorientation, headache, muscle cramps, and spasms. If you have any of these side effects, you should let your doctor know. He may advise you to quit taking the drug.

Special warnings:

- Your doctor should prescribe trimethobenzamide to children very cautiously.

Pregnancy and nursing mothers:

Not known if drug is safe to use while you're pregnant. Not known if drug is safe to use while nursing.

Possible food and drug interactions:

- Avoid alcohol while taking trimethobenzamide.
- You should be very cautious about taking trimethobenzamide and other depressants such as tranquilizers, sleeping pills and antihistamines at the same time.

Helpful hints:

- You shouldn't drive a car or operate heavy machinery until you are sure the medicine isn't making you drowsy or less than alert.
- Make sure you drink plenty of fluids and eat a balanced diet to replace lost fluids and minerals.

ULCER DRUGS

Cimetidine

Brand name: *Tagamet*

What this drug does for you:

Like ranitidine, nizatidine, and famotidine, cimetidine decreases the amount of acid your stomach produces. It helps stomach ulcers heal, treats gastroesophageal reflux disease (severe heartburn), controls bleeding in the stomach or intestines, and treats Zollinger-Ellison disease, a condition in which your stomach produces too much acid.

Possible side effects of this drug:

- Common side effects are headache, diarrhea, sleepiness, and dizziness. Some people, usually very ill people, experience confusion, hallucinations, depression, and anxiety. Cimetidine may cause enlargement of breasts in men and impotence.
- Side effects that involve your heart, such as an irregular heartbeat and heart block, are very rare. Liver, kidney, and urinary problems are rare.
- Even though it is very rare, cimetidine can lower the number of blood cells you have. If you don't have enough white blood cells, your immunity is down, and you can get a fever, sore throat, or pneumonia. If you are lacking red blood cells, you can become anemic, and that makes you tired and weak. Not having enough blood platelets makes you bruise easily and keeps your blood from clotting properly when you're injured. Be on the lookout for any of these symptoms.
- Cimetidine may cause itching or peeling skin. Very rare reactions are serious skin disorders in which dark red rings or raised spots erupt on your skin (Stevens-Johnson syndrome) or parts of your skin deteriorate.

Special warnings:

- Don't take cimetidine if you are allergic to any anti-ulcer drugs.
- Take this drug cautiously if you have liver or kidney problems.

Pregnancy and nursing mothers:

Category B. See page 9 for description of categories. Drug is present in mother's milk.

Possible food and drug interactions:

- Don't take antacids when you take your dose of cimetidine. Antacids decrease the absorption of cimetidine.
- Cimetidine may increase levels, effects, or toxicity of nifedipine, the anti-anxiety drugs chlordiazepoxide and diazepam, the analgesic lidocaine, the antibiotic metronidazole, the seizure drug phenytoin, the beta-blocker propanolol, the asthma drug theophylline, and the anticoagulant warfarin.

Helpful hint:

- The usual adult dosage for ulcers is 800 mg taken at bedtime.

Famotidine

Brand name: *Pepcid*

What this drug does for you:

Like cimetidine, ranitidine, and nizatidine, famotidine decreases the amount of acid your stomach produces. It helps stomach ulcers heal, treats gastroesophageal reflux disease (severe heartburn), controls bleeding in the stomach or intestines, and treats Zollinger-Ellison disease, a condition in which your stomach produces too much acid.

Possible side effects of this drug:

- Common side effects are headache, diarrhea, constipation, and dizzi-

ness. Some people experience confusion, hallucinations, depression, and anxiety. Very rarely, famotidine may cause enlargement of breasts in men and impotence.
- Side effects that involve your heart, such as an irregular heartbeat and heart block, are very rare. Liver, kidney, and urinary problems are rare.
- Even though it is very rare, famotidine can lower the number of blood cells you have. If you don't have enough white blood cells, your immunity is down, and you can get a fever, sore throat, or pneumonia. If you are lacking red blood cells, you can become anemic, and that makes you tired and weak. Not having enough blood platelets makes you bruise easily and keeps your blood from clotting properly when you're injured. Be on the lookout for any of these symptoms.
- Famotidine may cause itching or peeling skin. A very rare reaction is a serious skin disorder in which parts of your skin deteriorate.

Special warnings:
- Don't take famotidine if you are allergic to any anti-ulcer drugs.
- Your doctor may need to adjust your dosage if you have liver or kidney problems.

Pregnancy and nursing mothers:
Category B. See page 9 for description of categories. Drug is present in mother's milk.

Possible food and drug interaction:
- You can take antacids along with famotidine.

Helpful hints:
- The usual starting dosage for adults with active ulcers is 40 mg taken at bedtime.
- Shake the oral suspension form vigorously for five to 10 seconds before you use it. Unused constituted oral suspension should be thrown away after 30 days.

Misoprostol

Brand name: *Cytotec*

What this drug does for you:
Misoprostol is used to prevent stomach ulcers in certain people who take nonsteroidal anti-inflammatory drugs (NSAIDs).

Possible side effects of this drug:
- Diarrhea and stomach pain are the most common side effects. Other common side effects that usually go away after you've taken the drug for a while are nausea, gas, constipation, indigestion, and headache. If you have severe diarrhea or side effects that last longer than eight days, call your doctor.
- Women taking misoprostol may experience menstrual problems such as excessive or painful menstruation, spotting or cramps, or post-menopausal vaginal bleeding.

Special warnings:

- People allergic to prostaglandins should not use this drug.
- Your doctor should watch you closely if you have inflammatory bowel disease.

Pregnancy and nursing mothers:

Category X. See page 9 for description of categories. Misoprostol may cause miscarriage. Discuss any plans for pregnancy before taking this drug, and inform your doctor immediately if you become pregnant during treatment.

A pregnancy test should be done not more than two weeks before treatment is started. The drug should be started on the second or third day of the next menstrual period, and effective contraception should be used throughout treatment. Misoprostol should not be taken during nursing as it may cause severe diarrhea in babies.

Helpful hints:

- To help prevent diarrhea while taking this drug, take your doses after meals and at bedtime. Also, don't take magnesium-containing antacids when you take your dose.
- The usual adult dose is 200 mcg four times daily with food.

Nizatidine

Brand name: *Axid Pulvules*

What this drug does for you:

Like ranitidine, cimetidine, and famotidine, nizatidine decreases the amount of acid your stomach produces. It helps stomach ulcers heal, treats gastroesophageal reflux disease (severe heartburn), controls bleeding in the stomach or intestines, and treats Zollinger-Ellison disease, a condition in which your stomach produces too much acid.

Possible side effects of this drug:

- Some possible side effects are hives, anemia, damage to your liver, irregular heartbeat, sweating, rash, confusion, headache, diarrhea, and dizziness.

Special warnings:

- Don't take nizatidine if you are allergic to any anti-ulcer drugs.
- Your doctor may have to adjust your dosage if you have liver or kidney problems.

Pregnancy and nursing mothers:

Category C. See page 9 for description of categories. Drug is present in mother's milk.

Possible food and drug interactions:

- No significant interactions have been reported.

Helpful hint:

- The usual adult dosage for active ulcers is 300 mg taken at bedtime.

Omeprazole

Brand name: *Prilosec*

What this drug does for you:

Omeprazole decreases the amount of acid your stomach produces. It helps stomach ulcers heal, treats gastroesophageal reflux disease (severe heartburn), controls bleeding in the stomach or intestines, and treats Zollinger-Ellison disease, a condition in which your stomach produces too much acid.

Possible side effects of this drug:

- Some possible side effects are headache, diarrhea, stomach pain, nausea, dizziness, rash, constipation, cough, weakness, liver damage, chest pain, irregular heartbeats, and back pain.
- Even though it is very rare, omeprazole may lower the number of blood cells you have. If you don't have enough white blood cells, your immunity is down, and you can get a fever, sore throat, or pneumonia. If you are lacking red blood cells, you can become anemic, and that makes you tired and weak. Not having enough blood platelets makes you bruise easily and keeps your blood from clotting properly when you're injured. Be on the lookout for any of these symptoms of bone marrow depression.
- Another very rare reaction may be serious skin disorders in which dark red rings or raised spots erupt on your skin (Stevens-Johnson syndrome) or parts of your skin deteriorate.

Special warning:

- Animal studies have shown that long-term (two year) therapy with omeprazole could possibly cause the growth of cancerous tumors. More human studies need to be done.

Pregnancy and nursing mothers:

Category C. See page 9 for description of categories. Not known if drug is present in mother's milk.

Possible food and drug interactions:

- This drug may increase levels or effects of the anticoagulant warfarin, the tranquilizer diazepam, and the seizure drug phenytoin.

Helpful hints:

- Take your medicine before you eat.
- Swallow the capsules whole. Don't crush, chew, or open.
- For gastroesophageal reflux disease and ulcer, the usual adult dose is 20 mg once daily.

Ranitidine

Brand name: *Zantac*

What this drug does for you:

Like cimetidine, nizatidine, and famotidine, ranitidine decreases the amount of acid your stomach produces. It helps stomach ulcers heal, treats gastroesophageal reflux disease (severe heartburn), controls bleeding in the stomach or intestines, and treats Zollinger-Ellison disease, a condition in which your stomach produces too much acid.

Possible side effects of this drug:

- Common side effects are headache, diarrhea, sleepiness, and dizziness. Some people, usually very ill people, experience confusion, hallucinations, depression, and anxiety. Ranitidine may cause enlargement of breasts in men and impotence.
- Side effects that involve your heart, such as an irregular heartbeat and heart block, are very rare. Liver, kidney, and urinary problems are rare.
- Even though it is very rare, ranitidine can lower the number of blood cells you have. If you don't have enough white blood cells, your immunity is down, and you can get a fever, sore throat, or pneumonia. If you are lacking red blood cells, you can become anemic, and that makes you tired and weak. Not having enough blood platelets makes you bruise easily and keeps your blood from clotting properly when you're injured. Be on the lookout for any of these symptoms.
- Ranitidine may cause itching or peeling skin. Very rare reactions are serious skin disorders in which dark red rings or raised spots erupt on your skin (Stevens-Johnson syndrome) or parts of your skin deteriorate.

Special warnings:

- Don't take ranitidine if you are allergic to any anti-ulcer drugs.
- Your doctor may need to adjust your dosage if you have liver or kidney problems.
- People with a group of disorders called porphyria should not use ranitidine.

Pregnancy and nursing mothers:

Category B. See page 9 for description of categories. Drug is present in mother's milk.

Possible food and drug interactions:

- No significant interactions have been reported.

Helpful hints:

- You can take antacids while you take ranitidine.
- The usual adult dosage for active ulcers is 150 mg taken twice a day or 300 mg taken after the evening meal or at bedtime.

Sucralfate

Brand name: *Carafate*

What this drug does for you:

Sucralfate is used to treat stomach and duodenal ulcers.

Possible side effects of this drug:

- This drug may cause constipation, nausea, vomiting, diarrhea, stomach pain, gas, indigestion, dry mouth, headache, sleepiness, insomnia, dizziness, back pain. If you are allergic to the drug, you may experience rash, swelling and breathing difficulty.

Special warning:

- People with kidney failure and those on dialysis should use this drug cautiously. If you have kidney problems, make sure you avoid aluminum-containing antacids. Your body could absorb too much aluminum.

Pregnancy and nursing mothers:

Category B. See page 9 for description of categories. Not known if drug is present in mother's milk.

Possible food and drug interactions:

- Sucralfate may decrease your body's absorption of ciprofloxacin, ketoconazole, the seizure drug phenytoin, the ulcer drugs cimetidine and ranitidine, the heart drug digoxin, the antibiotic tetracycline, and the asthma drug theophylline.

Helpful hints:

- The recommended adult dosage is 1 gm twice a day.
- Take your medicine on an empty stomach at least one hour before meals.
- You can take antacids while you take sucralfate, but don't take the antacids within 30 minutes of taking your dose of sucralfate.

DRUGS FOR SPASTIC COLON

Dicyclomine

Brand name: *Bentyl*

What this drug does for you:

This drug treats stomach disorders such as irritable bowel syndrome (IBS) by relieving cramps or spasms of the stomach, intestines, and bladder.

Possible side effects of this drug:

- Dicyclomine may cause dry mouth, nausea, vomiting, constipation, bloated feeling, abdominal pain, loss of taste, loss of appetite, dizziness, tingling, headache, drowsiness, weakness, nervousness, numbness, confusion, excitement, involuntary muscle movements, difficulty speaking, insomnia, blurred vision, double vision, abnormal dilation of pupils, increased pressure in the eye, rash, itching, difficulty urinating, rapid heartbeat, palpitations, difficulty breathing, decreased sweating, nasal congestion, sneezing, impotence, and suppression of breast milk production.

Special warnings:

- People with the following conditions should not use this drug: allergy to anticholinergic drugs; kidney disease; any obstructive disease of the stomach, intestines, or urinary tract; severe ulcerative colitis or ulcerative colitis complicated by dilation of the colon; a disease of the muscles called myasthenia gravis; reflux esophagitis; unstable heart problems; and glaucoma.

- People with the following conditions should use this drug very cautiously: disease of the autonomic nervous system; liver or kidney disease; ulcerative colitis; overactive thyroid; high blood pressure; coronary heart disease; congestive heart failure; irregular, rapid heartbeat; hiatal hernia; and prostate disease.
- This drug can make you become overheated if you are exposed to hot weather. Watch yourself for signs of heatstroke or fever.

Pregnancy and nursing mothers:

Category B. See page 9 for description of categories. Drug is present in mother's milk.

Possible food and drug interactions:

- The following drugs may increase the effects of dicyclomine: the antiparkinson drug amantadine, the heartbeat regulating drug quinidine, antihistamines, the antipsychosis drug phenothiazine, the antianxiety drug benzodiazepine, the antidepressant drugs called monoamine oxidase (MAO) inhibitors, narcotic painkillers, and other drugs with anticholinergic qualities.
- Dicyclomine may interact with glaucoma medication and the anti-nausea drug metoclopramide.
- This drug may increase the levels of the heart drug digoxin in the blood.
- Antacids may decrease levels of this drug in the blood. You shouldn't take antacids within several hours of taking your dose of dicyclomine.

Helpful hint:

- You shouldn't drive a car or operate heavy machinery until you are sure the medicine isn't causing blurred vision or making you drowsy or less than alert.

Hyoscyamine Sulfate

Brand names: *Anaspaz, Cystospaz-M, Levsin, Levsin/SL, Levsinex*

What this drug does for you:

This drug relieves the spasms of many stomach and intestinal disorders including diverticulitis, peptic ulcer, pancreatitis, colitis, and irritable bowel syndrome (IBS). Hyoscyamine also treats bladder spasms, certain cases of heart block, and helps dry out a runny nose. This drug also controls tremors and muscle rigidity in Parkinson's disease.

Possible side effects of this drug:

- Hyoscyamine may cause dry mouth, impotence, difficulty urinating, headache, nervousness, increased pressure within the eye, blurred vision, rapid heartbeat, palpitations, hives, abnormal dilation of pupils, drowsiness, and a decrease in lactation in nursing mothers.

Special warnings:

- People with the following conditions should not take this drug: kidney disease; obstructive diseases of the stomach, intestines, or bladder; severe ulcerative colitis or ulcerative colitis complicated by dilation of the colon; liver disease; paralysis of the intestines; the elderly or debilitated with reduced muscle tone in the intestines; the nerve/muscle disease called myasthenia gravis; rapid heartbeat; angina; and some kinds of glaucoma (consult your doctor).

- People with the following conditions should take this drug very cautiously: overactive thyroid, diseases of the autonomic nervous system, congestive heart failure, coronary heart disease, high blood pressure, irregular heartbeat, enlarged prostate, chronic lung disease, asthma, allergies, hiatal hernia with stomach acid that washes back up into the esophagus, obstruction of the intestines, and glaucoma.
- This drug can make you become overheated if you are exposed to hot weather. Watch yourself for signs of heatstroke or fever.

Pregnancy and nursing mothers:

Category C. See page 9 for description of categories. Drug is present in mother's milk.

Possible food and drug interactions:

- You have an added risk of negative side effects if you take hyoscyamine along with any of the following drugs: the psychosis drug haloperidol, the antiparkinson drug amantadine, tranquilizers called phenothiazines, antidepressant drugs called monoamine oxidase (MAO) inhibitors, and tricyclic antidepressants.
- Antacids may reduce the effectiveness of this drug. Take the hyoscyamine before meals and antacids after meals.

Helpful hints:

- You shouldn't drive a car or operate heavy machinery until you are sure the medicine isn't causing blurred vision or making you drowsy or less than alert.
- You can chew the hyoscyamine tablets.
- Adults should not take more than 12 tablets or 12 teaspoonfuls in 24 hours.

Natural Alternatives

DIARRHEA

◀ Frequent bathroom breaks
◀ Loose, watery stools

Dealing with diarrhea

When diarrhea gets you down, you want to deal with the problem as quickly as possible. However, that's probably not best for your body. Diarrhea is Mother Nature's way of disposing of something disagreeable, whether it's a virus, food poisoning, or some food that just didn't agree with you. Your best option is to let your body take care of itself. Here are some suggestions to make you more comfortable and help Nature do her job.

Stay away from medicine right at first. Diarrhea usually doesn't last very long, and you shouldn't try to stop it right away. You may be interfering with your body's effort to get rid of an infection. Diarrhea that drags on or is severe needs treatment. Of course, if your doctor prescribes medicine, you should follow his directions exactly.

Swallow plenty of clear liquids such as Gatorade or Pedialyte. Diarrhea places both adults and children at risk for dehydration. Symptoms of dehydration are dry skin that may feel leathery, dry lips or sticky mouth, dark circles under sunken eyes, weakness, irritability, lack of tears when crying, and less urine. Urine may have a strong smell or be darker than usual.

Children under 2 years old definitely need an oral rehydration solution such as Pedialyte. It contains the right mix of salt, sugar, potassium, and other elements. Gatorade is usually OK for older children and adults. Adults with diarrhea need to be sure to drink at least eight to 10 glasses of water a day. Don't drink anything with caffeine. Caffeine makes you lose even more salt and water.

Get back to regular foods quickly. After you get some liquids down, you need nutritious, high-calorie foods. Breast milk or regular-strength formula is good for babies. You may have heard that you should water down the baby's formula, but recent studies show that regular-strength formula is better for your child.

Some children will not want to drink or eat at all. Very young children may want to eat too much. Both undereating and overeating may aggravate diarrhea.

Older children and adults should eat carbohydrate-rich foods such as rice, cereal, bananas, noodles, bread, and potatoes. You or your child should eat nutritious foods that appeal to you.

Avoid sugary foods and drinks — ice cream, juice, soda pop, and candy can make diarrhea worse.

Load up on yogurt. If antibiotics have disrupted the natural bacteria in your digestive system, you may be able to set matters straight by eating some yogurt.

Find out if fruit juice is your friend or foe. You can get too much of a good thing. Too much fruit juice, 12 ounces or more a day, may cause bouts of diarrhea. This is especially true for children. Apple juice in particular contains diarrhea-causing compounds that children's bodies can't absorb in large quantities. Pear and prune juices can be hard to absorb too.

Limit lactose. An ingredient in milk, lactose causes digestive problems, including diarrhea, in some people. See the What if milk is the culprit? section under General Gastrointestinal Upset later in this chapter for more information on dealing with lactose intolerance.

Stay away from sorbitol. This alcohol sugar, often found in chewing gum, can cause diarrhea, so it certainly won't be helpful now.

Pour up some Pepto-Bismol. In a recent study, children admitted to a hospital with severe diarrhea improved faster and were released sooner when they were given bismuth subsalicylate, the ingredient in Pepto-Bismol. There are no negative side effects if you use the recommended dose. Higher doses don't provide faster or better results, so follow package directions.

Normally, diarrhea runs its course within a few days, and you'll be feeling back in the pink quite soon.

However, if diarrhea lasts more than two days in a child or more than a week in an adult, consult your doctor. You should also see a doctor immediately if your diarrhea appears black or red, which indicates the presence of blood.

Sources —
American Family Physician (51,5:1115)
Athens Regional Medical Center Parent's Information Handbook and Pediatrics' Unit Teaching Tool: Gastroenteritis, Athens, Ga., 1994
Medical Abstracts Newsletter (13,8:4)
Nutrition Research Newsletter (12,2:21)
Pediatrics (92,2:241 and 93,3:438)
The New England Journal of Medicine (328,23:1653)

DIVERTICULOSIS AND DIVERTICULITIS

◄ Constipation

◄ Mild abdominal cramping, especially on the left side

◄ Nausea

◄ Fever

◄ Mucus and occasional blood in the stools

◄ Severe abdominal cramping, sometimes disabling

Eight ways to ease diverticulosis

If you love crisp, tart apples, sweet juicy oranges, or luscious, lovely blackberries, you're in luck. If you don't love 'em, you should at least learn to like 'em — that is if you want to help heal your diverticula. And no doubt you do, if you're experiencing the pain of diverticulosis or diverticulitis.

Diverticula are small sac-like growths that develop on the lower part of the colon. If you have diverticulosis, these small pouches can cause cramps, pain, tenderness in the left side of the abdomen, and gas. A bowel movement or passing gas may bring temporary relief. Bowel movements may be small and hard, alternating with attacks of diarrhea. Diverticulosis can turn into a more serious condition called diverticulitis if these sac-like swellings become inflamed.

To relieve the crampy, painful symptoms of diverticulosis, follow these eight easy steps:

Eat more fiber. The most important prevention measure and treatment is a high-fiber diet. Dietary fiber is the part of plants that cannot be broken down by digestive processes. Symptoms of diverticulosis usually disappear within a week or two after you start eating whole-grain breads, oatmeal and bran cereals, and fresh fruits and vegetables.

It's especially important to eat fresh fruits because they stimulate the growth of good microbes in the intestines. These microbes increase bowel movements and keep food waste moving through your system, which helps prevent diverticula problems. High-fiber fruits, listed with fiber grams per serving, include:

◁ Blackberries, 6.6 grams of fiber per cup
◁ Raspberries, 5.8 grams per cup
◁ Blueberries, 4.4 grams per cup
◁ Dates, 4.2 grams per 10 dates
◁ Pear, 4.1 grams per medium fruit
◁ Apple, 3 grams per medium fruit
◁ Banana, 2 grams per medium fruit
◁ Orange, 2 grams per medium fruit

Beans and peas are good sources of vegetable fiber to add to your diet. But increase your fiber intake slowly, or bloating and gas may occur.

Eat less red meat and fat. A diet low in fat and red meat is the second way to prevent diverticulosis. According to a recent study of nearly 50,000 doctors aged 40 to 75, men who ate a lot of fatty, red meat and little fiber were most likely to experience crippling forms of diverticulosis.

Medical researchers believe that red meat causes intestinal bacteria to produce substances that weaken the colon, so diverticula form more readily. Eating chicken and fish does not increase your risk of diverticulosis. Fats from meats are more likely to lead to diverticulosis than those from dairy products.

Do a lot of drinking. Of water, that is. Drink eight glasses of water each day. This will help soften stools so they are easier to pass.

Establish regular bathroom habits. Try to have a bowel movement around the same time every day. Don't strain, and allow plenty of time.

Try heat for relief. To help ease the pain of mild abdominal cramps, place a heating pad on your stomach.

Keep your heart healthy. Maintaining good cardiovascular fitness is one more thing you can do to help prevent diverticular disease, which seems to be associated with vascular disorders.

If you experience constant abdominal pain, fever, nausea, or pass blood with your bowel movements, see your doctor immediately. If your diverticula have become infected and you've developed diverticulitis, your doctor may need to prescribe antibiotics. So take your medicine correctly, get plenty of bed rest, and you'll be back in fine form soon.

Sources —
American Family Physician (51,2:419)
Cecil Textbook of Medicine, 19th ed., W.B. Saunders Co., Pa., 1992
Complete Guide to Symptoms, Illness & Surgery, Putnam Berkley Group, New York, 1995

The American Journal of Clinical Nutrition (60,5:737)
The American Medical Association Family Medical Guide, Random House, New York, 1982

GENERAL GASTROINTESTINAL UPSET

◀ Diarrhea
◀ Gas, pain, and bloating
   in stomach and intestines
◀ Vomiting

◀ Feeling of fullness in stomach
◀ Nausea
◀ Pain and burning in stomach

Oust indigestion!

You have that icky, achy feeling in your stomach, just a little painful, just a little queasy. You don't know if it's due to the stress at your office or the spicy pizza you ate for dinner. Whatever the cause, you just want some relief. Head off that yucky feeling with the tips listed below:

Avoid high-fat foods. Fatty meats, such as sausage, pepperoni, hot dogs, and bacon are not good for your digestive system (or any other part of your body). The same is true for fried foods and high-fat dairy products. Do your stomach a favor and forego fat.

Eliminate alcohol and caffeine. They can irritate your stomach, and so can decaffeinated drinks.

Watch out for gassy vegetables. Beans, broccoli, cauliflower, cabbage, onions, soybeans, and turnips can all cause a buildup of gas and discomfort in your intestines.

Rule out raw. In spite of the fact that you need fiber in your diet, you may find that raw fruits and vegetables don't agree with your digestive system. Try cooked ones instead, and get your fiber from other sources, such as the bran in whole-grain bread, rice, and pasta.

Abstain from acidic and spicy foods. Tomatoes, citrus fruit and juice, vinegar, spicy foods, and carbonated drinks can cause digestive problems for some people.

Change the form. If fresh onions and garlic irritate your stomach, try using them in powdered form instead. One teaspoon of onion powder equals one-half of a fresh onion, and one-eighth teaspoon of garlic powder equals one clove.

Take your medicine carefully. Be sure to follow all your doctor's instructions about taking prescription drugs, whether with food or on an empty stomach, and how often to take them. For over-the-counter drugs, follow directions exactly.

Eat your meals slowly. Savor your food, and try to relax for at least 30 minutes after each meal, instead of rushing off to other activities.

Sip some chamomile tea. Chamomile works to stop stomach cramps and puts the brakes on intestinal gas. If you have an upset stomach, drink a cup of chamomile tea between meals and before going to bed.

If you're allergic to ragweed, asters, or chrysanthemums, you're more likely to be allergic to chamomile and may want to think twice about using it. However, very few people are allergic to the herb.

Don't use chamomile at the same time that you're taking prescription drugs because chamomile can interfere with the absorption of some medicines. And don't overdo it — large quantities of chamomile can cause vomiting.

How to calm a churning stomach

Sometimes a churning stomach just can't be controlled and you end up tossing your cookies (and everything else you ate recently).

However unpleasant and unwelcome it may be, vomiting happens to everybody once in a while. It can be a symptom of many different illnesses, but it can also be the result of severe indigestion. Consult your doctor if the vomiting occurs in someone elderly, a person with heart disease, or an infant who is crying continually. Also call your doctor if vomiting continues for more than two days.

In the meantime:

◁ Limit liquids. Too much liquid can make vomiting worse. Small amounts of liquid every few minutes work best.

◁ Eat dry, low-fat crackers, just a little bit at a time.

◁ Sip on some ginger ale.

◁ Avoid all dairy products and spicy or fatty foods until you're feeling better.

If your child is vomiting, try giving one teaspoon of oral rehydration solution (available over-the-counter) every few minutes. Then when he's able to keep the drink down, slowly increase the amount.

What if milk is the culprit?

Lactose intolerance can be a major pain in the stomach. You could be suffering from frequent indigestion that's actually lactose intolerance, and not even know that you have it.

Lactose is the sugar found in milk and dairy products. Lactose intolerance can make you extremely uncomfortable, but it's not a disease or even a food allergy. It means that your digestive system is not producing enough of the enzyme lactase, which you need to break down milk sugar. This condition is more likely to occur as you get older, since your enzymes decrease as you age.

If you are lactose intolerant, after you eat a serving of dairy food, a large amount of undigested milk sugar moves through your digestive system, upsetting normal processes along the way. Within a few minutes to several hours after eating the dairy product, you may feel bloating, cramping, gas, diarrhea, pain, and nausea.

But there's hope, even in a world filled with dairy products. Here are some easy ways to cope with lactose intolerance:

Try hard cheeses and skim-milk cheeses. Many hard cheeses (like cheddar, Swiss, and Jarlsberg) and some skim-milk cheeses (like low-fat cream cheese and part-skim mozzarella) are usually low in lactose. Try these cheeses to see if you can enjoy them.

Never drink milk or eat ice cream on an empty stomach. Products containing lactose may not bother you if you eat them along with plenty of other food.

Substitute yogurt for other dairy foods. Yogurt with live and active cultures contains helpful bacteria that digest the lactose in the yogurt for you. Be sure to check your brand for the "live and active cultures" seal.

Try lactose-reduced milk. This milk has been treated so that the milk sugar has already been broken down. It usually has 70 percent less lactose than regular milk and may not upset your digestive system. Lactose-reduced cottage cheese and American cheese are also available.

Buy lactase tablets at your drugstore. You can add the enzyme capsule directly to the dairy product and break down the milk sugar before you eat or drink it. However, this chemical process increases the amount of other sugars in the food and tends to make the food unusually sweet.

Another method is to take the tablets yourself when you eat dairy food. These pills (Dairy Ease, Lactaid, Lactrase) can be found in grocery stores and pharmacies and are very convenient to use. Just follow the directions supplied with the pills. They can reduce the symptoms of pain and bloating that many people experience.

Train yourself to tolerate dairy products. Tests conducted by nutritional scientists show that even people with severe lactose intolerance can learn to drink milk without digestive problems.

You start with a small amount of milk that doesn't hurt your stomach. Stay at that level for two to four days. Then increase your milk intake slightly and see if you remain symptom-free. If you feel no discomfort after two to four days at that new level, increase it again by a slight amount.

If you feel digestive discomfort at any time, reduce the milk you drink to the previously tolerated level and remain there for a few days. Then begin the gradual increase once again.

Avoid milk and any foods made with milk. Avoiding milk is the most drastic way to deal with lactose intolerance. If you do this, you'll need to find alternative sources of calcium, especially if you are a woman. To avoid milk, read product labels carefully and watch out for these ingredients: lactose, dry milk solids, and whey.

There are two reasons why avoiding milk may be a bad idea:

1) Your lactose intolerance may just be a passing condition: a temporary reaction to a medicine, the result of an illness, or some other reason.
2) The longer you avoid dairy products, the less you'll be able to tolerate that occasional bowl of ice cream. Drinking a small amount of milk regularly may help keep your lactose-digesting bacteria strong.

A few people — about one in every 200 — are allergic to milk and need to avoid milk completely. When you are allergic to milk, you may get rashes, hives, wheezing, runny eyes, and a stuffy nose when you drink it.

The best way to beat the discomfort of gastrointestinal distress is to simply avoid it. Watch carefully what you eat and how it affects you; eat sensible, well-balanced meals; and you and your stomach should be able to avoid that icky, achy feeling most of the time.

Sources —
Age Page, National Institute on Aging Information Center, P.O. Box 8057,
Gaithersburg, Md. 20898-8057
Before You Call the Doctor, Random House, New York, 1992
Dairy Council Digest (65,2:7)
Inside Tract, Glaxo Institute for Digestive Health, P.O. Box 899, West Caldwell, N.J.,
07007-0899
Postgraduate Medicine (95,1:113)
The American Journal of Clinical Nutrition (58,6:879)
The Physician and Sportsmedicine (21,3:59)

HEARTBURN

◀ Choking
◀ Foul taste in mouth
◀ Shortness of breath
◀ Upset stomach

◀ Coughing
◀ Pain or discomfort in the upper
abdomen

Divine digestion

Mark Twain always had a way of turning clichés inside out to reveal a whole
new truth. If you've ever had heartburn, no doubt you'll agree with Twain's
twisted truism "To eat is human, to digest is divine."

Heartburn occurs when the food and digestive juices in your stomach accidentally flow backward into your esophagus, the tube which connects your
throat to your stomach. Doctors call this gastroesophageal reflux, and it's
sometimes accompanied by involuntary belching. But whether you belch or
not, you definitely feel the pain. Try the tips below to help ease your discomfort.

Prop up the head of your bed frame with blocks about 4 to 6 inches high.
Or support your entire upper body with a pillow or a foam wedge. This keeps
juices flowing downward instead of upward as you sleep. In fact, Dr. Malcolm
Robinson, the medical director of the Oklahoma Foundation for Digestive
Research, believes that elevating the head of your bed may be one of the most
important ways to control reflux.

Try the "beer-belly" maneuver. If you have a lot of heartburn, you may
have a hiatal hernia, a condition in which part of your stomach slides up into
your chest area and causes the burning sensation of heartburn. You may be
able to get relief by letting your stomach hang out for a few minutes.

Dr. Veronica D. Jenkins of Temple Hills, Md., recommends trying what she
calls the "beer-belly" maneuver. Stand with your feet slightly spread apart,
and let your stomach relax so that it hangs over your belt. Hold this position
for two or three minutes.

This technique relieves heartburn by taking the pressure off your stomach
contents. It may even help a hiatal hernia slide back into place.

Chuck the cigarettes. Smoking increases the production of acid. It also
relaxes a little valve between your esophagus and stomach, making it easier
for extra acid to back up into and burn your esophagus.

Shed your nicotine patch at bedtime. For people trying to kick the smoking habit, that nicotine patch can cause heartburn, especially at night. The nicotine in the patch relaxes the small valve between the stomach and the lower end of the esophagus. This allows stomach acid to back up into your esophagus, causing irritation and burning similar to the pain associated with heart disease. How can you avoid it? Take off your patch each night at bedtime.

Avoid straining and heavy lifting. Your abdominal muscles contract and squeeze the contents of your stomach up and out into your esophagus.

Get rid of that spare tire around your midsection, and wear loose-fitting clothes. Being overweight and wearing tight clothes can actually force your stomach's contents up into your esophagus.

Take your medicines with plenty of water. Don't lie down right after swallowing a pill. Stand or sit up when taking medicines so gravity can help the pill get to your stomach. These precautions are even more important if you're taking theophylline, calcium channel blockers, progesterone, potassium chloride, or nonsteroidal anti-inflammatory drugs (NSAIDs).

At the heart of heartburn

Of course, what you put into your stomach has the greatest effect on digestion. Here's some advice on eating to prevent heartburn:

Avoid stuffing yourself with a large meal. Use moderation when you eat, and you'll be thankful later. Also, don't bend over immediately after a meal.

Eat four to six small meals a day. Several small meals may sit easier on your stomach than two to three large meals.

Resist bedtime snacks, and don't lie down for at least three to four hours after eating. With your body in a horizontal position, it's much easier for food

---

Tight pants can stress your stomach

If you've been having unexplained stomach or chest pains lately, the reason could be right under your nose — your pants could be too small. Minor abdominal or chest pain sometimes results from wearing pants which are at least 3 inches too small in the waist. People with this problem, which is called "tight pants syndrome," usually experience pain shortly after meals, due to increased pressure on the abdominal area.

The name "tight pants syndrome" may sound amusing, but the problem itself can be serious. The abdominal pressure, if not remedied, could lead to a hiatal hernia, a condition in which part of the stomach pushes up into the chest. Hiatal hernias can cause serious heartburn when your acidic stomach contents sloshes back up into your esophagus.

If you've gained a little weight, or if you've just given birth, wear loose, comfortable clothing until you can fit into your favorite clothes again.

Sources —
  Archives of Internal Medicine (153,11:1396)
  The Journal of the American Medical Association (271,20:1628)

to go into reverse and give you problems.

Cut down on alcohol, coffee, and carbonated beverages. Coffee and other drinks with caffeine tend to irritate your stomach lining.

Which beverages cause the most heartburn? Researchers at the Glaxo Institute for Digestive Health questioned 400 heartburn sufferers to find out. They asked the participants about 17 juices or citrus drinks, 11 soft drinks, three alcoholic beverages, coffee, tea, four milk products, and water.

Grapefruit juice caused more heartburn than any other juice, although orange juice and tomato-containing juices were close runners-up. The high acid level of these juices seemed to be the problem, but the low acid level of soft drinks caused trouble too.

Alcohol, coffee, tea, chocolate drinks, and lemonade all caused reflux. Only the fattier milks caused heartburn; skim milk seems safe.

Satisfy your sweet tooth with something other than chocolate, spearmint, or peppermint. They make matters worse for many heartburn sufferers. Sucking on other types of sugarless candy during the day may relieve heartburn.

Stimulate some saliva. A little extra saliva will actually help soothe a burning esophagus. Easy ways to stimulate saliva include chewing gum and eating a sweet pickle.

Limit the amount of acid-rich foods you eat, such as citrus fruits, fruit drinks, and spicy foods. Tomato-based foods like spaghetti sauce can irritate your stomach. Onions and fatty foods contribute to heartburn too. Keep a food/heartburn diary to help you discover which foods cause problems for you.

Drink plenty of water. This will wash any acid out of your esophagus and give your stomach a fighting chance to do its job properly.

Eat slowly. Take small bites and chew your food thoroughly. This gives your stomach a head start on digestion.

Go easy on the antacids. Even though antacids can help, you can get too much of a good thing. The antacids you can buy at the drugstore are usually safe and effective. You should let your doctor know how many you're taking, just in case the antacids are masking a serious stomach problem that needs to be treated.

Antacids containing calcium are a good way to boost your calcium intake, but you have to be careful not to take too many. Taking calcium antacids for several days in a row can also cause "acid rebound," which means your stomach produces more acid than ever and makes your heartburn worse.

Take heart. If you try these tips, you should see a difference in your heartburn problem. If the pain is lower and stays with you for a few days, however, you may be suffering from a stomach ulcer. If this is the case, you need to see your doctor immediately.

Sources —
American Family Physician (47,6:1407)
British Journal of Clinical Practice (48,6:333)
Emergency Medicine (26,14:45)

Gastroenterology (108,1:125)
Patient Care (23,15:30)
Postgraduate Medicine (95,2:88)
U.S. Pharmacist (17,10:21 and 19,2:119)

IRRITABLE BOWEL SYNDROME (SPASTIC COLON, COLITIS, OR MUCOUS COLITIS)

◀ Anxiety
◀ Depression
◀ Difficulty concentrating
◀ Fatigue
◀ Headache
◀ Nausea, bloating, and gas

◀ Backache
◀ Diarrhea or constipation, usually alternating
◀ Painful cramps in the lower abdomen, usually relieved by bowel movement

Bran gets the boot for irritable bowel syndrome

If you've had to deal with a case of irritable bowel syndrome (IBS), you've probably followed the advice of doctors and nutritionists who told you to include plenty of bran in your diet. And like most people who followed that recommendation, you've probably also had to deal with a new set of problems: painful stomach cramps and a more irritated bowel than ever.

If you've been wondering whether boosting your intake of dietary fiber was worth it, you're not alone. New research shows that it's time to rethink the use of bran to treat IBS.

Give bran the boot. A study of 100 people with IBS by researchers at England's University Hospital of South Manchester confirms what many IBS sufferers have known for a long time. Too much bran in the diet may make IBS worse, not better.

Stick with fresh fruits and veggies. The good news is the study uncovered evidence that other kinds of dietary fiber produce better results with far less chance of abdominal pain and bowel disturbance. People with IBS should stick with the dietary fiber found in fresh fruits and vegetables.

However, the study also specifically identified citrus fruits as having the same results as bran and suggested avoiding citrus in favor of other fiber sources.

Get sold on psyllium. Researchers also said they were told by some study participants that psyllium, found in many fiber supplements (such as Metamucil), produced good results for them. Experiment to see if psyllium works for you.

Other natural ways to help

Here are some additional measures you can take to help keep your IBS under control:

Avoid foods and drinks that hurt. Spicy, ethnic foods and gas-producing vegetables should be avoided. Coffee and milk are culprits for some people too. Figure out which foods trigger your attacks, and don't eat them.

The gastrointestinal imposter

Are you a woman whose stomach pain remains a mystery to your doctor? The suspect could be part of an inside job called intestinal endometriosis. In this condition, tissue like that attached to the inner lining of the uterus attaches and grows on the intestines.

Doctors often overlook intestinal endometriosis because the signs are the same for more common digestive diseases. Symptoms include severe lower stomach pain, nausea, bloody urine or bowel movements, back pain, and cramping for several weeks.

Endometriosis can occur in women of any age, but it is most common in those 20 to 30 years old who have not had children, have irregular menstrual cycles, and have a family history of endometriosis.

Although intestinal endometriosis can be severely painful, it is not life-threatening. Surgery is not always necessary and mild cases can be treated with medicine.

So if after your medical line-up, your stomach pain remains a mystery, ask your doctor about endometriosis. It could be the clue that closes the case.

Sources —

Archives of Internal Medicine (155,9:77)
Complete Guide to Symptoms, Illness and Surgery, Putnam Berkley Group, New York, 1995

Eat small meals, but be sure to eat regularly.

Don't smoke or drink. Nicotine may contribute to the problem. And keep alcohol consumption to a minimum, since it can cause difficulties too.

Try a heating pad for pain relief. Place it on your stomach to help ease discomfort.

Work out. Keeping your body in good physical condition is good for bowel function and helps reduce stress.

Stop stress. Keeping stress under control is one of the best ways to help prevent symptoms of IBS. Try to learn new, healthier ways of dealing with stress, such as relaxation techniques, meditation, and biofeedback. Don't let yourself get too tired — fatigue causes more stress.

Taking good care of yourself will help you have a healthier life and keep your IBS under control.

Sources —

American Family Physician (50,5:1072)
Complete Guide to Symptoms, Illness & Surgery, Putnam Berkley Group, New York, 1995
Journal Watch (14,3:20)
The Atlanta Journal/Constitution (Oct. 13, 1994, H9)
The Lancet (344,8914:3,39)

MOTION SICKNESS

◀ **Cold sweats**   ◀ **Dizziness**
◀ **Drowsiness**   ◀ **Excess saliva**
◀ **Headache**   ◀ **Nausea**
◀ **Vomiting**   ◀ **Yawning**

The world is in motion

You're not sick if you suffer from motion sickness. The fact is, you could be sick if you don't.

Under the right conditions, most people would suffer from motion sickness. For some people, just a little movement is enough to set them off. For others, it might take a severe storm on the high seas. If you've never experienced it, count yourself lucky.

Doctors actually consider motion sickness a natural reaction to an unnatural situation, such as flying or sailing. People who don't experience motion sickness under any circumstances may have an inner ear disorder.

Chances are, if you suffer from motion sickness, you know it. What concerns you most is how to prevent it, without drugs whenever possible. Here's how:

Rely on rest to feel your best. Make sure you are completely rested before you begin a trip you think might cause motion sickness.

Avoid alcohol before and during your trip.

Focus on the horizon or some nearby object. You get motion sickness when your inner ear and your eyes don't agree. For example, many people experience seasickness on a rolling ship, when the wave motion their eyes perceive doesn't match the movement of the ship that the inner ear detects. Focusing on the horizon in front of you will help your inner ear and eyes agree.

Try not to be anxious. This may sound nearly impossible, especially if you think you're on the verge of vomiting. But if you let yourself get anxious, you'll feel even worse because anxiety causes some of the same undesirable symptoms in your body as motion sickness.

Let in the fresh air. Try to avoid unpleasant odors, such as cigarette smoke.

Don't stuff yourself full of food. Eat small meals and try to avoid fatty foods.

Take slow, deep breaths if you begin to feel queasy.

Put on some pressure — acupressure, that is. Hold your hand with the palm up, and look for a point on your forearm that is three finger widths from the crease of your wrist, between the two tendons and in line with your middle finger. Apply steady pressure to this spot with your thumb or finger until the symptoms of motion sickness fade.

Ease into the situation if possible. It's easier to adapt to the motion of a rocking boat, for example, if it is rocking only slightly at first. Then, as the motion increases, you can get used to it gradually.

Go for some ginger. Ginger may not prevent the dizziness or headache that accompanies motion sickness, but it seems to suppress vomiting pretty well. People taking a 940-milligram capsule of ginger experienced fewer episodes of vomiting during spins in a tilting chair than those who took Dramamine.

Another option is candied or crystallized ginger sold at Oriental food markets. A 1-inch square piece equals about 500 milligrams of powdered ginger. You might also try sipping some ginger ale, which was originally a tonic for stomach upset.

Consider behavior therapy. For people whose work exposes them to motion all the time, such as pilots, sailors, or truck drivers, techniques of behavior modification may be helpful. This may take a lot of time and effort, however, so it isn't the best approach if you only have to cope with motion sickness occasionally. If you're interested in this type of therapy, call a local counseling center and ask if anyone in your area offers behavior therapy training for motion sickness.

Whatever method you use to cope with your motion sickness, don't be discouraged. Motion sickness can lessen with repeated exposure over time, so the next time you're on a ship in a storm, you may have smooth sailing after all.

Sources —
Before You Call the Doctor, Random House, New York, 1992
Popular Nutritional Practices, Dell Publishing, New York, 1988
Postgraduate Medicine (89,6:139)
The American Medical Association Encyclopedia of Medicine, Random House, New York, 1989

ULCERATIVE COLITIS

◀ Abdominal cramps
◀ Bloody diarrhea
◀ Loss of appetite
◀ Sweating and dehydration
◀ Bloated abdomen
◀ Fever
◀ Nausea
◀ Weight loss

Taking care of colitis

Ulcerative colitis is an inflammatory disease of the colon. It is more severe than irritable bowel syndrome (also called colitis), and has the added difficulties of bloody diarrhea and fever. There is also the chance of severe blood loss.

If you have ulcerative colitis, there's a good chance that your doctor has prescribed steroids or other medications to ease the inflammation in your colon. But in addition to your doctor's care, there are some things you can do to care for yourself.

Favor some fish oil. This potential cure is certainly not new to the medical community, having been tossed around as a possible treatment for just about every disorder under the sun. But now, fish oil is back as a treatment for colitis.

Dr. William F. Stenson, a gastroenterologist at the Washington University School of Medicine, tested the effects of fish oil for four months on 24 people diagnosed with ulcerative colitis. He divided the people into two groups. One group took 18 capsules of Max-EPA brand fish oil capsules every day, and the other group took a placebo of peanut oil.

After two to three months of testing, Stenson found that the group given fish oil had less rectal bleeding and that on average the steroid medicine they were taking had been cut in half. Some people were able to stop the steroids completely.

You might want to consider trying fish oil supplements or adding fatty fish, such as salmon, anchovies, herring, mackerel, and albacore tuna, to your diet to help ease your irritated colon.

Keep a food diary. Find out which foods trigger symptoms, and avoid them. Watch out for milk products, especially, if you think you might have lactose intolerance. See the *What if milk is the culprit?* section under ***General Gastrointestinal Upset*** earlier in this chapter for more information on dealing with lactose intolerance.

Check on vitamins. See if your doctor thinks you need to take vitamin or mineral supplements, especially iron. Diarrhea and bleeding can deplete your system of these nutrients.

Don't use aspirin. It increases the risk of bleeding.

Avoid raw fruits and vegetables if you experience cramping. Eat canned or cooked ones instead.

Stay away from spicy foods, caffeine, alcohol, and fiber, especially when you have diarrhea. These may all be irritants you should eliminate from your diet.

See the *Other natural ways to help* section under ***Irritable Bowel Syndrome*** earlier in this chapter for additional self-help tips.

If you have ulcerative colitis, you and your doctor should work as a team. At certain times, you need his treatment, but the things you can do to help yourself make a big difference in staving off attacks.

However, if you experience fever, chills, increased bleeding, a bloated abdomen, jaundice, vomiting, or increased pain, call your doctor right away.

Sources —
> *Complete Guide to Symptoms, Illness & Surgery,* Putnam Berkley Group, New York, 1995
> *The Atlanta Journal/Constitution* (Sept. 14, 1995, H12)

ULCERS

◀ Burning, cramping, or gnawing sensation in the stomach

◀ Pain comes in waves, for three to four days at a time, subsiding completely for months

◀ Worst pain occurs when stomach is empty, such as before meals and at bedtime

New ulcer cure works four times out of five

Got a stomach that's plagued by ulcers? More likely than not your doctor will treat it by prescribing a drug like Tagamet or Zantac or a foul-tasting antacid to stop the flow of acid in your stomach. If this doesn't work, your doctor may want you to have an operation to remove a large part of your stomach.

Even if these drugs help and you don't have to have an operation, your doctor may not tell you that you'll probably have to take stomach-acid reducers for the rest of your life. These drugs often reduce symptoms of chronic stomachache and ulcers without curing them.

But a lifetime of taking these drugs can cost you a lot of money. Zantac costs from $64.99 to $98.51 a month, and Tagamet costs from $66.49 to $84.06 a month. Drug companies love these figures, but your pocketbook doesn't.

Get the permanent cure. Now there's a way to actually cure your ulcer instead of treating the symptoms for life. In the early 1980s, an Australian scientist began to believe that most ulcers are caused by a type of bacteria in your stomach, called *Helicobacter pylori*.

The medical world has been slow to accept the fact that most ulcers are caused by bacteria, but now the National Institutes of Health has even put out a recommendation about *H. pylori*. The NIH says if you have an ulcer and you are infected with the bacteria, you need to be treated for it.

A simple, cheap treatment will kill these bacteria and cure your ulcer.

Give your ulcer a triple punch. All you need is a two-week treatment with two antibiotics and bismuth subsalicylate, better known as Pepto-Bismol. Doctors using the triple therapy of Pepto-Bismol and the antibiotics metronidazole (Flagyl) and tetracycline are reporting a 90-percent cure rate for their patients with ulcers.

Recently, a group of researchers found they could heal most ulcers with just one week of antibiotic/bismuth therapy.

Pepto-Bismol, which you can buy without a doctor's prescription, may be all you need to cure simple indigestion. But for ulcers, Pepto-Bismol works best when taken briefly with two prescription antibiotics. Therefore, you'll need to get the cooperation of your doctor.

Test your blood for *H. pylori* antibodies. What if your doctor is skeptical and doesn't believe that something as simple and easy to cure as a bacterial infection could be the cause of a problem that has baffled doctors for decades?

The solution is simple. Ask your doctor about taking a blood test, designed specifically to test for the *Helicobacter pylori* bacteria. Be careful if you have been taking antibiotics, bismuth compounds, or omeprazole recently. They could give you a false positive test result. The newest blood tests for *H. pylori* are very accurate and very inexpensive.

Once the presence of *Helicobacter pylori* is verified, your doctor can feel comfortable about prescribing the antibiotics which will clear up the illness, usually in two weeks or less, for good.

Keep in mind, however, that this treatment probably won't work if you have ulcers caused by taking nonsteroidal anti-inflammatory drugs (NSAIDs).

How to live peacefully with ulcers

The wise ones of the world recommend that "if you can't beat 'em, join 'em." However, in the case of stomach ulcers, that's hardly sound advice. We'd like to suggest a slight modification. If you can't lick 'em, at least you can learn to live with them. Here's how:

◁ Limit alcohol and caffeine. Decaffeinated drinks can also irritate your stomach.

◁ Avoid nonsteroidal anti-inflammatory drugs (NSAIDs), like aspirin, Voltaren (diclofenac), Feldene (piroxicam), or Ansaid (flurbiprofen) whenever possible. Although ibuprofen is also an NSAID, it seems to cause fewer stomach problems than other NSAIDs.

◁ Stop smoking. Nicotine damages the lining of the stomach.

◁ Enjoy several small meals a day instead of two or three large ones. Try to space your mini-meals at regular intervals.

◁ Manage your stress. Experts agree that stress doesn't play the role in ulcer development they once thought it did, but excess stress can cause your stomach to produce excess stomach acid — not something you need if you have an ulcer.

◁ Antacids can spell relief (although most English teachers would disagree). Just don't overdo it. Over-the-counter antacids work well. If you've had a stroke or have high blood pressure, heart disease, diabetes, or glaucoma or need to restrict your salt intake for some other reason, avoid antacids that contain a lot of sodium. Be sure to let your doctor know you're using antacids.

Experiments have shown that licorice in very small amounts can help treat stomach ulcers. However, in many cases, side effects from licorice outweighed the benefits.

Talk with your doctor if you are interested in using licorice to treat your ulcer. He can help you decide if licorice therapy is a good option for you. Just remember that licorice can be a potent drug, and too much can cause headache, tiredness, sodium and water retention, high blood pressure, and even heart failure.

If your ulcer is caused by bacteria, and you can get rid of it, by all means do so. But if the cause is something else, use these tips to make your ulcer a little easier to live with. Take control of your ulcer, so that it doesn't control you.

Sources —
Before You Call the Doctor, Random House, New York, 1992
FDA Consumer (28,10:15)
Helicobacter Pylori in Peptic Ulcer Disease, National Institutes of Health, Office of Medical Applications of Research, Federal Building, Room 618, Bethesda, Md. 20892, 1994
Herbs of Choice: The Therapeutic Use of Phytomedicinals, by Varro E. Tyler, Ph.D., Haworth Press, New York, 1994
The American Journal of Medicine (97,3:265)
The American Medical Association Encyclopedia of Medicine, Random House, New York, 1989
The New England Journal of Medicine (332,3139)

HEART AND BLOOD VESSEL DISORDERS

Prescription Drugs

Natural Alternatives

Prescription Drugs ℞

ANGIOTENSIN CONVERTING ENZYME (ACE) INHIBITORS

Captopril

Brand name: *Capoten*

What this drug does for you:

Captopril is an Angiotensin Converting Enzyme (ACE) inhibitor. It is used to control high blood pressure, to treat congestive heart failure, to slow down further weakening of the heart after a heart attack, and to treat kidney problems in some people with diabetes. ACE inhibitors block an enzyme in the body that is necessary to produce a substance that causes blood vessels to tighten. As a result, they relax blood vessels. This lowers blood pressure and increases the supply of blood and oxygen to the heart.

Possible side effects of this drug:

- Common side effects are cough, rash, itching, very low blood pressure, and loss of ability to taste.
- Even though it is rare, captopril can lower the number of blood cells you have. If you don't have enough white blood cells, your immunity is down, and you can get a fever, sore throat, or pneumonia. If you are lacking red blood cells, you can become anemic, and that makes you tired and weak. Not having enough blood platelets makes you bruise easily and keeps your blood from clotting properly when you're injured. Be on the lookout for any of these symptoms.
- Another side effect you should watch for is swelling of the face, mouth, hands, feet, tongue, or larynx. Contact your doctor if you notice any swelling.
- If you develop jaundice (yellow eyes or skin), you should contact your doctor immediately.
- Serious skin disorders in which dark red rings or raised spots erupt on your skin (Stevens-Johnson syndrome) or parts of your skin deteriorate are another very rare reaction.

Special warnings:

- Don't use this drug if you are allergic to any of the ACE inhibitor heart medicines.
- If you have poor kidney function, diabetes, heart failure, arthritis or lupus, you should use this drug cautiously. If you have high blood pressure, heart failure, or poor kidney function, your kidneys should be tested regularly while you're taking this drug.
- People taking nerve-blocking drugs, diuretics, angina drugs, and people on dialysis should be watched closely by their doctors.

Pregnancy and nursing mothers:

Category C in first trimester. Category D in second and third trimesters. See page 9 for description of categories. Drug is present in mother's milk.

Possible food and drug interactions:

- If you take captopril along with the antipsychotic drug lithium, the combination may cause lithium to accumulate to toxic levels.
- Aspirin and other nonsteroidal anti-inflammatory drugs (NSAIDs), such as indomethacin, may decrease the effects of captopril.
- Captopril can be used safely with other blood pressure drugs like diuretics, but may cause too much fluid loss or very low blood pressure.

Helpful hints:

- Take captopril one hour before meals.
- Be careful in hot weather and during exercise. Sweating can cause loss of fluid, low blood pressure, and, therefore, lightheadedness.
- This drug can cause very low blood pressure, especially when you first begin to take it. Be careful when you rise quickly — you may feel lightheaded and dizzy.
- Never stop taking this drug without your doctor's approval.
- Captopril may cause dangerously high levels of potassium in the blood.

Don't use potassium-sparing diuretics or take potassium supplements without talking to your doctor. Very high levels of potassium can be fatal.

- The usual starting dose for adults is 25 mg two or three times a day.

Enalapril

Brand name: *Vasotec*

What this drug does for you:

This Angiotensin Converting Enzyme (ACE) inhibitor treats high blood pressure. ACE inhibitors block an enzyme in the body that is necessary to produce a substance that causes blood vessels to tighten. As a result, they relax blood vessels. This lowers blood pressure and increases the supply of blood and oxygen to the heart.

Possible side effects of this drug:

- The most common side effects are dizziness, headache, fatigue, and cough. You may also experience low blood pressure, diarrhea, headache, chest pain, abdominal pain, vomiting, nausea, itching, hives, fainting, rash, increased sweating, and difficulty breathing.
- Rare side effects are heart attack, embolism, heartbeat irregularities, loss of appetite, dry mouth, constipation, muscle cramps, mental depression, confusion, nervousness, hair loss, sensitivity to light, kidney failure, blurred vision, and ringing in the ears.
- Even though it is rare, enalapril can lower the number of blood cells you have. If you don't have enough white blood cells, your immunity is down, and you can get a fever, sore throat, or pneumonia. If you are lacking red blood cells, you can become anemic, and that makes you tired and weak. Not having enough blood platelets makes you bruise easily and keeps your blood from clotting properly when you're injured. Be on the lookout for any of these symptoms.
- Another side effect you should watch for is swelling. Mild swelling can occur in the throat, face, lips, tongue, mucous membranes, hands, or feet, but swelling of the throat can be extremely dangerous. Contact your doctor immediately.
- If you develop jaundice (yellow eyes or skin), you should contact your doctor immediately.

Special warnings:

- People with poor kidney function and people with heart failure and collagen vascular diseases should take this drug very cautiously.
- Enalapril may cause a severe drop in blood pressure after the first dose, particularly in people taking diuretics, on dialysis, or with congestive heart failure.

Pregnancy and nursing mothers:

Category C in first trimester. Category D in second and third trimesters. See page 9 for description of categories. Drug is present in mother's milk.

Possible food and drug interactions:

- If this drug is taken with the antipsychotic drug lithium, it may cause lithium to accumulate to toxic levels.
- Nonsteroidal anti-inflammatory drugs (NSAIDs) may decrease the blood-pressure-lowering effects of enalapril.
- You could have a dangerous drop in blood pressure if you drink alcohol or take barbiturates or narcotics with enalapril.

Helpful hints:

- Enalapril may cause dangerously high levels of potassium in the blood. Don't use potassium-sparing diuretics or take potassium supplements without talking to your doctor. Very high levels of potassium can be fatal.
- Be careful in hot weather and during exercise. Sweating can cause loss of fluid, low blood pressure, and, therefore, lightheadedness.
- This drug can cause very low blood pressure, especially when you first begin to take it. Be careful when you rise quickly — you may feel light-headed and dizzy.

Fosinopril

Brand name: *Monopril*

What this drug does for you:

This Angiotensin Converting Enzyme (ACE) inhibitor treats high blood pressure. ACE inhibitors block an enzyme in the body that is necessary to produce a substance that causes blood vessels to tighten. As a result, they relax blood vessels. This lowers blood pressure and increases the supply of blood and oxygen to the heart.

Possible side effects of this drug:

- The most common side effects are fatigue, dizziness, headache, cough, sexual dysfunction, diarrhea, and nausea.
- Less common side effects are heartburn, itching, tingling, rash, sensitivity to light, gout, dry mouth, gas, constipation, muscle pain or cramps, confusion, drowsiness, ringing in the ears, stuffy nose, sore throat, frequent urination, and irritated eyes.
- Even though it is rare, fosinopril can lower the number of blood cells you have. If you don't have enough white blood cells, your immunity is down, and you can get a fever, sore throat, or pneumonia. If you are lacking red blood cells, you can become anemic, and that makes you tired and weak. Not having enough blood platelets makes you bruise easily and keeps your blood from clotting properly when you're injured. Be on the lookout for any of these symptoms.
- Another side effect you should watch for is swelling. Mild swelling can occur in the throat, face, lips, tongue, mucous membranes, hands, or feet, but swelling of the throat can be extremely dangerous. Contact your doctor immediately.
- If you develop jaundice (yellow eyes or skin), you should contact your

doctor immediately.

Special warnings:

- People with poor kidney and liver functions should take this drug very cautiously.
- Fosinopril may cause a severe drop in blood pressure after the first dose, particularly in people taking diuretics, on dialysis, or with congestive heart failure.

Pregnancy and nursing mothers:

Category C in first trimester. Category D in second and third trimesters. See page 9 for description of categories. Drug is present in mother's milk.

Possible food and drug interactions:

- This drug may increase levels or effects of the anti-psychotic drug lithium, so lithium levels should be monitored while using this drug.
- Antacids can keep fosinopril from being absorbed properly, so don't take antacids within two hours of taking fosinopril.

Helpful hints:

- Fosinopril may cause dangerously high levels of potassium in the blood. Don't use potassium-sparing diuretics or take potassium supplements without talking to your doctor. Very high levels of potassium can be fatal.
- Be careful in hot weather and during exercise. Sweating can cause loss of fluid, low blood pressure, and, therefore, lightheadedness.
- This drug can cause very low blood pressure, especially when you first begin to take it. Be careful when you rise quickly — you may feel light-headed and dizzy. If you faint, stop taking the drug and immediately contact your doctor.
- Make sure you take in plenty of fluids to help prevent a drop in blood pressure.

Lisinopril

Brand names: *Prinivil, Zestril*

What this drug does for you:

This Angiotensin Converting Enzyme (ACE) inhibitor treats high blood pressure and helps manage heart failure. ACE inhibitors block an enzyme in the body that is necessary to produce a substance that causes blood vessels to tighten. As a result, they relax blood vessels. This lowers blood pressure and increases the supply of blood and oxygen to the heart.

Possible side effects of this drug:

- Possible side effects are fatigue, headache, cough, vomiting, diarrhea, and nausea.
- Rarer side effects are heartburn, itching, tingling, rash, sensitivity to light, gout, dry mouth, gas, constipation, muscle pain or cramps, confusion, drowsiness, ringing in the ears, stuffy nose, sore throat, frequent urination, and irritated eyes.

- Even though it is rare, lisinopril can lower the number of blood cells you have. If you don't have enough white blood cells, your immunity is down, and you can get a fever, sore throat, or pneumonia. If you are lacking red blood cells, you can become anemic, and that makes you tired and weak. Not having enough blood platelets makes you bruise easily and keeps your blood from clotting properly when you're injured. Be on the lookout for any of these symptoms.
- Another side effect you should watch for is swelling. Mild swelling can occur in the throat, face, lips, tongue, mucous membranes, hands, or feet, but swelling of the throat can be extremely dangerous. Contact your doctor immediately.

Special warnings:
- People with poor kidney and liver functions should take this drug very cautiously.
- Lisinopril may cause a severe drop in blood pressure after the first dose, particularly in people taking diuretics, on dialysis, or with congestive heart failure.

Pregnancy and nursing mothers:
Category C in first trimester. Category D in second and third trimesters. See page 9 for description of categories. Every effort should be made to find an alternative treatment when pregnancy is confirmed. Don't use while nursing.

Possible food and drug interactions:
- This drug may increase levels or effects of the antipsychotic drug lithium, so lithium levels should be monitored while using this drug.
- Nonsteroidal anti-inflammatory drugs (NSAIDs) may decrease the blood-pressure-lowering effects of lisinopril.

Helpful hints:
- Lisinopril may cause dangerously high levels of potassium in the blood. Don't use potassium-sparing diuretics or take potassium supplements without talking to your doctor. Very high levels of potassium can be fatal.
- Be careful in hot weather and during exercise. Sweating can cause loss of fluid, low blood pressure, and, therefore, lightheadedness.
- This drug can cause very low blood pressure, especially when you first begin to take it and when you're also taking diuretics. Be careful when you rise quickly — you may feel lightheaded and dizzy. If you faint, stop taking the drug and immediately contact your doctor.
- Make sure you take in plenty of fluids to help prevent a drop in blood pressure.

Quinapril

Brand name: *Accupril*

What this drug does for you:
This Angiotensin Converting Enzyme (ACE) inhibitor treats high blood

pressure. ACE inhibitors block an enzyme in the body that is necessary to produce a substance that causes blood vessels to tighten. As a result, they relax blood vessels. This lowers blood pressure and increases the supply of blood and oxygen to the heart.

Possible side effects of this drug:

- Common side effects are dizziness, coughing, fatigue, nausea, chest pain, low blood pressure, diarrhea, headache, and back pain. Some other possible side effects are palpitations, rapid heartbeat, fluid retention, dry mouth, back pain, itching, sweating, fainting, constipation, sore throat, nasal congestion, mental depression, and nervousness.
- Even though it is rare, quinapril can lower the number of blood cells you have. If you don't have enough white blood cells, your immunity is down, and you can get a fever, sore throat, or pneumonia. If you are lacking red blood cells, you can become anemic, and that makes you tired and weak. Not having enough blood platelets makes you bruise easily and keeps your blood from clotting properly when you're injured. Be on the lookout for any of these symptoms.
- Another side effect you should watch for is swelling. Mild swelling can occur in the throat, face, lips, tongue, mucous membranes, hands, or feet, but swelling of the throat can be extremely dangerous. Contact your doctor immediately.
- If you develop jaundice (yellow eyes or skin), you should contact your doctor immediately.

Special warnings:

- People with poor kidney and liver functions should take this drug very cautiously.
- Quinapril may cause a severe drop in blood pressure after the first dose, particularly in people taking diuretics, on dialysis, or with congestive heart failure.

Pregnancy and nursing mothers:

Category C in first trimester. Category D in second and third trimesters. See page 9 for description of categories. Not known if drug is present in mother's milk.

Possible food and drug interactions:

- Quinapril may increase levels of the antipsychotic drug lithium, possibly to toxic levels.
- Quinapril may decrease levels of the antibiotic tetracycline.

Helpful hints:

- Quinapril may cause dangerously high levels of potassium in the blood. Don't use potassium-sparing diuretics or take potassium supplements without talking to your doctor. Very high levels of potassium can be fatal.
- Be careful in hot weather and during exercise. Sweating can cause loss of fluid, low blood pressure, and, therefore, lightheadedness.
- This drug can cause very low blood pressure, especially when you first

begin to take it and when you're also taking diuretics. Be careful when you rise quickly — you may feel lightheaded and dizzy. If you faint, stop taking the drug and immediately contact your doctor.

- Make sure you take in plenty of fluids to help prevent a drop in blood pressure.

Ramipril

Brand name: *Altace*

What this drug does for you:
This Angiotensin Converting Enzyme (ACE) inhibitor treats high blood pressure. ACE inhibitors block an enzyme in the body that is necessary to produce a substance that causes blood vessels to tighten. As a result, they relax blood vessels. This lowers blood pressure and increases the supply of blood and oxygen to the heart.

Possible side effects of this drug:
- Common side effects are coughing, headache, dizziness, fatigue, and nausea. Less common side effects are palpitations, rapid heartbeat, fluid retention, dry mouth, back pain, itching, sweating, fainting, constipation, nasal congestion, mental depression, and nervousness.
- Even though it is rare, ramipril can lower the number of blood cells you have. If you don't have enough white blood cells, your immunity is down, and you can get a fever, sore throat, or pneumonia. If you are lacking red blood cells, you can become anemic, and that makes you tired and weak. Not having enough blood platelets makes you bruise easily and keeps your blood from clotting properly when you're injured. Be on the lookout for any of these symptoms.
- Another side effect you should watch for is swelling. Mild swelling can occur in the throat, face, lips, tongue, mucous membranes, hands, or feet, but swelling of the throat can be extremely dangerous. Contact your doctor immediately.

Special warnings:
- People with poor kidney and liver functions should take this drug very cautiously.
- Ramipril may cause a severe drop in blood pressure after the first dose, particularly in people taking diuretics, on dialysis, or with congestive heart failure.

Pregnancy and nursing mothers:
Category C in first trimester. Category D in second and third trimesters. See page 9 for description of categories. Not known if drug is present in mother's milk.

Possible food and drug interaction:
- This drug may increase levels of the antipsychotic drug lithium, possibly to toxic levels.

Helpful hints:

- Ramipril may cause dangerously high levels of potassium in the blood. Don't use potassium-sparing diuretics or take potassium supplements without talking to your doctor. Very high levels of potassium can be fatal.
- Be careful in hot weather and during exercise. Sweating can cause loss of fluid, low blood pressure, and, therefore, lightheadedness.
- This drug can cause very low blood pressure, especially when you first begin to take it and when you're also taking diuretics. Be careful when you rise quickly — you may feel lightheaded and dizzy. If you faint, stop taking the drug and immediately contact your doctor.
- Make sure you take in plenty of fluids to help prevent a drop in blood pressure.

ANGINA DRUGS

Isosorbide Dinitrate

Brand names: *Dilatrate-SR, Isordil, Sorbitrate* **(Generic available)**

What this drug does for you:

Isosorbide dinitrate prevents angina (chest pain).

Possible side effects of this drug:

- This drug may cause headache, low blood pressure, flushing, weakness, and dizziness. Less common side effects are nausea, vomiting, rash, and sweating.

Special warning:

- If you have low blood pressure, have had a recent heart attack, or are sensitive to nitrates or nitrites, take this drug very cautiously.

Pregnancy and nursing mothers:

Category C. See page 9 for description of categories. Not known if drug is present in mother's milk.

Possible food and drug interaction:

- Don't drink alcohol while you take this drug. The combination may cause very low blood pressure.

Helpful hints:

- Take your medicine regularly, as prescribed, and keep it easily available at all times.
- You can take an additional dose before a stressful time or at bedtime if you have angina at night. Discuss these options with your doctor.
- Since this drug can cause very low blood pressure and dizziness, sit or stand up slowly and be careful on stairs.

Nitroglycerin

Brand names: *Deponit, Minitran, Nitro-Bid IV, Nitro-Dur, Nitrodisc, Nitrogard, Nitroglyn, Nitrolingual Spray, Nitrostat, Transderm-Nitro* (Generic available)

What this drug does for you:

Nitroglycerin prevents angina (chest pain) caused by coronary artery disease.

Possible side effects of this drug:

- A common side effect of nitroglycerin is very low blood pressure, especially when you stand up. Other side effects are fainting, a worsening of your angina, frequent headaches, and lightheadedness.

Special warnings:

- People with allergies to nitrates or adhesives should not take this drug.
- People with low blood pressure, a recent heart attack, or heart failure should take nitroglycerin with extreme caution.
- Nitroglycerin can cause very low blood pressure, leading to a slow heartbeat and a worsening of your angina.

Pregnancy and nursing mothers:

Category C. See page 9 for description of categories. Not known if drug is present in mother's milk.

Possible food and drug interaction:

- Don't drink alcohol while you take this drug. The combination may cause very low blood pressure.

Helpful hints:

- You can become physically dependent on nitroglycerin, so don't stop taking it suddenly. You may experience withdrawal symptoms.
- Have your nitroglycerin within easy reach at all times. Take your dose regularly, as your doctor has prescribed.
- You can take an additional dose before a stressful time or at bedtime if you have angina at night. Discuss these options with your doctor.
- Since this drug can cause very low blood pressure and dizziness, sit or stand up slowly and be careful on stairs.
- Take tablets on an empty stomach, one or two hours before meals.

ANTICOAGULANTS

Warfarin

Brand name: *Coumadin*

What this drug does for you:

Warfarin reduces the ability of the blood to form clots. It is also used to prevent or treat various kinds of clots, especially in people who may be at risk of heart attack or stroke. Warfarin also protects against blood clots after a heart attack.

Possible side effects of this drug:

- Rare but serious side effects are bleeding under the skin or in an organ and death or gangrene of skin or other tissues.
- A painful, continuous erection of the penis is another serious side effect you should let your doctor know about immediately.
- Other side effects are nausea, vomiting, diarrhea, stomach cramps, red-orange discoloration of urine, swelling, hair loss, and hives. You could also have liver problems such as jaundice. Look for yellow eyes and skin.
- Fever and skin rash signal a bad reaction to the drug. Tell your doctor immediately.

Special warnings:

- People with blood diseases, intestinal or other bleeding, people who have just had or about to have surgery, and pregnant women shouldn't take this drug.
- People with the following conditions should use this drug with caution: poor liver or kidney function, high blood pressure, diabetes, "protein C" deficiency, heart failure, trauma, or infectious disease.
- Factors that may influence the actions of anticoagulants include the general level of health of the person, other drugs being taken, changes in eating habits or environment, and travel.

Pregnancy and nursing mothers:

Category X. See page 9 for description of categories. Don't take this drug while you are nursing.

Possible food and drug interactions:

- If you take warfarin with the anticoagulant ticlopidine, you can get hepatitis.
- The following drugs may increase the effects of warfarin: acetaminophen, the gout drug allopurinol, aspirin, the ulcer drug cimetidine, blood fat-reducer clofibrate, the antidiabetic drug chlorpropamide, the pain drug diflunisal, the anti-alcoholic drug disulfiram, the anticoagulant heparin, the blood fat-reducer lovastatin, monoamine oxidase (MAO) inhibitors, the blood pressure drug methyldopa, the antibiotic metronidazole, the antifungal miconazole, narcotics, nonsteroidal anti-inflammatory drugs (NSAIDs), the seizure drug phenytoin, the heartbeat regulator quinidine, the cancer drug tamoxifen, the antidiabetic drug tolbutamide, and thyroid drugs.
- The following drugs may decrease the effects of warfarin: antacids, antihistamines, corticosteroids, barbiturates, birth control pills, the seizure drug carbamazepine, the anti-anxiety drug chlordiazepoxide, the antifungal drug griseofulvin, the anti-anxiety drug meprobamate, the seizure drug primidone, the tuberculosis drug rifampin, and the antidepressant trazodone.

Helpful hints:

- You should have regular tests to measure clotting time while you're taking this drug.
- Take your warfarin dose at the same time every day.
- Watch yourself for bleeding gums, bruises on your arms or legs, nosebleeds, and blood in your urine. Tell your doctor if you have any of these side effects.
- Eat plenty of leafy green vegetables every day to get a regular, unchanging diet of vitamin K.

ANTIHYPERTENSIVES

Benazepril

Brand name: *Lotensin*

What this drug does for you:
Benazepril controls high blood pressure.

Possible side effects of this drug:

- Common side effects are headache, dizziness, fatigue, drowsiness, nausea, and cough.
- Less common side effects are low blood pressure, angina, palpitations, constipation, vomiting, rash, sensitivity to light, anxiety, insomnia, arthritis, asthma, sinus problems, and sweating.
- Rare reactions are heart attack, stroke, and breast enlargement in males and females.
- One serious side effect you should watch for is swelling, an allergic reaction to the drug. Mild swelling can occur in the throat, face, lips, tongue, mucous membranes, hands, or feet, but swelling of the throat can be extremely dangerous. Contact your doctor immediately.
- Even though it is very rare, benazepril can lower the number of blood cells you have. If you don't have enough white blood cells, your immunity is down, and you can get a fever, sore throat, or pneumonia. If you are lacking red blood cells, you can become anemic, and that makes you tired and weak. Not having enough blood platelets makes you bruise easily and keeps your blood from clotting properly when you're injured. Be on the lookout for any of these symptoms of bone marrow depression.

Special warning:

- People with poor kidney function, diabetes, liver disease, heart failure, rheumatoid arthritis, or lupus should take this drug with caution.

Pregnancy and nursing mothers:
Category C in first trimester. Category D in second and third trimesters. See page 9 for description of categories. Drug is present in mother's milk.

Possible food and drug interactions:

- Taken with diuretics, benazepril can cause very low blood pressure as well as a dangerous buildup of potassium in the body.

- Taken with the antipsychotic drug lithium, benazepril may cause dangerous buildup of lithium, especially if you are also taking a diuretic.

Helpful hint:
- Benazepril may cause dangerously high levels of potassium in your blood. Don't use potassium-sparing diuretics or take potassium supplements or salt substitutes containing potassium without talking to your doctor.

Clonidine Hydrochloride

Brand name: *Catapres* **(Generic available)**

What this drug does for you:
Clonidine controls high blood pressure.

Possible side effects of this drug:
- Common side effects are dry mouth, drowsiness, dizziness, and constipation.
- Less common side effects are nausea, vomiting, weakness, nervousness, and impotence.
- Rare side effects are loss of appetite, liver problems, elevated blood sugar, mental depression, headache, nightmares or vivid dreams, restlessness, anxiety, hallucinations, palpitations, rapid or slow heartbeat, numbness or tingling of extremities, congestive heart failure, heart block, rash, itching, hives, frequent urination during the night, difficulty urinating, muscle cramps in legs, dry eyes, blurry vision, dry nose, and fever.

Special warning:
- People with severe heart problems, recent heart attack, disease of blood vessels in the brain, or kidney failure should take this drug with caution.

Pregnancy and nursing mothers:
Category C. See page 9 for description of categories. Drug is present in mother's milk.

Possible food and drug interactions:
- Some antidepressants may decrease the effectiveness of clonidine.
- If you take clonidine along with a drug that depresses your nervous system, such as tranquilizers, alcohol, antihistamines, or muscle relaxers, the combination may dangerously depress your nervous system.
- This drug may increase your sensitivity to alcohol.

Helpful hints:
- You shouldn't drive a car or operate heavy machinery until you are sure the medicine isn't making you drowsy, dizzy, or less than alert. After you've been taking the drug for a while, drowsiness should be less of a problem.
- Don't stop taking this drug without consulting your doctor. Quitting suddenly could cause dangerous withdrawal symptoms.

- This drug can cause very low blood pressure, especially when you first begin to take it. Be careful when you rise quickly — you may feel light-headed and dizzy.

Doxazosin

Brand name: *Cardura*

What this drug does for you:

Doxazosin controls high blood pressure by relaxing and expanding blood vessel walls.

Possible side effects of this drug:

- Very low blood pressure is a common side effect. This can cause dizziness after standing up, lightheadedness, and fainting.
- A rapid heartbeat, sometimes very rapid, can be a dangerous side effect.
- Other side effects are heart palpitations, weakness, headache, drowsiness, nausea, constipation, diarrhea, fluid retention, difficulty breathing, frequent urination, blurred vision, rash, dry mouth, and stuffy nose.
- Rare side effects are hallucinations, stomach pain, very rapid heartbeat, abnormal liver function, inflammation of the pancreas, impotence, incontinence, itchy skin eruptions, profuse sweating, and hair loss.

Special warning:

- You should take this drug cautiously if you are taking other blood-pressure-lowering drugs or if you have poor liver function.

Pregnancy and nursing mothers:

Category C. See page 9 for description of categories. Drug is present in mother's milk.

Possible food and drug interactions:

- If you take doxazosin with other blood pressure drugs, you're more likely to experience very low blood pressure and fainting.
- Alcohol can make your blood pressure drop even further while you're taking this drug.

Helpful hints:

- Doxazosin may cause you to have very low blood pressure when you first start taking it. Your blood pressure can drop so low that you faint or lose consciousness. This is known as the "first-dose" effect. It can also occur if your dose is increased quickly, if your treatment is restarted after you've missed several doses, or if you begin taking another antihypertensive drug.
- Don't drive or do any other potentially hazardous task for 24 hours after you take the first dose. Even after you've been taking the drug for a while, drive with caution. It may cause dizziness, lightheadedness, and palpitations at any time.
- Taking the first dose at bedtime may help reduce the "first-dose" effect.
- Move slowly and carefully when you get up from a sitting or lying position.

Guanfacine

Brand name: *Tenex*

What this drug does for you:
Guanfacine lowers your blood pressure and heart rate. Many people take it along with a thiazide diuretic.

Possible side effects of this drug:
- The most common side effects are dry mouth, constipation, sleepiness, insomnia, weakness, dizziness, headache, and impotence. These side effects often go away after you've been taking guanfacine for a while. You may also experience nausea and low blood pressure when you stand up.
- If you develop a skin rash or "rebound hypertension," a rise in your blood pressure after two to four days on the drug, you should quit taking guanfacine under your doctor's supervision.

Special warning:
- People with severe heart disease, a recent heart attack, chronic liver or kidney failure, or cerebrovascular disease should use this drug cautiously.

Pregnancy and nursing mothers:
Category B. See page 9 for description of categories. Not known if drug is present in mother's milk.

Possible food and drug interactions:
- Taking guanfacine with alcohol or other depressants such as tranquilizers or sleeping pills may cause dangerous depressant effects.
- Phenobarbital and phenytoin reduce the effectiveness of guanfacine.

Helpful hints:
- Don't stop taking guanfacine suddenly. You may feel nervous and anxious, and your blood pressure may skyrocket.
- Be careful when you drive, especially when you first start taking guanfacine. The drug can cause you to feel sedated or drowsy.
- The usual adult starting dose is 1 mg daily.
- Take the medicine at bedtime to minimize the sleepiness side effect.

Hydralazine

Brand name: *Apresoline* (Generic available)

What this drug does for you:
Hydralazine dilates blood vessels and quickly reduces very high blood pressure.

Possible side effects of this drug:
- Possible side effects are nausea, vomiting, diarrhea, constipation, difficult urination, difficulty breathing, numbness or tingling, angina, rapid heartbeat, palpitations, flushing, edema, dizziness, tremors, depression, anxiety, disorientation, headache, conjunctivitis, tearing, nasal conges-

tion, hoarseness, loss of appetite, low blood pressure, and muscle cramps.
- One rare side effect of this drug is a lupus-like reaction. Watch yourself for sore throat, fever, muscle and joint aches, and skin rash. Call your doctor immediately if you develop any of these signs.
- Even though it is rare, hydralazine can lower the number of blood cells you have. If you don't have enough white blood cells, your immunity is down, and you can get a fever, sore throat, or pneumonia. If you are lacking red blood cells, you can become anemic, and that makes you tired and weak. Not having enough blood platelets makes you bruise easily and keeps your blood from clotting properly when you're injured. Be on the lookout for any of these symptoms of bone marrow depression.
- Another rare side effect is hepatitis. You should have regular liver function tests while you are taking this drug.

Special warnings:
- This drug should not be used by people with coronary artery disease or rheumatic heart disease.
- Use this drug with caution if you have kidney damage or cerebral vascular problems.

Pregnancy and nursing mothers:
Category C. See page 9 for description of categories. Not known if drug is present in mother's milk.

Possible food and drug interactions:
- If you are taking antidepressant drugs called monoamine oxidase (MAO) inhibitors, take hydralazine cautiously.
- If you take hydralazine with other high blood pressure drugs, you may develop very low blood pressure.

Helpful hints:
- This drug can cause very low blood pressure, especially when you first begin to take it. Be careful when you rise quickly — you may feel light-headed and dizzy.
- Take the oral form with meals to increase absorption.

Methyldopa

Brand name: *Aldomet* **(Generic available)**

What this drug does for you:
Methyldopa controls high blood pressure.

Possible side effects of this drug:
- Some common side effects are sleepiness, decreased mental sharpness, low blood pressure when you stand up, stuffy nose, dry mouth, weight gain, and drug fever.
- Other possible side effects of methyldopa are vomiting, diarrhea, constipation, gas, inflammation of the pancreas, "black" tongue, inflammation of the salivary glands, angina, fluid retention, slow heartbeat, conges-

tive heart failure, inflammation of the tissue around the heart, involuntary muscle movements, Bell's palsy, nightmares, headache, a prickling or tingling sensation, joint or muscle pain, weakness, dizziness, rash, enlargement of breasts in men and women, impotence, and menstrual irregularities.

- Methyldopa can lower the number of blood cells you have. If you don't have enough white blood cells, your immunity is down, and you can get a fever, sore throat, or pneumonia. If you are lacking red blood cells, you can become anemic, and that makes you tired and weak. Not having enough blood platelets makes you bruise easily and keeps your blood from clotting properly when you're injured. Be on the lookout for any of these symptoms of bone marrow depression.
- Methyldopa can cause liver damage, including hepatitis and jaundice. Look for yellow eyes and skin.

Special warnings:
- People who are allergic to methyldopa or who have ever developed liver problems from using methyldopa, or who currently have liver disease should not take this drug.
- If you have a history of liver problems, take this drug with caution. You should have regular liver function tests while you're taking methyldopa.

Pregnancy and nursing mothers:
Category B. See page 9 for description of categories. Drug is present in mother's milk.

Possible food and drug interactions:
- Methyldopa may increase the effects of other high blood pressure drugs and anesthesia.
- Methyldopa may decrease your body's removal of the antipsychotic drug lithium, allowing the lithium to build up to toxic levels.

Helpful hints:
- This drug can cause very low blood pressure, especially when you first begin to take it. Be careful when you rise quickly — you may feel light-headed and dizzy.
- You shouldn't drive a car or operate heavy machinery until you are sure the medicine isn't making you drowsy, dizzy, or less than alert.

Minoxidil

Brand names: *Loniten, Rogaine* (Generic available)

What this drug does for you:
Minoxidil is used to control severe high blood pressure when other treatments haven't worked. Minoxidil lowers blood pressure by relaxing the muscles within the walls of small arteries throughout the body. It is usually used together with a diuretic.

Minoxidil is also applied to the scalp to treat male-pattern baldness. It may improve blood flow in the scalp and restore small hair follicles.

Possible side effects of this drug:

- Minoxidil may cause various heart problems, such as a rapid heartbeat and angina. Your doctor may prescribe a beta blocker for this side effect. Minoxidil may also cause fluid to accumulate in the cavity around the heart, especially in people with fluid retention or congestive heart failure. If this happens, your doctor may take you off the drug for a while.
- Minoxidil may cause thickening, lengthening, and darkening of your body hair. Other possible side effects are nausea, vomiting, headache, fatigue, rash, and fluid and salt retention. A rare side effect is breast tenderness.
- It is very rare, but minoxidil can lower the number of white blood cells you have. If you don't have enough white blood cells, your immunity is down, and you can get a fever, sore throat, or pneumonia. It can also lower the number of blood platelets you have. Not having enough blood platelets makes you bruise easily and keeps your blood from clotting properly when you're injured. Be on the lookout for any of these symptoms.
- Another very rare reaction is a serious skin disorder in which dark red rings or raised spots erupt on your skin (Stevens-Johnson syndrome).

Special warnings:

- People who have recently had a heart attack should not use minoxidil.
- Minoxidil should not be taken by people with pheochromocytoma, a type of tumor that may be stimulated to grow larger by this drug.
- People with kidney problems may need smaller doses.

Pregnancy and nursing mothers:

Category C. See page 9 for description of categories. Drug is present in mother's milk.

Possible food and drug interaction:

- If you take minoxidil with the blood pressure drug guanethidine, the combination may cause dangerously low blood pressure.

Helpful hint:

- Retaining too much fluid can lead to congestive heart failure, particularly if you're not taking diuretics. Swelling and gaining weight could be signs that you're retaining water. You should weigh yourself at least once a week and report to your doctor any weight gain over five pounds.

Prazosin

Brand name: *Minipress* (Generic available)

What this drug does for you:

Prazosin controls high blood pressure by relaxing and expanding blood vessel walls.

Possible side effects of this drug:

- Very low blood pressure is a common side effect. This can cause dizziness after standing up, lightheadedness, and fainting.

- A rapid heartbeat, sometimes very rapid, can be a dangerous side effect.
- Other side effects are heart palpitations, weakness, headache, drowsiness, nausea, constipation, diarrhea, fluid retention, difficulty breathing, frequent urination, blurred vision, rash, dry mouth, and stuffy nose.
- Rare side effects are hallucinations, stomach pain, very rapid heartbeat, abnormal liver function, inflammation of the pancreas, impotence, incontinence, itchy skin eruptions, profuse sweating, and hair loss.

Special warning:
- You should take this drug cautiously if you are taking other blood-pressure-lowering drugs or if you have poor liver function.

Pregnancy and nursing mothers:
Category C. See page 9 for description of categories. Drug is present in mother's milk.

Possible food and drug interactions:
- Don't drink alcohol while taking this drug.
- If you take prazosin with other blood pressure drugs, you're more likely to experience very low blood pressure and fainting.

Helpful hints:
- Prazosin may cause you to have very low blood pressure when you first start taking it. Your blood pressure can drop so low that you faint or lose consciousness. This is known as the "first-dose" effect. It can also occur if your dose is increased quickly, if your treatment is restarted after you've missed several doses, or if you begin taking another antihypertensive drug.
- Don't drive or do any other potentially hazardous task for 24 hours after you take the first dose. Even after you've been taking the drug for a while, drive with caution. It may cause dizziness, lightheadedness, and palpitations at any time.
- Taking the first dose at bedtime may help reduce the "first-dose" effect.
- Move slowly and carefully when you get up from a sitting or lying position.

Terazosin

Brand name: *Hytrin*

What this drug does for you:
Terazosin controls high blood pressure by relaxing and expanding blood vessel walls.

Possible side effects of this drug:
- Very low blood pressure is a common side effect. This can cause dizziness after standing up, lightheadedness, and fainting.
- A rapid heartbeat, sometimes very rapid, can be a dangerous side effect.
- Other side effects are heart palpitations, weakness, headache, drowsiness, nausea, constipation, diarrhea, fluid retention, difficulty breathing, frequent urination, blurred vision, rash, dry mouth, and stuffy nose.

- Rare side effects are hallucinations, stomach pain, very rapid heartbeat, abnormal liver function, inflammation of the pancreas, impotence, incontinence, itchy skin eruptions, profuse sweating, and hair loss.

Special warning:

- You should take this drug cautiously if you are taking other blood-pressure-lowering drugs or if you have poor liver function.

Pregnancy and nursing mothers:

Category C. See page 9 for description of categories. Not known if drug is present in mother's milk.

Possible food and drug interactions:

- Don't drink alcohol while taking this drug.
- If you take terazosin with other blood pressure drugs, you're more likely to experience very low blood pressure and fainting.

Helpful hints:

- Terazosin may cause you to have very low blood pressure when you first start taking it. Your blood pressure can drop so low that you faint or lose consciousness. This is known as the "first-dose" effect. It can also occur if your dose is increased quickly, if your treatment is restarted after you've missed several doses, or if you begin taking another antihypertensive drug.
- Don't drive or do any other potentially hazardous task for 24 hours after you take the first dose. Even after you've been taking the drug for a while, drive with caution. It may cause dizziness, lightheadedness, and palpitations at any time.
- Taking the first dose at bedtime may help reduce the "first-dose" effect.
- Move slowly and carefully when you get up from a sitting or lying position.

ANTIPLATELETS

Dipyridamole

Brand name: *Persantine* **(Generic available)**

What this drug does for you:

Dipyridamole is used to prevent clotting after heart valve replacement surgery. It is often used along with warfarin.

Possible side effects of this drug:

- Common side effects are dizziness, headache, rash, and upset stomach. You may also experience vomiting, diarrhea, flushing, and itching. These side effects are usually mild and usually go away after you've been taking the drug for a while.
- Rare side effects are angina pectoris and liver problems.

Pregnancy and nursing mothers:

Category B. See page 9 for description of categories. Drug is present in mother's milk.

Possible food and drug interactions:
No significant interactions have been reported.

Helpful hint:
- The recommended adult dose is 75 to 100 mg four times daily along with the usual warfarin therapy.

Ticlopidine

Brand name: *Ticlid*

What this drug does for you:
Ticlopidine helps prevent strokes caused by blood clots. It is meant for people who have already had a stroke or are at high risk of stroke and cannot take aspirin.

Possible side effects of this drug:
- Possible side effects are diarrhea, indigestion, nausea, gas, rash, itching, hives, dizziness, loss of appetite, nosebleed, intestinal bleeding, bleeding of the conjunctiva of the eye, blood in the urine, headache, ringing in the ears, and weakness.
- Ticlopidine can lower the number of blood cells you have. If you don't have enough white blood cells, your immunity is down, and you can get a fever, sore throat, or pneumonia. If you are lacking red blood cells, you can become anemic, and that makes you tired and weak. Not having enough blood platelets makes you bruise easily and keeps your blood from clotting properly when you're injured. Be on the lookout for any of these symptoms of bone marrow depression. You should have regular blood counts while you're taking ticlopidine and before you begin taking the drug.
- This drug can also cause hepatitis with jaundice. Watch yourself for yellow eyes and skin, skin rashes, light-colored stools, or dark urine.
- Ticlopidine can raise your cholesterol and triglyceride levels.
- Rare reactions are lupus joint disease, muscle inflammation, and serum sickness.

Special warnings:
- People with blood or bleeding disorders or severe liver problems should not take this drug.
- People with poor kidney function or any condition which may increase the risk of internal bleeding should take this drug cautiously.

Pregnancy and nursing mothers:
Category B. See page 9 for description of categories. Not known if drug is present in mother's milk.

Possible food and drug interactions:
- Don't take aspirin while taking this drug.
- Ticlopidine may increase levels of the asthma drug theophylline and the liver-function-testing drug antipyrine.

- Ticlopidine may decrease levels of the heart drug digoxin.
- The ulcer drug cimetidine may increase levels of ticlopidine.
- Antacids may decrease levels of ticlopidine. Don't take antacids within two hours of taking your dose of ticlopidine.

Helpful hint:
- Take your medicine after meals or with food to help avoid stomach upset.

BETA-BLOCKERS

Acebutolol

Brand name: *Sectral*

What this drug does for you:
Acebutolol is a beta blocker. It controls high blood pressure and regulates heart rhythm by blocking certain actions of the sympathetic nervous system.

Possible side effects of this drug:
- Acebutolol may cause fatigue, dizziness, headache, difficulty breathing, diarrhea, constipation, nausea, gas, frequent urination, insomnia, chest pain, swelling, depression, abnormal dreams, rash, and stuffy nose.
- Less common side effects are low blood pressure, slow heartbeat, anxiety, increased or decreased sensitivity to touch, impotence, itching, vomiting, stomach pain, painful urination, need to urinate at night, sore throat, wheezing, cold hands and feet, fever, eye pain, unusual bleeding or bruising, and pain in joints, muscles, or back.
- Potential serious side effects include severe depression, congestive heart failure, allergic reaction, and asthma.

Special warnings:
- Acebutolol should not be used by people with congestive heart failure, heart block, cardiogenic shock, or slow heartbeat.
- Acebutolol should be used with caution by people with angina, diseases of the arteries, bronchitis, emphysema, and liver or kidney problems.
- If you have diabetes, you should use this drug cautiously because beta-blockers can mask the signs of low blood sugar.
- Acebutolol can also mask signs of an overactive thyroid.

Pregnancy and nursing mothers:
Category B. See page 9 for description of categories. Drug is present in mother's milk.

Possible food and drug interactions:
- Aspirin and other nonsteroidal anti-inflammatory drugs (NSAIDs) may lower the effects of acebutolol.
- The effects of acebutolol may be increased by other high blood pressure medicines, cold medicines, and nose drops.

Helpful hints:
- Never quit taking this drug without talking to your doctor. It could increase your risk of angina and heart attack.
- Discuss your medication with your doctor before having surgery. He may want to discontinue the drug before your surgery.
- You shouldn't drive a car or operate heavy machinery until you are sure the medicine isn't making you drowsy or less than alert.

Atenolol

Brand name: *Tenormin* (Generic available)

What this drug does for you:
Atenolol is used to treat and control high blood pressure and angina. It also aids in recovery from some kinds of heart attacks by controlling nerve impulses to the heart.

Possible side effects of this drug:
- Atenolol may cause slow heartbeat, low blood pressure, leg pain, dizziness, mental depression, difficulty breathing, fatigue, diarrhea, nausea, wheezing, drowsiness, and cold, tingling fingers and toes.
- Atenolol can raise your cholesterol and triglyceride levels.
- Rare reactions are liver abnormalities, headache, impotence, rash, discoloration of the skin, hair loss, decrease in blood platelets (easy bruising and bleeding), and lupus.
- Very rarely, this drug can cause a potentially fatal allergic reaction. Symptoms can include low blood pressure, bronchospasm, slow heartbeat, hives, and swelling around the heart.

Special warnings:
- People with abnormally slow heartbeat, congestive heart failure, heart block, or cardiogenic shock should not take atenolol.
- People with circulatory disorders, bronchitis, emphysema, or liver or kidney problems should take atenolol with caution.
- If you have diabetes, you should use this drug cautiously because beta-blockers can mask the signs of low blood sugar.
- Atenolol can also mask signs of an overactive thyroid.

Pregnancy and nursing mothers:
Category D. See page 9 for description of categories. Drug is present in mother's milk.

Possible food and drug interactions:
- If you take both atenolol and the high blood pressure drug clonidine, you may have serious, even fatal, increases in blood pressure called rebound hypertension when you stop taking clonidine.
- Taking atenolol and the high blood pressure drug reserpine together may cause very low blood pressure.

Helpful hints:
- Never quit taking this drug without talking to your doctor. It could in-

crease your risk of angina and heart attack.

- You shouldn't drive a car or operate heavy machinery until you are sure the medicine isn't making you drowsy or less than alert.
- Tell your doctor immediately if you have any signs of congestive heart failure such as night cough; swelling of your legs, feet, or hands; or difficulty breathing, especially when lying down or after physical exertion.

Betaxolol

Brand names: *Betoptic, Betoptic S, Kerlone*

What this drug does for you:

Betaxolol is a beta blocker. It controls high blood pressure and regulates heart rhythm by blocking certain actions of the sympathetic nervous system. It expands blood vessel walls and slows down the contractions of the heart.

Possible side effects of this drug:

- Side effects include fatigue, dizziness, headache, difficulty breathing, diarrhea, constipation, nausea, gas, frequent urination, insomnia, chest pain, swelling, depression, abnormal dreams, rash, and stuffy nose.
- Less common side effects are low blood pressure, slow heartbeat, anxiety, increased or decreased sensitivity to touch, impotence, itching, vomiting, abdominal pain, painful urination, need to urinate at night, sore throat, wheezing, cold hands and feet, fever, eye pain, unusual bleeding or bruising, and pain in joints, muscles, or back.
- Potential serious side effects include severe depression, congestive heart failure, allergic reaction, and asthma.

Special warnings:

- Betaxolol should not be used by people with congestive heart failure, heart block, cardiogenic shock, or slow heartbeat.
- People with angina, diseases of the arteries, bronchitis, emphysema, or liver or kidney problems should use betaxolol with caution.
- If you have diabetes, you should use this drug cautiously because beta blockers can mask the signs of low blood sugar.
- Betaxolol can also mask signs of an overactive thyroid.

Pregnancy and nursing mothers:

Category C. See page 9 for description of categories. Drug is present in mother's milk.

Possible food and drug interactions:

- Betaxolol may decrease the effects of the allergic reaction drug epinephrine.
- Taking betaxolol with the blood pressure drugs diltiazem, nifedipine, reserpine, and verapamil may increase the effects of betaxolol and lead to very low blood pressure.

Helpful hints:

- You shouldn't drive a car or operate heavy machinery until you are sure the medicine isn't making you drowsy or less than alert.

- Discuss your medication with your doctor before having surgery. He may want to discontinue the drug before your surgery.
- Tell your doctor immediately if you have any signs of congestive heart failure such as night cough; swelling of your legs, feet, or hands; or difficulty breathing, especially when lying down or after physical exertion.
- Never quit taking this drug without talking to your doctor. It could increase your risk of angina and heart attack.

Labetalol

Brand names: *Normodyne, Trandate*

What this drug does for you:

Labetalol is an alpha/beta blocker. It controls high blood pressure and regulates heart rhythm by blocking certain actions of the sympathetic nervous system. It expands blood vessel walls and slows down the contractions of the heart.

Labetalol can be used alone or with other blood pressure-lowering drugs, particularly thiazide and loop diuretics.

Possible side effects of this drug:

- This drug may cause headache, indigestion, weakness, vertigo, and stuffy nose.
- Less common side effects are fatigue, dizziness, nausea, low blood pressure, fainting, slow heartbeat, heart block, fever, lupus, jaundice, hepatitis, tingling of the scalp, dry eyes, muscle cramps, spasms of the breathing tubes (especially for people with asthma), rash, and difficulty urinating.
- Rarely, may cause allergic reaction including fluid retention, vomiting, diarrhea, difficulty breathing, prickling or tingling sensation, drowsiness, sweating, itching, and hives or a rash.

Special warnings:

- Labetalol should not be used by people with severely slow heartbeat, greater than first degree heart block, heart failure, or asthma.
- Take labetalol with extreme caution if you have a history of heart failure, poor liver function, emphysema, or bronchitis.
- If you have diabetes, you should use this drug cautiously because beta blockers can mask the signs of low blood sugar. Labetalol may also reduce the effects of insulin. Diabetics may need to have their insulin dosages adjusted.
- Labetalol can also mask signs of an overactive thyroid.

Pregnancy and nursing mothers:

Category C. See page 9 for description of categories. Drug is present in mother's milk.

Possible food and drug interactions:

- The ulcer drug cimetidine may increase levels of labetalol.
- Taking labetalol while you're taking the anesthesia drug halothane or

the angina drug nitroglycerin may cause dangerously low blood pressure.

Helpful hints:
- You shouldn't drive a car or operate heavy machinery until you are sure the medicine isn't making you drowsy or less than alert.
- Discuss your medication with your doctor before having surgery. He may want to discontinue the drug before your surgery.
- Tell your doctor immediately if you have any signs of congestive heart failure such as night cough; swelling of your legs, feet, or hands; or difficulty breathing, especially when lying down or after physical exertion.
- Never quit taking this drug without talking to your doctor. It could increase your risk of angina and heart attack.

Metoprolol

Brand names: *Lopressor, Toprol-XL* **(Generic available)**

What this drug does for you:
Metoprolol is a beta blocker. It controls high blood pressure and regulates heart rhythm by blocking certain actions of the sympathetic nervous system. It expands blood vessel walls and slows down the contractions of the heart.

Possible side effects of this drug:
- Possible side effects are tiredness, dizziness, memory loss, depression, mental confusion, nightmares, insomnia, palpitations, numbness or tingling in hands or feet, slow heartbeat, headache, fainting, chest pain, rash, itching, blurred vision, muscle pain, and ringing in the ears.
- Tell your doctor immediately if you have any signs of congestive heart failure such as night cough; swelling of your legs, feet, or hands; or difficulty breathing, especially when lying down or after physical exertion. This drug can worsen congestive heart failure.
- Rare side effects are hair loss, dry eyes, and a low white blood cell count. A low number of white blood cells means your immunity is down and your risk of infection is up.

Special warnings:
- This drug should not be taken by people with emphysema, bronchitis, heart block, cardiac shock, heart failure, or slow heartbeat. This drug can aggravate asthma symptoms.
- If you have diabetes, you should use this drug cautiously because beta blockers can mask the signs of low blood sugar.
- Metoprolol can also mask signs of an overactive thyroid.
- People with poor liver function should take this drug cautiously.

Pregnancy and nursing mothers:
Category C. See page 9 for description of categories. Drug is present in mother's milk.

Possible food and drug interactions:
- Taking metoprolol with the blood pressure drug reserpine can cause

your blood pressure to drop to a very low level.
- Metoprolol may decrease the effects of the asthma drug epinephrine.

Helpful hints:
- Take metoprolol with or after meals.
- You shouldn't drive a car or operate heavy machinery until you are sure the medicine isn't making you drowsy or less than alert.
- Discuss your medication with your doctor before having surgery. He may want to discontinue the drug before your surgery.
- Never quit taking this drug without talking to your doctor. It could increase your risk of angina and heart attack.

Nadolol

Brand names: *None available* **(Generic available)**

What this drug does for you:
Nadolol is a beta blocker. It is used to treat and control high blood pressure and angina.

Possible side effects of this drug:
- Nadolol may cause slow heartbeat, low blood pressure, leg pain, dizziness, mental depression, difficulty breathing, fatigue, diarrhea, nausea, wheezing, drowsiness, and cold, tingling fingers and toes.
- Nadolol can raise your cholesterol and triglyceride levels.
- Rare reactions are liver abnormalities, headache, impotence, rash, discoloration of the skin, hair loss, decrease in blood platelets (easy bruising and bleeding), and lupus.
- Very rarely, this drug can cause a potentially fatal allergic reaction. Symptoms can include low blood pressure, bronchospasm, slow heartbeat, hives, and swelling around the heart.

Special warnings:
- People with abnormally slow heartbeat, congestive heart failure, heart block, or cardiogenic shock should not take nadolol.
- People with circulatory disorders, bronchitis, emphysema, or liver or kidney problems should take nadolol with caution.
- If you have diabetes, you should use this drug cautiously because beta-blockers can mask the signs of low blood sugar.
- Nadolol can also mask signs of an overactive thyroid.

Pregnancy and nursing mothers:
Category C. See page 9 for description of categories. Drug is present in mother's milk.

Possible food and drug interactions:
- Taking nadolol and the high blood pressure drug reserpine together may cause very low blood pressure.
- Nadolol may increase the effects of anesthesia.
- Nadolol may decrease the effects of the asthma drug epinephrine.

Helpful hints:
- Never quit taking this drug without talking to your doctor. It could increase your risk of angina and heart attack.
- You shouldn't drive a car or operate heavy machinery until you are sure the medicine isn't making you drowsy or less than alert.
- Tell your doctor immediately if you have any signs of congestive heart failure such as night cough; swelling of your legs, feet, or hands; or difficulty breathing, especially when lying down or after physical exertion.

Penbutolol

Brand name: *Levatol*

What this drug does for you:
Penbutolol is used to treat and control high blood pressure.

Possible side effects of this drug:
- Penbutolol may cause nausea, diarrhea, indigestion, headache, weakness, dizziness, hallucinations, abnormal dreams, prickling or tingling sensation, slow heartbeat, insomnia, chest pain, cough, difficulty breathing, wheezing, and sweating.
- Impotence is a rare side effect.

Special warnings:
- Penbutolol should not be taken by people with very slow heartbeat, heart failure, heart block, shock, bronchitis, emphysema, or asthma. The drug may worsen heart failure, heart disease, or angina. Penbutolol can also make asthma symptoms worse.
- If you have diabetes, you should use this drug cautiously because beta-blockers can mask the signs of low blood sugar.
- Penbutolol can also mask signs of an overactive thyroid.

Pregnancy and nursing mothers:
Category C. See page 9 for description of categories. Not known if drug is present in mother's milk.

Possible food and drug interactions:
- Avoid alcohol while taking penbutolol.
- Penbutolol may decrease the effects of the asthma drug epinephrine and the heart rhythm drug lidocaine.
- Nonsteroidal anti-inflammatories (NSAIDs), such as indomethacin, may decrease effects of penbutolol.

Helpful hints:
- Never quit taking this drug without talking to your doctor. It could increase your risk of angina and heart attack.
- You shouldn't drive a car or operate heavy machinery until you are sure the medicine isn't making you drowsy or less than alert.
- Tell your doctor immediately if you have any signs of congestive heart failure such as night cough; swelling of your legs, feet, or hands; or difficulty breathing, especially when lying down or after physical exertion.

Pindolol

Brand name: *Visken* **(Generic available)**

What this drug does for you:
Pindolol is a beta blocker. It treats and controls high blood pressure by slowing down the contractions of the heart and expanding blood vessel walls.

Possible side effects of this drug:
- Possible side effects are insomnia, muscle pain, joint pain, nausea, stomach pain, chest pain, strange dreams, prickling or tingling sensation, and itching.
- Rare side effects are rash, hallucinations, and heart palpitations.
- Tell your doctor immediately if you have any signs of congestive heart failure such as night cough; swelling of your legs, feet, or hands; or difficulty breathing, especially when lying down or after physical exertion.

Special warnings:
- People with asthma, very slow heartbeat, heart block, shock, or heart failure should not take this drug.
- You should take pindolol cautiously if you have bronchitis, emphysema, or poor liver or kidney function.
- If you have diabetes, you should use this drug cautiously because beta-blockers can mask the signs of low blood sugar.
- Pindolol can also mask signs of an overactive thyroid.

Pregnancy and nursing mothers:
Category B. See page 9 for description of categories. Drug is present in mother's milk.

Possible food and drug interactions:
- Pindolol may increase effects of the antipsychotic drug thioridazine.
- Pindolol may decrease the effectiveness of the asthma drug theophylline.
- Effects of pindolol may be increased by the blood pressure drug reserpine and birth control pills.
- Nonsteroidal anti-inflammatory drugs (NSAIDs), such as aspirin, may decrease the effects of pindolol.

Helpful hints:
- Never quit taking this drug without talking to your doctor. It could increase your risk of angina and heart attack.
- You shouldn't drive a car or operate heavy machinery until you are sure the medicine isn't making you drowsy or less than alert.
- Discuss your medication with your doctor before having surgery. He may want to discontinue the drug before your surgery.

Propranolol

Brand names: *Inderal, Inderal LA* **(Generic available)**

What this drug does for you:

Propranolol is a beta blocker. It controls high blood pressure by expanding the blood vessel walls and slowing down the contractions of the heart. It is also used to treat angina, various heart rhythm problems, and some kinds of muscle tremors.

Propranolol is used after heart attacks to prevent further heart attacks. This drug is also used to treat and to prevent migraine headaches.

Possible side effects of this drug:

- Propranolol may cause low blood pressure, prickling or tingling of the hands, lightheadedness, slow heartbeat, mental depression, abnormal vision, hallucinations, disorientation, short-term memory loss, vivid dreams, hair loss, dry eyes, impotence, nausea, diarrhea, colitis, and constipation.
- Lupus is a rare side effect. Some signs of lupus are sore throat, fever, muscle and joint aches, and skin rash. Call your doctor immediately if you develop any of these signs.
- Tell your doctor immediately if you have any signs of congestive heart failure such as night cough; swelling of your legs, feet, or hands; or difficulty breathing, especially when lying down or after physical exertion.
- Even though it is very rare, propranolol can lower the number of blood cells you have. If you don't have enough white blood cells, your immunity is down, and you can get a fever, sore throat, or pneumonia. If you are lacking red blood cells, you can become anemic, and that makes you tired and weak. Not having enough blood platelets makes you bruise easily and keeps your blood from clotting properly when you're injured. Be on the lookout for any of these symptoms.

Special warnings:

- People with heart failure, heart block, or asthma should not take propranolol. Propranolol can aggravate asthma symptoms.
- If you have diabetes, you should use this drug cautiously because beta-blockers can mask the signs of low blood sugar.
- Propranolol can also mask signs of an overactive thyroid.
- Propranolol may decrease pressure in the eyes, which can alter glaucoma tests.
- People with poor liver or kidney function, bronchitis, or emphysema should take this drug with caution.

Pregnancy and nursing mothers:

Category C. See page 9 for description of categories. Drug is present in mother's milk.

Possible food and drug interactions:

- Propranolol may increase the effects of antipyrine (drug that tests liver function) and the heart drug lidocaine.

- Propranolol may decrease the effects of the hormone thyroxine and the asthma drug theophylline.
- Effects of propranolol may be increased by the ulcer drug cimetidine and the antipsychotic drug chlorpromazine.
- Effects of propranolol may be decreased by alcohol, aluminum hydroxide gel (antacid), the seizure drug phenytoin, and the tuberculosis drug rifampin.
- If you take propranolol with the blood pressure drug reserpine, the combination may cause very low blood pressure, very slow heartbeat, or fainting.
- If you take propranolol with the antipsychotic drug haloperidol, the combination may cause very low blood pressure and heart attack.
- If you take propranolol with the angina drug verapamil, the combination may cause further weakening of the heart.

Helpful hint:
- Never quit taking this drug without talking to your doctor. It could increase your risk of angina and heart attack.

CALCIUM CHANNEL BLOCKERS

Amlodipine

Brand name: *Norvasc*

What this drug does for you:
Amlodipine is a calcium channel blocker. It lowers blood pressure and treats some forms of angina. It works by affecting the movement of calcium into the cells of the heart and blood vessels. It relaxes blood vessels and increases the supply of blood and oxygen to the heart.

Possible side effects of this drug:
- The most common side effects are swollen ankles and feet, headache, and flushing. You may also experience heart palpitations, tiredness, and nausea.
- Less common side effects are abnormal heart rhythms, chest pain, vertigo, loss of appetite, constipation, back pain, weight gain, depression, abnormal dreams, eye pain, and dry mouth.
- Rare reactions are heart failure, skin discoloration, muscle weakness, increased appetite, and cold, clammy skin.
- When you withdraw from the drug, you may experience rebound angina. In other words, your chest pain may get worse for a while.

Special warning:
- People with liver disease, narrowing of the aorta, or congestive heart failure, and people who have had heart attacks should use this drug with caution.

Pregnancy and nursing mothers:
Category C. See page 9 for description of categories. Not known if drug is

present in mother's milk.

Possible food and drug interactions:

- The ulcer drug cimetidine may increase the effects of amlodipine.
- Using amlodipine with beta blockers may result in very low blood pressure or heart irregularities. Don't suddenly stop taking beta blockers before or during treatment with calcium channel blockers.

Helpful hints:

- Tell your doctor immediately if you have any signs of congestive heart failure such as night cough; swelling and fluid retention in your legs, feet, or hands; or difficulty breathing, especially when lying down or after physical exertion.
- Have your blood pressure checked regularly while you're taking this drug.
- Don't stop taking your medicine without your doctor's approval, even if you feel better.
- The usual adult dose is 5 mg once daily, with a maximum dose of 10 mg once daily.

Diltiazem

Brand names: *Cardizem, Dilacor XR* **(Generic available)**

What this drug does for you:

Diltiazem is a calcium channel blocker. It lowers blood pressure and treats some forms of angina. It works by affecting the movement of calcium into the cells of the heart and blood vessels. It relaxes blood vessels and increases the supply of blood and oxygen to the heart.

Possible side effects of this drug:

- The most common side effects are weakness, swelling of the hands or feet, headache, dizziness, slow or irregular heartbeat, flushing, nausea, and rash.
- Other possible side effects are insomnia, drowsiness, nervousness, depression, confusion, low blood pressure, congestive heart failure, constipation, diarrhea, frequent urination (especially at night), sexual difficulties, and sensitivity of your skin to light.
- Rare side effects are swollen and bleeding gums, liver damage, and uncontrollable muscle movements.
- Even though it is very rare, diltiazem may lower the number of blood cells you have. If you don't have enough white blood cells, your immunity is down, and you can get a fever, sore throat, or pneumonia. If you are lacking red blood cells, you can become anemic, and that makes you tired and weak. Not having enough blood platelets makes you bruise easily and keeps your blood from clotting properly when you're injured. Be on the lookout for any of these symptoms.

Special warnings:

- Diltiazem should not be used by people with various heart conditions including sick sinus syndrome, very low blood pressure, and some forms of irregular heartbeat.

- Diltiazem should be used with caution by people with liver disease, kidney disease, congestive heart failure, or people already taking beta-blockers.

Pregnancy and nursing mothers:

Category C. See page 9 for description of categories. Drug is present in mother's milk.

Possible food and drug interactions:

- Diltiazem may increase the effects of anesthetics and the immuno-suppressant cyclosporine.
- The ulcer drug cimetidine may increase the effects of diltiazem.
- Using diltiazem with the beta blocker propanolol may result in various heartbeat irregularities. Don't suddenly stop taking beta blockers before or during treatment with this drug.

Helpful hint:

- The usual starting dose for adults with high blood pressure is 180 to 240 mg once daily. The usual starting dose for adults with angina is 120 or 180 mg once daily.

Felodipine

Brand name: *Plendil*

What this drug does for you:

Felodipine is a calcium channel blocker. It is used to lower blood pressure. It works by affecting the movement of calcium into the cells of the heart and blood vessels. It relaxes blood vessels and increases the supply of blood and oxygen to the heart.

Possible side effects of this drug:

- The most common side effects of felodipine are headaches, flushing, and swollen feet, ankles, and hands.
- You may also experience dizziness, common cold symptoms, weakness, cough, prickling or tingling sensation, upset stomach, chest pain, nausea, muscle cramps, heart palpitations, constipation, diarrhea, sore throat, back pain, swollen gums, and rash.
- Rare side effects are hallucinations, amnesia, thirst, dry mouth, low blood pressure, fainting, irregular heart rhythms, urinary problems, sexual problems, wheezing, difficulty breathing, nervousness, sleepiness, insomnia, anxiety, gas, nosebleed, flu, bronchitis, irritability, bruising, and redness of the skin.

Special warning:

- Your doctor should be cautious when prescribing this drug to you if you have heart failure or liver disease or are older than 65.

Pregnancy and nursing mothers:

Category C. See page 9 for description of categories. Not known if drug is present in mother's milk.

Possible food and drug interactions:

- If you take felodipine with beta-blockers, the combination may cause very low blood pressure or heart irregularities. Don't suddenly stop taking beta-blockers before or during treatment with calcium-channel blockers.
- If you take felodipine with the pain drug fentanyl, the combination may cause dangerously low blood pressure.
- Felodipine may increase the effects of the heart drug digitalis.
- Felodipine may decrease the effects of the asthma drug theophylline.
- Levels or effects of felodipine may be increased by the ulcer drugs cimetidine and ranitidine and the antibiotic erythromycin.
- Levels or effects of felodipine may be decreased by barbiturates and the seizure drug carbamazepine.

Helpful hints:

- Tablets should be swallowed whole. Don't crush or chew.
- Felodipine can cause your gums to swell and bleed. Brushing, flossing, and visiting your dentist regularly will make this side effect less severe.
- You shouldn't drive a car or operate heavy machinery until you are sure the medicine isn't making you drowsy, dizzy, or less than alert.
- Don't stop taking this drug suddenly. It can cause chest pain.

Isradipine

Brand name: *DynaCirc*

What this drug does for you:

Isradipine is a calcium channel blocker. It is used to lower blood pressure. It works by affecting the movement of calcium into the cells of the heart and blood vessels. It relaxes blood vessels and increases the supply of blood and oxygen to the heart.

Possible side effects of this drug:

- Common side effects are headache, fluid retention, flushing, dizziness, nausea, diarrhea, rash, fatigue, and palpitations.
- Rare side effects are drowsiness, impotence, depression, numbness or tingling in hands or feet, foot or leg cramps, throat pain, itching, hives, dry mouth, low blood pressure, heart attack, and heart failure.

Special warning:

- Take isradipine with caution if you have congestive heart failure.

Pregnancy and nursing mothers:

Category C. See page 9 for description of categories. Not known if drug is present in mother's milk.

Possible food and drug interactions:

- If you take isradipine along with blood pressure drugs called beta blockers, you may experience very low blood pressure or heart irregularities.
- You may also have severe low blood pressure if you take isradipine along with the pain drug fentanyl.

Helpful hints:

- Tell your doctor immediately if you have any signs of congestive heart failure such as night cough; swelling and fluid retention in your legs, feet, or hands; or difficulty breathing, especially when lying down or after physical exertion.
- If you stop taking calcium channel blockers suddenly, you could have rebound angina. Stop taking the drug gradually under your doctor's supervision.

Nicardipine

Brand names: *Cardene, Cardene I.V., Cardene SR*

What this drug does for you:

Nicardipine is a calcium channel blocker. It lowers blood pressure and treats some forms of angina. It works by affecting the movement of calcium into the cells of the heart and blood vessels. It relaxes blood vessels and increases the supply of blood and oxygen to the heart.

Possible side effects of this drug:

- Possible side effects are headache, dizziness, weakness, swelling of the feet, flushing, worsening of angina, indigestion, nausea, palpitations, dry mouth, rash, muscle pain, rapid heartbeat, fluid retention or swelling, and a prickling or tingling sensation.
- Rare side effects are fainting, constipation, tremors, nervousness, low blood pressure, sleepiness, frequent urination, sore throat, inflammation of the sinuses, ringing in the ears, joint pain, blurred vision, confusion, anxiety, hot flashes, vertigo, and impotence.

Special warnings:

- People with narrowing of the aorta should not take this drug.
- Your doctor should prescribe this drug cautiously and monitor you carefully if you have heart failure, poor liver or kidney function, decreased blood supply to the brain (cerebral infarction), or hemorrhage in the brain.

Pregnancy and nursing mothers:

Category C. See page 9 for description of categories. Not known if drug is present in mother's milk.

Possible food and drug interactions:

- If you take nicardipine with beta blockers or the anesthetic fentanyl, the combination may cause very low blood pressure or heart irregularities.
- This drug may increase levels or effects of the immunosuppressant cyclosporine and the heart drug digoxin.
- The ulcer drug cimetidine may increase the levels or effects of nicardipine.

Helpful hints:

- If you stop taking calcium channel blockers suddenly, your angina could get worse. Stop taking the drug gradually under your doctor's supervision.
- Your angina may get worse when you first start taking this drug or anytime your doses are increased.

Nifedipine

Brand names: *Adalat, Adalat CC, Procardia, Procardia XL* **(Generic available)**

What this drug does for you:

Nifedipine is a calcium channel blocker. It is used to treat angina. It works by affecting the movement of calcium into the cells of the heart and blood vessels. It relaxes blood vessels and increases the supply of blood and oxygen to the heart.

Possible side effects of this drug:

- The most common side effects are headache, dizziness, weakness, nervousness, heart palpitations, wheezing and shortness of breath, heartburn, and muscle cramps.
- Other possible side effects are flushing, giddiness, nausea, tremors, swelling of the hands and feet, cough, stuffy nose, low blood pressure, gas, diarrhea, constipation, joint pain, chills, fever, itching, hives, and sweating.
- Rare side effects are depression, anemia, fainting, hepatitis, and temporary blindness.
- Even though it is very rare, nifedipine can lower the number of blood cells you have. If you don't have enough white blood cells, your immunity is down, and you can get a fever, sore throat, or pneumonia. If you are lacking red blood cells, you can become anemic, and that makes you tired and weak. Not having enough blood platelets makes you bruise easily and keeps your blood from clotting properly when you're injured. Be on the lookout for any of these symptoms.

Special warning:

- Your doctor should prescribe this drug cautiously and monitor you carefully if you have liver disease or kidney disease.

Pregnancy ad nursing mothers:

Category C. See page 9 for description of categories. Drug is present in mother's milk.

Possible food and drug interactions:

- If you take nifedipine with the anesthetic fentanyl, the combination may cause very low blood pressure.
- The ulcer drug cimetidine may increase the levels or effects of nifedipine.
- Nifedipine may increase the levels or effects of anticoagulants and the

heart drug digoxin.

- Don't suddenly stop taking beta-blockers before or during treatment with calcium-channel blockers. It can make your angina worse.

Helpful hints:

- Your angina may get worse when you first start taking this drug or anytime your doses are increased.
- Tell your doctor immediately if you have any signs of congestive heart failure such as night cough; swelling and fluid retention in your legs, feet, or hands; or difficulty breathing, especially when lying down or after physical exertion.
- You should have your blood pressure tested regularly, especially when you first start taking nifedipine.

Verapamil

Brand names: *Calan, Calan SR, Isoptin, Isoptin SR, Verelan* **(Generic available)**

What this drug does for you:

Verapamil is a calcium channel blocker. It is used to treat angina and irregular heart rhythms. It works by affecting the movement of calcium into the cells of the heart and blood vessels. It relaxes blood vessels and increases the supply of blood and oxygen to the heart.

Possible side effects of this drug:

- Common side effects are headache, dizziness, tiredness, nausea, upset stomach, constipation, low blood pressure, fluid retention and swelling, and slow or irregular heartbeat.
- Less common side effects are flushing, rash, joint or muscle pain, sweating, frequent urination, impotence, enlargement of breasts in men, itching, prickling or tingling in hands or feet, hair loss, blurred vision, dry mouth, diarrhea, and fainting.
- In rare instances, verapamil may cause congestive heart failure. Tell your doctor immediately if you have any signs of congestive heart failure such as night cough; swelling and fluid retention in your legs, feet, or hands; or difficulty breathing, especially when lying down or after physical exertion.
- Liver damage is a rare side effect.

Special warnings:

- People with the following conditions should not use verapamil: sick sinus syndrome (unless using a pacemaker), low blood pressure, heart block (unless using a pacemaker), severe heart failure, dysfunction of the left ventricle of the heart, or atrial fibrillation.
- Your doctor should prescribe this drug cautiously and monitor you carefully if you have heart failure, poor liver or kidney function, or Duchenne's muscular dystrophy.

Pregnancy and nursing mothers:

Category C. See page 9 for description of categories. Drug is present in mother's milk.

Possible food and drug interactions:

- Don't take the heartbeat regulator disopyramide within 48 hours of taking verapamil.
- Taking verapamil along with beta blockers, ACE inhibitors, or diuretics may cause very low blood pressure or heart irregularities. Don't suddenly stop taking beta blockers before or during treatment with calcium-channel blockers. It can make your angina worse.
- Verapamil may increase the levels or effects of muscle relaxers, the seizure drug carbamazepine, the antibiotic cyclosporin, and the heart drug digitalis.
- Verapamil may decrease levels or effects of the heartbeat regulator quinidine.
- Levels or effects of verapamil may be decreased by the seizure drug phenobarbital and the tuberculosis drug rifampin.

Helpful hints:

- You should have your blood pressure tested regularly, especially when you first start taking verapamil.
- If you stop taking calcium channel blockers suddenly, your angina could get worse. Stop taking the drug gradually under your doctor's supervision.
- You should have your blood pressure tested regularly, especially when you first start taking verapamil. When you are also taking other drugs to lower your blood pressure, regular tests are even more important.
- You should have regular liver function tests while you're taking verapamil.

CHOLESTEROL-REDUCING DRUGS

Cholestyramine

Brand name: *Questran*

What this drug does for you:

Cholestyramine is used to reduce blood cholesterol levels. It works by attaching to certain substances in the intestine. Since cholestyramine is not absorbed into the body, the substances also pass out of the body without being absorbed.

Possible side effects of this drug:

- Constipation is a very common side effect.
- Less common side effects are stomach pain, gas, nausea, diarrhea, indigestion, belching, loss of appetite, flaky skin, osteoporosis (bone loss), rash, and skin irritation.
- Cholestyramine may reduce your body's absorption of the fat-soluble vit-

amins — A, D, E, K, and folic acid. A shortage of vitamin K can cause bruising and longer bleeding times.

Special warnings:
- People with bile duct obstruction should not use this drug.

Pregnancy and nursing mothers:
Category C. See page 9 for description of categories. Not known if safe to use while breast-feeding.

Possible food and drug interactions:
- Cholestyramine may decrease the absorption of other drugs you take including the anti-inflammatory phenylbutazone, the anticoagulant warfarin, the blood pressure drugs chlorothiazide and propanolol, some antibiotics, the sedative phenobarbital, some thyroid drugs, the heart drug digitalis, and phosphate supplements. You should take other drugs one to two hours before or four to six hours after taking cholestyramine. Ask your doctor about dosing schedules.

Helpful hints:
- You may need vitamin supplements while taking this drug.
- Increase your fluid and fiber intake to help avoid constipation.

Colestipol

Brand name: *Colestid*

What this drug does for you:
Colestipol is used to reduce blood cholesterol levels. It works by attaching to certain substances in the intestine. Since colestipol is not absorbed into the body, the substances also pass out of the body without being absorbed.

Possible side effects of this drug:
- Colestipol frequently causes constipation. It may aggravate hemorrhoids.
- Other side effects include stomach pain and bloating, belching, gas, nausea, and diarrhea.
- Rare side effects are itching, skin irritation, muscle or joint pain, arthritis, headache, dizziness, anxiety, drowsiness, loss of appetite, fatigue, weakness, and shortness of breath.
- Colestipol may reduce your body's absorption of the fat-soluble vitamins — A, D, E, K, and folic acid. A shortage of vitamin K can cause bruising and longer bleeding times.

Pregnancy and nursing mothers:
Not known if safe to use while pregnant. Not known if safe to use while breast-feeding.

Possible food and drug interactions:
- Colestipol may decrease the absorption of other drugs you take such as the beta-blocker propanolol, the diuretics furosemide and chlorothiazide, the antibiotics tetracycline and penicillin G, the heart drugs

digitoxin and digoxin, and the antilipemic gemfibrozil. You should take other drugs one to two hours before or four to six hours after taking colestipol. Ask your doctor about dosing schedules.

Helpful hints:

- Be careful while handling the dry powder form of this drug. Always mix with a liquid. You may use water, carbonated beverages (although this may give you a stomachache) or other liquids, soups, or pulpy fruits such as crushed pineapple. Rinse the glass with additional beverage to make sure you get all the medicine.
- Increase your fluid and fiber intake to help avoid constipation.

Gemfibrozil

Brand names: *Gemcor, Lopid* **(Generic available)**

What this drug does for you:

Gemfibrozil tablets decrease triglyceride levels and very low density lipoprotein (VLDL) cholesterol levels, and they increase high density lipoprotein (HDL) cholesterol levels. HDL cholesterol is the "good" cholesterol. This effect on lipid levels seems to lower the risk of heart attack.

Gemfibrozil is meant to help people at risk for pancreatitis and heart disease who haven't been able to lower their very high triglyceride levels through diet, exercise, and weight loss. Very high triglyceride levels are typically over 2000 mg/dL. HDL levels below 35 mg/dL are a risk factor for heart disease.

Possible side effects of this drug:

- The most common side effects of gemfibrozil are indigestion, stomachache, and diarrhea.
- You may also experience nausea, an irregular heartbeat, itchy and inflamed skin, rash, dizziness, constipation, and headache.
- Other possible side effects are blurred vision, sleepiness, decreased sex drive, depression, impotence, muscle pain, and anemia (low number of red blood cells).
- Notify your doctor immediately if you develop any pain, tenderness, or weakness in your muscles. Gemfibrozil can cause severe muscle disease.

Special warnings:

- People with gallbladder disease, poor liver function, or poor kidney function should not use gemfibrozil. You should quit taking the drug (under your doctor's supervision) if you develop gallstones.

Pregnancy and nursing mothers:

Category C. See page 9 for description of categories. Not known if drug is present in mother's milk.

Possible food and drug interactions:

- Using gemfibrozil with the lipid-lowering drug lovastatin can cause severe muscle and kidney damage.
- Gemfibrozil may increase the effects of anticoagulants, so your dosage of

the anticoagulant may need to be reduced.

Helpful hints:

- It is very important to try to improve your triglyceride and HDL levels with a low-fat diet and exercise while you are taking gemfibrozil.
- Your blood counts, kidney function, and liver function should be checked regularly while you're taking gemfibrozil.
- The usual adult dosage is 1200 mg a day.
- If you are prescribed 1200 mg a day, take one tablet a half-hour before you eat breakfast and one tablet a half-hour before your evening meal.

Lovastatin

Brand name: *Mevacor*

What this drug does for you:

Lovastatin is used to reduce total cholesterol and LDL cholesterol levels. It works by blocking an enzyme that your body needs to make cholesterol.

Possible side effects of this drug:

- Possible side effects are nausea, diarrhea, heartburn, constipation, gas, stomach pain or cramps, headache, joint pain, itching, rash, blurred vision, weakness, altered sense of taste, and decreased sexual ability.
- Some serious possible side effects are hepatitis, stomach ulcers, and the dangerous disease that destroys muscle tissue called rhabdomyolysis. Contact your doctor if you develop any muscle pain, tenderness, or weakness, especially if accompanied by fever.

Special warnings:

- Lovastatin should not be used by people with liver disease or suspected liver problems.
- Use lovastatin with caution if you have a history of high alcohol consumption, or poor kidney function.
- This drug can also lead to kidney failure (caused by the rhabdomyolysis) in people with severe infections, uncontrolled seizures, low blood pressure, any kind of trauma such as major surgery, or severe metabolic, electrolyte, or endocrine disorders.

Pregnancy and nursing mothers:

Category X. See page 9 for description of categories. Don't take this drug during pregnancy. Not known if drug is present in mother's milk.

Possible food and drug interactions:

- Lovastatin may increase effects of the anticoagulant warfarin.
- The following drugs may increase the risk of rhabdomyolysis (a muscle-destroying disease) when you take them with lovastatin: the immuno-suppressant cyclosporine, the antibiotic erythromycin, the vitamin niacin, and the blood-fat reducer gemfibrozil.

Helpful hint:

- Take lovastatin with your evening meal.

Niacin

Brand names: *Niacin-Time, Niacinol, Nicolar, Slo-Niacin*

What this drug does for you:
Niacin, or vitamin B3, controls cholesterol or triglyceride levels in some people when diet and exercise are not effective. It is a potent medicine, not just a vitamin.

Possible side effects of this drug:
- Possible side effects are low blood pressure, rapid or irregular heartbeat, weakened vision, headache, abnormal pigmentation of the skin, dry skin, inflammatory disease of the skin called acanthosis nigricans, flushing, itching, diarrhea, vomiting, and indigestion.
- Niacin may cause stomach ulcer or aggravate diabetes or gout.
- Time-release forms of niacin may cause severe liver damage. Some signs of hepatitis with jaundice are yellow eyes and skin, dark-colored urine, and light-colored stools. Contact your doctor if you notice any of these signs.

Special warnings:
- Niacin should not be used by alcoholics or people with poor liver function, bleeding from an artery, or stomach ulcer.
- Niacin may cause the dangerous and sometimes fatal disease that destroys muscle tissue called rhabdomyolysis.
- People with gallbladder disease, diabetes, heart disease, gout, jaundice, liver disease, or stomach ulcer should take niacin with extreme caution.
- People with angina or people who have had a recent heart attack should take niacin with caution.

Pregnancy and nursing mothers:
Category C. See page 9 for description of categories. Not known if safe to use in pregnancy and nursing.

Possible food and drug interactions:
- If you take niacin with the cholesterol-lowering drug lovastatin, your risk of rhabdomyolysis is increased.
- Niacin combined with blood pressure-lowering drugs may cause very low blood pressure.
- Aspirin may increase levels or effects of niacin.
- Avoid alcohol and hot drinks as these may increase some side effects including itching and flushing.

Helpful hints:
- Take niacin with meals to reduce upset stomach, itching, and flushing.
- Liver function and blood sugar levels should be checked frequently.

Pravastatin

Brand name: *Pravachol*

What this drug does for you:

Pravastatin is used to reduce total cholesterol and LDL cholesterol levels. It works by blocking an enzyme that your body needs to make cholesterol.

Possible side effects of this drug:

- Possible side effects are nausea, chest pain, rash, diarrhea, stomach pain, heartburn, gas, constipation, headache, inflammation of nasal passages, dizziness, and flu-like symptoms.
- Rare side effects are hair loss, enlargement of breasts in men, worsening of cataracts, memory loss, mental depression, tremors, joint pain, prickling or tingling sensation, sensitivity to light, fever, and chills.
- Some serious possible side effects are stomach ulcers and the dangerous disease that destroys muscle tissue called rhabdomyolysis. Contact your doctor if you develop any muscle pain, tenderness, or weakness, especially if accompanied by fever.
- Pravastatin may cause severe liver damage. Some signs of hepatitis with jaundice are yellow eyes and skin, dark-colored urine, and light-colored stools. Contact your doctor if you notice any of these signs.

Special warnings:

- Pravastatin should not be used by people with liver disease or suspected liver problems.
- Use pravastatin with caution if you have a history of liver disease or high alcohol consumption, or poor kidney function.
- Pravastatin may alter some hormone levels.
- This drug can also lead to kidney failure (caused by the rhabdomyolysis) in people with severe infections, uncontrolled seizures, low blood pressure, any kind of trauma such as major surgery, or severe metabolic, electrolyte, or endocrine disorders.

Pregnancy and nursing mothers:

Category X. See page 9 for description of categories. Discuss pregnancy with your doctor before beginning treatment with this drug. If you become pregnant while taking this drug, inform your doctor immediately. Drug is present in mother's milk.

Possible food and drug interactions:

- The following drugs may increase the risk of rhabdomyolysis (a muscle-destroying disease) when you take them with pravastatin: the blood fat-reducer gemfibrozil, the antibiotic erythromycin, or the ulcer drug cimetidine.

Helpful hint:

- You should have regular liver function tests while you're taking this drug.

Probucol

Brand name: *Lorelco*

What this drug does for you:

Probucol is used to reduce cholesterol levels, particularly LDL cholesterol, in people who have not been able to lower their cholesterol through diet, exercise, and weight loss.

Possible side effects of this drug:

- The most common side effects are nausea, gas, stomach pain, diarrhea, increased sweating, and swelling of face, mouth, hands, or feet.
- Probucol may also cause irregular heartbeat, fainting, prickling or tingling in hands or feet, dizziness, headache, ringing in the ears, blurred vision, insomnia, impotence, rash, itching, body odor, and loss of appetite.
- Even though it is very rare, probucol can lower the number of blood cells you have. If you don't have enough white blood cells, your immunity is down, and you can get a fever, sore throat, or pneumonia. If you are lacking red blood cells, you can become anemic, and that makes you tired and weak. Not having enough blood platelets makes you bruise easily and keeps your blood from clotting properly when you're injured. Be on the lookout for any of these symptoms of bone marrow depression.

Special warnings:

- People with the following conditions should not take probucol: poor heart function, serious irregular heartbeat, unexplained fainting or fainting associated with cardiovascular disorders, or certain electrocardiogram (ECG) abnormalities. An ECG should be done before beginning and during treatment.
- Before you take this drug, your doctor should treat any diseases you have that contribute to high cholesterol levels, such as diabetes, underactive thyroid, and obstructive liver disease.

Pregnancy and nursing mothers:

Category B. See page 9 for description of categories. Don't get pregnant for at least six months after treatment. Not known if drug is present in mother's milk.

Possible food and drug interactions:

- Don't take with the cholesterol-reducer clofibrate.
- If you take probucol with antidepressants, heart rhythm regulators, or phenothiazines (tranquilizers), the combination may worsen irregular heartbeat.

Helpful hint:

- Take probucol with meals.

Simvastatin

Brand name: *Zocor*

What this drug does for you:

Simvastatin is used to reduce total cholesterol and LDL cholesterol levels. It works by blocking an enzyme that your body needs to make cholesterol.

Possible side effects of this drug:

- Possible side effects are headache, stomach pain, upper respiratory infection (such as a cold), nausea, gas, indigestion, constipation, diarrhea, and weakness.
- A serious possible side effect is the dangerous disease that destroys muscle tissue called rhabdomyolysis. Contact your doctor if you develop any muscle pain, tenderness, or weakness, especially if accompanied by fever.
- Simvastatin may cause severe liver damage.

Special warnings:

- Simvastatin should not be used by people with liver disease or suspected liver problems.
- Use simvastatin with caution if you have a history of liver disease or high alcohol consumption, or poor kidney function.
- Simvastatin may alter some hormone levels.
- This drug can also lead to kidney failure (caused by the rhabdomyolysis) in people with severe infections, uncontrolled seizures, low blood pressure, any kind of trauma such as major surgery, or severe metabolic, electrolyte, or endocrine disorders.

Pregnancy and nursing mothers:

Category X. See page 9 for description of categories. Discuss plans for pregnancy with your doctor. If you become pregnant while taking this drug, inform your doctor immediately. Not known if drug is present in mother's milk.

Possible food and drug interactions:

- The following drugs may increase the risk of rhabdomyolysis (a muscle-destroying disease) when you take them with simvastatin: the blood fat-reducer gemfibrozil, the antibiotic erythromycin, immunosuppressant drugs, and niacin.
- Simvastatin may increase the effects of the anticoagulant warfarin.

Helpful hint:

- You should have regular liver function tests while you're taking this drug.

DIGITALIS PREPARATIONS

Digoxin

Brand names: *Lanoxicaps, Lanoxin* **(Generic available)**

What this drug does for you:
Digoxin treats congestive heart failure and certain heart rhythm irregularities. It makes your heart stronger and improves your blood circulation.

Possible side effects of this drug:
- Possible side effects are nausea, vomiting, headache, visual disturbances, hallucinations, breast enlargement in both men and women, confusion, depression, drowsiness, disorientation, weakness, seizures, heart rhythm irregularities, and loss of appetite and diarrhea, sometimes with stomach pain or discomfort.

Special warnings:
- People with cardiovascular disease or thyroid problems should take digoxin with caution.
- If you have kidney problems, your doctor may need to carefully adjust your dosage of digoxin.

Pregnancy and nursing mothers:
Category C. See page 9 for description of categories. Drug is present in mother's milk.

Possible food and drug interactions:
- Effects of digoxin may be decreased by antacids, the anti-inflammatory drug sulfasalazine, the cholesterol-lowering drugs colestipol and cholestyramine, and the antibiotic neomycin.
- Effects of digoxin may be increased by the ulcer drug propantheline, the angina drug verapamil, the antispasmodic diphenoxylate, and the heartbeat regulators amiodarone, propafenone, and quinidine.
- If you take digoxin along with drugs that decrease potassium levels in the blood such as diuretics and the steroid prednisone, the combination may cause a dangerous loss of potassium.

Helpful hints:
- Digoxin can quickly reach toxic levels. You should watch yourself carefully for any side effects.
- Digoxin should not be used to treat obesity. It can cause dangerous irregular heartbeats which can be fatal.
- It is important to maintain correct levels of potassium, calcium, and magnesium as these minerals also affect the heart. Talk to your doctor about a proper diet.

DIURETICS

Acetazolamide

Brand name: *Diamox*

What this drug does for you:

Acetazolamide is a diuretic. It treats some kinds of glaucoma, fluid retention in congestive heart failure, epilepsy, and altitude sickness by helping the body to release excess fluids.

Diuretics work on the kidneys to increase urination. That helps your body get rid of water and salt.

Possible side effects of this drug:

- Side effects include confusion, weakness, fatigue, drowsiness, frequent urination, fever, rash, loss of appetite, nausea, and tingling of extremities.
- Even though it is very rare, acetazolamide can lower the number of blood cells you have. If you don't have enough white blood cells, your immunity is down, and you can get a fever, sore throat, or pneumonia. If you are lacking red blood cells, you can become anemic, and that makes you tired and weak. Not having enough blood platelets makes you bruise easily and keeps your blood from clotting properly when you're injured. Be on the lookout for any of these symptoms of bone marrow depression.
- Serious skin disorders in which dark red rings or raised spots erupt on your skin (Stevens-Johnson syndrome) or parts of your skin deteriorate are another very rare reaction.
- Acetazolamide can also cause liver and kidney damage and kidney stones. You should have regular liver and kidney tests while you're taking this drug.
- Acetazolamide may raise blood sugar levels.

Special warnings:

- People with liver or kidney problems should not use acetazolamide.
- This drug may mask symptoms of some forms of glaucoma.

Pregnancy and nursing mothers:

Category C. See page 9 for description of categories. Drug may be present in mother's milk.

Possible food and drug interactions:

- Acetazolamide can increase the effects of the heart drug quinidine.
- If you take acetazolamide with high doses of aspirin, you could experience loss of appetite, rapid breathing, coma, and death.

Helpful hints:

- You shouldn't drive a car or operate heavy machinery until you are sure the medicine isn't making you drowsy or less than alert.
- Since acetazolamide can cause you to lose sodium and potassium, eat extra potassium-rich foods like bananas.
- Weigh daily so you'll know if you're losing too much fluid. Losing too

much fluid can cause dehydration and possibly blood clots. Warning signs of dehydration include dry mouth, thirst, drowsiness, weakness, loss of appetite, restlessness, nausea, vomiting, low blood pressure, heart rhythm abnormalities, and muscle pains or cramps. Quit using the drug and contact your doctor if you stop urinating.

Amiloride

Brand name: *Midamor*

What this drug does for you:

This diuretic is used to treat high blood pressure and congestive heart failure by eliminating excess fluids from the body. Unlike some diuretics, it does not cause a loss of potassium.

Diuretics work on the kidneys to increase urination. That helps your body get rid of water and salt.

Possible side effects of this drug:

- The most common side effects are headache, nausea, loss of appetite, and diarrhea. Also common are stomach pain, constipation, mild skin rash, weakness, muscle cramps, dizziness, cough, and impotence.
- Less common reactions are muscle or joint pain, angina, palpitations, jaundice, heartburn, gas pain, thirst, dry mouth, itching, insomnia, depression, shortness of breath, stuffy nose, vision problems, and frequent urination.
- Even though it is very rare, amiloride can lower the number of blood cells you have. If you don't have enough white blood cells, your immunity is down, and you can get a fever, sore throat, or pneumonia. If you are lacking red blood cells, you can become anemic, and that makes you tired and weak. Not having enough blood platelets makes you bruise easily and keeps your blood from clotting properly when you're injured. Be on the lookout for any of these symptoms of bone marrow depression.
- Stomach ulcer and liver damage are also possible serious reactions.
- This drug can cause dangerously high levels of potassium in your body. Some warning signs are a prickling or tingling sensation, muscle weakness, tiredness, and slow heartbeat. Very high levels of potassium can be fatal.

Special warning:

- People with diabetes, liver problems, or kidney problems should take this drug with caution.

Pregnancy and nursing mothers:

Category B. See page 9 for description of categories. Not known if drug is present in mother's milk.

Possible food and drug interactions:

- Anti-inflammatory drugs may lessen the effectiveness of amiloride.
- Amiloride is often used with other blood pressure drugs for beneficial effects, but some combinations may put you at risk for high levels of po-

tassium in the blood. Amiloride should not be used with other potassium-sparing drugs.
- This drug may cause the antipsychotic drug lithium to accumulate to toxic levels in the body.

Helpful hints:
- Take this drug with food to avoid upset stomach.
- Weigh daily so you'll know if you're losing too much fluid. Losing too much fluid can cause dehydration and possibly blood clots. Warning signs of dehydration include dry mouth, thirst, drowsiness, weakness, loss of appetite, restlessness, nausea, vomiting, low blood pressure, heart rhythm abnormalities, and muscle pains or cramps. Contact your doctor immediately if you stop urinating.

Bumetanide

Brand name: *Bumex*

What this drug does for you:
Bumetanide is a diuretic. It is used to reduce excess fluid in the body that may be associated with high blood pressure, congestive heart failure, or liver or kidney disease.

Diuretics work on the kidneys to increase urination. That helps your body get rid of water and salt.

Possible side effects of this drug:
- Possible side effects are muscle cramps or spasms, dizziness, headache, low blood pressure, and nausea.
- Less common side effects are impaired hearing, itching, hives, rash, arthritic pain, and vomiting.
- Rarely, this drug may cause chest pain, vertigo, fatigue, impotence, ear discomfort, dehydration, diarrhea, and kidney failure.
- Very rarely, bumetanide may lower the number of blood platelets you have. That can make you bruise easily and keep you blood from clotting properly when you're injured.
- Bumetanide may increase levels of uric acid in the blood (this puts you at risk for gout) and may worsen symptoms of lupus.

Special warnings:
- Contact your doctor immediately if you experience allergic symptoms or stop urinating.
- People with liver problems who take this drug may experience irreversible hearing loss, increased sensitivity to light, impaired central nervous system function, or coma.
- If you have diabetes, bumetanide may raise your blood sugar levels.

Pregnancy and nursing mothers:
Category C. See page 9 for description of categories. Not known if drug is present in mother's milk.

Possible food and drug interactions:

- The effects of bumetanide may be decreased by the gout drug probenecid and nonsteroidal anti-inflammatory drugs (NSAIDs) such as indomethacin and aspirin.
- Bumetanide should not be used with thiazide diuretics as this can cause severe fluid loss and serious electrolyte problems.
- Bumetanide should not be used with the antipsychotic drug lithium as it may cause lithium to accumulate to toxic levels.

Helpful hints:

- Bumetanide can cause dangerously low levels of potassium and other electrolytes. Eat extra potassium-rich foods like bananas.
- Weigh daily so you'll know if you're losing too much fluid. Losing too much fluid can cause dehydration and possibly blood clots. Warning signs of dehydration include dry mouth, thirst, drowsiness, weakness, loss of appetite, restlessness, nausea, vomiting, low blood pressure, heart rhythm abnormalities, and muscle pains or cramps. Contact your doctor immediately if you stop urinating.
- If you have high blood pressure, avoid using over-the-counter cold remedies or diet pills which can increase blood pressure.

Chlorothiazide

Brand name: *Diuril*

What this drug does for you:

This diuretic treats high blood pressure and the fluid retention and swelling associated with congestive heart failure, cirrhosis of the liver, kidney disease, estrogen therapy, and steroid therapy.

Diuretics work on the kidneys to increase urination. That helps your body get rid of water and salt.

Possible side effects of this drug:

- Chlorothiazide may cause weakness, low blood pressure, jaundice, diarrhea, vomiting, breathing problems, muscle spasms, dizziness, tingling, skin irritation, blurred vision, kidney failure, and impotence.
- Chlorothiazide may increase levels of uric acid in the blood (this puts you at risk for gout) and may worsen symptoms of lupus.
- This drug may cause excess levels of calcium in the blood and may raise blood sugar levels.
- This diuretic may cause dangerously low levels of potassium and other electrolytes. Contact your doctor if you experience any of the symptoms of potassium loss: unusual thirst, tiredness, drowsiness, restlessness, muscle pains or cramps, nausea, or rapid heart rate.
- Even though it is very rare, chlorothiazide can lower the number of blood cells you have. If you don't have enough white blood cells, your immunity is down, and you can get a fever, sore throat, or pneumonia. If you are lacking red blood cells, you can become anemic, and that makes you tired and weak. Not having enough blood platelets makes you bruise

easily and keeps your blood from clotting properly when you're injured. Be on the lookout for any of these symptoms of bone marrow depression.

Special warnings:
- Don't use this drug if you are allergic to diuretics or sulfonamide drugs.
- People with poor kidney function or liver disease should use this drug with caution.
- People with moderate or high cholesterol levels should use this drug with caution. This drug may increase cholesterol levels.

Pregnancy and nursing mothers:
Category C. See page 9 for description of categories. New mothers who want to breast-feed should not take chlorothiazide. It may cause serious adverse reactions in nursing infants.

Possible food and drug interactions:
- Nonsteroidal anti-inflammatory drugs (NSAIDs) such as aspirin may decrease the effects of chlorothiazide.
- If you take chlorothiazide with alcohol, depressants, narcotics, or other high blood pressure medicines, the combination may cause very low blood pressure.
- Corticosteroids combined with chlorothiazide may cause dangerous loss of potassium from the blood.
- Chlorothiazide can increase the effects of muscle relaxers.

Helpful hints:
- This drug can cause dangerously low levels of potassium and other electrolytes. Eat extra potassium-rich foods like bananas.
- Weigh daily so you'll know if you're losing too much fluid. Losing too much fluid can cause dehydration and possibly blood clots. Warning signs of dehydration include dry mouth, thirst, drowsiness, weakness, loss of appetite, restlessness, nausea, vomiting, low blood pressure, heart rhythm abnormalities, and muscle pains or cramps. Contact your doctor immediately if you stop urinating.
- If you have high blood pressure, avoid using over-the-counter cold remedies or diet pills which can increase blood pressure.

Chlorthalidone

Brand names: *Hygroton, Thalitone*

What this drug does for you:
This diuretic treats high blood pressure and the fluid retention and swelling associated with congestive heart failure, cirrhosis of the liver, kidney disease, estrogen therapy, and steroid therapy.

Diuretics work on the kidneys to increase urination. That helps your body get rid of water and salt.

Possible side effects of this drug:
- Chlorthalidone may cause loss of appetite, upset stomach, nausea, cramping, diarrhea, constipation, jaundice, pancreas problems, dizzi-

ness, tingling, headache, vision problems, sensitivity to light, rash, hives and other skin problems, very low blood pressure, muscle spasm, weakness, restlessness, and impotence.

- Chlorthalidone may increase levels of uric acid in the blood (this puts you at risk for gout), may worsen symptoms of lupus, and may raise your blood sugar.
- This diuretic may cause dangerously low levels of potassium and other electrolytes. Contact your doctor if you experience any of the symptoms of potassium loss: unusual thirst, tiredness, drowsiness, restlessness, muscle pains or cramps, nausea, or rapid heart rate.
- Even though it is very rare, chlorthalidone can lower the number of blood cells you have. If you don't have enough white blood cells, your immunity is down, and you can get a fever, sore throat, or pneumonia. If you are lacking red blood cells, you can become anemic, and that makes you tired and weak. Not having enough blood platelets makes you bruise easily and keeps your blood from clotting properly when you're injured. Be on the lookout for any of these symptoms of bone marrow depression.

Special warnings:
- Don't use chlorthalidone if you are allergic to diuretics or sulfonamide drugs.
- If you have poor kidney function or liver disease, use this drug with caution.

Pregnancy and nursing mothers:
Category B. See page 9 for description of categories. Drug is present in mother's milk.

Possible food and drug interactions:
- Avoid alcohol while taking this drug.
- Taking chlorthalidone along with other high blood pressure drugs may cause very low blood pressure.
- Chlorthalidone may increase or decrease the effects of insulin.
- If used with the antipsychotic drug lithium, chlorthalidone may cause lithium to accumulate to toxic levels.

Helpful hints:
- This drug can cause dangerously low levels of potassium and other electrolytes. Eat extra potassium-rich foods like bananas.
- Weigh daily so you'll know if you're losing too much fluid. Losing too much fluid can cause dehydration and possibly blood clots. Warning signs of dehydration include dry mouth, thirst, drowsiness, weakness, loss of appetite, restlessness, nausea, vomiting, low blood pressure, heart rhythm abnormalities, and muscle pains or cramps. Contact your doctor immediately if you stop urinating.
- If you have high blood pressure, avoid using over-the-counter cold remedies or diet pills which can increase blood pressure.

Furosemide

Brand name: *Lasix* **(Generic available)**

What this drug does for you:

This diuretic is used to reduce fluid retention associated with congestive heart failure, liver or kidney disease and to reduce high blood pressure.

Diuretics work on the kidneys to increase urination. That helps your body get rid of water and salt.

Possible side effects of this drug:

- Furosemide may cause muscle cramps or involuntary muscle spasms, low blood pressure when you stand up, bladder spasms, weakness, restlessness, dizziness, headache, nausea, loss of appetite, stomach and mouth irritation, cramping, diarrhea, constipation, jaundice, inflammation of the pancreas, tingling sensations, vision problems, hearing loss, and rash. This drug may make your skin extra-sensitive to sunlight.
- Rarely, this drug may raise blood sugar levels and cause diabetes.
- Furosemide may increase levels of uric acid in the blood (this puts you at risk for gout) and may worsen symptoms of lupus.
- This diuretic may cause dangerously low levels of potassium and other electrolytes. Contact your doctor if you experience any of the symptoms of potassium loss: unusual thirst, tiredness, drowsiness, restlessness, muscle pains or cramps, nausea, or rapid heart rate.
- Even though it is very rare, furosemide can lower the number of blood cells you have. If you don't have enough white blood cells, your immunity is down, and you can get a fever, sore throat, or pneumonia. If you are lacking red blood cells, you can become anemic, and that makes you tired and weak. Not having enough blood platelets makes you bruise easily and keeps your blood from clotting properly when you're injured. Be on the lookout for any of these symptoms of bone marrow depression.

Special warnings:

- Diabetics should use this drug with caution because it can raise your blood sugar levels.
- Use furosemide with caution if you have kidney disease.

Pregnancy and nursing mothers:

Category C. See page 9 for description of categories. Drug is present in mother's milk.

Possible food and drug interactions:

- Don't use furosemide with antibiotics called aminoglycosides or the diuretic ethacrynic acid because of potential damage to hearing.
- Furosemide may increase levels of the antipsychotic drug lithium and blood pressure drugs called beta-blockers.
- Furosemide may decrease effects of norepinephrine.
- The anti-inflammatory indomethacin may decrease effects of furosemide.

Helpful hints:
- This drug can cause dangerously low levels of potassium and other electrolytes. Eat extra potassium-rich foods like bananas.
- Weigh daily so you'll know if you're losing too much fluid. Losing too much fluid can cause dehydration and possibly blood clots. Warning signs of dehydration include dry mouth, thirst, drowsiness, weakness, loss of appetite, restlessness, nausea, vomiting, low blood pressure, heart rhythm abnormalities, and muscle pains or cramps. Contact your doctor immediately if you stop urinating.
- If you have high blood pressure, avoid using over-the-counter cold remedies or diet pills which can increase blood pressure.

Hydrochlorothiazide

Brand names: *Esidrix, HydroDIURIL, Oretic* **(Generic available)**

What this drug does for you:
This diuretic is used to reduce blood pressure and to treat fluid retention associated with kidney disease, congestive heart failure, cirrhosis of the liver, estrogen therapy, and corticosteroid therapy. Diuretics work on the kidneys to increase urination. That helps your body get rid of water and salt.

Possible side effects of this drug:
- Side effects may include low blood pressure, loss of appetite, sensitivity to light, nausea, stomach pain or cramps, diarrhea, constipation, inflammation of salivary glands, tingling sensations, blurred vision, jaundice, inflammation of the pancreas, hives, rash, dizziness, headache, weakness, restlessness, and muscle cramps or spasms.
- Hydrochlorothiazide may increase levels of uric acid in the blood (this puts you at risk for gout), may worsen symptoms of lupus, and may raise blood sugar levels.
- This diuretic may cause dangerously low levels of potassium and other electrolytes. Contact your doctor if you experience any of the symptoms of potassium loss: unusual thirst, tiredness, drowsiness, restlessness, muscle pains or cramps, nausea, or rapid heart rate.
- Even though it is very rare, hydrochlorothiazide can lower the number of blood cells you have. If you don't have enough white blood cells, your immunity is down, and you can get a fever, sore throat, or pneumonia. If you are lacking red blood cells, you can become anemic, and that makes you tired and weak. Not having enough blood platelets makes you bruise easily and keeps your blood from clotting properly when you're injured. Be on the lookout for any of these symptoms of bone marrow depression.

Special warning:
- Take hydrochlorothiazide with caution if you have poor kidney function or liver disease.

Pregnancy and nursing mothers:
Category B. See page 9 for description of categories. Drug is present in mother's milk.

Possible food and drug interactions:
- Hydrochlorothiazide may increase the effects of the heart drug digitalis and the muscle relaxer tubocurarine.
- Hydrochlorothiazide may increase blood levels of the anti-psychotic drug lithium to toxic levels.
- Hydrochlorothiazide may decrease the effects of the blood pressure drug norepinephrine.
- Nonsteroidal anti-inflammatory drugs (NSAIDs) may decrease the effectiveness of this drug.

Helpful hints:
- This drug can cause dangerously low levels of potassium and other electrolytes. Eat extra potassium-rich foods like bananas.
- Weigh daily so you'll know if you're losing too much fluid. Losing too much fluid can cause dehydration and possibly blood clots. Warning signs of dehydration include dry mouth, thirst, drowsiness, weakness, loss of appetite, restlessness, nausea, vomiting, low blood pressure, heart rhythm abnormalities, and muscle pains or cramps. Contact your doctor immediately if you stop urinating.
- If you have high blood pressure, avoid using over-the-counter cold remedies or diet pills which can increase blood pressure.

Indapamide

Brand name: *Lozol*

What this drug does for you:
This diuretic is used to reduce blood pressure and fluid retention associated with congestive heart failure.

Diuretics work on the kidneys to increase urination. That helps your body get rid of water and salt.

Possible side effects of this drug:
- Side effects may include anxiety, nervousness, weakness, headache, dizziness, blurred vision, drowsiness, depression, stomach pain, diarrhea, vomiting, constipation, frequent urination, impotence, dry mouth, rash, itching, and hives.
- Indapamide may increase levels of uric acid in the blood (this puts you at risk for gout), may worsen symptoms of lupus, and may raise blood sugar levels.
- This diuretic may cause dangerously low levels of potassium and other electrolytes. Contact your doctor if you experience any of the symptoms of potassium loss: unusual thirst, tiredness, drowsiness, restlessness, muscle pains or cramps, nausea, or rapid heart rate.

Special warnings:
- People with poor kidney function or liver disease should use this drug with caution.
- Your doctor should check your electrolyte balances frequently if you have heart failure, kidney disease, or liver disease. Your electrolyte bal-

ances should also be watched carefully if you get sick and are vomiting or have diarrhea.

Pregnancy and nursing mothers:

Category B. See page 9 for description of categories. Not known if drug is present in mother's milk.

Possible food and drug interactions:

- Taking indapamide with the antipsychotic drug lithium may cause lithium to accumulate to toxic levels.
- Indapamide may increase the effects of other high blood pressure drugs.
- Indapamide may decrease the effects of the heart drug norepinephrine.
- Since indapamide may raise blood sugar levels, people with diabetes may need adjustments to their doses of insulin or other glucose-lowering agents if they begin taking indapamide.

Helpful hints:

- Weigh daily so you'll know if you're losing too much fluid. Losing too much fluid can cause dehydration and possibly blood clots. Warning signs of dehydration include dry mouth, thirst, drowsiness, weakness, loss of appetite, restlessness, nausea, vomiting, low blood pressure, heart rhythm abnormalities, and muscle pains or cramps. Contact your doctor immediately if you stop urinating.
- If you have high blood pressure, avoid using over-the-counter cold remedies or diet pills which can increase blood pressure.

Methyclothiazide

Brand names: *Aquatensen, Enduron* **(Generic available)**

What this drug does for you:

This diuretic reduces blood pressure. It is also used with other drugs to treat swelling and fluid retention associated with congestive heart failure, cirrhosis of the liver, kidney disease, estrogen therapy, and corticosteroid therapy.

Diuretics work on the kidneys to increase urination. That helps your body get rid of water and salt.

Possible side effects of this drug:

- This drug may cause inflammation of the pancreas, loss of appetite, constipation, nausea, stomach pain or cramps, diarrhea, blurred vision, jaundice, sensitivity to light, hives, rash, dizziness, headache, weakness, low blood pressure, restlessness, muscle cramps or spasms, and tingling sensations.
- Methyclothiazide may increase levels of uric acid in the blood (this puts you at risk for gout), may worsen symptoms of lupus, and may raise blood sugar levels.
- This diuretic may cause dangerously low levels of potassium and other electrolytes. Contact your doctor if you experience any of the symptoms of potassium loss: unusual thirst, tiredness, drowsiness, restlessness, muscle pains or cramps, nausea, or rapid heart rate.

- Even though it is very rare, methyclothiazide can lower the number of blood cells you have. If you don't have enough white blood cells, your immunity is down, and you can get a fever, sore throat, or pneumonia. If you are lacking red blood cells, you can become anemic, and that makes you tired and weak. Not having enough blood platelets makes you bruise easily and keeps your blood from clotting properly when you're injured. Be on the lookout for any of these symptoms of bone marrow depression.

Special warnings:
- Don't take methyclothiazide if you are allergic to thiazides or sulfonamide-derived drugs.
- People with poor liver or kidney function should take methyclothiazide with caution.
- Your doctor should check your electrolyte balances frequently if you have heart failure, kidney disease, or liver disease, or if you are taking ACTH or corticosteroids. Your electrolyte balances should also be watched carefully if you get sick and are vomiting or have diarrhea.
- Take methyclothiazide with caution if you have moderate or high cholesterol levels. This drug may increase cholesterol and triglyceride levels.

Pregnancy and nursing mothers:
Category B. See page 9 for description of categories. Drug is present in mother's milk.

Possible food and drug interactions:
- Methyclothiazide may increase the effects of the muscle relaxer tubocurarine.
- Methyclothiazide may decrease the effects of the blood pressure-raising drug norepinephrine.
- Methyclothiazide may decrease the excretion of the antipsychotic drug lithium which can build up to toxic levels.
- If you take methyclothiazide with the heart drug digitalis, steroids, or the hormone ACTH, the combination may lower your potassium levels.
- Since methyclothiazide may raise blood sugar levels, people with diabetes may need adjustments to their doses of insulin or other glucose-lowering agents if they begin taking methyclothiazide.

Helpful hints:
- Weigh daily so you'll know if you're losing too much fluid. Losing too much fluid can cause dehydration and possibly blood clots. Warning signs of dehydration include dry mouth, thirst, drowsiness, weakness, loss of appetite, restlessness, nausea, vomiting, low blood pressure, heart rhythm abnormalities, and muscle pains or cramps. Contact your doctor immediately if you stop urinating.
- If you have high blood pressure, avoid using over-the-counter cold remedies or diet pills which can increase blood pressure.

Metolazone

Brand name: *Zaroxolyn*

What this drug does for you:

This diuretic is used to reduce blood pressure and the swelling and fluid retention associated with congestive heart failure and kidney disease.

Diuretics work on the kidneys to increase urination. That helps your body get rid of water and salt.

Possible side effects of this drug:

- Metolazone may cause inflammation of the pancreas, muscle or joint pain, muscle spasms, jaundice, hepatitis, constipation, vomiting, diarrhea, nausea, loss of appetite, bloating, headache, fainting, vertigo, weakness, tingling sensation, low blood pressure, palpitations, chest pain, and skin problems including rash, hives, and sensitivity to light.
- Metolazone may increase levels of uric acid in the blood (this puts you at risk for gout) and may worsen symptoms of lupus.
- This diuretic may cause dangerously low levels of potassium and other electrolytes. Contact your doctor if you experience any of the symptoms of potassium loss: unusual thirst, tiredness, drowsiness, restlessness, muscle pains or cramps, nausea, or rapid heart rate.
- Even though it is very rare, metolazone can lower the number of blood cells you have. If you don't have enough white blood cells, your immunity is down, and you can get a fever, sore throat, or pneumonia. If you are lacking red blood cells, you can become anemic, and that makes you tired and weak. Not having enough blood platelets makes you bruise easily and keeps your blood from clotting properly when you're injured. Be on the lookout for any of these symptoms of bone marrow depression.

Special warnings:

- Don't use metolazone if you are allergic to thiazides or sulfonamide-derived drugs.
- Don't interchange this drug with the related diuretic called Mykrox.
- People with poor kidney function should use metolazone with caution.
- Your doctor should check your electrolyte balances frequently if you have heart failure, kidney disease, or liver disease, or if you are taking ACTH or corticosteroids. Your electrolyte balances should also be watched carefully if you get sick and are vomiting or have diarrhea.

Pregnancy and nursing mothers:

Category B. See page 9 for description of categories. Drug is present in mother's milk.

Possible food and drug interactions:

- Metolazone may increase the effects of other blood pressure lowering drugs.
- Metolazone may decrease the excretion of the antipsychotic drug lithium, which can build up to toxic levels.
- Effects of metolazone may be decreased by the urinary antiseptic meth-

enamine and some nonsteroidal anti-inflammatory drugs (NSAIDs), such as aspirin.

- If you take metolazone along with alcohol or a drug that depresses your nervous system, such as tranquilizers, antihistamines, or muscle relaxers, the combination may dangerously depress your nervous system.
- If you take metolazone with the heart drug digitalis, the combination may cause irregular heartbeat.
- If you take metolazone with corticosteroids, the combination may increase potassium loss and cause salt and water retention.
- If you take metolazone with the muscle relaxer tubocurarine, the combination may cause respiratory depression.
- Since metolazone may raise blood sugar levels, people with diabetes may need adjustments to their doses of insulin or other glucose-lowering agents if they begin taking metolazone.

Helpful hints:

- This drug can cause dangerously low levels of potassium and other electrolytes. Eat extra potassium-rich foods like bananas.
- Weigh daily so you'll know if you're losing too much fluid. Losing too much fluid can cause dehydration and possibly blood clots. Warning signs of dehydration include dry mouth, thirst, drowsiness, weakness, loss of appetite, restlessness, nausea, vomiting, low blood pressure, heart rhythm abnormalities, and muscle pains or cramps. Contact your doctor immediately if you stop urinating.
- If you have high blood pressure, avoid using over-the-counter cold remedies or diet pills which can increase blood pressure.

Spironolactone

Brand names: *Aldactazide, Aldactone* **(Generic available)**

What this drug does for you:

This diuretic helps control high blood pressure. It is also used to help stabilize potassium levels in people taking digitalis and to reduce fluid retention and swelling in conditions such as cirrhosis of the liver, congestive heart failure, and kidney disease. Doctors may use spironolactone to diagnose an overactive adrenal gland. Diuretics work on the kidneys to increase urination. That helps your body get rid of water and salt.

Possible side effects of this drug:

- This drug may cause vomiting, stomach cramps, diarrhea, bleeding or ulcer-ation in the stomach, menstrual problems, postmenopausal bleeding, inability to achieve or maintain an erection, breast tumors, unusual hair growth, deepening of the voice, enlargement of breasts in men, confusion, headache, lack of coordination, tiredness, drowsiness, drug fever, rash, and hives.
- This drug can cause dangerously high levels of potassium in your body. Some warning signs are a prickling or tingling sensation, muscle weakness, tiredness, and slow heartbeat. Very high potassium levels can

cause serious heart rhythm problems and death.

Special warnings:

- People with kidney problems should not take this drug.

Pregnancy and nursing mothers:

Use with extreme caution in pregnancy and only if the potential benefits to the mother outweigh the risks to the baby. Drug is present in mother's milk.

Possible food and drug interactions:

- No significant interactions reported.

Helpful hints:

- Weigh daily so you'll know if you're losing too much fluid. Losing too much fluid can cause dehydration and possibly blood clots. Warning signs of dehydration include dry mouth, thirst, drowsiness, weakness, loss of appetite, restlessness, nausea, vomiting, low blood pressure, heart rhythm abnormalities, and muscle pains or cramps. Contact your doctor immediately if you stop urinating.
- If you have high blood pressure, avoid using over-the-counter cold remedies or diet pills which can increase blood pressure.
- Don't take supplements that contain potassium unless your doctor tells you otherwise.
- Your doctor should regularly check your electrolyte levels (levels of salt, potassium, etc.).
- You shouldn't drive a car or operate heavy machinery until you are sure the medicine isn't making you drowsy or less than alert.

Triamterene and Hydrochlorothiazide

Brand names: *Dyazide, Maxzide* **(Generic available)**

What this drug does for you:

This drug combines two products for people who need a thiazide diuretic but can't afford to risk potassium loss. It is used to treat swelling and high blood pressure. Diuretics work on the kidneys to increase urination. That helps your body get rid of water and salt.

Possible side effects of this drug:

- This drug can cause dangerously high levels of potassium in your body. Some warning signs are a prickling or tingling sensation, muscle weakness, tiredness, and slow heartbeat. Very high levels of potassium can be fatal.
- This drug may cause kidney stones and other kidney disorders, high blood sugar, low blood pressure and dizziness when you change positions, allergic shock reaction, a decrease in folic acid levels, jaundice, nausea, diarrhea, rash, sensitivity to light, headache, drowsiness, insomnia, restlessness, shortness of breath, rapid heartbeat, dry mouth, muscle cramps, decreased sexual performance, and weakness.
- Hydrochlorothiazide may increase levels of uric acid in the blood (this puts you at risk for gout).

- Even though it is very rare, this drug may lower the number of blood cells you have. If you don't have enough white blood cells, your immunity is down, and you can get a fever, sore throat, or pneumonia. If you are lacking red blood cells, you can become anemic, and that makes you tired and weak. Not having enough blood platelets makes you bruise easily and keeps your blood from clotting properly when you're injured. Be on the lookout for any of these symptoms of bone marrow depression.

Special warning:
- People with kidney problems should not take this drug.

Pregnancy and nursing mothers:
Category C. See page 9 for description of categories. This drug is present in mother's milk. If you must take this drug, you should not breast-feed.

Possible food and drug interactions:
- You shouldn't take potassium-containing salt substitutes or eat a potassium-enriched diet while you're taking this drug.
- This drug may increase levels of the antipsychotic drug lithium, possibly to toxic levels.
- You should not take this drug if you are taking other drugs that increase or maintain potassium levels.
- Taking this drug and nonsteroidal anti-inflammatory drugs (NSAIDs) at the same time may cause kidney failure.
- Taking this drug along with an ACE inhibitor may increase your risk of dangerously high potassium levels.

Helpful hints:
- Weigh daily so you'll know if you're losing too much fluid. Losing too much fluid can cause dehydration and possibly blood clots. Warning signs of dehydration include dry mouth, thirst, drowsiness, weakness, loss of appetite, restlessness, nausea, vomiting, low blood pressure, heart rhythm abnormalities, and muscle pains or cramps. Contact your doctor immediately if you stop urinating.
- If you have high blood pressure, avoid using over-the-counter cold remedies or diet pills which can increase blood pressure.
- Your doctor should monitor your potassium levels and test your blood, kidney, and liver functions while you are taking this drug.

HEART RHYTHM REGULATORS

Amiodarone

Brand name: *Cordarone*

What this drug does for you:
Amiodarone is an antiarrhythmic. It is used to correct irregular heartbeats to a normal rhythm. It works by slowing nerve impulses in the heart and acting directly on the heart tissues.

Possible side effects of this drug:

- Many people experience nausea, vomiting, increased sensitivity to the sun, lack of coordination, and constipation.
- Less frequent side effects are insomnia, headache, sleep disturbances, decreased sex drive, congestive heart failure, abdominal pain, liver problems, flushing, and altered taste and smell.
- Rare side effects are a blue-gray discoloration of the skin, low blood pressure, overactive or underactive thyroid, stomach pain, liver disorders, and inflammation of the lungs.

Special warnings:

- Toxic effects can be very severe, even fatal. Amiodarone should only be used as a last resort, after other heart-rhythm regulators have been tried.
- People with some types of heart rhythm disorders should not use this drug, for instance, people with second- or third-degree AV block not being treated with a pacemaker or people with a slow heartbeat that has caused fainting.

Pregnancy and nursing mothers:

Category D. See page 9 for description of categories. Drug is present in mother's milk.

Possible food and drug interactions:

- Amiodarone may increase the effects of anticoagulants and the effects of other drugs that regulate the rhythm of the heart.
- Amiodarone may cause toxic levels of the heart drug digoxin to build up in the blood.

Helpful hint:

- Amiodarone will increase your skin's sensitivity to the sun. Always use a sunscreen and wear protective clothes when you will be exposed to the sun for a while.

Disopyramide

Brand name: *Norpace* **(Generic available)**

What this drug does for you:

Disopyramide is an antiarrhythmic. It is used to correct irregular heartbeats to a normal rhythm. It works by slowing nerve impulses in the heart and acting directly on the heart tissues.

Possible side effects of this drug:

- Disopyramide may cause dry mouth, constipation, blurred vision, gas, bloating, frequent urination, weakness, headache, impotence, low blood pressure and dizziness when you stand up, congestive heart failure, fluid retention, weight gain, chest pain, loss of appetite, vomiting, diarrhea, itching, nervousness, rash, and dry nose, eyes, and throat.
- Rare side effects are tingling, insomnia, painful urination, and depression.

Special warnings:
- People with some types of heart rhythm disorders should not use this drug, for instance, people with second- or third-degree AV block not being treated with a pacemaker.
- People with the following conditions should take this drug very cautiously: congestive heart failure, low blood pressure, urinary retention, the nerve/muscle disorder called myasthenia gravis, or glaucoma.
- You may need a lower drug dosage if you have poor liver or kidney function.
- You should have your blood sugar levels tested regularly if you have liver disease or congestive heart failure or if you are taking any other drugs which may affect your blood sugar levels.
- Men with enlarged prostates have an increased risk of urinary retention while taking disopyramide.
- Disopyramide may stimulate uterine contractions in pregnant women.

Pregnancy and nursing mothers:
Category C. See page 9 for description of categories. Drug is present in mother's milk.

Possible food and drug interactions:
- Other antiarrhythmic drugs such as procainamide, quinidine, or lidocaine may increase levels or effects of this drug.
- The seizure drug phenytoin may decrease levels of this drug.

Helpful hints:
- Take your medicine on time and exactly as your doctor prescribes.
- Eat a high-fiber diet and drink plenty of liquids to improve constipation, one of disopyramide's side effects.
- You shouldn't drive a car or operate heavy machinery until you are sure the medicine isn't making you drowsy or less than alert or causing blurred vision.

Flecainide

Brand name: *Tambocor*

What this drug does for you:
Flecainide is an antiarrhythmic. It is used to correct irregular heartbeats to a normal rhythm. It works by slowing nerve impulses in the heart and acting directly on the heart tissues.

Possible side effects of this drug:
- Flecainide may cause dizziness, difficulty breathing, headache, nausea, fatigue, blurred vision, palpitations, chest pain, loss of strength, tremors, constipation, fluid retention, and stomach pain.
- Less common side effects are indigestion, vomiting, loss of appetite, diarrhea, fever, rapid or irregular heartbeat, double vision, ringing in the ears, tingling, sweating, insomnia, depression, and anxiety.
- Rare side effects are chest pain, worsened irregular heartbeats, high or

low blood pressure, hives, itching, hair loss, eye irritation, intolerance of light, dry mouth, muscle twitching or pain, difficulty urinating, impotence, and swelling of lips, mouth, or tongue.

- Even though it is very rare, flecainide can lower the number of blood cells you have. If you don't have enough white blood cells, your immunity is down, and you can get a fever, sore throat, or pneumonia. If you are lacking red blood cells, you can become anemic, and that makes you tired and weak. Not having enough blood platelets makes you bruise easily and keeps your blood from clotting properly when you're injured. Be on the lookout for any of these symptoms of bone marrow depression.

Special warnings:

- People with some types of heart rhythm disorders should not use this drug, for instance, people with second- or third-degree AV block not being treated with a pacemaker. People with cardiogenic shock and people who have recently had a heart attack should not take this drug either.
- People with poor liver function should take this drug with extreme caution.
- People with the following conditions should take this drug cautiously: the heart condition called sick sinus syndrome, a history of congestive heart failure, severe kidney disease, or the use of a pacemaker. This drug may worsen irregular heartbeats or cause heart failure in people with poor heart function.
- Any potassium imbalance should be corrected before beginning treatment because high or low potassium levels can alter the effects of this drug on the heart.

Pregnancy and nursing mothers:

Category C. See page 9 for description of categories. Drug is present in mother's milk.

Possible food and drug interactions:

- Flecainide may increase levels of the heart drug digoxin.
- Taking flecainide along with the beta-blocker propranolol may increase the effects of both drugs.
- Levels of flecainide may be increased by the ulcer drug cimetidine, the seizure drugs carbamazepine and phenytoin, the sedative phenobarbital, and the heart drug amiodarone.

Helpful hints:

- You shouldn't drive a car or operate heavy machinery until you are sure the medicine isn't making you drowsy or less than alert or causing blurred vision.
- Take your medicine on time and exactly as your doctor prescribes.

Mexiletine

Brand name: *Mexitil*

What this drug does for you:

Mexiletine is an antiarrhythmic. It is used to correct irregular heartbeats to a normal rhythm. It works by slowing nerve impulses in the heart and acting directly on the heart tissues.

Possible side effects of this drug:

- The most common side effects are upset stomach (nausea, vomiting, and heartburn), dizziness and lightheadedness, shakiness, and lack of coordination. You may also experience diarrhea, constipation, dry mouth, fever, swelling, difficulty breathing, chest pain, fatigue, weakness, headache, ringing in the ears, visual disturbances, confusion, depression, numbness or tingling, sleep disorders, rash, and joint pain. Mexiletine may make some cases of irregular heartbeat worse.
- Rare side effects are difficulty urinating, impotence, decreased libido, hot flashes, hiccups, fainting, high blood pressure, hair loss, liver damage, short-term memory loss, and loss of consciousness.
- Even though it is very rare, mexiletine can lower the number of blood cells you have. If you don't have enough white blood cells, your immunity is down, and you can get a fever, sore throat, or pneumonia. If you are lacking red blood cells, you can become anemic, and that makes you tired and weak. Not having enough blood platelets makes you bruise easily and keeps your blood from clotting properly when you're injured. Be on the lookout for any of these symptoms of bone marrow depression.
- Serious skin disorders in which dark red rings or raised spots erupt on your skin (Stevens-Johnson syndrome) or parts of your skin deteriorate are another very rare reaction.

Special warnings:

- People with some types of heart rhythm disorders should not use this drug.
- Because mexiletine can make some arrhythmias worse, it should only be used for serious arrhythmias.
- Your doctor should prescribe mexiletine to you very cautiously and monitor you very carefully if you have heart problems such as heart disease, heart block or congestive heart failure, if you have low blood pressure, or if you have poor liver function.

Pregnancy and nursing mothers:

Category C. See page 9 for description of categories. Drug is present in mother's milk.

Possible food and drug interactions:

- Mexiletine may increase the effects of the asthma drug theophylline.
- Levels or effects of mexiletine may be decreased by the tuberculosis drug rifampin, the seizure drug phenytoin, and the sedative phenobarbital.

Helpful hint:
- You should have regular liver function tests and blood counts while you're taking this drug.

Procainamide

Brand name: *Procan SR* **(Generic available)**

What this drug does for you:
Procainamide is an antiarrhythmic. It is used to correct irregular heart-beats to a normal rhythm. It works by slowing nerve impulses in the heart and acting directly on the heart tissues.

Possible side effects of this drug:
- Possible side effects include low blood pressure, nausea, diarrhea, loss of appetite, stomach pain, bitter taste, enlargement of the liver, swelling, flushing, itching, hives, rash, weakness, dizziness, depression, and psychosis with hallucinations. Procainamide may make some cases of irregular heartbeat worse.
- At least 20 percent of the people who take procainamide eventually get lupus erythematosus-like syndrome. Some symptoms are fever, skin eruptions, and joint and muscle pains. Call your doctor immediately if you have any of these symptoms.
- Even though it is very rare, procainamide can lower the number of blood cells you have. If you don't have enough white blood cells, your immunity is down, and you can get a fever, sore throat, or pneumonia. If you are lacking red blood cells, you can become anemic, and that makes you tired and weak. Not having enough blood platelets makes you bruise easily and keeps your blood from clotting properly when you're injured. Be on the lookout for any of these symptoms of bone marrow depression. You should have blood counts taken weekly for the first three months and then periodically throughout treatment.

Special warnings:
- Procainamide should not be used by people with complete heart block, the irregular heart rhythm called "torsade de pointes," asthma, allergic reaction, or lupus.
- Use procainamide with caution if you have heart disease, heart block, heart failure, poor kidney or liver function, or myasthenia gravis (muscle weakness disease).

Pregnancy and nursing mothers:
Category C. See page 9 for description of categories. Drug is present in mother's milk.

Possible food and drug interactions:
- Procainamide may increase the effects of neuromuscular blocking agents.
- If you take procainamide with the heartbeat regulators quinidine or disopyramide, the combination may cause very low blood pressure or

worsen irregular heartbeat.

Helpful hint:
- Take your medicine on time and exactly as your doctor prescribes.

Quinidine

Brand names: *Cardioquin, Quinidex* **(Generic available)**

What this drug does for you:
Quinidine is an antiarrhythmic. It is used to correct irregular heartbeats to a normal rhythm. It works by slowing nerve impulses in the heart and acting directly on the heart tissues.

Possible side effects of this drug:
- Possible side effects include stomach pain, nausea, diarrhea, low blood pressure, confusion, excitement, fainting, dizziness, headache, fever, ringing in the ears, visual abnormalities, and liver damage. Quinidine may make some cases of irregular heartbeat worse.
- This drug may cause allergic reactions including skin rash, swelling, itching, hives, and difficulty breathing.
- Even though it is very rare, quinidine can lower the number of blood cells you have. If you don't have enough white blood cells, your immunity is down, and you can get a fever, sore throat, or pneumonia. If you are lacking red blood cells, you can become anemic, and that makes you tired and weak. Not having enough blood platelets makes you bruise easily and keeps your blood from clotting properly when you're injured. Be on the lookout for any of these symptoms of bone marrow depression.

Special warnings:
- Quinidine should not be used by people with certain kinds of heart problems, people with the nerve/muscle weakness disease called myasthenia gravis, and by those who have previously had allergic reactions to quinidine.
- Quinidine may mask an allergic reaction, especially in people with asthma. A test dose should be given before beginning treatment to determine if there is an allergy. Blood counts and liver and kidney function tests should be done periodically. This drug may cause fainting or loss of consciousness. People with severe heart failure, those on digitalis treatment, and people with poor kidney function or low blood pressure should use this drug with extreme caution.

Pregnancy and nursing mothers:
Use in pregnancy only if the potential benefits to the mother outweigh the risks to the baby. Drug is present in mother's milk.

Possible food and drug interactions:
- Quinidine may increase the levels of the heart drug digoxin, possibly to toxic levels.
- Quinidine may increase effects of heart rhythm drugs, anticoagulants, and muscle relaxers.

- Effects of quinidine may be decreased by the anticonvulsant drugs phe nobarbital and phenytoin.

Helpful hints:

- Take tablets with plenty of water or fluid and swallow the tablets whole.
- Never use discolored (brownish) quinidine solution.
- Take your medicine with meals to help prevent stomach problems.
- You should have regular kidney and liver function tests and blood counts while you are taking this drug.

INTERMITTENT CLAUDICATION DRUGS

Pentoxifylline

Brand name: *Trental*

What this drug does for you:

Pentoxifylline makes the blood less sticky and improves the flow of blood through blood vessels. It eases calf pain caused by poor blood circulation. The drug makes it possible to walk farther before having to rest.

Possible side effects of this drug:

- Pentoxifylline may cause indigestion, nausea, dizziness, headache, chest pain, belching, gas, bloating, tremors, fluid retention, blurred vision, nervousness, irregular heartbeat, and flushing.
- Rare side effects include earache, loss of appetite, confusion, anxiety, mental depression, itching, rash, hives, sore throat, dry mouth, nasal congestion, constipation, and difficulty breathing.

Special warnings:

- Pentoxifylline should not be used by people allergic to methylxanthines (such as caffeine, theophylline, theobromine).
- Use pentoxifylline with caution if you have any condition in which there is a risk of bleeding: stomach ulcers, rectal bleeding, recent stroke, or recent surgery.

Pregnancy and nursing mothers:

Category C. See page 9 for description of categories. Drug is present in mother's milk.

Possible food and drug interactions:

- Pentoxifylline may increase the effects of the anticoagulant warfarin, which may increase the risk of hemorrhaging.

Helpful hints:

- Swallow the tablet whole. Don't crush, break, or chew before swallowing.
- Take the medicine with meals to help avoid stomach upset.

Natural Alternatives

HEART DISEASE

- ◄ Burning or heavy sensation in the chest
- ◄ Heart attack
- ◄ Shortness of breath
- ◄ Tightness and squeezing in the chest

- ◄ Difficulty breathing
- ◄ Irregular heartbeat
- ◄ Swollen ankles
- ◄ Tingling or ache in left arm, neck, jaw, or shoulder blade

21 ways to fight off heart disease

"How can you mend a broken heart?" asks the popular song. Both poets and doctors have debated this question for centuries. Human nature being what it is, poets are still wondering. But medical science has come a long way toward understanding the physical heart and what makes it tick.

The best thing you can do for your heart is to practice preventive measures to keep it well. But even if you've already been diagnosed with heart disease, there are many things you can do to make your heart healthier.

In addition to the tips listed below, be sure to see the **High blood pressure** and **High cholesterol** sections later in this chapter for more helpful suggestions.

Try the Ornish Program. Similar to the Pritikin Program of the 1970's, Ornish's program promises to make a real difference in your life and your health. Dr. Ornish has developed a program, detailed in his book *Dr. Dean Ornish's Program for Reversing Heart Disease*, that focuses on stress management, diet, and exercise as the keys to preventing and reversing heart disease.

In one of the recent programs Ornish conducted, 82 percent of the participants experienced a significant reversal in their coronary artery disease within the first year — all without drugs or surgery. Here are some of the main points of Dr. Ornish's program:

◁ Connect with others in your family or community. Feeling isolated contributes to health-destroying behaviors such as smoking, drinking alcohol, overeating, and putting yourself under constant stress.

◁ Learn techniques for managing stress. Learning to relax and deal with stress can help you head off potential health problems and perform more effectively.

◁ Learn to communicate your feelings and wants clearly and effectively. Don't expect a big "thank you" for everything you do, and don't expect other people or yourself to be perfect. However, be kind and giving to others. Studies have shown that helpful people live 2 1/2 times longer than ungiving people.

◁ Adopt a heart-healthy diet. For people who have been diagnosed with heart disease, Ornish recommends a vegetarian diet that is less than 10 percent fat. The diet includes fruits, vegetables, grains, legumes, and soybean products. There are a few high-fat vegetarian choices you should avoid, such as avocados, olives, coconut, nuts, seeds, and cocoa products.

You should also avoid all animal products with the exception of egg whites and one cup of nonfat yogurt or milk a day. Limit alcohol to two ounces per day or less and try to stay away from caffeine, which may worsen irregular heartbeats or provoke stress.

◁ Exercise regularly. Dr. Ornish recommends walking 30 minutes daily or one hour every other day. Walking is the exercise of choice for many people because it poses the least risk of injury.

Have a healthy workout. You already know that aerobic exercise is healthy for your heart. Recent studies have shown that strength training on Nautilus equipment has many of the same advantages for people with heart disease risk factors.

You should always check with your doctor before beginning any exercise pro-

Coenzyme Q10: A natural cure for heart disease?

Researchers around the world have come up with evidence linking a deficiency of the nutrient ubiquinone, or Coenzyme Q10 (CoQ10, for short) to a variety of heart problems. Scientists studying these people consistently found levels of CoQ10 far below those of healthy people. Supplementing with CoQ10, in some cases, has actually reversed severe heart disease symptoms, and prolonged the lives of people thought to be terminally ill.

Scientists at the University of Texas at Austin tried CoQ10 on 154 people with congestive heart failure. Half of these people were deemed hopeless. But after taking CoQ10 regularly, 95 percent of these "dying" people were still alive three years later.

CoQ10 has also been used to lower high blood pressure and correct heart arrhythmias.

A variety of foods contain CoQ10, but only organ meats, like beef hearts, contain substantial amounts. Luckily, the human body has the ability to synthesize CoQ10 from the foods you eat, but your body can only synthesize nutrients into the CoQ10 form if your diet has adequate levels of all the trace elements and vitamins you need.

While no serious side effects have ever been associated with taking CoQ10 supplements, you should discuss CoQ10 with your doctor before using it. The best way to make sure you have enough CoQ10 is to eat a nutritious, varied, and balanced diet.

Sources —
  American Journal of Clinical Nutrition (61,35:621S)
  Drug Topics (135,5:42)
  The American Journal of Cardiology (65:521 and 66:504)
  The Clinical Investigator (1993,71:S140)
  The Journal of Clinical Pharmacology (1990,30:596)
  The Journal of Optimal Nutrition (2,3:264 and 3,3:115)
  The Journal of the American Dietetic Association (92,10:1213)
  The Journal of Thoracic and Cardiovascular Surgery (107,1:242)
  The Miracle Nutrient CoenzymeQ10, Bantam Books, New York, 1989

gram, however. Lifting too much weight or doing too many repetitions can be just as harmful as pushing yourself too far in the advanced aerobics class or trying to run a marathon after just two days of training.

Take advantage of aspirin. Recent studies have shown that aspirin can save thousands of lives every year by preventing heart attacks and strokes. Aspirin can also reduce severity and long-term damage caused by heart attacks. And for people with atrial fibrillation, it reduces the risk of stroke 50 to 80 percent.

Doctors and scientists are now strongly recommending that everyone who has experienced a heart attack, stroke, bypass surgery, or angioplasty, or who has experienced angina (chest pain) or transient ischemic attacks ("mini-strokes") could benefit from taking an aspirin a day. Aspirin helps keep the blood from getting "sticky" and forming clots that could lead to a fatal heart attack or stroke.

For some people, it seems that baby aspirin (75 mg) provides as much protection as regular aspirin (325 mg) without some of the side effects that come with larger doses. Talk with your doctor about daily aspirin therapy.

Make your Monday mornings heart safe. On Monday mornings, you have a one-third greater chance of suffering a heart attack than at any other time of the week. Physical or mental stress on Monday mornings, changes in hormone levels, changes in behavior patterns over the weekend, and changes in the food and drink you consume on weekends all contribute to the higher rate of heart attacks. Follow these tips to make Monday morning safer for your heart:

◁ Don't be a couch potato. The sudden change from inactivity to hard work is one of the causes of Monday morning heart attacks. You can minimize that factor by staying physically active on weekends.

◁ Take it easy Monday morning. Schedule stressful meetings or heavy labor later in the day or week. Ease yourself back into the routine of work. Don't pick Monday morning to begin an exercise routine.

◁ Don't get up too quickly. Bolting out of bed, or even sitting up quickly, can stress your heart. This is especially true for people who have heart disease. So don't feel guilty about hitting that snooze alarm a couple of times on Monday.

◁ But don't stop your morning exercise routine. You don't have to wait until afternoon or evening to exercise, even if you have heart disease. If you enjoy exercising in the morning, keep it up, but use moderation.

Walk away from intermittent claudication. If you have intermittent claudication, it means your heart isn't pumping enough blood to your legs, and it's a symptom of serious artery disease. Intermittent claudication can hurt so badly that the last thing you want to do is walk. But that's exactly what you need to do to get relief.

You need to walk until you bring on the pain, then rest for a minute or two until the pain subsides, then start walking again. Keep this up for one hour. If you walk for one hour three times a week, you should get your leg pain under control within two or three months. If you don't do your walking exercises, you may find yourself confined to your armchair at home as your leg pain gets worse and worse.

See your doctor for regular "AAA screenings." Intermittent claudication is a common sign of an "abdominal aortic aneurysm," or AAA, a weakness in the wall of the artery which supplies blood to your stomach, liver, and spleen. This is a serious condition and you need to know if you have it.

Make the switch to a Mediterranean diet. This is especially important if you've already had one heart attack. In a study of 584 people in Lyons, France, the risk of a second heart attack or death was 70 percent lower for people who followed a Mediterranean diet, compared to those who followed a diet recommended by the American Heart Association.

The AHA diet uses lean meat and fish as its basic components and adds on vegetables, fruits, and grains, with 30 percent of calories coming from total fat. The Mediterranean diet uses fruits and vegetables as its basis, with chicken and fish added on to make a meal.

A recent study reported that the risk of cardiac arrest can be reduced by 50 to 70 percent, even in those who have already had one heart attack. The trick is to eat one serving of fatty fish each week. Cooked fresh salmon, albacore tuna, and cod are good sources for the heart-helping substances called fatty acids.

Ease the ache of angina. It feels like a heart attack, but your doctor has told you not to worry — that the pain usually goes away with rest and angina doesn't permanently damage your heart. But angina is still a warning sign that your heart isn't getting enough oxygen, and you could have a heart attack someday soon if you don't take care of yourself.

When you've been diagnosed with angina, you need to make a few lifestyle changes to control your condition. Here's what you can do:

◁ Schedule regular 30-minute walks. Start gradually and increase to a level that feels comfortable. If you exercise in extremely hot or cold weather, dress appropriately, and limit the amount of time spent outdoors.

◁ Give your heart a break — stop smoking! Smoking makes it harder for the heart to do its work — namely, to pump blood throughout your body.

◁ Get a handle on stress. Try to avoid tight deadlines and overcrowded schedules. Ask for help instead of trying to do everything yourself. If you can't get rid of your stressors, learn stress management. Here are two ways to beat stress: Relax all your muscles for 20 minutes twice a day. Breathe deeply and concentrate on a pleasant thought when something stressful comes your way.

◁ Control your blood pressure. Take the blood-pressure medicine your doctor has prescribed for you, and see our tips in the ***High blood pressure*** section.

◁ Eat small meals. Large meals make your digestive system and your heart work harder. Eat several smaller meals rather than three big meals a day. Take it easy after eating, and try not to overdo it.

◁ Shed pounds and you may shed your angina too. If you've always wanted to, now is the time to lose weight. Sometimes losing weight can make angina go away altogether.

All-natural way to stop a racing heart

Although tachycardia (rapid heartbeat) is not usually serious, it can be very uncomfortable and even scary for your heart rate to suddenly rise to 160 beats per minute. The normal heart rate for healthy adults is about 50 to 100 beats per minute.

If you occasionally experience tachycardia, here are some natural ways to return your heart to its normal rhythm:

◁ Place your hands over your eyes and put mild pressure on your eyelids.

◁ Massage the arteries in your neck.

◁ Soak a towel in ice water and hold the towel to your face.

◁ Prepare a large bowl of ice water and plunge your face into it.

A word of warning: Check with your doctor about the wisdom of using the cold-water techniques. People who have chest pain or angina that becomes worse in cold weather should avoid these methods of slowing the heart rate.

Source —
Emergency Medicine (27,3:64 and 23,21:95)

◁ Drink alcohol only in moderation. Too much alcohol raises your heart rate, a definite no-no for angina sufferers.

◁ Carry your nitroglycerin with you wherever you go. If you think that a particular activity may trigger angina, take nitroglycerin before you begin. As always, carefully follow your doctor's instructions about medicines prescribed for your angina.

Connect socially and spiritually for your health and survival. After having heart surgery, people with religious beliefs that give them strength and comfort have a much better chance of survival. The same is true for people who regularly see family or friends. People with both religious and social support survive the longest.

The course of action you take to "mend your broken heart" is up to you. Along with the advice of your doctor and our helpful hints, you can do a lot to improve the health of your heart. You have many healthy years yet to live with a song in your heart!

Sources —

Age Page, National Institute on Aging Information Center, P.O. Box 8057, Gaithersburg, Md. 20898-8057, 1994

American Heart Association news release (July 18, 1994)

Archives of Internal Medicine (154,1:37)

Atherosclerosis and Thrombosis (14,11:1746)

Blood Pressure: Take Control, Baylor College of Medicine, One Baylor Plaza, Room 176B, Houston, Texas 77030

Circulation (90,1:87; 90,1:121 and 90;4:1866)

Dr. Dean Ornish's Program for Reversing Heart Disease, Random House, New York, 1990

Heart and Stroke Facts and *Controlling Your Risk Factors for Heart Attack*, American Heart Association, 7272 Greenville Ave., Dallas, Texas 75231-4596, 1993

Ischemic Heart Disease: Angina Pectoris, Scientific American Medicine, New York, 1991

Medical Tribune (35,2:1)

Medical Tribune for the Family Physician (35,13:18)

Medical World News (35,2:25)

Metabolism (42,2:177)

National Institute of Neurological Disorders and Stroke, Office of Scientific and Health Reports, Building 31 Room 8A-16, 31 Center Drive MSC 2540, Bethesda, Md. 20892-2540, 1994

Science (263,5143:24)

Science News (143,15:239 and 147,8:124)

The American Journal of Epidemiology (141,5:451)

The Atlanta Journal/Constitution (Sept. 14, 1994, D6; and Sept. 28, 1995, A6)

The Food Guide Pyramid, United States Department of Agriculture

The Journal of the American Medical Association (272,10:781 and 273,15:1211)

The New Pritikin Program, Pocket Books, New York, 1990

The Wall Street Journal (July 9, 1993, B1)

The Wellness Encyclopedia: The Comprehensive Family Resource for Safeguarding Health and Preventing Illness, Houghton Mifflin, Boston, 1991

U.S. Pharmacist (9,7:38)

Understanding Angina, American Heart Association, 7272 Greenville Ave., Dallas, Texas 75231, 1991

HIGH BLOOD PRESSURE

◀ Confusion

◀ Drowsiness

◀ Memory loss

◀ Numbness and tingling
   in hands and feet

◀ Coughing up blood

◀ Headache

◀ Nosebleeds

◀ Severe shortness of breath

12-step program lowers blood pressure

The force with which your heart pumps blood through your body is blood pressure, and it is measured in two numbers. The top one (systolic) represents the pressure of your blood during the beat of your heart. The bottom one (diastolic) represents the pressure of your blood between beats. Blood pressure is expressed as systolic "over" diastolic.

The healthiest blood pressure is 120 over 80 or less. While low blood pressure can be a problem, too high is more dangerous than too low. High blood pressure or hypertension is defined as 140 or more over 90 or more. Many people have high blood pressure and aren't aware of it. High blood pressure can lead to stroke, heart disease, kidney failure, and other health problems.

Your blood pressure is influenced by many factors in your life, most of which you can control. Keeping your blood pressure low is an important part of staying heart-healthy. Here are some tips to help you:

Get it checked regularly. If your blood pressure is in the high-to-normal range (130/85 to 139/89), you should have it checked by your doctor at least once every year. Drugstore and supermarket blood pressure monitors are OK to use, but don't depend only on them. Their readouts are wrong as much as 60 percent of the time.

People who have higher blood pressure need to follow a rigorous schedule of follow-up blood pressure checks. Seek your doctor's advice about follow-up vis·its, and make notes on your calendar to remind you when it's time to have your blood pressure checked.

Aim for a moderate decrease in blood pressure. People with very large and very small drops in blood pressure face three to four times the risk of heart attack compared to people with moderate declines, says a study from Albert Einstein College of Medicine in New York City.

Researchers say many more people eventually had severe or fatal heart attacks following blood pressure treatment that resulted in drops of less than six points or more than 18 points. Those whose diastolic blood pressure dropped from seven to 17 points had the fewest heart attacks.

Use your diet to lower blood pressure naturally. In the 1970s, The Pritikin Program made news with a plan to stop high blood pressure and high cholesterol with a low-fat, low-calorie, low-salt diet, and moderate daily exercise. In the 1980s, Dr. Dean Ornish developed a similar plan with equally beneficial results. (See more details under the *Heart disease* section of this chapter.)

The idea of Pritikin's diet program is to eat lots of fresh, unprocessed food, eliminate fat and cholesterol, cut calories, and say goodbye to most sugar and salt. All this is combined with moderate exercise for a total improvement in your health.

When a team of researchers from Loma Linda University studied people who used the program, they found that people lost weight, lowered cholesterol levels, and reduced their need for medication. Eighty-three percent of those who had been taking high blood pressure medicine were able to stop taking these drugs with their doctors' permission.

Try weight loss instead of drugs. In a smaller study at the University of Minnesota, researchers found that people with mild high blood pressure who had been taking prescription blood pressure-lowering drugs could keep their blood pressures down without drugs. They did it simply by losing weight and reducing the amount of salt and alcohol in their diets.

Try going on a diet with your spouse. Studies show that the success rate is higher for couples who support each other in a weight loss program.

Walk your way to better health. One of the best exercises for people with high blood pressure is walking. Not only will it help with your weight loss program, but it will not temporarily raise blood pressure as some more strenuous exercises do.

Manage it with magnesium. Before turning to a prescription drug to lower blood pressure, talk to your doctor about the possibility of a natural alternative — magnesium. Women in one study who received 485 mg of magnesium a day for six months lowered their systolic blood pressures an average of 2.7 points and their diastolic pressures an average of 3.4 points. Evidence continues to mount that the mineral can lower blood pressure safely.

Catch up on calcium. Calcium may also fight high blood pressure, and it has no side effects. People who have high blood pressure caused by eating too

Music therapy for heart problems

Since ancient times, people have recognized music as a powerful healing tool. New research supports many of these ancient claims.

Dr. Helen Bonny, a Baltimore psychotherapist, used tapes of her favorite music to help regain her health after coronary bypass surgery. When she tried her musical healing theory on other hospital patients, they experienced significant drops in heart rate and blood pressure, were less agitated, slept better, needed less pain medicine, and developed a more positive outlook.

Researchers from the State University of New York at Buffalo found that listening to your favorite music while performing stressful jobs can keep your blood pressure and heartbeat from rising and improve performance and concentration. Listening to favorite music can also help relieve childbirth or surgical pain and even chronic pain.

To promote healing in your body or relieve stress, choose music that has an easy, flowing melody and a rhythm of 72 beats per minute or less. This rhythm is similar to the resting heart rate.

For more serious health problems, consider consulting a music therapist. They treat health problems ranging from mental disorders to stroke. To find a qualified music therapist in your area or for more in-depth information about music therapy, contact the National Association for Music Therapy at 301-589-3300.

Sources —
The Healing Forces of Music, Amity House, Warwick, N.Y., 1988
The Journal of the American Medical Association (272,11:882)

much salt seem to get the most benefits from calcium.

If you have high blood pressure and you eat a lot of salt, make sure you eat a calcium-rich diet. If you're pregnant, eating a high-calcium diet may also help cut down on pregnancy-related high blood pressure.

Of course, you can overdo anything. Taking too many calcium or vitamin D supplements can lead to excess calcium in the blood, and that can cause high blood pressure.

Protect with potassium. Many scientific studies suggest that a diet high in potassium can help protect against high blood pressure.

But don't run out and buy potassium supplements. Too much potassium in the blood is much more serious and life-threatening than low potassium. A diet that includes fresh fruits and vegetables, rather than canned or processed ones, will automatically raise your potassium intake and lower your sodium intake. Bananas are an excellent source of potassium, and multivitamins may also contain potassium.

Several medications can cause a buildup of excess potassium in the blood, including potassium-sparing diuretics, ACE inhibitors, beta-blockers, heparin, and NSAIDs, such as aspirin and ibuprofen. People using these medications or people with diabetes or kidney disease should use extreme caution in eating large amounts of potassium-rich foods or taking potassium supplements.

Strengthen with vitamin C. Two studies have shown that people with high levels of vitamin C in their blood tend to have low blood pressure. The current recommended daily allowance for vitamin C is 60 mg per day, although some scientists think that number should be higher. Some natural sources of vitamin C are citrus fruits and dark-green vegetables like broccoli.

Be careful with over-the-counter pain medicines. Massachusetts researchers recently found that people older than 65 who used nonsteroidal anti-inflammatory drugs (NSAIDs) were about one-and-a-half times more likely to need treatment for high blood pressure than people who weren't using NSAIDs. Over-the-counter naproxen (sold as Aleve), ibuprofen (sold as Advil, Nuprin, and Motrin), and aspirin (such as Anacin, Bayer, and Excedrin), as well as dozens of prescription drugs, fall into the NSAIDs category.

People who have had heart attacks or strokes often take a low dose of aspirin every day. It's when people take high doses of NSAIDs that problems such as high blood pressure tend to develop. If you take NSAIDs, use the lowest effective dose for the shortest possible period of time.

Don't mix coffee and exercise. If you have high blood pressure, you may be better off not drinking coffee before you exercise. In a study of men between the ages of 30 and 45, the heart rates of the men with high blood pressure rose higher during exercise after they drank coffee than when they didn't drink it. Caffeine didn't have the same effect on men with normal blood pressures. During exercise, caffeine may place additional stress on the cardiovascular systems of men with hypertension.

Take your medicine correctly. If you have to take medication for your blood pressure, take it at the same time every day to set a regular routine that you can easily remember. If you should miss one day of medication, don't double the dosage the next day. Call your doctor for instructions.

Slash salt intake to lower blood pressure

A low-sodium diet is one of the best natural ways to lower high blood pressure, but many people are hesitant because they think that a salt-free diet is bland. However, researchers at the University of Minnesota discovered that your desire for salt decreases when you stick to a low-salt diet.

Cut back to 500 mg a day. Getting salt down into the range of 500 milligrams (mg) per day (1/4 teaspoon of salt = 500 mg) seems to be the most effective. Since most Americans consume between 6,000 and 12,000 mg of salt each day, it shouldn't be too difficult to cut back some.

Any food that comes in a can, frozen package, or box is likely to have salt added as a preservative or flavor enhancer. Check the labels on the foods you buy. The higher salt appears on the ingredients list, the higher the content. A slice of bread may contain over 200 mg of salt, a bowl of cornflakes over 300 mg, a bowl of canned soup over 1,000 mg, a chicken dinner from a fast food restaurant over 2,000 mg, and a large dill pickle over 1,000 mg.

Eat less salt without sacrificing flavor. Here's how:
◁ Avoid processed foods and store-bought mixes. Use fresh or frozen vegetables instead of canned.

◁ Try using half the amount of salt a recipe recommends.

◁ Remove the salt shaker from your table and put out lemon slices to use instead.

◁ Learn about the many natural herbs, spices, and fruit peels that are available. Use fresh onion and garlic as seasonings.

◁ Don't use potassium chloride salt substitutes. They can increase potassium levels in your body and perhaps even cause heart rhythm abnormalities.

◁ Beware of Oriental food. It can be high in MSG (monosodium glutamate), which is high in sodium.

◁ To spice up chicken dishes, add fruits such as mandarin oranges or pineapples. Marinate chicken, fish, beef, or poultry in orange juice or lemon juice. Add a honey glaze.

◁ Be sure to keep meals attractive and include a variety of colors and textures. Most people are more tempted to add salt when a meal appears bland.

◁ Drink water with your meals and avoid soft drinks. Soft drinks are high in sugar, which dulls your taste buds and makes it more difficult to give up salt. Also, many carbonated drinks are high in sodium. Even some sugar-free soft drinks contain sodium as sodium saccharin, an artificial sweetener.

A few very rare people are salt-resistant, and a low-salt diet may actually be harmful for these people. If your blood pressure isn't lower after two months on a low-salt diet, talk with your doctor.

Sources —
American Family Physician (47,1:210)
Archives of Internal Medicine (115,10:753; 153,2:154; 155,5:450)
Circulation (90,1:225)
Hypertension (19,6:749; 24,1:83)
Medical Tribune for the Internist and Cardiologist (35,14:4)
Recommended Dietary Allowances, 10th ed., National Academy Press, Washington, D.C., 1989
The American Journal of Clinical Nutrition (60,1:129)
The Fifth Report of the Joint National Committee on Detection, Evaluation and Treatment of High Blood Pressure (Jan. 25, 1993)
The Food Guide Pyramid, United States Department of Agriculture
The Journal of Optimal Nutrition (3,1:34)
The Journal of the American Medical Association (262,13:1801)
The New Pritikin Program, Pocket Books, New York, 1990
The Newnan Times/Herald (Oct. 25, 1995, 7B)
The Real Vitamin and Mineral Book: Going Beyond the RDA for Optimum Health, Avery Publishing, Garden City Park, N.Y., 1990

HIGH CHOLESTEROL

◄ High levels of fat in your blood
◄ No visible, physical symptoms

Take control of cholesterol

Atherosclerosis is a condition in which cholesterol, fat, and other substances build up inside the walls of arteries. As arteries narrow, the flow of blood is lessened and can even be cut off to the heart (heart attack) or to the brain (stroke). If you already have heart disease, it is even more important for you to control your cholesterol level and keep these arteries from getting clogged.

Your cholesterol reading is broken down into LDL (low-density lipoprotein) and HDL (high-density lipoprotein). You want to see a low level of LDL cholesterol, the "bad" lipoprotein that carries cholesterol from the liver to the bloodstream, where excess can accumulate in arteries. HDL is the "good" lipoprotein because it carries cholesterol to the liver for removal. You want to see a high level of HDL.

Most people can lower or maintain their cholesterol levels just by making a few additions and substractions to their diets. Here are several ideas for dietary changes:

Know that all fat is not created equal. Strangely enough, eating cholesterol doesn't raise blood cholesterol nearly as much as eating a type of fat called saturated fat. Like cholesterol, saturated fat is found mainly in animal products, like cheese, butter, cream, whole milk, ice cream, lard, and marbled meats.

Some vegetable oils — palm oil, palm kernel oil, coconut oil, and cocoa butter — are also high in saturated fat. These oils are often used in commercially baked goods, coffee creamers, and nondairy whipped toppings, so read all labels. Unsaturated fats, both polyunsaturated and monounsaturated, have been shown to reduce blood cholesterol levels. They are found in many vegetable oils, including corn oil, olive oil, and canola oil. These are the oils to use.

Buy the leanest cuts of meat, and regularly substitute poultry (without skin) and fish, which are lower in saturated fat, for red meat. Switch to low-fat cottage cheese and yogurt, reduced-fat hard cheeses, and skim or 1-percent milk.

Avoid egg yolks. One third of Americans are "cholesterol responders." Their blood cholesterol goes up when they eat cholesterol, such as that found in egg yolks. Since you probably don't know if you're a cholesterol responder, the American Heart Association says play it safe — don't eat more than four egg yolks a week. Or try substituting two egg whites for each egg yolk.

Forget frying. Buying low-fat foods is only the first step. You need to use low-fat cooking methods to keep fat from creeping back in. Trim all fat off meat before cooking. Remove fatty skin from chicken and turkey.

Don't fry foods. Roast, bake, broil, or poach them instead. Use fat-free basting or marinating liquids, such as wine, tomato juice, or lemon juice.

If you use oil for sautéing or baking, use olive or canola. Use diet, tub, or squeeze margarines instead of regular. Watch out for the term "hydrogenated," which means some of the fat has been made saturated.

Eat your vegetables and complex carbohydrates. The lowest-fat foods of all are vegetables, fruits, grains (rice, barley, and pasta), beans, and legumes. Substitute these for meat and high-fat dairy products.

Don't douse your pasta in butter or your baked potato in sour cream. Use tomato-based sauces instead of cream-based. Use lemon juice, low-sodium soy sauce, or herbs to season vegetables. Make chili with extra beans and seasonings, and leave out the meat.

Go a little nutty. If you like nuts, especially walnuts or almonds, add them to your cereal, muffins, pancakes, casseroles, or stir-fries. In one study, eating about three ounces of walnuts a day was shown to decrease blood cholesterol levels by 10 percent more than an already low-fat, low-cholesterol diet. Another study showed that about three ounces of almonds lowered LDL cholesterol by 9 percent. Be sure to decrease other sources of fat to allow for extra calories from the nuts.

Even some chocolate is OK. Studies indicate that the primary type of saturated fat in chocolate, stearic acid, has no effect on cholesterol levels. When a chocolate bar was substituted for a high-carbohydrate snack on a low-fat, low-cholesterol diet, the chocolate did not increase LDL cholesterol (the bad type), and even seemed to raise HDL cholesterol (the good type), according to one study. But chocolate is high in fat and calories, so take it easy.

Quench your thirst with fruit juice. A low rate of heart disease in France — despite a high-fat diet — led researchers to investigate the French habit of drinking red wine with meals. They found that both purple grape juice and red wine lower the level of fat in your blood. The cholesterol-lowering effect comes from a naturally occurring compound that helps grapes resist mold. The darker the grape juice, the better.

Grapefruit juice can also lower the level of cholesterol in your blood, and improves the ratio of good cholesterol to bad. Grapefruit juice may also help you get rid of a fatty substance called plaque that can build up in your arteries and cause a heart attack.

Eat more garlic. The cholesterol-lowering effects of garlic have been repeatedly demonstrated in people with normal and high cholesterol, so don't hold back. Garlic seems to raise your good HDL levels too. If the odor bothers you, try it in tablets. These have been shown to be almost as effective as the cooked or raw cloves.

Fill up on fiber. Scientists generally believe that soluble fiber, the kind found in oat bran, helps lower LDL cholesterol and raise HDL cholesterol. Other sources of soluble fiber are barley, beans, peas, and many other vegetables. Corn fiber is also a good cholesterol reducer.

Pectin, a soluble fiber found in fruits such as apples and prunes, and psyllium, the fiber you'll find in many breakfast cereals and bulk laxatives, seem to lower cholesterol even better than oat bran. To get the best cholesterol-lowering results from a bulk laxative containing psyllium, mix it with your food instead of taking it between meals.

Serve up some soy. You can substitute soy protein for the animal proteins you normally eat. Soy proteins are high in polyunsaturated fat, low in saturated fat, and don't contain cholesterol, unlike animal proteins which are high in saturated fat and cholesterol. Polyunsaturated fat, when eaten in moderation, can help lower your cholesterol level. Soy proteins are also full of good quality nutrients.

Tofu is the most common kind of soy protein you'll find in the grocery stores. It comes in cake-like form, has a chewy texture, and takes on the flavor of foods and sauces that are cooked with it. You can stir-fry it, or use it in lasagna and chili. Soft tofu can go in salad dressings, dips, and even milkshakes.

Take time for tea. Green tea, and possibly black tea, may lower your cholesterol and improve your HDL to LDL ratio.

Five vitamins and minerals that help keep cholesterol in check

Niacin works, but be careful. Niacin, one of the B vitamins, is proven to lower total cholesterol and raise HDL. It is one of the cheapest and most effective cholesterol-lowering drugs around.

But without a doctor's supervision, it may not be safe. Doses high enough to lower cholesterol have been shown to cause very high blood sugar or lead to liver damage. In one study, liver problems developed at 1500 mg a day. If you have very high cholesterol, check with your doctor about this treatment.

Vitamin E looks promising. Several studies have documented the good effects vitamin E has on cholesterol. Most say that you need up to 800 international units (IU) a day — which is far more than you can get in your diet alone. Large amounts of vitamin E appear to be safe, but some researchers want to see more long-term studies before they are sure it's safe to take large doses for years. New research has showed that even much smaller amounts of vitamin E (25 IU) may be beneficial.

Calcium can help. In one study, when 56 people took a calcium carbonate supplement, their total cholesterol went down 4 percent and their HDL (good) cholesterol went up 4 percent. They took 400 mg of calcium three times a day. No side effects were reported.

Don't forget the C. Vitamin C, the No. 1 immune-system booster, also drives up your good cholesterol. In a recent study, the people who took in more than 60 mg of vitamin C a day (60 mg is the recommended dietary allowance) had the highest HDL levels.

Count on copper; zero in on zinc. The trace element zinc prevents copper from being absorbed by the body. A copper deficiency in the body can lower HDL (good) cholesterol levels and raise LDL (bad) levels. If you have a problem with cholesterol, you probably should not take zinc supplements, and look for the smallest amount of zinc in the multivitamins that you buy.

Simple lifestyle changes lead to lower cholesterol

Lose weight. People who are overweight usually have high cholesterol levels. Most can lower their LDL (bad) cholesterol and raise their HDL (good) cholesterol by dropping a few pounds.

Include the family. Your children can join you in the low-fat lifestyle; it certainly makes planning meals and cooking much simpler. Eating habits carry into adulthood, so get your kids started on a healthy eating pattern early. But don't start them before age 2. Babies need extra fat calories to develop properly.

Snack to your heart's content. Don't be afraid to snack several times a day on low-fat foods, such as yogurt, fruit, vegetables, bagels, and whole-grain breads and cereals. As a matter of fact, evidence points to lower cholesterol levels in people who eat small meals several times a day. Eating often keeps hormones like insulin from rising and signaling your body to make cholesterol. Just make sure your total intake of calories doesn't go up when you eat more often.

Keep moving. Evidence shows that exercise can lower LDL cholesterol and boost HDL cholesterol. But exercise alone can't perform this magic. People who exercise and still eat high-fat diets or who are overweight may not reap the cholesterol-lowering benefits.

Both aerobic exercise — walking, jogging, swimming, bicycling, cross-country skiing, and strength training (lifting weights or using weight machines) lower cholesterol levels. An analysis of 11 studies on weight training shows that this exercise lowers LDL cholesterol by 13 percent and raises HDL cholesterol by 5 percent. If you lift weights, use light to moderate weights and do many repetitions.

Sources —
ACP Journal (119,3:68)
American Heart Association news release (April 12, 1993)
Archives of Family Medicine (2,2:130)
Archives of Internal Medicine (153,17:2050)
Arteriosclerosis, Thrombosis, and Vascular Biology (15,3:325)
British Medical Journal (303,6805:785)
Cholesterol and Your Heart, American Heart Association, 7272, Greenville Ave., Dallas, Texas 75231-4596
Cholesterol in Children: Healthy Eating is a Family Affair, National Institutes of Health, 9000 Rockville Pike, Bethesda, Md. 20892
Food, Nutrition and Health (18,2:1 and 18,4:3)
HerbalGram (30,11)
Journal of the American Dietetic Association (94,4:425 and 94,1:65)
Medical Tribune (35,2:12 and 36,8:21)
Nutrition Forum (10,3:22)
Nutrition Research Newsletter (12,11/12:122)
Nutrition Today (28,3:30)
So You Have High Blood Cholesterol, Eating to Lower Your High Blood Cholesterol and National Cholesterol Education Program's Report of the Expert Panel on Blood Cholesterol Levels in Children and Adolescents, National Institutes of Health, National Heart, Lung and Blood Institute, National Cholesterol Education Program, NHLBI Information Center, P.O. Box 30105, Bethesda, Md. 20824 - 0105
The American Journal of Clinical Nutrition, (57,6:868; 58,4:501; 59,1:66; 59,5:1055; and 60,1:100)
The Atlanta Journal/Constitution (June 16, 1993; Nov. 11, 1993; March 16, 1995, H12; and March 30, 1995, H7)
The Journal of Nutrition (124,1:78)
The Lancet (341,8843:454 and 341,8836:27)

The New England Journal of Medicine (328,9:603)
The Physician and Sportsmedicine (21,10:103 and 22,7:15)
The Wall Street Journal (March 2, 1994, B9)
U.S. Pharmacist (18,9:100)

> Please check with your doctor for approval before taking or discontinuing
> any prescription drug or using a natural healing alternative.

HORMONAL DISORDERS

Prescription Drugs

Natural Alternatives

Prescription Drugs

FEMALE HORMONES

Estradiol

Brand name: *Estrace*

What this drug does for you:

Estradiol is the most potent estrogen, a female hormone. It is used to treat symptoms of menopause, such as vaginal dryness and hot flashes. It is also used to help prevent osteoporosis (loss of bone mass).

Possible side effects of this drug:

- Possible side effects include nausea, change in appetite or weight, breast tenderness, headache, eye problems, diarrhea, fluid retention, dizziness, depression, vaginal discharge or bleeding, breast lumps, nipple discharge, rash, joint pain, increased skin sensitivity to sunlight, a spotty darkening of the skin, and an increased risk of blood clots.
- Drugs containing estrogen cause some people's gums to bleed, swell, and become tender. You can help prevent this side effect by brushing and flossing your teeth regularly and massaging your gums.

Special warnings:

- Smoking increases your chances of developing serious side effects, such as stroke, heart attacks, and blood clots.
- If you experience any signs of a blood clot — shortness of breath, pain in your chest or legs, a severe headache, dizziness, or faintness — call your doctor immediately.
- Taking estrogen for a number of years may increase your risk of endometrial cancer (cancer of the lining of the uterus). Adding progestin (another female hormone) to your estrogen dose reduces that increased risk. Of course, if you have had your uterus removed, you will not develop endometrial cancer. Taking estrogen does not seem to increase your risk of breast cancer.

Pregnancy and nursing mothers:

Category X. See page 9 for description of categories. Estrogen therapy decreases the quantity and quality of breast milk.

Possible food and drug interaction:

- Check with your doctor if you are taking phenobarbital, warfarin, phenytoin, rifampin, amitriptyline, or imipramine.

Helpful hints:

- Take this drug after meals or with a snack if you experience nausea.
- Wear a sunscreen when you go outdoors if your skin burns more easily.
- If you forget to take a dose, take it as soon as you remember. If you don't remember until the following day, skip that dose and resume your regular schedule. Don't take two doses at the same time.
- Try to take your medicine at the same time every day to reduce side effects and help it work better.

Estradiol Transdermal System

Brand name: *Estraderm*

What this drug does for you:

Estradiol is the most potent estrogen, a female hormone. This patch you wear on your skin is used to treat symptoms of menopause, such as vaginal dryness and hot flashes. It is also used to help prevent osteoporosis (loss of bone mass).

Possible side effects of this drug:

- Side effects include nausea, vomiting, change in appetite or weight, breast tenderness, headache, eye problems, diarrhea, fluid retention, dizziness, depression, vaginal discharge or bleeding, breast lumps, nipple discharge, rash, joint pain, increased skin sensitivity to sunlight, a spotty darkening of the skin, and an increased risk of blood clots.
- Drugs containing estrogen cause some people's gums to bleed, swell, and become tender. You can help prevent this side effect by brushing and flossing your teeth regularly and massaging your gums.

Special warnings:
- Smoking increases your chances of developing serious side effects, such as stroke, heart attacks, and blood clots.
- If you experience any signs of a blood clot — shortness of breath, pain in your chest or legs, a severe headache, dizziness, or faintness — call your doctor immediately.
- Taking estrogen for a number of years may increase your risk of endometrial cancer (cancer of the lining of the uterus). Adding progestin (another female hormone) to your estrogen dose reduces that increased risk. Of course, if you have had your uterus removed, you will not develop endometrial cancer. Taking estrogen does not seem to increase your risk of breast cancer.

Pregnancy and nursing mothers:
Category X. See page 9 for description of categories. Estrogen therapy decreases the quantity and quality of breast milk.

Possible food and drug interaction:
- Check with your doctor if you are taking phenobarbital, warfarin, phenytoin, rifampin, amitriptyline, or imipramine.

Helpful hints:
- Take this drug after meals or with a snack if you experience nausea.
- Wear a sunscreen when you go outdoors if your skin burns more easily.
- Place adhesive side of patch on clean, dry skin of the buttocks or stomach. Avoid the waistline area since clothing may rub the patch off. Change the site of the patch weekly to help prevent skin irritation. If the patch falls off, reapply the same patch or use a new one.

Estrogens, Conjugated

Brand names: *PMB, Premarin*

What this drug does for you:
This female hormone is used to treat symptoms of menopause, such as vaginal dryness and hot flashes. It is also used to help prevent osteoporosis (loss of bone mass).

Possible side effects of this drug:
- Side effects include nausea, vomiting, change in appetite or weight, breast tenderness, headache, eye problems, diarrhea, fluid retention, dizziness, depression, vaginal discharge or bleeding, breast lumps, nipple discharge, rash, joint pain, increased skin sensitivity to sunlight, a spotty darkening of the skin, and an increased risk of blood clots.
- Drugs containing estrogen cause some people's gums to bleed, swell, and become tender. You can help prevent this side effect by brushing and flossing your teeth regularly and massaging your gums.

Special warnings:
- Smoking increases your chances of developing serious side effects, such

as stroke, heart attacks, and blood clots.

- If you experience any signs of a blood clot — shortness of breath, pain in your chest or legs, a severe headache, dizziness, or faintness — call your doctor immediately.
- Taking estrogen for a number of years may increase your risk of endometrial cancer (cancer of the lining of the uterus). Adding progestin (another female hormone) to your estrogen dose reduces that increased risk. Of course, if you have had your uterus removed, you will not develop endometrial cancer. Taking estrogen does not seem to increase your risk of breast cancer.

Pregnancy and nursing mothers:

Category X. See page 9 for description of categories. Drug is present in mother's milk. Estrogen therapy decreases the quantity and quality of breast milk.

Possible food and drug interaction:

- Check with your doctor if you are taking phenobarbital, warfarin, phenytoin, rifampin, amitriptyline, or imipramine.

Helpful hints:

- Take this drug after meals or with a snack if you experience nausea.
- Wear a sunscreen when you go outdoors if your skin burns more easily.
- If you forget to take a dose, take it as soon as you remember. If you don't remember until the following day, skip that dose and resume your regular schedule. Don't take two doses at the same time.
- Try to take your medicine at the same time every day to reduce side effects and help it work better.

Estropipate

Brand name: *Ogen*

What this drug does for you:

This drug is a form of estrogen, a female hormone. It is used to treat symptoms of menopause, such as vaginal dryness and hot flashes. It is also used to help prevent osteoporosis (loss of bone mass).

Possible side effects of this drug:

- Side effects include nausea, vomiting, change in appetite or weight, breast tenderness, headache, eye problems, diarrhea, fluid retention, dizziness, depression, vaginal discharge or bleeding, breast lumps, nipple discharge, rash, joint pain, increased skin sensitivity to sunlight, a spotty darkening of the skin, and an increased risk of blood clots.
- Drugs containing estrogen cause some people's gums to bleed, swell, and become tender. You can help prevent this side effect by brushing and flossing your teeth regularly and massaging your gums.

Special warnings:

- Smoking increases your chances of developing serious side effects, such as stroke, heart attacks, and blood clots.

- If you experience any signs of a blood clot — shortness of breath, pain in your chest or legs, a severe headache, dizziness, or faintness — call your doctor immediately.
- Taking estrogen for a number of years may increase your risk of endometrial cancer (cancer of the lining of the uterus). Adding progestin (another female hormone) to your estrogen dose reduces that increased risk. Of course, if you have had your uterus removed, you will not develop endometrial cancer. Taking estrogen does not seem to increase your risk of breast cancer.

Pregnancy and nursing mothers:

Category X. See page 9 for description of categories. Estrogen therapy decreases the quantity and quality of breast milk.

Possible food and drug interaction:

- Check with your doctor if you are taking phenobarbital, warfarin, phenytoin, rifampin, amitriptyline, or imipramine.

Helpful hints:

- Take this drug after meals or with a snack if you experience nausea.
- Wear a sunscreen when you go outdoors if your skin burns more easily.
- If you forget to take a dose, take it as soon as you remember. If you don't remember until the following day, skip that dose and resume your regular schedule. Don't take two doses at the same time.
- Try to take your medicine at the same time every day to reduce side effects and help it work better.

Ethinyl Estradiol and Ethynodiol Diacetate

Brand name: *Demulen*

What this drug does for you:

This drug, an oral contraceptive, is mainly used to prevent pregnancy by changing the hormone balance of the body. It contains a higher-than-average dose of estrogen and progestin.

Possible side effects of this drug:

- Side effects include changes in appetite, acne, headache, nausea, breakthrough bleeding and spotting, breast tenderness or enlargement, stomach cramps, changes in weight, depression, vaginal discharge or bleeding, breast lumps, nipple discharge, rash, joint pain, a spotty darkening of the skin, and an increased risk of blood clots.
- Drugs containing estrogen cause some people's gums to bleed, swell, and become tender. You can help prevent this side effect by brushing and flossing your teeth regularly and massaging your gums. Estrogen-containing oral contraceptives may also cause a healing problem called dry socket after a tooth has been removed. If you are going to have a tooth removed, tell your dentist that you are taking oral contraceptives.

Special warnings:

- Smoking increases your chances of developing serious side effects, such as stroke, heart attacks, and blood clots.

- If you experience any signs of a blood clot — shortness of breath, pain in your chest or legs, a severe headache, dizziness, or faintness — call your doctor immediately.
- Oral contraceptives should be used with caution if you are over 40, or if you have any of the following conditions: thyroid disease, high blood pressure, heart disease, high cholesterol, asthma, liver disease, diabetes, epilepsy, kidney or gallbladder disease, or the blood disorder porphyria.
- If you wear contact lenses and begin to have problems with them, check with your doctor.

Pregnancy and nursing mothers:

Category X. See page 9 for description of categories. Drug is present in mother's milk. It may cause jaundice or enlarged breasts in nursing infant.

Possible food and drug interaction:

- Check with your doctor if you are taking phenobarbital, warfarin, phenytoin, rifampin, amitriptyline, or imipramine.

Helpful hints:

- Take this drug at the same time every day so you are less likely to forget to take it.
- If you forget to take one pill, take it as soon as you remember. If you forget to take more than one pill, do not take the missed pills. Instead, resume your normal medication schedule, but use another method of contraception for the remainder of the cycle.

Ethinyl Estradiol and Desogestrel

Brand names: *Desogen, Ortho-Cept*

What this drug does for you:

This drug, an oral contraceptive, is mainly used to prevent pregnancy by changing the hormone balance of the body. It contains both estrogen and progestin.

Possible side effects of this drug:

- Side effects include changes in appetite, acne, headache, nausea, breakthrough bleeding and spotting, breast tenderness or enlargement, stomach cramps, changes in weight, depression, vaginal discharge or bleeding, breast lumps, nipple discharge, rash, joint pain, a spotty darkening of the skin, and an increased risk of blood clots.
- Drugs containing estrogen cause some people's gums to bleed, swell, and become tender. You can help prevent this side effect by brushing and flossing your teeth regularly and massaging your gums. Estrogen-containing oral contraceptives may also cause a healing problem called dry socket after a tooth has been removed. If you are going to have a tooth removed, tell your dentist that you are taking oral contraceptives.

Special warnings:
- Smoking increases your chances of developing serious side effects, such as stroke, heart attacks, and blood clots.
- If you experience any signs of a blood clot — shortness of breath, pain in your chest or legs, a severe headache, dizziness, or faintness — call your doctor immediately.
- Oral contraceptives should be used with caution if you are over 40, or if you have any of the following conditions: thyroid disease, high blood pressure, heart disease, high cholesterol, asthma, liver disease, diabetes, epilepsy, kidney or gallbladder disease, or the blood disorder porphyria.
- If you wear contact lenses and begin to have problems with them, check with your doctor.

Pregnancy and nursing mothers:
Category X. See page 9 for description of categories. Drug is present in mother's milk. It may cause jaundice or enlarged breasts in nursing infant.

Possible food and drug interaction:
- Check with your doctor if you are taking phenobarbital, warfarin, phenytoin, rifampin, amitriptyline, tetracycline, or imipramine.

Helpful hints:
- Take this drug at the same time every day so you are less likely to forget to take it.
- If you forget to take one pill, take it as soon as you remember. If you forget to take more than one pill, do not take the missed pills. Instead, resume your normal medication schedule, but use another method of contraception for the remainder of the cycle.

Ethinyl Estradiol and Levonorgestrel

Brand names: *Levlen, Tri-Levlen, Triphasil*

What this drug does for you:
This drug, an oral contraceptive, is mainly used to prevent pregnancy by changing the hormone balance of the body. It contains both estrogen and progestin.

Possible side effects of this drug:
- Side effects include changes in appetite, acne, headache, nausea, breakthrough bleeding and spotting, breast tenderness or enlargement, stomach cramps, changes in weight, depression, vaginal discharge or bleeding, breast lumps, nipple discharge, rash, joint pain, a spotty darkening of the skin, and an increased risk of blood clots.
- Drugs containing estrogen cause some people's gums to bleed, swell, and become tender. You can help prevent this side effect by brushing and flossing your teeth regularly and massaging your gums. Estrogen-containing oral contraceptives may also cause a healing problem called dry socket after a tooth has been removed. If you are going to have a tooth

removed, tell your dentist that you are taking oral contraceptives.

Special warnings:

- Smoking increases your chances of developing serious side effects, such as stroke, heart attacks, and blood clots.
- If you experience any signs of a blood clot — shortness of breath, pain in your chest or legs, a severe headache, dizziness, or faintness — call your doctor immediately.
- Oral contraceptives should be used with caution if you are over 40, or if you have any of the following conditions: thyroid disease, high blood pressure, heart disease, high cholesterol, asthma, liver disease, diabetes, epilepsy, kidney or gallbladder disease, or the blood disorder porphyria.
- If you wear contact lenses and begin to have problems with them, check with your doctor.

Pregnancy and nursing mothers:

Category X. See page 9 for description of categories. Drug is present in mother's milk. It may cause jaundice or enlarged breasts in nursing infant.

Possible food and drug interaction:

- Check with your doctor if you are taking phenobarbital, warfarin, phenytoin, rifampin, amitriptyline, tetracycline, or imipramine.

Helpful hints:

- Take this drug at the same time every day so you are less likely to forget to take it.
- If you forget to take one pill, take it as soon as you remember. If you forget to take more than one pill, do not take the missed pills. Instead, resume your normal medication schedule, but use another method of contraception for the remainder of the cycle.

Ethinyl Estradiol and Norethindrone

Brand names: *Modicon, Ortho-Novum 1/35, Ortho-Novum 7/7/7, Ortho-Novum 10/11*

What this drug does for you:

This drug, an oral contraceptive, is mainly used to prevent pregnancy by changing the hormone balance of the body. It contains both estrogen and progestin.

Possible side effects of this drug:

- Side effects include changes in appetite, acne, headache, nausea, breakthrough bleeding and spotting, breast tenderness or enlargement, stomach cramps, changes in weight, depression, vaginal discharge or bleeding, breast lumps, nipple discharge, rash, joint pain, a spotty darkening of the skin, and an increased risk of blood clots.
- Drugs containing estrogen cause some people's gums to bleed, swell, and become tender. You can help prevent this side effect by brushing and flossing your teeth regularly and massaging your gums. Estrogen-con-

taining oral contraceptives may also cause a healing problem called dry socket after a tooth has been removed. If you are going to have a tooth removed, tell your dentist that you are taking oral contraceptives.

Special warnings:

- Smoking increases your chances of developing serious side effects, such as stroke, heart attacks, and blood clots.
- If you experience any signs of a blood clot — shortness of breath, pain in your chest or legs, a severe headache, dizziness, or faintness — call your doctor immediately.
- Oral contraceptives should be used with caution if you are over 40, or if you have any of the following conditions: thyroid disease, high blood pressure, heart disease, high cholesterol, asthma, liver disease, diabetes, epilepsy, kidney or gallbladder disease, or the blood disorder porphyria.
- If you wear contact lenses and begin to have problems with them, check with your doctor.

Pregnancy and nursing mothers:

Category X. See page 9 for description of categories. Drug is present in mother's milk. It may cause jaundice or enlarged breasts in nursing infant.

Possible food and drug interaction:

- Check with your doctor if you are taking phenobarbital, warfarin, phenytoin, rifampin, amitriptyline, tetracycline, or imipramine.

Helpful hints:

- Take this drug at the same time every day so you are less likely to forget to take it.
- If you forget to take one pill, take it as soon as you remember. If you forget to take more than one pill, do not take the missed pills. Instead, resume your normal medication schedule, but use another method of contraception for the remainder of the cycle.

Ethinyl Estradiol, Norethindrone Acetate and Ferrous Fumarate

Brand name: *Loestrin Fe*

What this drug does for you:

This drug, a low-dose oral contraceptive, is mainly used to prevent pregnancy by changing the hormone balance of the body. The active tablets contain estrogen and progestin, and the inactive tablets contain iron.

Possible side effects of this drug:

- Side effects include changes in appetite, acne, headache, nausea, breakthrough bleeding and spotting, breast tenderness or enlargement, stomach cramps, changes in weight, depression, vaginal discharge or bleeding, breast lumps, nipple discharge, rash, joint pain, a spotty darkening of the skin, and an increased risk of blood clots.
- Drugs containing estrogen cause some people's gums to bleed, swell, and become tender. You can help prevent this side effect by brushing and

flossing your teeth regularly and massaging your gums. Estrogen-containing oral contraceptives may also cause a healing problem called dry socket after a tooth has been removed. If you are going to have a tooth removed, tell your dentist that you are taking oral contraceptives.

Special warnings:

- Smoking increases your chances of developing serious side effects, such as stroke, heart attacks, and blood clots.
- If you experience any signs of a blood clot — shortness of breath, pain in your chest or legs, a severe headache, dizziness, or faintness — call your doctor immediately.
- Oral contraceptives should be used with caution if you are over 40, or if you have any of the following conditions: thyroid disease, high blood pressure, heart disease, high cholesterol, asthma, liver disease, diabetes, epilepsy, kidney or gallbladder disease, or the blood disorder porphyria.
- If you wear contact lenses and begin to have problems with them, check with your doctor.

Pregnancy and nursing mothers:

Category X. See page 9 for description of categories. Drug is present in mother's milk. It may cause jaundice or enlarged breasts in nursing infant.

Possible food and drug interaction:

- Check with your doctor if you are taking phenobarbital, warfarin, phenytoin, rifampin, amitriptyline, tetracycline, or imipramine.

Helpful hints:

- Take this drug at the same time every day so you are less likely to forget to take it.
- If you forget to take one pill, take it as soon as you remember. If you forget to take more than one pill, do not take the missed pills. Instead, resume your normal medication schedule, but use another method of contraception for the remainder of the cycle.

Ethinyl Estradiol and Norgestrel

Brand name: *Lo/Ovral*

What this drug does for you:

This drug, an oral contraceptive, is mainly used to prevent pregnancy by changing the hormone balance of the body. It contains a low dose of estrogen and progestin.

Possible side effects of this drug:

- Side effects include changes in appetite, acne, headache, nausea, breakthrough bleeding and spotting, breast tenderness or enlargement, stomach cramps, changes in weight, depression, vaginal discharge or bleeding, breast lumps, nipple discharge, rash, joint pain, a spotty darkening of the skin, and an increased risk of blood clots.
- Drugs containing estrogen cause some people's gums to bleed, swell, and

become tender. You can help prevent this side effect by brushing and flossing your teeth regularly and massaging your gums. Estrogen-containing oral contraceptives may also cause a healing problem called dry socket after a tooth has been removed. If you are going to have a tooth removed, tell your dentist that you are taking oral contraceptives.

Special warnings:
- Smoking increases your chances of developing serious side effects, such as stroke, heart attacks, and blood clots.
- If you experience any signs of a blood clot — shortness of breath, pain in your chest or legs, a severe headache, dizziness, or faintness — call your doctor immediately.
- Oral contraceptives should be used with caution if you are over 40, or if you have any of the following conditions: thyroid disease, high blood pressure, heart disease, high cholesterol, asthma, liver disease, diabetes, epilepsy, kidney or gallbladder disease, or the blood disorder porphyria.
- If you wear contact lenses and begin to have problems with them, check with your doctor.

Pregnancy and nursing mothers:
Category X. See page 9 for description of categories. Drug is present in mother's milk. It may cause jaundice or enlarged breasts in nursing infant.

Possible food and drug interaction:
- Check with your doctor if you are taking phenobarbital, warfarin, phenytoin, rifampin, amitriptyline, tetracycline, or imipramine.

Helpful hints:
- Take this drug at the same time every day so you are less likely to forget to take it.
- If you forget to take one pill, take it as soon as you remember. If you forget to take more than one pill, do not take the missed pills. Instead, resume your normal medication schedule, but use another method of contraception for the remainder of the cycle.

Medroxyprogesterone

Brand names: *Amen, Cycrin, Depo-Provera, Provera* **(Generic available)**

What this drug does for you:
This female hormone prevents ovulation and thins the lining of the uterus. It is also used to treat endometriosis, certain forms of endometrial or kidney cancers, abnormal uterine bleeding, and some menstrual disorders. Women may also receive an injection of Depo-Provera every three months to prevent pregnancy.

Possible side effects of this drug:
- Common side effects include rash, itching, hives, skin eruptions, hair loss, blood clots, menstrual abnormalities, fluid retention and swelling, nausea, fever, mental depression, and jaundice (yellow eyes and skin, dark urine).

- Rare side effects include lactation or breast tenderness.

Special warnings:

- This drug should not be used by people with a history of any type of clotting disorder, brain hemorrhage, liver problems, breast cancer, or unexplained vaginal bleeding.
- A complete physical examination including a pap smear should be done before treatment begins.
- Drug may be stopped if vision problems occur.
- Changes in menstruation may occur, and if treatment is prolonged, menstruation may stop.
- If you have heart or kidney problems, asthma, epilepsy or migraines, use with caution as water retention (a side effect of the drug) can adversely affect these conditions.

Pregnancy and nursing mothers:

Don't take this drug while you are pregnant because it can cause birth defects. Drug is present in mother's milk.

Possible food and drug interaction:

- The effects of this drug may be decreased by the cancer drug aminoglutethimide.

Nafarelin

Brand name: *Synarel*

What this drug does for you:

This drug is used to treat endometriosis.

Possible side effects of this drug:

- Side effects include hot flashes, headache, acne, muscle pain, insomnia, vaginal dryness, nasal irritation, decreased sex drive, reduction in breast size, and emotional instability.

Special warnings:

- Do not use this drug if you have any abnormal, undiagnosed vaginal bleeding.
- If you smoke, drink, have a family history of osteoporosis, or use any other drugs, such as corticosteroids or anticonvulsants that may cause bone loss, you should use this drug with caution.
- This drug may cause cysts to form on the ovaries. Notify your doctor if regular menstrual periods persist.
- Avoid sneezing while using this spray or immediately afterwards as the drug may not be absorbed correctly.

Pregnancy and nursing mothers:

Category X. See page 9 for description of categories. Do not use during pregnancy or nursing. Pregnancy should be ruled out before this drug is taken, and appropriate birth control should be used throughout treatment. Not known if drug is present in mother's milk.

Possible food and drug interaction:
- Do not use a spray decongestant within two hours of this drug.

Norethindrone

Brand names: *Micronor, Nor-QD*

What this drug does for you:
This drug, a progestin-only oral contraceptive, is mainly used to prevent pregnancy by changing the hormone balance of the body.

Possible side effects of this drug:
- Side effects include changes in appetite, acne, headache, nausea, break-through bleeding and spotting, breast tenderness or enlargement, stomach cramps, changes in weight, depression, vaginal discharge or bleeding, breast lumps, nipple discharge, rash, joint pain, a spotty darkening of the skin, and an increased risk of blood clots.

Special warnings:
- Smoking increases your chances of developing serious side effects, such as stroke, heart attacks, and blood clots.
- If you experience any signs of a blood clot — shortness of breath, pain in your chest or legs, a severe headache, dizziness, or faintness — call your doctor immediately.
- Oral contraceptives should be used with caution if you are over 40, or if you have any of the following conditions: thyroid disease, high blood pressure, heart disease, high cholesterol, asthma, liver disease, diabetes, epilepsy, kidney or gallbladder disease, or the blood disorder porphyria.

Pregnancy and nursing mothers:
Category X. See page 9 for description of categories. Drug is present in mother's milk. It may cause jaundice or enlarged breasts in nursing infant.

Possible food and drug interactions:
- Check with your doctor if you are taking phenobarbital, warfarin, phenytoin, rifampin, amitriptyline, tetracycline, or imipramine.

Helpful hints:
- Take this drug at the same time every day so you are less likely to forget to take it.
- If you forget to take one pill, take it as soon as you remember. If you forget to take more than one pill, do not take the missed pills. Instead, resume your normal medication schedule, but use another method of contraception for the remainder of the cycle.

THYROID DRUGS

Levothyroxine

Brand names: *Levothroid, Levoxine, Synthroid* **(Generic available)**

What this drug does for you:
This drug is used to replace thyroid hormones when the thyroid gland does not produce enough. It is also used to suppress the release of thyroid stimulating hormone from the pituitary gland for people with some forms of goiter and thyroid cancer.

Possible side effects of this drug:
- Side effects are rare, but overdose may occur. Symptoms of overdose include diarrhea, nervousness, stomach cramps, rapid heartbeat, headache, weight loss, palpitations, fever, sweating, chest pain, insomnia, and irregular heartbeat.

Special warnings:
- This drug should not be used by people with abnormal adrenal or thyroid glands.
- If you have heart or blood vessel abnormalities, such as angina, or if you have diabetes or adrenal gland abnormalities, you should use this drug with extreme caution.
- Diabetics may need their dosage of antidiabetic medication adjusted.
- Periodic lab tests should be done to reassess thyroid function and speed of blood clotting.
- Call your doctor if you have any signs of overdose.

Pregnancy and nursing mothers:
Category A. See page 9 for description of categories. Drug is present in mother's milk.

Possible food and drug interactions:
- This drug may increase the effects of the anticoagulant warfarin and decrease the levels or effects of insulin in diabetics.
- Levels of this drug may be reduced by the cholesterol reducers cholestyramine and colestipol.

Liothyronine

Brand names: *Cytomel, Triostat*

What this drug does for you:
This drug is used to replace thyroid hormones when the thyroid gland does not produce enough. It is also used to suppress the release of thyroid stimulating hormone from the pituitary gland for people with some forms of goiter and thyroid cancer.

Possible side effects of this drug:
- Side effects are rare, but overdose may occur. Symptoms of overdose

include diarrhea, nervousness, stomach cramps, rapid heartbeat, headache, weight loss, palpitations, fever, sweating, chest pain, insomnia, and irregular heartbeat.

Special warnings:
- You should not use this drug if you have abnormal adrenal or thyroid gland function.
- If you have heart or blood vessel abnormalities, such as angina, or diabetes or adrenal gland abnormalities, you should use with extreme caution.
- Diabetics may need their dosage of antidiabetic medication adjusted.
- Periodic lab tests should be done to reassess thyroid function and speed of blood clotting.
- Call your doctor if you have any signs of overdose.

Pregnancy and nursing mothers:
Category A. See page 9 for description of categories. Drug is present in mother's milk.

Possible food and drug interactions:
- This drug may increase the effects of the anticoagulant warfarin and decrease the levels or effects of insulin in diabetics.
- Levels of this drug may be reduced by the cholesterol reducers cholestyramine and colestipol.
- Taking this drug along with the asthma drug epinephrine may cause heart problems.

Thyroid, desiccated

Brand names: *Armour Thyroid, S-P-T* (Generic available)

What this drug does for you:
This drug is used to replace thyroid hormones when the thyroid gland does not produce enough. It is also used to suppress the release of thyroid stimulating hormone from the pituitary gland for people with some forms of goiter and thyroid cancer.

Possible side effects of this drug:
- Side effects are rare, but overdose may occur. Symptoms of overdose include diarrhea, nervousness, stomach cramps, rapid heartbeat, headache, weight loss, palpitations, fever, sweating, chest pain, insomnia, and irregular heartbeat.

Special warnings:
- You should not use this drug if you have abnormal adrenal or thyroid gland function.
- If you have heart or blood vessel abnormalities, such as angina, or diabetes or adrenal gland abnormalities, you should use with extreme caution.
- Diabetics may need their dosage of antidiabetic medication adjusted.
- Periodic lab tests should be done to reassess thyroid function and speed

of blood clotting.
- Call your doctor if any signs of overdose occur.

Pregnancy and nursing mothers:

Category A. See page 9 for description of categories. Drug is present in mother's milk.

Possible food and drug interactions:

- This drug may increase the effects of the anticoagulant warfarin and decrease the levels or effects of insulin in diabetics.
- Levels of this drug may be reduced by the cholesterol reducers cholestyramine and colestipol.
- Taking this drug along with the asthma drug epinephrine may cause heart problems.

Natural Alternatives

HYPERTHYROIDISM

- ◀ Bulging eyeballs
- ◀ Frequent bowel movements
- ◀ Hyperactivity
- ◀ Insomnia
- ◀ Menstrual problems
- ◀ Sensitivity to heat
- ◀ Fast pulse
- ◀ Goiter
- ◀ Inability to gain weight
- ◀ Irritability
- ◀ Nervousness

Taming your energy

Everyone is searching for ways to get extra energy. But what do you do if your body wants to go at a faster pace than you want it to? An overactive thyroid, called hyperthyroidism, can produce too high a rate of metabolism, sending your body into fast forward. Besides medical treatment, there are several things you can do to press pause and slow things down.

Read the label. Many nutritional supplements contain animal thyroid hormones which can send your gland into overdrive. Several case studies highlight people seeking medical help for hyperthyroidism. All were taking large doses of nutritional supplements containing animal thyroid hormone at the time. When they stopped taking the tablets, their glands returned to normal.

Read the label to see if your supplement contains thyroid or desiccated thyroid. Don't exceed the recommended daily dosage since excess hormones can be toxic.

Relax. Stress can cause your body to secrete more thyroid hormones.

Eat a high-protein diet. Tissue mass can be lost from thyroid overactivity. To fight the decline, eat protein-rich foods like meats, cheese, dry beans, peas, and whole-grain breads.

Give yourself an A vitamin. In studies of countries with high rates of goiter, or an enlarged thyroid, people had low levels of vitamin A. The difference was most significant in young adults. Eating foods rich in vitamin A could reduce your risk of a problem thyroid.

Monitor your treatment. Radioactive iodine and surgery are commonly used to treat an overactive thyroid. This usually leads to an underactive thyroid, or hypothyroidism. Be sure and talk to your doctor about any side effects you are experiencing. For mild cases of hyperthyroidism, anti-thyroid drug therapy can be used.

Having a hyper gland can make you feel like your life is a movie going by in a blur. Some people suffering from hyperthyroidism report feeling "wired" or "always on edge." By adding relaxation and healthy eating to your thyroid therapy, you can help put your body and your life back in focus.

Sources —
> *Complete Guide to Symptoms, Illness and Surgery*, Putnam Berkley Group, New York, 1995
> *Encyclopedia of Natural Medicine*, Prima Publishing, Rocklin, Calif., 1991
> *FDA Consumer* (26,10:34)
> *International Journal for Vitamin & Nutrition Research* (58,2:155)
> *Journal of Family Practice* (38,3:287)

HYPOTHYROIDISM

◄ Constipation
◄ Difficulty losing weight
◄ Fatigue
◄ Low body temperature
◄ Muscle and joint pain
◄ Sensitivity to cold

◄ Depression
◄ Dry skin
◄ Headaches
◄ Menstrual problems
◄ Recurrent infections

Energize your life

Feel like your body is running in slow motion? You could attribute it to aging, but it may be just a gland gone wrong. An underactive thyroid condition, called hypothyroidism, can zap your energy as easily as Father Time. While hormone treatments may be necessary, there are several things you can do to help speed things up again.

Make your own energy. Numerous studies show that exercise increases your metabolism and tissue's sensitivity to thyroid hormones. Also, dieting can slow down your metabolism, so work out to keep up your energy.

Emphasize high-fiber foods. Eating plenty of fresh fruits and vegetables plus whole grains will help prevent the constipation that often accompanies hypothyroidism.

Shed extra pounds. An underactive thyroid decreases your body's use of fat, causing you to gain more weight. Another reason to watch your food intake is that even mild hypothyroidism can raise your cholesterol level significantly.

Eat your iodine. You only need a small daily amount of iodine, so don't take supplements unless directed by your doctor. Instead, eat foods that are rich in iodine like seafood, dairy products, and vegetables.

Take your vitamins. The vitamins A, B, C, and E, as well as zinc, help the thyroid function. Taking a daily multivitamin could also help with some of the side effects of hypothyroidism, such as dry skin.

Avoid excess iron. Stay away from iron supplements or multivitamins with iron. In a Canadian study, 14 people suffering from hypothyroidism were given iron supplements and thyroid medicine. After 12 weeks, nine people had an increase in hypothyroidism. Scientists think that iron may bind to the thyroid hormones and reduce their effectiveness.

Avoid foods with goitrogens. Foods such as turnips, cabbage, soybeans, and peanuts contain substances called goitrogens which prevent the utilization of iodine by your body.

Watch your dosage. Synthetic hormones are often used to restore thyroid balance, but need to be closely monitored. Too high a dosage can put your thyroid into overdrive, causing hyperthyroidism.

An underactive gland can be caused by many things including infection, iodine deficiency, or even giving birth. While it may take some extra hormones to get you moving, staying active and eating right should get you back up to the speed of life.

Sources —
Annals of Internal Medicine (117,12:1010)
Complete Guide to Symptoms, Illness and Surgery, Putnam Berkley Group, New York, 1995
Encyclopedia of Natural Medicine, Prima Publishing, Rocklin, Calif., 1991
FDA Consumer (26,10:34)

MENOPAUSE

◀ Chills
◀ Dizziness
◀ Fatigue
◀ Headache
◀ Hot flashes
◀ Irritability
◀ Mood swings
◀ Nervousness
◀ Urinary tract disturbances

◀ Depression
◀ Excitability
◀ Gastrointestinal disorders
◀ Heart tremors
◀ Insomnia
◀ Lack of interest in previously enjoyable activities
◀ Numbness, tingling

Beyond hormone therapy: Natural alternatives for menopause

"Free at last! Free at last! Thank God Almighty, we are free at last!"

Even though menopause wasn't what Martin Luther King had in mind when he uttered those historic words, they certainly seem appropriate to women experiencing the liberation of menopause.

Finally, you're free from the worry of an unplanned pregnancy, difficult deci-

---

Four ways to fend off a hot flash

◁ Dress in layers. When you feel a hot flash coming on, remove as many layers as are socially acceptable until you feel cooler.

◁ Drink a glass of cold water or juice.

◁ Keep an ice pack or a thermos of ice water beside your bed at night to fight off nighttime hot flashes.

◁ Choose cotton. Cotton sheets, lingerie, and clothing absorb excess moisture while letting your skin breathe.

Source —
Menopause, National Institutes of Health, NIH Publication No. 92-3466

---

sions concerning contraception, painful periods, PMS symptoms, and a host of other uncomfortable problems that often accompany a woman's reproductive years.

Children are moving out, leaving more time for you, your friends, your hobbies, and your spouse. But like every great opportunity, menopause poses some special challenges.

Know the three stages of menopause. Menopause actually occurs in three stages. Premenopause begins in your early 40s. Your ovaries gradually produce less estrogen, and your periods become irregular, often alternating between light and heavy.

Actual menopause occurs when you have your last menstrual period, usually around age 52. You've reached the third and final stage, postmenopause, when you've gone for 12 full months without a period. During these transition years, many women opt for hormone replacement therapy (HRT) to help them cope with hot flashes, vaginal dryness, mood swings, and insomnia.

In addition to relieving the troublesome symptoms of menopause, HRT provides protection against heart disease and osteoporosis. (If you're taking estrogen to prevent osteoporosis, see the Osteoporosis section of this chapter for more self-help.)

Other women, for health or personal reasons, seek other answers to menopause. These answers are often hard to find at your typical doctor's office.

Discover your alternatives. A 1993 Gallup Poll reported that less than 2 percent of doctors consulted about menopause mentioned alternative therapies. In fact, many doctors doubt the effectiveness of such remedies.

But Dr. Susan Lark, author of The Estrogen Decision, believes women should be aware of all their options, including alternative therapies. Even for women who decide to have HRT, the alternative therapies Lark describes in her book can make sailing through menopause a much smoother ride.

Lark outlines a plan emphasizing diet, exercise, and stress management that can help you relieve your symptoms of menopause, no matter how slight or severe.

Center your diet around beans, peas, grains, raw seeds and nuts, fruits, vegetables, and fish high in Omega-3. These foods contain essential nutrients that help your body cope naturally with menopause. Some fish rich in Omega-3 are Atlantic mackerel, lake trout, and bluefin tuna.

Add soybeans to your diet. Women in Asian countries who eat lots of soybean products have a lower rate of the health hazards that can come with menopause. Tofu, one soy product, is available in many supermarkets. It can be scrambled like eggs and used in stir-fry recipes, lasagna, or chili, or pureed into dips and salad dressings. Other soy products are soy milk, miso, and tempeh.

Limit caffeine, alcohol, sugar, salt, meat, fatty dairy products, and saturated oils, such as coconut and palm-kernel oil. These foods will either make your menopausal symptoms worse or increase your risk of developing disorders that often occur during the postmenopausal period, including arthritis, cancer, diabetes, heart disease, and stroke.

Include a daily multivitamin. The supplement should provide 100 percent of the recommended daily allowance (RDA) for most nutrients. Dr. Lark recommends supplements because even a healthy diet usually will not include all the nutrients your body needs to completely relieve your menopausal symptoms. Keep in mind, however, that supplements won't do you much good if you don't also follow the healthy diet outlined above.

Get herbal relief. Dr. Lark suggests that herbs, when used wisely, are a healthy addition to a nutritious diet. She has developed three different special menopause formulas, which you can purchase at an herb shop or make at home by combining small amounts of the herbs listed for each formula.

Formula 1. This combination of herbs helps relieve hot flashes and vaginal dryness. Mix the following herbs together in equal amounts: black cohosh, don quai, false unicorn root, fennel, anise, and blessed thistle.

Formula 2. This formula helps relieve tiredness and weakness. Mix the following herbs together in equal amounts: ginger, oat straw, ginkgo biloba, and Siberian ginseng.

Formula 3. These herbs help combat anxiety, insomnia, and irritability. Mix the following herbs together in equal amounts: valerian root, catnip, chamomile, and hops.

Dr. Lark recommends that you add the herbs to tea or take with meals. Don't take more than one to two herbal capsules or drink more than one to two cups of herbal tea daily. Although Lark considers all of these herbs safe, you should stop using them if you have any symptoms that make you uncomfortable.

Be sure to let your doctor know you are using herbs. They can sometimes react with other medicines you may be taking.

Practice stress management. During menopausal years, women often find that their unstable hormones lead to more extreme responses to stress. Relaxation techniques practiced for 10 to 20 minutes a day will help you feel calmer and more in control.

Deep breathing is an especially helpful relaxation exercise you can practice anytime, anywhere: Close your eyes and focus on moving your stomach in and out as you breathe through your nose. Breathe in and out 10 times or until you begin to feel yourself relax.

Beat vaginal dryness with water-based lubricants. To combat the vaginal dryness that often accompanies menopause and makes sexual intercourse uncomfortable, use a water-soluble surgical jelly (not petroleum jelly). Water-soluble lubricants help prevent infection, and they aren't as likely to irritate as petroleum-based lubricants.

Take care with personal care. To lower your increased risk of infections after menopause and reduce your chances of having to take antibiotics, follow these steps:

◁ Urinate before and after sexual intercourse.
◁ Take regular bathroom breaks. (You don't want your bladder to remain full for long periods of time.)
◁ Keep your genital area very clean. (However, douching won't prevent infection.)

Exercise your symptoms away. Regular exercise will relieve your hot flashes, improve bladder control, help you concentrate better, think clearer, and solve problems more effectively. You'll also reduce your risk of osteoporosis and heart disease.

Start slowly if you haven't exercised in a while. Aim to exercise at least three times a week for 30 minutes at a time. Try to set aside a regular time to exercise. Aerobic exercise, such as walking, dancing, swimming, or bicycling, is especially helpful.

Say yes to yoga. Through a series of gentle exercises and stretches, yoga restores balance to your muscles, cells, and tissues, which helps your body cope with the hormone changes of menopause. In her book, Dr. Lark recommends specific yoga exercises for the different symptoms of menopause.

For example, the Locust stretch helps control irregular or excessive menstrual bleeding, relieves hot flashes, and helps improve bladder control. You can find more information on yoga at your local library.

Try some hands-on healing. Lark suggests acupressure, an ancient Oriental therapy which involves applying finger pressure to different parts of the body to treat different ailments. She says that many women she has treated for menopause have found this technique helpful for relieving hot flashes, insomnia, mood swings, and tiredness.

Here's an easy acupressure technique you can try at home to relieve hot flashes and emotional tension: Sit in a chair. Press the first three fingers of your right hand on the area between your eyebrows, right at the top of your nose. Apply steady pressure for one to three minutes.

If you greet the changes of menopause with good health habits and a few simple lifestyle changes, you'll be in great shape to glide through it gracefully. Enjoy your newfound freedom!

Sources —

Age Page: Should You Take Estrogen, National Institute on Aging, Federal Building, 6th Floor, Bethesda, Md., 20892, 1988

Medical Tribune for the Internist and Cardiologist (36,7:11)

Menopause, National Institutes of Health, NIH Publication No. 92-3466

The Estrogen Decision, Westchester Publishing, Los Altos, Calif., 1994

Prevent fractures; fall-proof your home

Osteoporosis is responsible for about 1.3 million bone fractures a year. Take these steps to protect yourself from potentially dangerous falls and fractures:

◁ Install night lights along the path to your bathroom. Most serious falls in older people occur during nighttime trips to the bathroom. A lighted path reduces your chances of stumbling.

◁ Tape down rugs and use only nonskid floor wax.

◁ Add handrails in halls and grab bars in bath tubs and showers.

◁ Keep floors clear of items which could trip you up.

◁ Stand up slowly after meals. Blood pressure tends to drop after a meal, which can make you dizzy, so be especially careful after eating.

Sources —
Medical Tribune (33,24:2)
The Physician and Sportsmedicine (20,11:147)

OSTEOPOROSIS

◀ Backache
◀ Bone fractures from minor injury (common sites include spine, wrist, and hip)
◀ Curving of the spine (sometimes called dowager's hump)
◀ Loss of height

How to outwit osteoporosis

Seem to be shrinking? As startling as it may seem, you could be. Even though human beings generally arrive preshrunk and with at least a 20-year growth guarantee, sometimes something called osteoporosis gets the best of you, and you actually start to shrink.

In fact, osteoporosis affects quite a few adults. One in four women over age 60 and half of all men and women over 75 suffer from osteoporosis. Osteoporosis causes your bones to lose calcium and other minerals very slowly, over many years. The bones aren't diseased or abnormal in any way. They're just not as dense as they were when you were younger. Women going through menopause lose even more bone than normal as their bodies produce less and less estrogen.

In addition to making you look shrunken or humped, these thin, weak bones are easily broken, especially in the spine, wrist, or hip. But you don't have to settle for shrinking or let osteoporosis slow you down. You can outwit osteoporosis. Here's how:

Get moving! Inactivity increases bone loss. Try to engage in weight-bearing exercises such as walking, bicycling, or aerobics three to four hours a week. Exercising and strengthening your back muscles can help correct or prevent "dowager's hump." Exercise will also strengthen your muscles, making falls less likely.

New research suggests that weight lifting may be the most effective way to build bones. A group of elderly women increased bone density in their spines after nine months of weight training, while another group lost spine density after a year of brisk walking.

A combined program of aerobic and weight-training exercise is your best bet for beating osteoporosis. Talk with a certified fitness instructor at a local gym about helping you set up a program, or get some books from your local library and develop a program yourself. Remember to start slowly and work up gradually.

Keep up the calcium. You probably already know how important calcium is for healthy bones. Most people need at least 1,000 milligrams (mg) of calcium a day, but older people should increase their intake to 1,200 to 1,500 mg per day.

Your body absorbs calcium from food better than from supplements. So try to get most of your calcium from your meals. Calcium-rich foods include milk, cheese, salmon, canned sardines, oysters, dried beans, and dark green vegetables such as broccoli. Fortified orange juice and yogurt are also excellent sources that your body absorbs better than calcium supplements or antacids.

You can get a full-day's supply of calcium by consuming one cup of milk with breakfast, two cups of cottage cheese, or a cup of yogurt with lunch and two cups of greens or broccoli with dinner.

Limit protein. Too much protein interferes with your body's ability to use calcium. Try to keep pure protein intake at around three ounces (about 85 grams) a day or slightly less.

Remember your potassium and vitamin D. Potassium and vitamin D both work to regulate acid levels in your blood. This affects how much calcium your body soaks up and uses to build strong bones. Potassium, vitamin D, and calcium work together, so make sure you get plenty of each.

The average adult needs about 2,000 mg of potassium a day. If you eat plenty of fresh fruits and vegetables (2 to 4 fruit servings and 3 to 5 vegetable servings), you should easily ingest enough potassium. People over 25 should get about 200 International Units (IU) of vitamin D a day, but older people need 400 to 800 IU daily.

Sunlight helps your body produce vitamin D. If you're light skinned, you can get a full-day's supply of vitamin D just by spending 15 minutes in direct sunlight. (Don't put on sunscreen that has a sun protection factor (SPF) of eight or more, or you will prevent your body from making vitamin D).

If you're dark-skinned, you may need to spend up to three hours in the sun to get a full-day's dose of vitamin D. Keep in mind, however, that one day's exposure to sunlight will be enough to help your body produce vitamin D for some days afterward, so don't fret if you don't see the sun for several days. Normally, your body also stores enough vitamin D in your fat tissue to see you through the bleak winter months.

You can also find vitamin D in fortified milk, liver, and fatty fish like sardines and salmon.

Bone up calcium intake with trace minerals. Certain trace minerals aid in bone formation, so check your supplement label. Recommended minerals include 15 mg of zinc, 2.5 mg of copper, and 5 mg of manganese daily.

Stop smoking and reduce your intake of alcohol and caffeine. All these habits reduce your body's ability to absorb calcium. Smoking also lowers estrogen levels, and heavy drinking (more than two drinks a day) may affect your bones' proper growth and function. If you're a caffeinated coffee lover, make sure you drink at least a glass of milk a day to offset any possible risk of bone loss.

Talk with your doctor about potassium bicarbonate. Early research indicates you can absorb calcium better by taking a daily dose of potassium bicarbonate (bicarbonate of soda). Let your doctor know you're interested in this treatment, so that if it does become more widely available, you can be first in line.

Keep an eye out for fluoride updates. You already know that fluoride helps prevent tooth decay. Now it may also help prevent bone decay. Fluoride treatment is still in the experimental stages, but it may offer hope for the future.

It's never too late to start taking care of your bones and begin the healthy habits that will keep them strong for the rest of your life. Try some of these suggestions, and stand tall again.

Sources —

Age Page on Osteoporosis: The Bone Thinner, National Institutes of Health
Consultant (35,3:339)
Food, Nutrition, and Health (18,5:1)
Medical Tribune for the Internist and Cardiologist (35,14:18)
Osteoporosis, Clinical Center Communications, National Institute of Arthritis and Musculoskeletal and Skin Diseases, NIH Publication No. 91-3216, 1991
Osteoporosis, Clinical Center Communications, National Institutes of Health, NIH Publication No. 89-2893, 1989
Patient Care (22,9:131)
Science News (145,26:405)
The New England Journal of Medicine (330,25:1776)

PREMENSTRUAL SYNDROME

◀ Anger
◀ Bloating
◀ Cramps
◀ Dizziness or fainting
◀ Headache
◀ Nervousness

◀ Backache
◀ Constipation or diarrhea
◀ Depression
◀ Food cravings
◀ Irritability
◀ Swelling in the feet, ankles, hands, face, breasts

Breaking the PMS cycle

Long thought to be just an invention of women's minds, doctors now recognize what women have known forever. Premenstrual syndrome is real. Its symptoms are many, and its impact can be crippling. In fact, PMS has been used successfully as a legal defense in the United States, Canada, Great Britain, and France, where it is recognized as a form of insanity.

Birth control pills can cause vitamin deficiency

Take birth control pills? If you do, watch for signs that may signal a B6 deficiency. Symptoms include depression, irritability, weakness, cracked lips, or a swollen mouth or tongue.

For relief, try increasing your intake of foods rich in vitamin B6 such as liver, chicken, pork, fish, whole grains, wheat germ, bananas, potatoes, and dried beans.

If you don't experience any improvement within a couple of weeks, talk with your doctor. A simple B6 supplement of 10 to 50 milligrams (mg) usually provides relief.

If you experience tingling or numbness in your hands or feet, you may be taking too much vitamin B6. Overdoses of this vitamin can cause permanent nerve damage, so don't use any more than your doctor recommends, and be sure to report any suspicious symptoms immediately.

Sources —

Complete Guide to Vitamins, Minerals & Supplements, Fisher Books, Tucson, Ariz., 1988

The American Medical Association Encyclopedia of Medicine, Random House, New York, 1989

The Doctor's Complete Guide to Vitamins and Minerals, Dell Publishing, New York, 1994

The medical literature on menstrual disorders goes all the way back to Hippocrates, a Greek physician often called the father of medicine. The term "hysteria" was used to describe menstrual dysfunction, thought to be due to the uterus wandering through a woman's body and causing trouble wherever it lodged.

In the figurative sense, that's not too far off base. Researchers have documented more than 150 symptoms, ranging from dizziness and migraines to forgetfulness and suicidal tendencies. It's been estimated that 70 to 90 percent of women of reproductive age have some symptoms associated with their periods, and 40 percent of them have true PMS to some degree. About one in 10 have symptoms severe enough to disrupt their normal routines.

On the bright side, one researcher found that 66 percent of women reported at least one positive premenstrual symptom, such as more energy, increased creativity, a greater tendency to get things done, or a higher sex drive.

A disorder that affects both the body and the emotions, PMS can respond to a variety of treatments. Many women find a large measure of comfort in education, emotional support, and reassurance. The knowledge that PMS is a disorder of their reproductive system, instead of a psychological problem, gives women a sense of control. Stress management classes and PMS support groups can be helpful.

Some doctors may recommend birth control pills to control PMS. They work by tightly controlling the menstrual cycle. Progesterone supplements are also given to women to help combat PMS. These drug treatments may or may not work for you. There's no cure for PMS, but it can be managed. Here are some suggestions to help control the symptoms naturally:

Get plenty of sleep. PMS sufferers sometimes experience what's called an altered circadian rhythm, leading to insomnia and other sleep disturbances. Try to go to bed and get up at about the same time every day.

Exercise. Women who exercise regularly tend to have fewer PMS symptoms. Exercise also cuts down on fluid retention. Try adding 30 minutes a day to your workout the week before your period starts. (This should also help you get to sleep more easily.)

Watch what you eat and drink. Stick to a low-fat, low-salt diet, and stay away from caffeine, which is a stimulant and can increase tension, irritability, and sleeplessness. Alcohol and illegal drugs can also make you more emotionally unstable.

Try a vitamin supplement with calcium, magnesium, and vitamin B6. Doctors aren't sure why, but 1 mg of calcium a day has reportedly reduced both the physical and emotional symptoms of PMS, including depression, irritability, headache, mood swings, back pain, and bloating. Drink an extra glass of milk if you don't want to take a calcium supplement.

Magnesium and B6 have been shown to help with reducing water retention and fatigue, as well as the emotional symptoms. A daily dose of 250 to 360 mg of magnesium and 25 to 50 mg (no more) of vitamin B6 per day should help improve your mood and reduce water retention.

Don't get married. Or plan any other major stressful event for the time of the month when your PMS symptoms are at their height. If there's one plus to PMS, it's that you usually know when it's going to hit and can plan around it.

Relax. Deep breathing, yoga, and visualization are all relaxation techniques. They're used frequently by people who experience panic attacks, spastic colons, and other stress-related disorders, as well as by women in labor.

Select a quiet, private place for a time out, where you can calm yourself, and put on some soothing music. Breathe in slowly through your nose, hold your breath for a few seconds, and breathe out slowly through your mouth. Think of a relaxing place and picture it in your mind.

Educate the people in your life. Women with PMS don't suffer alone. The disorder has helped to ruin some people's personal lives and careers. In varying degrees, your family, friends, and co-workers need to know what's happening.

Coping with PMS brings an extra element of challenge to your life. Realize that you are not alone, and are not imagining your symptoms. Use the self-help tips above to make a real and positive difference in the way you experience life. You're up to the challenge!

Sources —
American Family Physician (50,6:1309)
Journal of the American College of Nutrition (12,4:442)
Medical Tribune for the Family Physician (35,18:16)
The Doctor's Complete Guide to Vitamins and Minerals, Dell Publishing, New York, 1994

Unusual Bleeding

◀ **Excessively heavy menstrual bleeding**
◀ **Irregular bleeding or spotting**

Find a cause to find the cure

One of the drawbacks to being a woman is "that time of the month." Everyone learns to deal with the special problems associated with menstruation. But what happens when you experience abnormal bleeding?

Abnormal uterine bleeding is defined as any uterine bleeding that does not result from a normal menstrual period. This includes any bleeding which occurs between periods and excessive bleeding during periods. Although flow varies from woman to woman, if you soak 25 pads or 30 tampons of any size during a period, it is probably abnormal. (A pad is considered "soaked" when a stain is beginning to show through.)

There are a number of possible reasons for abnormal uterine bleeding, but the most common ones are pregnancy, injury, and medication complications. If you aren't pregnant, and haven't experienced any type of injury which could be responsible for your bleeding, you should consider any medications you are currently taking when you discuss your problem with your doctor.

The medications and devices which most often cause unusual uterine bleeding are:

◁ **Contraceptives.** Oral contraceptives as well as intrauterine devices (IUDs) are the most common cause of abnormal bleeding.

◁ **Tranquilizers**

◁ **Cimetidine (Tagamet)**

◁ **Metoclopramide HCl (Reglan)**

◁ **Phenothiazines**

◁ **Antidepressants**

◁ **Anticoagulants**

◁ **Corticosteroids**

If you have abnormal bleeding, be sure to see your doctor so he can find the cause. If you are taking any of the medications listed above, be sure to point this out as a possible contributing factor.

Sources —
Encyclopedia of Natural Medicine, Prima Publishing, Rocklin, Calif., 1991
FDA Consumer (26,10:34)

Please check with your doctor for approval before taking or discontinuing
any prescription drug or using a natural healing alternative.

INFECTIONS

Prescription Drugs

Natural Alternatives

Prescription Drugs

ANTIBIOTICS AND OTHER DRUGS TO FIGHT INFECTIONS

Acyclovir

Brand name: *Zovirax*

What this drug does for you:
This antiviral is used to treat the fever, pain, and other symptoms of Herpes Simplex Virus types 1 and 2 (genital herpes), shingles, chickenpox, and Epstein-Barr virus. It is not a cure for herpes simplex infections.

Possible side effects of this drug:
- This drug may cause skin rash, bleeding gums, headache, dizziness, and nausea.
- Rare side effects include sore throat, leg or joint pain, loss of appetite, vomiting, and diarrhea.
- The ointment may cause burning, stinging, and itching. Let your doctor know if these side effects continue to bother you.

Special warning:
- You can transmit the virus to others while you're being treated. Avoid sexual intercourse if you can still see blisters and inflammation.

Pregnancy and nursing mothers:

Category C. See page 9 for description of categories. Drug is present in mother's milk.

Possible food and drug interactions:

- The effects of acyclovir may be increased by the gout drug probenecid.
- If used with the AIDS drug zidovudine, acyclovir may cause intense tiredness and drowsiness.
- Interactions with kidney drugs may cause kidney problems.

Helpful hints:

- You shouldn't drive a car or operate heavy machinery until you are sure the medicine isn't making you drowsy or less than alert.
- Use a finger cot or a rubber glove to apply the ointment so that you won't spread the infection. A one-half inch of ointment usually covers about four square inches.
- If you miss a dose, take it as soon as possible. If several hours have passed or it's almost time for your next dose, don't try to catch up by doubling the dose (unless your doctor tells you to).

Amoxicillin/Clavulanate Potassium

Brand name: *Augmentin*

What this drug does for you:

This penicillin antibiotic is used to treat a wide variety of infections of the ears, nose, throat, skin, lungs, and bladder by killing the bacteria that cause the infections. Penicillins you take by mouth treat mild to moderate infections. The drug will only kill the bacteria completely if enough of the drug reaches the blood or tissue where the bacteria is. The clavulanic acid makes the amoxicillin more effective.

Possible side effects of this drug:

- This drug may cause nausea, vomiting, diarrhea, and rash.
- Rare side effects include dizziness, anxiety, insomnia, and hyperactivity.
- Even though it is very rare, amoxicillin/clavulanate can lower the number of blood cells you have. If you don't have enough white blood cells, your immunity is down, and you can get a fever, sore throat, or pneumonia. If you are lacking red blood cells, you can become anemic, and that makes you tired and weak. Not having enough blood platelets makes you bruise easily and keeps your blood from clotting properly when you're injured. Be on the lookout for any of these symptoms of bone marrow depression.
- Call your doctor if you develop rash, itching, or fever. You may be having an allergic reaction to the drug.

Special warnings:

- This drug should not be used by people allergic to penicillin or cephalosporin antibiotics.

- People with diabetes may have false-positive sugar tests.

Pregnancy and nursing mothers:
It is not known if drug is safe to use during pregnancy. Drug is present in mother's milk.

Possible food and drug interaction:
- This drug may decrease the ability of birth control pills to prevent pregnancy.

Helpful hints:
- Take all of the prescription, even after the infection goes away.
- Most penicillins shouldn't be taken with food, but you can take amoxicillin with food to help prevent upset stomach.

Amoxicillin Trihydrate

Brand names: *Amoxil, Trimox, Wymox* **(Generic available)**

What this drug does for you:
This penicillin antibiotic is used to treat a wide variety of infections of the ears, nose, throat, skin, lungs, and bladder by killing the bacteria that cause the infections. Penicillins you take by mouth treat mild to moderate infections. The drug will only kill the bacteria completely if enough of the drug reaches the blood or tissue where the bacteria is.

Possible side effects of this drug:
- This drug may cause nausea, vomiting, diarrhea, and rash.
- Rare side effects include dizziness, anxiety, insomnia, and hyperactivity.
- Even though it is very rare, amoxicillin can lower the number of blood cells you have. If you don't have enough white blood cells, your immunity is down, and you can get a fever, sore throat, or pneumonia. If you are lacking red blood cells, you can become anemic, and that makes you tired and weak. Not having enough blood platelets makes you bruise easily and keeps your blood from clotting properly when you're injured. Be on the lookout for any of these symptoms of bone marrow depression.
- Call your doctor if you develop rash, itching, or fever. You may be having an allergic reaction to the drug.

Special warnings:
- This drug should not be used by people allergic to penicillin or cephalosporin antibiotics.
- People with diabetes may have false-positive sugar tests.

Pregnancy and nursing mothers:
It is not known if drug is safe to use during pregnancy. Drug may be present in mother's milk.

Possible food and drug interaction:
- This drug may decrease the ability of birth control pills to prevent pregnancy.

Helpful hints:
- Take all of the prescription, even after the infection goes away.
- Most penicillins shouldn't be taken with food, but you can take amoxicillin with food to help prevent upset stomach.

Ampicillin

Brand names: *Omnipen* **(Generic available)**

What this drug does for you:
This penicillin antibiotic is used to treat a wide variety of infections of the ears, nose, throat, skin, lungs, and bladder by killing the bacteria that cause the infections. Penicillins you take by mouth treat mild to moderate infections. The drug will only kill the bacteria completely if enough of the drug reaches the blood or tissue where the bacteria is.

Possible side effects of this drug:
- This drug may cause a mild rash, nausea, vomiting, and diarrhea.
- Call your doctor if you develop rash, itching, or fever. You may be having an allergic reaction to the drug.
- Even though it is very rare, ampicillin can lower the number of blood cells you have. If you don't have enough white blood cells, your immunity is down, and you can get a fever, sore throat, or pneumonia. If you are lacking red blood cells, you can become anemic, and that makes you tired and weak. Not having enough blood platelets makes you bruise easily and keeps your blood from clotting properly when you're injured. Be on the lookout for any of these symptoms of bone marrow depression.

Special warnings:
- This drug should not be used by people allergic to penicillin or cephalosporin antibiotics.
- People with diabetes may have false-positive sugar tests.

Pregnancy and nursing mothers:
Category B. See page 9 for description of categories. Drug is present in mother's milk and may cause diarrhea in infants.

Possible food and drug interaction:
- This drug may decrease the ability of birth control pills to prevent pregnancy.

Helpful hints:
- Take all of the prescription, even after the infection goes away.
- To improve absorption of the drug, take it on an empty stomach — at least one hour before or two hours after a meal.

Azithromycin

Brand name: *Zithromax*

What this drug does for you:

This antibiotic is used to treat some infections of the respiratory system and skin and some sexually transmitted diseases by killing the bacteria that cause them.

Possible side effects of this drug:

- This drug may cause nausea, diarrhea, stomach pain, inflammation of the vagina or the kidneys, palpitations, chest pain, headache, dizziness, sleepiness, indigestion, gas, black and tarry feces, rash, and sensitivity to sunlight.
- Rare side effects include jaundice (yellow skin and eyes, white-colored stools, dark urine), water retention, swelling, and colitis. Colitis is inflammation of the colon, and symptoms include bloody diarrhea, stomach cramps, and fever. Tell your doctor immediately if you have any of these symptoms.

Special warnings:

- Do not use if allergic to any macrolide-type antibiotics, such as erythromycin.
- This drug should be used with caution by people with liver or kidney problems, and it should not be used to treat syphilis or gonorrhea.

Pregnancy and nursing mothers:

Category B. See page 9 for description of categories. Not known if drug is present in mother's milk.

Possible food and drug interaction:

- Antacids may decrease the levels of this drug.

Helpful hints:

- Take one hour before or two hours after a meal. Do not take with food.
- Do not take aluminum-containing or magnesium-containing antacids with azithromycin.
- Take all of your prescription, even after your symptoms have disappeared.
- If you miss a dose, take it as soon as possible. If several hours have passed or it is nearing time for the next dose, don't try to catch up by doubling up your dose unless your doctor tells you to.

Carbenicillin

Brand name: *Geocillin*

What this drug does for you:

This penicillin antibiotic is used to treat infections of the skin, urinary tract, and prostate by killing the bacteria that cause the infections. Penicillins you take by mouth treat mild to moderate infections. The drug will only kill the bacteria completely if enough of the drug reaches the blood or tissue where the bacteria is.

Possible side effects of this drug:

- This drug may cause nausea, bad taste in the mouth, diarrhea, gas, and inflammation of the tongue.
- Rare side effects include stomach cramps, dry mouth, furry tongue, rectal bleeding, loss of appetite, stomach pain, itching, high fever, headache, itchy eyes, and vaginal itch.
- Even though it is very rare, carbenicillin can lower the number of blood cells you have. If you don't have enough white blood cells, your immunity is down, and you can get a fever, sore throat, or pneumonia. If you are lacking red blood cells, you can become anemic, and that makes you tired and weak. Not having enough blood platelets makes you bruise easily and keeps your blood from clotting properly when you're injured. Be on the lookout for any of these symptoms of bone marrow depression.
- Call your doctor if you develop a rash, fever, or chills. You could be having an allergic reaction to the drug.

Special warnings:

- Do not use this drug if you are allergic to penicillin, as severe allergic reaction can occur.
- Long-term use may lead to development of resistant bacteria in the body.
- People with kidney problems, liver problems, and blood disorders should take this drug with caution.

Pregnancy and nursing mothers:

Category B. See page 9 for description of categories. Drug is present in mother's milk.

Possible food and drug interaction:

- Levels of this drug may be increased by probenecid, a drug used to treat gout.

Helpful hints:

- To improve absorption of the drug, take it on an empty stomach — at least one hour before or two hours after a meal.
- Take all of the medication, even after you feel better.

Cefaclor

Brand names: *Ceclor*

What this drug does for you:

This antibiotic is used to treat infections of the lungs, urinary tract, skin, and ears.

Possible side effects of this drug:

- This drug may cause diarrhea and colitis. Colitis is inflammation of the colon, and symptoms include bloody diarrhea, stomach cramps, and fever.

- Rare side effects include nausea, jaundice, hyperactivity, nervousness, insomnia, confusion, muscle or blood vessel cramps, dizziness, and sleepiness. Call your doctor if you develop a rash.
- Even though it is very rare, cefaclor can lower the number of blood cells you have. If you don't have enough white blood cells, your immunity is down, and you can get a fever, sore throat, or pneumonia. If you are lacking red blood cells, you can become anemic, and that makes you tired and weak. Not having enough blood platelets makes you bruise easily and keeps your blood from clotting properly when you're injured. Be on the lookout for any of these symptoms of bone marrow depression.

Special warnings:

- Do not use if allergic to related antibiotics.
- People with impaired kidney function or a history of gastrointestinal disease, particularly colitis, should use with caution.

Pregnancy and nursing mothers:

Category B. See page 9 for description of categories. Drug is present in mother's milk.

Possible food and drug interactions:

- This drug may cause a false-positive urine glucose test, and it may increase the effects of anticoagulant drugs.
- Probenecid, a drug used to treat gout, can increase the effects of cefaclor.
- If taken with some other antibiotics, cefaclor may increase the side effects of those drugs.

Helpful hints:

- Take the full course of the antibiotic. Don't stop after symptoms go away.
- You can take this drug with meals.
- You can store the reconstituted suspension in the refrigerator for 14 days.
- If you miss a dose, take it as soon as possible. If several hours have passed or it is nearing time for the next dose, don't try to catch up by doubling up your dose unless your doctor tells you to.

Cefadroxil Monohydrate

Brand name: *Duricef*

What this drug does for you:

This antibiotic is used to treat infections of the lungs, urinary tract, skin, and ears.

Possible side effects of this drug:

- This drug may cause diarrhea and colitis. Colitis is inflammation of the colon, and symptoms include bloody diarrhea, stomach cramps, and fever.
- Rare side effects include nausea, jaundice, hyperactivity, nervousness, insomnia, confusion, muscle or blood vessel cramps, dizziness, sleepiness, anemia, and blood clotting problems. Call your doctor if you devel-

op a skin rash.

Special warnings:
- Do not use if allergic to related antibiotics.
- People who have impaired kidney function or a history of gastrointestinal disease, particularly colitis, should use with caution.

Pregnancy and nursing mothers:
Category B. See page 9 for description of categories. Drug is present in mother's milk.

Possible food and drug interactions:
- This drug may cause a false-positive urine glucose test, and it may increase the effects of anticoagulant drugs.
- Probenecid, a drug used to treat gout, can increase the effects of cefadroxil.
- If taken with some other antibiotics, cefadroxil may increase the side effects of those drugs.

Helpful hints:
- Take the full course of the antibiotic. Don't stop after symptoms go away.
- You can take this drug with food or milk if it irritates your stomach.
- If you miss a dose, take it as soon as possible. If several hours have passed or it is nearing time for the next dose, don't try to catch up by doubling up your dose unless your doctor tells you to.

Cefixime

Brand name: *Suprax*

What this drug does for you:
This antibiotic is used to treat infections of the ears, throat, tonsils, lungs, and urinary tract. It is also used to treat gonorrhea.

Possible side effects of this drug:
- This drug may cause diarrhea and colitis. Colitis is inflammation of the colon, and symptoms include bloody diarrhea, stomach cramps, and fever.
- Rare side effects include nausea, vomiting, itching, hives, drug fever, headache, dizziness, and vaginal and genital itching. Call your doctor if you develop a skin rash.

Special warnings:
- Do not use this drug if you are allergic to related antibiotics.
- People who have impaired kidney function or a history of gastrointestinal disease, particularly colitis, should use with caution.

Pregnancy and nursing mothers:
Category B. See page 9 for description of categories. Not known if drug is present in mother's milk.

Possible food and drug interaction:
- This drug may cause a false-positive urine glucose test.

Helpful hints:
- Take the full course of the antibiotic. Don't stop after symptoms go away.
- You can keep the reconstituted suspension in a tightly closed container for 14 days.
- You can take your medicine with food or milk.
- If you miss a dose, take it as soon as possible. If several hours have passed or it is nearing time for the next dose, don't try to catch up by doubling up your dose unless your doctor tells you to.

Cefpodoxime Proxetil

Brand name: *Vantin*

What this drug does for you:
This drug is used to treat infections of the skin, urinary tract, and upper and lower respiratory tract. It is also used to treat sexually transmitted diseases.

Possible side effects of this drug:
- This drug may cause diarrhea, nausea, yeast infection, stomach pain, rash, and headache.
- Rare side effects include chest pain, skin fungus, peeling skin, irregular menstruation, itching of genitals, gas, decreased salivation, decreased appetite, weakness, fever, dizziness, anxiety, insomnia, flushing, nightmares, cough, nosebleed, abnormal taste sensation, and eye itching.
- Another rare side effect is colitis. Colitis is inflammation of the colon, and symptoms include bloody diarrhea, stomach cramps, and fever.

Special warnings:
- Do not use if you are allergic to related antibiotics. Allergic reactions can be life-threatening.
- People who have impaired kidney function or a history of gastrointestinal disease, particularly colitis, should use with caution.

Pregnancy and nursing mothers:
Category B. See page 9 for description of categories. Drug is present in mother's milk.

Possible food and drug interactions:
- Antacids can decrease the effects of this drug.
- Probenecid, a drug used to treat gout, can increase the effects of this drug.
- This drug may cause a false-positive result for the Coombs' test.

Helpful hints:
- Take with food to avoid upset stomach.
- Take the full course of the antibiotic. Don't stop after symptoms go away.
- If you miss a dose, take it as soon as possible. If several hours have passed or it is nearing time for the next dose, don't try to catch up by

doubling up your dose unless your doctor tells you to.

Cefprozil

Brand name: *Cefzil*

What this drug does for you:
This antibiotic is used to treat infections of the skin, tonsils, throat, ears, and lungs.

Possible side effects of this drug:
- Cefprozil may cause diarrhea, nausea, stomach pain, and dizziness.
- Rare side effects include rash, hives, headache, nervousness, insomnia, confusion, and sleepiness.

Special warnings:
- Do not use if you are allergic to related antibiotics. Allergic reactions can be life-threatening.
- People who have impaired kidney function or a history of gastrointestinal disease, particularly colitis, should use with caution.

Pregnancy and nursing mothers:
Category B. See page 9 for description of categories. Not known if drug is present in mother's milk.

Possible food and drug interactions:
- Probenecid, a drug used to treat gout, can increase the effects of this drug.
- Using this drug with some antibiotics may cause kidney damage.
- This drug may cause a false-positive urine glucose test.

Helpful hints:
- Take the full course of the antibiotic. Don't stop after symptoms go away.
- Shake suspension well before using.
- You can take your medicine with food or milk.
- If you miss a dose, take it as soon as possible. If several hours have passed or it is nearing time for the next dose, don't try to catch up by doubling up your dose unless your doctor tells you to.

Ceftriaxone Sodium

Brand name: *Rocephin*

What this drug does for you:
This antibiotic injection is used to treat infections of the lungs, skin, urinary tract, bones and joints, as well as other infectious diseases.

Possible side effects of this drug:
- This drug may cause diarrhea, vomiting, rash, hives, and pain at site of injection.
- This drug may cause a severe case of colitis. Colitis is inflammation of the colon, and symptoms include bloody diarrhea, stomach cramps, and

fever. Call your doctor immediately if you have any of these symptoms.

- Even though it is rare, ceftriaxone can lower the number of blood cells you have. If you don't have enough white blood cells, your immunity is down, and you can get a fever, sore throat, or pneumonia. If you are lacking red blood cells, you can become anemic, and that makes you tired and weak. Not having enough blood platelets makes you bruise easily and keeps your blood from clotting properly when you're injured.

- Taking an antibiotic for a long time can cause bacteria or fungus to overgrow, leading to another infection (such as a yeast infection of the mouth or skin). If you get one of these "superinfections," you may need to start taking another antibiotic for the second infection.

Special warnings:

- Do not use if allergic to cephalosporin antibiotics. People with any known allergic reactions to antibiotics should use with caution.
- People with kidney or liver problems, a history of colitis, or gallbladder disease should use with caution.

Pregnancy and nursing mothers:

Category B. See page 9 for description of categories. Drug is present in mother's milk.

Cefuroxime Axetil

Brand names: *Ceftin*

What this drug does for you:

This antibiotic is used to treat infections of the urinary tract, skin, bones, joints, tonsils, throat, ears, and lungs. It is also used to treat gonorrhea.

Possible side effects of this drug:

- This drug may cause diarrhea, nausea, vomiting, and colitis. Colitis is inflammation of the colon, and symptoms include bloody diarrhea, stomach cramps, and fever.
- Rare side effects include rash, vaginal itching, hives, headache, and dizziness.

Special warnings:

- Do not use if allergic to related antibiotics.
- People with impaired kidney function or a history of gastrointestinal disease, particularly colitis, should use with caution.

Pregnancy and nursing mothers:

Category B. See page 9 for description of categories. Drug is present in mother's milk.

Possible food and drug interactions:

- This drug may cause a false-positive urine glucose test.

Helpful hints:

- Take with food to enhance absorption.
- Take the full course of the antibiotic. Don't stop after symptoms go away.

- If you miss a dose, take it as soon as possible. If several hours have passed or it is nearing time for the next dose, don't try to catch up by doubling up your dose unless your doctor tells you to.

Cephalexin

Brand names: *Biocef, Keflex* **(Generic available)**

What this drug does for you:
This cephalosporin antibiotic is used to treat infections of the ears, lungs, skin, bones, urinary tract, and genitals.

Possible side effects of this drug:
- This drug may cause diarrhea, stomach pains, jaundice, rash, hives, genital, vaginal, or anal itching, dizziness, fatigue, headache, agitation, confusion, hallucinations, and arthritis.
- Even though it is rare, cephalexin can lower the number of blood cells you have. If you don't have enough white blood cells, your immunity is down, and you can get a fever, sore throat, or pneumonia. If you are lacking red blood cells, you can become anemic, and that makes you tired and weak. Not having enough blood platelets makes you bruise easily and keeps your blood from clotting properly when you're injured.
- Taking an antibiotic for a long time can cause bacteria or fungus to overgrow, leading to another infection (such as a yeast infection of the mouth or skin). If you get one of these "superinfections," you may need to stop taking cephalexin and start taking another antibiotic for the second infection.
- Kidney damage is a rare side effect.

Special warnings:
- Do not use if allergic to related antibiotics.
- People with impaired kidney function or a history of intestinal disease, particularly colitis, should use with caution.

Pregnancy and nursing mothers:
Category B. See page 9 for description of categories. Drug is present in mother's milk.

Possible food and drug interaction:
- This drug may cause a false-positive urine glucose test.

Helpful hints:
- Take with food or milk to help prevent upset stomach.
- Take the full course of the antibiotic. Don't stop after symptoms go away.
- If you miss a dose, take it as soon as possible. If several hours have passed or it is nearing time for the next dose, don't try to catch up by doubling up your dose unless your doctor tells you to.

Cephalexin Hydrochloride

Brand name: *Keftab*

What this drug does for you:

This antibiotic is used to treat infections of the lungs, skin, bones, urinary tract, and genitals.

Possible side effects of this drug:

- This drug may cause diarrhea, stomach pains, jaundice, rash, hives, genital or anal itching, dizziness, fatigue, headache, agitation, confusion, hallucinations, and arthritis.
- Even though it is rare, cephalexin can lower the number of blood cells you have. If you don't have enough white blood cells, your immunity is down, and you can get a fever, sore throat, or pneumonia. If you are lacking red blood cells, you can become anemic, and that makes you tired and weak. Not having enough blood platelets makes you bruise easily and keeps your blood from clotting properly when you're injured.
- Taking an antibiotic for a long time can cause bacteria or fungus to overgrow, leading to another infection (such as a yeast infection of the mouth or skin). If you get one of these "superinfections," you may need to stop taking cephalexin and start taking another antibiotic for the second infection.
- Kidney damage is a rare side effect.

Special warnings:

- Do not use if you are allergic to related antibiotics.
- People with impaired kidney function or a history of intestinal disease, particularly colitis, should use with caution.

Pregnancy and nursing mothers:

Category B. See page 9 for description of categories. Drug is present in mother's milk.

Possible food and drug interaction:

- This drug may cause a false-positive urine glucose test.

Helpful hints:

- Take the full course of the antibiotic. Don't stop after symptoms go away.
- Take with food or milk to help prevent upset stomach.
- If you miss a dose, take it as soon as possible. If several hours have passed or it is nearing time for the next dose, don't try to catch up by doubling up your dose unless your doctor tells you to.

Chloramphenicol

Brand name: *Chloromycetin*

What this drug does for you:

This antibiotic is used to treat serious infections. It is potentially harmful, so you should only use it when safer drugs wouldn't be effective. The cream form is used to treat minor skin infections or prevent infections when you have a cut, scrape, or splinter.

Possible side effects of this drug:

- This drug may cause nausea, inflammation of the tongue, diarrhea, headache, mild depression, confusion, vision problems, fever, rash, swelling, and hives.
- This drug, like many antibiotics, can cause colitis. Colitis is inflammation of the colon, and symptoms include bloody diarrhea, stomach cramps, and fever.
- Chloramphenicol can lower the number of blood cells you have. This side effect can be serious, even fatal. If you don't have enough white blood cells, your immunity is down, and you can get a fever, sore throat, or pneumonia. If you are lacking red blood cells, you can become anemic, and that makes you tired and weak. Not having enough blood platelets makes you bruise easily and keeps your blood from clotting properly when you're injured. Be on the lookout for any of these symptoms of bone marrow depression.
- Taking an antibiotic for a long time can cause bacteria or fungus to overgrow, leading to another infection. If you get one of these "superinfections," you may need to quit taking chloramphenicol and start taking another antibiotic for the second infection.

Special warning:

- People with liver or kidney problems should use with caution.

Pregnancy and nursing mothers:

Category C. See page 9 for description of categories. Not known if safe to use while breast-feeding.

Possible food and drug interactions:

- The sedative effects of barbiturates may be increased when you take this drug.
- Phenytoin may build up to toxic levels in your blood.
- This drug may decrease the effectiveness of iron in the treatment of anemia, and it may decrease levels of vitamin B-12.

Helpful hints:

- You should have your blood, liver function, and kidney function checked weekly while taking this drug.
- Take on an empty stomach unless the drug upsets your stomach.

Ciprofloxacin

Brand names: *Ciloxan (for eyes), Cipro* **(tablets and injections)**

What this drug does for you:

This fluoroquinolone antibiotic is used to treat lower respiratory infections, bone and joint infections, urinary tract infections, skin infections, and infectious diarrhea. The ophthalmic solution is used to treat eye infections.

Possible side effects of this drug:

- Ciprofloxacin tablets and injections may cause nausea, diarrhea, stomach pain, headache, restlessness, and rash.
- This drug may cause mild to severe colitis. Colitis is inflammation of the colon, and symptoms include bloody diarrhea, stomach cramps, and fever.
- The ophthalmic solution may cause eye itching and irritation. Rarely, it may cause a bad taste in your mouth and nausea.
- Rare side effects of the tablets or injections include heart palpitations, irregular heartbeat, high blood pressure, angina, heart attack, blood clot in the brain, dizziness, insomnia, nightmares, hallucinations, irritability, tremors, lack of coordination, seizure, tiredness, loss of appetite, depression, mouth pain, difficulty swallowing, intestinal bleeding, jaundice, joint or back pain, flare-up of gout, kidney problems, difficulty urinating, bleeding from the urinary tract, vaginal itch, nosebleed, hiccups, coughing up blood, sensitivity of skin to light, flushing, fever, chills, changes in skin pigmentation, and skin eruptions on the legs.
- Taking an antibiotic for a long time can cause bacteria or fungus to overgrow, leading to another infection (such as a yeast infection of the mouth or skin). If you get one of these "superinfections," you may need to quit taking ciprofloxacin and start taking another antibiotic for the second infection.

Special warnings:

- Do not use if you have any allergies to drugs in the quinolone class. Dangerous sensitivity reactions can occur, causing symptoms such as swelling of the face or throat, difficult breathing (such as an asthma attack), itching, hives, tingling, or loss of consciousness. Call your doctor at the first sign of rash or allergic reaction.
- People with any condition which increases the risk of seizures should use with caution.
- The dose may need to be adjusted for people who have poor kidney function. Kidney and liver function tests and certain blood tests should be done periodically while on this drug.

Pregnancy and nursing mothers:

Category C. See page 9 for description of categories. Drug is present in mother's milk.

Possible food and drug interactions:

- Ciprofloxacin may increase the effects of caffeine, the asthma drug theophylline, and the anticoagulant warfarin.
- Antacids, some iron pills, and multivitamins containing zinc may decrease absorption of this drug.
- Probenecid, a drug used to treat gout, may increase levels of ciprofloxacin in the blood.

Helpful hints:

- Although this drug may be taken with food, it is best taken two hours

after you eat.
- Drink plenty of fluids while taking this drug.
- Use caution while driving. Ciprofloxacin may cause dizziness or light-headedness.
- This drug may make your skin extra-sensitive to sunlight, so protect your skin if you'll be outdoors in sunny weather.
- If you miss a dose, take it as soon as possible. If several hours have passed or it is nearing time for the next dose, don't try to catch up by doubling up your dose unless your doctor tells you to.

Clarithromycin

Brand name: *Biaxin*

What this drug does for you:
This antibiotic is used to treat mild to moderate infections of the skin and the respiratory tract.

Possible side effects of this drug:
- This drug may cause diarrhea, nausea, abnormal sense of taste, indigestion, stomach pain, and headache.
- This drug may cause mild to severe colitis. Colitis is inflammation of the colon, and symptoms include bloody diarrhea, stomach cramps, and fever. Tell your doctor if you have any of these symptoms.

Special warnings:
- Do not use if allergic to any of the macrolide antibiotics.
- People with severe kidney problems should use with caution.

Pregnancy and nursing mothers:
Category C. See page 9 for description of categories. Not known if drug is present in mother's milk.

Possible food and drug interaction:
- This drug may increase levels of carbamazepine, a drug used to treat seizures, and the asthma drug theophylline.

Helpful hints:
- Take all the medicine you are prescribed, even after you begin to feel better.
- You can take this drug with or without food. Take each dose with fluids, preferably more than six ounces.
- If you miss a dose, take it as soon as possible. If several hours have passed or it is nearing time for the next dose, don't try to catch up by doubling up your dose unless your doctor tells you to.
- Do not refrigerate suspension. After mixing, store at room temperature away from light and use within 14 days.

Clindamycin Phosphate

Brand names: *Cleocin, Cleocin T, Clinda-Derm*

What this drug does for you:

This drug is used to treat infections of the skin, lungs, digestive system, and female genitals. The gel is used to treat acne and, occasionally, rosacea.

Possible side effects of this drug:

- This drug may cause stomach pain, inflammation of the esophagus, nausea, diarrhea, rash, itching, and jaundice (yellow eyes and skin).
- This drug may cause severe or fatal colitis. Colitis is inflammation of the colon, and symptoms include bloody diarrhea, stomach cramps, and fever.
- Taking an antibiotic for a long time can cause bacteria or fungus to overgrow, leading to another infection (fungal infections of the mouth, anus, or vagina). If you get one of these "superinfections," you may need to quit taking clindamycin and start taking another antibiotic for the second infection.
- Rare side effects include skin eruptions and inflammation of joints.
- Even though it is very rare, clindamycin can lower the number of blood cells you have. If you don't have enough white blood cells, your immunity is down, and you can get a fever, sore throat, or pneumonia. If you are lacking red blood cells, you can become anemic, and that makes you tired and weak. Not having enough blood platelets makes you bruise easily and keeps your blood from clotting properly when you're injured. Be on the lookout for any of these symptoms of bone marrow depression.

Special warnings:

- People with kidney disease, liver disease, or a history of intestinal diseases, such as colitis, should not use this drug. Call your doctor immediately if severe diarrhea develops.
- Apply the gel or solution form cautiously if you have a history of skin allergies.

Pregnancy and nursing mothers:

Not known if safe to use in pregnancy. Drug is present in mother's milk.

Possible food and drug interaction:

- This drug may increase the effects of muscle relaxers.

Helpful hint:

- Take this drug with a glass of water to avoid irritating the esophagus.
- For the gel or solution, apply a thin layer to the affected area twice daily. If the drug comes in contact with your eye, bathe your eye in water for several minutes.

Dicloxacillin

Brand name: *Pathocil*

What this drug does for you:
This penicillin antibiotic is used to treat a wide variety of infections by killing the bacteria that cause the infections. Penicillins you take by mouth treat mild to moderate infections. The drug will only kill the bacteria completely if enough of the drug reaches the blood or tissue where the bacteria is.

Possible side effects of this drug:
- This drug may cause nausea, stomach pain, gas, and loose stools.

Special warning:
- Don't use this drug if you are allergic to penicillin or other antibiotics. It may cause a dangerous allergic reaction which can be fatal. Notify your doctor if you develop nausea, vomiting, severe diarrhea, fever, rash, hives, itching, wheezing, shortness of breath, sore throat, black tongue, swollen joints, or any unusual bleeding or bruising.

Pregnancy and nursing mothers:
Not known if drug is safe to use in pregnancy. Not known if drug is safe to use while nursing.

Possible food and drug interactions:
- The antibiotics neomycin and tetracycline may reduce the effects of this drug.
- This drug may interact with beta-blockers and the antibiotics chloramphenicol and erythromycin.
- The effects of oral contraceptives and some other penicillins may be reduced.
- This drug can cause a false-positive urine glucose test, a false-positive Coombs' test, and a false-positive protein test.

Helpful hints:
- Take all of the prescription, even after the infection goes away.
- To improve absorption of the drug, take it on an empty stomach — at least one hour before or two hours after a meal.

Doxycycline Hyclate

Brand names: *Doryx, Vibramycin, Vibra-Tabs* **(Generic available)**

What this drug does for you:
This antibiotic is used to treat a variety of infections.

Possible side effects of this drug:
- This drug may cause nausea, diarrhea or loose stools, loss of appetite, sore throat or hoarseness, inflammation of the mouth or tongue, difficulty swallowing, rash, sensitivity of skin to light, blue-gray discoloration of the skin and mucous membranes, liver or kidney problems,

worsening of lupus, hives, fluid retention, fever, rash, and joint pain
- Doxycycline may cause increased pressure on the brain in adults. Signs of this high pressure include headache, nausea, and visual disturbances. Let your doctor know immediately if you develop these symptoms. Doxycycline may also cause bulging "soft spots" on babies' heads.
- This drug may cause colitis. Colitis is inflammation of the colon, and symptoms include bloody diarrhea, stomach cramps, and fever.
- This drug may cause permanent tooth discoloration and may slow bone growth in children under 8 years old.
- Even though it is rare, doxycycline can lower the number of blood cells you have. If you don't have enough white blood cells, your immunity is down, and you can get a fever, sore throat, or pneumonia. If you are lacking red blood cells, you can become anemic, and that makes you tired and weak. Not having enough blood platelets makes you bruise easily and keeps your blood from clotting properly when you're injured. Be on the lookout for any of these symptoms of bone marrow depression.
- Taking an antibiotic for a long time can cause bacteria or fungus to overgrow, leading to another infection (such as fungal infections of the mouth, anus, or vagina). If you get one of these "superinfections," you may need to quit taking doxycycline and start taking another antibiotic for the second infection.

Special warnings:
- Do not use if allergic to tetracycline antibiotics.
- Discontinue use if allergic skin reaction appears after exposure to sunlight.
- If you have kidney problems, tetracyclines can accumulate to toxic levels in your body.

Pregnancy and nursing mothers:
Category D. See page 9 for description of categories. Drug is present in mother's milk.

Possible food and drug interactions:
- The effectiveness of birth control pills may be reduced, resulting in unplanned pregnancy.
- This drug may increase the levels or effects of anticoagulants, and it may interfere with the actions of penicillin antibiotics.
- Antacids and iron-containing products may reduce absorption of this drug.

Helpful hints:
- Take with food or milk to avoid irritation of the stomach. Make sure you wash down the drug with plenty of liquid to help prevent ulcers and irritation of the esophagus and throat, especially if you will be lying down afterward.
- This drug may make your skin extra-sensitive to sunlight, so protect your skin if you'll be outdoors in sunny weather.
- If you miss a dose, take it as soon as possible. If several hours have passed or it is nearing time for the next dose, don't try to catch up by

doubling up your dose unless your doctor tells you to.

Erythromycin

Brand names: *A / T / S, Akne-mycin, E.E.S., E-Mycin, Emgel, ERYC, Erycette, Erygel, Erymax, EryPed, Erythra-Derm, Ery-Tab, Erythrocin Stearate, Ilotycin, PCE Dispertab, T-Stat, Theramycin* **(Generic available)**

What this drug does for you:

This antibiotic is used to treat a variety of infections, including respiratory tract and skin infections, conjunctivitis in newborns, pneumonia in infants, whooping cough, diphtheria, urinary and genital infections during pregnancy, pelvic inflammatory disease, syphilis, rheumatic fever, and Legionnaires' disease.

The gel and ointment forms are used to treat acne.

Possible side effects of this drug:

- This drug may cause nausea, loss of appetite, diarrhea, stomach cramps and discomfort, itching, skin eruptions (such as hives), or irregular heartbeat.
- Abnormal liver function including jaundice (yellow eyes and skin, dark urine) is a rare side effect. If you have jaundice or feel unusually tired, contact your doctor.
- Taking an antibiotic for a long time can cause bacteria or fungus to overgrow, leading to another infection (such as fungal infections of the mouth, anus, or vagina). If you get one of these "superinfections," you may need to quit taking erythromycin and start taking another antibiotic for the second infection.
- The gel and ointment forms may cause flushing, red or flaking skin, burning or tenderness, dry and itchy skin, oily skin, or eye irritation.

Special warning:

- People with liver disease should not take this drug.

Pregnancy and nursing mothers:

Category B. See page 9 for description of categories. Drug is present in mother's milk.

Possible food and drug interactions:

- This drug may cause rhabdomyolysis (a disease that destroys muscle tissue) in people who are taking the cholesterol-reducer lovastatin.
- This drug may increase the levels or effects of anticoagulants, the seizure drug carbamazepine, the heart drug digoxin, the migraine drug ergotamine, the asthma drug theophylline, and the insomnia drug triazolam.
- Taking terfenadine and erythromycin together can cause life-threatening heart rhythm disturbances.

Helpful hints:

- The effectiveness of erythromycin is decreased in some people when they take it with food. Take it with food if it upsets your stomach, but

if it doesn't, take it on an empty stomach — one hour before or two hours after meals.
- Take all of the prescription, even after you begin to feel better.
- Take each dose at evenly spaced intervals throughout the day with at least six ounces of fluids.
- Shake the oral suspension well before using it, and refrigerate it to make it taste better.
- For the gel and ointment forms, wash with soap and warm water, rinse well, and pat dry before applying the drug. Apply in the morning and evening, and wash your hands after applying.

Iodoquinol

Brand name: *Yodoxin*

What this drug does for you:
This drug is used to treat infestation of the intestines by amoebas.

Possible side effects of this drug:
- Iodoquinol may cause rash, itching, hives, enlarged thyroid, fever, chills, headache, eye problems, stomach cramps, nausea, vomiting, diarrhea, itching around the anus, and dizziness.

Special warnings:
- This drug should not be used by people with liver damage.
- Avoid long-term treatment, as damage to the optic nerve of the eye may result.
- People with thyroid disease should use with caution.

Pregnancy and nursing mothers:
Category C. See page 9 for description of categories. Not known if drug is present in mother's milk.

Possible food and drug interaction:
- This drug may alter the results of some thyroid function tests.

Helpful hints:
- You can crush the tablets and mix them with a soft food such as applesauce if you prefer.
- Don't prepare food for others until the infection is completely cleared up.

Lomefloxacin

Brand name: *Maxaquin*

What this drug does for you:
This fluoroquinolone antibiotic is used to treat adults with mild to moderate infections of the lower respiratory tract and urinary tract. It is also used before surgery to protect against urinary tract infections that may develop after surgery.

Possible side effects of this drug:

- This drug may cause sensitivity to light, headache, nausea, dizziness, and diarrhea.
- Rare side effects include vision problems, eye pain, dizziness, prickling or tingling sensation, convulsions, vomiting, indigestion, gas, intestinal bleeding, difficulty swallowing, dry mouth, high or low blood pressure, fluid retention or swelling, irregular heartbeat, angina, heart attack, heart failure, fainting, muscle pain, chills, flu-like symptoms, ringing in the ears, gout, low blood sugar, loss of appetite, confusion, menstrual cycle abnormalities, itching, rash, hives, and difficulty urinating.
- Taking an antibiotic for a long time can cause bacteria or fungus to overgrow, leading to another infection. If you get one of these "superinfections," you may need to quit taking lomefloxacin and start taking another antibiotic for the second infection.
- This drug may cause mild to severe colitis. Colitis is inflammation of the colon, and symptoms include bloody diarrhea, stomach cramps, and fever.

Special warnings:

- Do not use if you have any allergies to quinolone antibiotics. Serious, sometimes fatal, allergic reactions can occur, with symptoms such as swelling or fluid retention in the face or throat, difficult breathing, itching, hives, tingling, or loss of consciousness.
- Severe sensitivity to light may occur in some people exposed to sunlight or ultraviolet light.
- If you have any disorders of the central nervous system, such as epilepsy, or any other condition which increases your risk of seizures, you should use with caution.

Pregnancy and nursing mothers:

Category C. See page 9 for description of categories. Not known if drug is present in mother's milk.

Possible food and drug interactions:

- This drug may increase the effects of the anticoagulant warfarin, and it may increase levels of the immunosuppressant cyclosporine.
- Levels of lomefloxacin may be increased by the ulcer drug cimetidine and the drug probenecid, used to treat gout.
- Take antacids or any products containing iron or zinc four hours before or two hours after taking this drug.

Helpful hints:

- Drink extra amounts of fluids while taking this drug.
- This drug may make your skin extra-sensitive to sunlight, so protect your skin if you'll be outdoors in sunny weather.
- Don't drive or operate dangerous machinery until you determine whether the drug makes you dizzy or drowsy.
- You may take this drug with or without meals.
- If you miss a dose, take it as soon as possible. If several hours have

passed or it is nearing time for the next dose, don't try to catch up by doubling up your dose unless your doctor tells you to.

Loracarbef

Brand name: *Lorabid*

What this drug does for you:

This cephalosporin antibiotic is used to combat infections of the respiratory tract, throat, tonsils, ears, urinary tract, and skin by killing the organisms that cause them.

Possible side effects of this drug:

- This drug may cause skin rash, diarrhea, stomach pain, nausea, headache, or inflammation of the vagina (vaginitis).
- Rare side effects include itching, hives, loss of appetite, insomnia, dizziness, and colitis. Colitis is inflammation of the colon, and symptoms include bloody diarrhea, stomach cramps, and fever.
- Even though it is rare, loracarbef can lower the number of blood cells you have. If you don't have enough white blood cells, your immunity is down, and you can get a fever, sore throat, or pneumonia. If you are lacking red blood cells, you can become anemic, and that makes you tired and weak. Not having enough blood platelets makes you bruise easily and keeps your blood from clotting properly when you're injured. Be on the lookout for any of these symptoms of bone marrow depression.

Special warnings:

- Do not use if you are allergic to cephalosporin antibiotics.
- If you are allergic to penicillin, you should use with caution. If an allergic reaction does occur, notify your doctor immediately.
- People who have impaired kidney function or a history of intestinal disease, particularly colitis, should use with caution. Tell your doctor if you have diarrhea, particularly if it is severe or it contains blood, pus, or mucus.

Pregnancy and nursing mothers:

Category B. See page 9 for description of categories. Not known if drug is present in mother's milk.

Possible food and drug interaction:

- The effects of this drug may be increased by the drug probenecid, which is used to treat gout.

Helpful hints:

- Take one hour before or two hours after food.
- Take the full course of the antibiotic. Don't stop even though symptoms might go away.
- If you miss a dose, take it as soon as possible. If several hours have passed or it is nearing time for the next dose, don't try to catch up by doubling up your dose unless your doctor tells you to.

Metronidazole

Brand names: *Flagyl, MetroGel, MetroGel-Vaginal, Protostat*
(Generic available)

What this drug does for you:

This drug is used to treat many serious bacterial infections, including endo-carditis, lower respiratory tract infections, bone and joint infections, skin and skin structure infections, certain stomach infections, cervical and vaginal infections, blood poisoning, and meningitis. The gel form is used to treat rosacea.

Possible side effects of this drug:

- This drug may cause headache, nausea, loss of appetite, diarrhea, constipation, stomach cramps, seizures, dizziness, insomnia, depression, confusion, irritability, cystitis, painful or frequent urination, incontinence, painful sexual intercourse, dark urine (deep red-brown), taste disturbances, inflammation of the rectum and anus, and joint pain.
- If you have an allergic reaction to the drug, you may experience rash, hives, nasal congestion, dry mouth or vagina, fever, and flushing.
- One possible side effect is the growth of a yeast infection in the mouth or vagina. A furry tongue or inflammation of the mouth or tongue may accompany the yeast infection in the mouth.
- Metronidazole may damage nerve tissues in your extremities. Symptoms include numbness or tingling in the hands or feet, lack of muscle coordination, and weakness.
- Like many other drugs, metronidazole may lower your red blood cell count and cause anemia, or it may lower your white blood cell count and therefore lower your immunity.

Special warnings:

- Metronidazole should not be used by anyone who has had an allergic reaction to a similar drug.
- If you have any disease of the central nervous system, Crohn's disease, or blood disorders, you should use this drug with caution.

Pregnancy and nursing mothers:

Category B. See page 9 for description of categories. Drug is present in mother's milk.

Possible food and drug interactions:

- Avoid alcohol while you're taking metronidazole. The combination may cause stomach cramps, vomiting, or headache.
- Metronidazole may increase levels of the anticoagulant warfarin and the seizure drug phenytoin.
- Metronidazole may decrease the excretion of the antipsychotic drug lithium which can build up to toxic levels.
- Levels or effects of metronidazole may be increased by the ulcer drug cimetidine.

Helpful hints:
- You can take this drug with or without food. If it upsets your stomach, take it with food.
- Don't be alarmed if the drug turns your urine a deep red-brown color or if you have a metallic taste in your mouth. These harmless side effects will go away when you quit taking the drug.
- Before applying the gel form, wash the area. Rub on a thin film twice daily. You should see results in approximately three weeks.

Minocycline

Brand names: *Dynacin, Minocin* **(Generic available)**

What this drug does for you:
This antibiotic is used to treat infections caused by various bacteria and microorganisms.

Possible side effects of this drug:
- Minocycline may cause itching, swelling, rash, joint pain, sensitivity of skin to light, loss of appetite, worsening of lupus, difficulty swallowing, nausea, diarrhea, and darkening of the skin.
- Minocycline may cause increased pressure on the brain in adults. Signs of this high pressure include headache, nausea, and visual disturbances. Let your doctor know immediately if you develop these symptoms. Minocycline may also cause bulging "soft spots" on babies' heads.
- This drug may cause colitis. Colitis is inflammation of the colon, and symptoms include bloody diarrhea, stomach cramps, and fever.
- Even though it is rare, minocycline can lower the number of blood cells you have. If you don't have enough white blood cells, your immunity is down, and you can get a fever, sore throat, or pneumonia. If you are lacking red blood cells, you can become anemic, and that makes you tired and weak. Not having enough blood platelets makes you bruise easily and keeps your blood from clotting properly when you're injured. Be on the lookout for any of these symptoms of bone marrow depression.
- Tooth discoloration is a rare side effect.
- Taking an antibiotic for a long time can cause bacteria or fungus to over-grow, leading to another infection (fungal infections of the mouth, anus, or vagina). If you get one of these "superinfections," you may need to quit taking minocycline and start taking another antibiotic for the second infection.

Special warnings:
- Do not use this drug if you are allergic to tetracycline.
- If you have liver or kidney problems, tetracyclines can accumulate to toxic levels in your body.

Pregnancy and nursing mothers:
Category D. See page 9 for description of categories. May cause tooth discoloration and retard bone formation in the developing baby. Drug is present

in mother's milk.

Possible food and drug interactions:
- Antacids may decrease absorption of this drug, so take this drug two hours before or after antacids.
- Iron-containing products also reduce absorption, so take these at least three hours before or two hours after taking this drug.
- This drug may increase the levels or effects of anticoagulants and decrease the effects of oral contraceptives.
- Do not take with the antibiotic penicillin.

Helpful hints:
- This drug may make your skin extra-sensitive to sunlight, so protect your skin if you'll be outdoors in sunny weather. Tell your doctor if you develop a severe sunburn or rash.
- People who have dizziness or lightheadedness as a side effect should be careful while driving.
- You can take this drug with or without food or milk.
- If you miss a dose, take it as soon as possible. If several hours have passed or it is nearing time for the next dose, don't try to catch up by doubling up your dose unless your doctor tells you to.

Ofloxacin

Brand names: *Floxin, Floxin I.V., Ocuflox*

What this drug does for you:
This antibiotic is used to treat infections of the lower respiratory tract, urinary tract, skin, and skin structures. It is also used to treat sexually transmitted diseases and an inflamed prostate gland.

Possible side effects of this drug:
- This drug may cause headache, nausea, diarrhea, dizziness, insomnia, itching, rash, vaginal itch, altered sense of taste, chest pain, dry mouth, nervousness, fever, sore throat, loss of appetite, gas, fatigue, and constipation.
- Rare side effects include high or low blood pressure, fluid retention, heart palpitations, chills, indigestion, muscle or joint pain, menstrual irregularities, seizures, depression, confusion, fainting, hallucinations, prickling or tingling in hands or feet, ringing in the ears, and difficulty urinating.
- Taking an antibiotic for a long time can cause bacteria or fungus to overgrow, leading to another infection. If you get one of these "superinfections," you may need to quit taking ofloxacin and start taking another antibiotic for the second infection.

Special warnings:
- This drug should not be taken by people with allergies to fluoroquinolones or quinolone medications. Serious, sometimes fatal, allergic reactions can occur, causing symptoms such as swelling of the face or

throat, difficulty breathing, itching, hives, tingling, or loss of consciousness.

- The safety of this drug in anyone under 18 years of age, pregnant women, and nursing mothers has not been established.
- If you have any disorders of the central nervous system, such as epilepsy, which may increase the risk of seizures, you should use with caution. People with diabetes or poor kidney or liver function should also use with caution.
- Blood glucose levels and liver and kidney functions should be checked periodically. If low blood sugar occurs in diabetics, stop taking the drug and call your doctor.

Pregnancy and nursing mothers:

Category C. See page 9 for description of categories. Drug is present in mother's milk.

Possible food and drug interactions:

- This drug may increase the effects of the anticoagulant warfarin and the immunosuppressant cyclosporine.
- Levels or effects of ofloxacin may be decreased by the antibacterial drug nitrofurantoin.
- Take antacids, vitamins, or any products containing iron or zinc four hours before or two hours after taking ofloxacin.
- If taken with nonsteroidal anti-inflammatory drugs (NSAIDs), ofloxacin may increase the risk of seizure.

Helpful hints:

- Take one hour before or two hours after meals.
- Sensitivity to light may occur even when sunscreens or sun blocks are used and may persist when treatment is stopped.
- You shouldn't drive a car or operate heavy machinery until you are sure the medicine isn't making you drowsy, dizzy, or less than alert.
- If you miss a dose, take it as soon as possible. If several hours have passed or it is nearing time for the next dose, don't try to catch up by doubling up your dose unless your doctor tells you to.

Penicillin V Potassium

Brand name: *Ledercillin VK, Pen-Vee K* **(Generic available)**

What this drug does for you:

This penicillin antibiotic is used to treat a wide variety of infections by killing the bacteria that cause the infections. Penicillins you take by mouth treat mild to moderate infections. The drug will only kill the bacteria completely if enough of the drug reaches the blood or tissue where the bacteria is.

Possible side effects of this drug:

- This drug may cause stomach pain or cramps, nausea, diarrhea, gas, black tongue, and skin eruptions.
- Even though it is rare, this antibiotic can lower the number of blood cells

you have. If you don't have enough white blood cells, your immunity is down, and you can get a fever, sore throat, or pneumonia. If you are lacking red blood cells, you can become anemic, and that makes you tired and weak. Not having enough blood platelets makes you bruise easily and keeps your blood from clotting properly when you're injured. Be on the lookout for any of these symptoms of bone marrow depression.

Special warnings:
- Do not use this drug if you are allergic to penicillin or other antibiotics. It is estimated that allergic reactions occur in as many as 10 percent of people taking penicillin, and they can be fatal. Call your doctor if you develop a rash, fever, or chills.
- If you are vomiting or have diarrhea, do not use this drug.

Possible food and drug interactions:
- This drug may decrease the effects of birth control pills.
- Levels or effects of this drug may be decreased by the antibiotics neomycin, erythromycin, chloramphenicol, and tetracycline.

Helpful hints:
- Take one hour before or two hours after meals.
- Take all of the prescription, even after the infection goes away.
- Most penicillins shouldn't be taken with food, but you can take penicillin V with food to help prevent upset stomach.

Pentamidine

Brand name: *NebuPent, Pentacarinat, Pentam 300*

What this drug does for you:
This drug is used to treat pneumocystis pneumonia (PCP) and to prevent the infection in certain people with HIV.

Possible side effects of this drug:
- Pentamidine may cause decreased appetite, dizziness, rash, fatigue, shortness of breath, congestion, cough, wheezing, nausea, chills, diarrhea, night sweats, sore throat, headache, muscle pain, swelling, and stomach pain.
- Rare side effects include anxiety, confusion, tremors, drowsiness, mental depression, memory loss, insomnia, itching, dry skin, hives, high or low blood sugar, high or low blood pressure, fainting, rapid heartbeat, eye pain, urinary incontinence, mouth ulcers, black and tarry feces, kidney failure, inflammation of the pancreas or colon, hepatitis, rapid breathing, and stuffy nose.

Pregnancy and nursing mothers:
Category C. See page 9 for description of categories. Not known if drug is present in mother's milk.

Special warnings:
- This drug should not be used by anyone who has had an allergic reaction

to any form of pentamidine.
- If you develop a fever, cough, or difficult breathing, see your doctor for a thorough medical exam.

Helpful hints:
- Use the aerosol device until the chamber is empty. This can take up to 45 minutes.
- This drug can cause low blood pressure and dizziness. You should lie down while someone gives you an injection.
- Store the solution at room temperature away from light. The solution is stable for 48 hours. After this time, throw away any unused medicine.

Sulfamethoxazole

Brand name: *Gantanol*

What this drug does for you:
This sulfa drug is used to treat various infections of the urinary tract, ears, and eyes. It is also used to treat meningitis, malaria, nocardiosis, and toxoplasmosis.

Possible side effects of this drug:
- This drug may cause nausea, diarrhea, loss of appetite, stomach pain, headache, depression, insomnia, drowsiness, convulsions, hallucinations, ringing in the ears, hearing loss, dizziness, lack of muscle coordination, joint pain, fever, chills, hair loss, inflammation of the mouth or tongue, inflammation of the intestines and colon, and sensitivity of skin to sunlight.
- Liver and kidney damage and allergic reactions such as rashes and other skin problems are some of the possible risks of taking this drug. Allergic reactions can be serious and even fatal. Discontinue drug and call your doctor if fever, rash, or other allergic reaction occurs.
- Rare side effects also include low blood sugar and loss of fluids through frequent urination.
- Even though it is rare, this antibiotic can lower the number of blood cells you have. If you don't have enough white blood cells, your immunity is down, and you can get a fever, sore throat, or pneumonia. If you are lacking red blood cells, you can become anemic, and that makes you tired and weak. Not having enough blood platelets makes you bruise easily and keeps your blood from clotting properly when you're injured. Be on the lookout for any of these symptoms of bone marrow depression.

Special warnings:
- People with poor liver or kidney function, asthma, or G6PD deficiency should use with caution. This drug may cause the destruction of red blood cells in people with G6PD.
- Blood and urine should be tested regularly during treatment.
- This drug may cause blood disorders in elderly people who are taking diuretics.

Pregnancy and nursing mothers:

Category C. See page 9 for description of categories. Drug is present in mother's milk.

Possible food and drug interactions:

- This drug may increase levels or effects of the seizure drug phenytoin and the anticoagulant warfarin.
- It may also cause the cancer drug methotrexate to build up to toxic levels.
- You should not use sulfamethoxazole with methenamine, a drug used to relieve discomfort of the lower urinary tract. Methenamine may increase your chances of dangerous, and possibly fatal, reactions to sulfa drugs. Sulfamethoxazole can also increase levels of methenamine in your body.

Helpful hints:

- To help prevent kidney stones, drink plenty of fluids while taking this drug.
- This drug may make your skin extra-sensitive to sunlight, so protect your skin if you'll be outdoors in sunny weather.
- Take all of the prescription, even after you begin to feel better.
- Take your medicine on an empty stomach with a full glass of water.
- Shake the oral suspensions well before using. Store in the refrigerator, and throw away any medicine you haven't used after 14 days.

Sulfamethoxazole and Trimethoprim

Brand names: *Bactrim, Bactrim DS, Septra, Septra DS* **(Generic available)**

What this drug does for you:

This combination drug is used to treat infections of the intestines (such as traveler's diarrhea), urinary tract, ears, and lungs (such as frequently recurring bronchitis).

Possible side effects of this drug:

- This drug may cause nausea, diarrhea, loss of appetite, stomach pain, inflammation of the mouth or tongue, inflammation of the intestines and colon, headache, depression, insomnia, drowsiness, convulsions, hallucinations, ringing in the ears, hearing loss, dizziness, lack of muscle coordination, joint pain, fever, chills, hair loss, and sensitivity of skin to sunlight.
- Liver and kidney damage and allergic reactions such as rashes and other skin problems are some of the possible risks of taking this drug. Allergic reactions can be serious and even fatal. Discontinue drug and call your doctor if you experience difficulty breathing, fever, chills, hallucinations, a skin rash or hives, tiredness, nervousness, muscle weakness, or low back pain.
- Rare side effects also include low blood sugar and loss of fluids through frequent urination.
- Even though it is rare, this antibiotic can lower the number of blood cells you have. If you don't have enough white blood cells, your immunity is

down, and you can get a fever, sore throat, or pneumonia. If you are lacking red blood cells, you can become anemic, and that makes you tired and weak. Not having enough blood platelets makes you bruise easily and keeps your blood from clotting properly when you're injured. Be on the lookout for any of these symptoms of bone marrow depression.

- Taking an antibiotic for a long time can cause bacteria or fungus to overgrow, leading to another infection. If you get one of these "superinfections," you may need to quit taking this drug and start taking another antibiotic for the second infection.

Special warnings:

- People with poor liver or kidney function, asthma, folate deficiency, malnutrition, or G6PD deficiency should use with caution. This drug may cause destruction of red blood cells in people with G6PD.
- Blood and urine should be tested regularly during treatment.

Pregnancy and nursing mothers:

Category C. See page 9 for description of categories. Drug is present in mother's milk.

Possible food and drug interactions:

- This drug may increase levels or effects of the seizure drug phenytoin and the anticoagulant warfarin. It may also increase levels of the cancer drug methotrexate to toxic levels.
- This drug may cause blood disorders in elderly people who are taking diuretics.

Helpful hints:

- To help prevent kidney stones, drink at least four to six glasses of water every day while taking this drug.
- Take with food or milk if this drug upsets your stomach. If it doesn't upset your stomach, take it one hour before or two hours after a meal.
- This drug may make your skin extra-sensitive to sunlight, so protect your skin if you'll be outdoors in sunny weather.

Sulfisoxazole

Brand name: *Gantrisin*

What this drug does for you:

This drug is used to treat various infections of the urinary tract, ears, and eyes. It is also used to treat meningitis, malaria, nocardiosis, and toxoplasmosis.

Possible side effects of this drug:

- This drug may cause nausea, diarrhea, loss of appetite, stomach pain, inflammation of the mouth or tongue, inflammation of the intestines and colon, headache, depression, insomnia, drowsiness, convulsions, hallucinations, ringing in the ears, hearing loss, dizziness, lack of muscle coordination, joint pain, fever, chills, hair loss, and sensitivity of skin to sunlight.
- Liver and kidney damage and allergic reactions including rashes and other skin problems are some of the possible risks of taking this drug.

Allergic reactions can be serious and even fatal. Discontinue drug and call your doctor if fever, rash, or other allergic reaction occurs.

- Rare side effects also include low blood sugar, goiter, and loss of fluids through frequent urination.
- Even though it is rare, this antibiotic can lower the number of blood cells you have. If you don't have enough white blood cells, your immunity is down, and you can get a fever, sore throat, or pneumonia. If you are lacking red blood cells, you can become anemic, and that makes you tired and weak. Not having enough blood platelets makes you bruise easily and keeps your blood from clotting properly when you're injured. Be on the lookout for any of these symptoms of bone marrow depression.

Special warnings:
- People who have poor liver or kidney functions, asthma, or G6PD deficiency should use with caution. This drug may cause destruction of red blood cells in people with G6PD.

Pregnancy and nursing mothers:
Category C. See page 9 for description of categories. Drug is present in mother's milk.

Possible food and drug interactions:
- This drug may increase levels or effects of the anesthetic thiopental and the anticoagulant warfarin. It may also increase levels of the cancer drug methotrexate to toxic levels.

Helpful hints:
- Blood and urine should be tested regularly during treatment.
- To help prevent kidney stones, drink plenty of fluids while taking this drug.
- This drug may make your skin extra-sensitive to sunlight, so protect your skin if you'll be outdoors in sunny weather.
- Take all of the prescription, even after you begin to feel better.
- Take your medicine on an empty stomach with a full glass of water.
- Shake the oral suspensions well before using. Store in the refrigerator, and throw away any medicine you haven't used after 14 days.

Tetracycline

Brand names: *Achromycin V, Topicycline* (Generic available)

What this drug does for you:
This antibiotic is used to treat many infections by various microorganisms.

Possible side effects of this drug:
- This drug may cause sensitivity to light, difficulty swallowing, loss of appetite, nausea, diarrhea, inflammation of the tongue, rash, itching, fluid retention or swelling of the hands or feet, dizziness, lupus, ringing in the ears, and abnormal liver function.
- Tetracycline may cause increased pressure on the brain in adults. Signs of this high pressure include headache, nausea, and blurred vision. Let

your doctor know immediately if you develop these symptoms. Tetracycline may cause bulging "soft spots" on babies' heads too.

- Rare side effects include ulcers, inflammation of the esophagus, and colitis. Colitis is inflammation of the colon, and symptoms include bloody diarrhea, stomach cramps, and fever.
- Even though it is rare, this antibiotic can lower the number of blood cells you have. If you don't have enough white blood cells, your immunity is down, and you can get a fever, sore throat, or pneumonia. If you are lacking red blood cells, you can become anemic, and that makes you tired and weak. Not having enough blood platelets makes you bruise easily and keeps your blood from clotting properly when you're injured. Be on the lookout for any of these symptoms of bone marrow depression.
- Taking an antibiotic for a long time can cause bacteria or fungus to overgrow, leading to another infection (fungal infections of the mouth, anus, or vagina). If you get one of these "superinfections," you may need to quit taking tetracycline and start taking another antibiotic for the second infection.

Special warning:
- Tetracycline may accumulate to toxic levels in people with kidney problems.

Pregnancy and nursing mothers:
Category D. See page 9 for description of categories. Tetracycline should not be used during pregnancy because it can cause tooth discoloration and slow down bone formation in the developing fetus. Drug is present in mother's milk.

Possible food and drug interactions:
- Tetracycline may increase the effects of anticoagulants.
- This drug may decrease the effects of the antibiotic penicillin.
- Levels of this drug may be decreased by antacids.

Helpful hints:
- Take on an empty stomach, with a full glass of water, one hour before or two hours after meals.
- Liver tests should be performed regularly during treatment.
- If you miss a dose, take it as soon as possible. If several hours have passed or it is nearing time for the next dose, don't try to catch up by doubling up your dose unless your doctor tells you to.

Vancomycin

Brand name: *Vancocin* **(Generic available)**

What this drug does for you:
This antibiotic is used to treat various forms of colitis. Colitis is inflammation of the colon often caused by antibiotics, and symptoms include bloody diarrhea, stomach cramps, and fever.

Possible side effects of this drug:
- This drug may cause blood abnormalities, nausea, and allergic reactions

such as skin rash and drug fever.
- Rare side effects include hearing loss, dizziness, and kidney failure. If you feel a sense of fullness in your ears or have ringing in your ears, tell your doctor immediately. Those sensations could indicate nerve damage that could lead to hearing loss.

Special warning:
- This drug should be used with caution by people who have poor kidney function, inflammatory disorders of the intestines, or hearing problems.
- Blood levels of this drug should be monitored because it can be very toxic to the kidneys.

Pregnancy and nursing mothers:
Category C. See page 9 for description of categories. Drug is present in mother's milk.

Possible food and drug interaction:
- Check with your doctor before taking this drug with other diarrhea medications.

Helpful hints:
- Take all of your medicine, even after you begin to feel better.
- Have hearing tests before you begin taking the drug and during long-term treatment. Also have regular blood counts.

DRUGS TO FIGHT FUNGAL INFECTIONS

Fluconazole

Brand name: *Diflucan*

What this drug does for you:
Fluconazole comes in tablets or oral suspension and is used to treat certain fungal infections including pneumonia, peritonitis, urinary tract infections, meningitis, and yeast infections of the mouth, throat and esophagus.

Possible side effects of this drug:
- This drug may cause nausea, diarrhea, stomach pain, headache, rash, seizures, and low white blood cell or platelet count.
- Rare side effects include dangerous skin rashes and, possibly, liver damage. If you develop a rash, tell your doctor.

Special warnings:
- If you are allergic to any other fungicides, you should use this drug with caution.
- People with impaired immune systems who develop rashes should be closely watched. Treatment may need to be stopped.
- People with poor kidney function may need a reduced dose.

Pregnancy and nursing mothers:
Category C. See page 9 for description of categories. Drug is present in

mother's milk.

Possible food and drug interactions:

- This drug may increase levels or effects of the immunosuppressant cyclosporine, the seizure drug phenytoin, the anticoagulant warfarin, and the diabetes drugs tolbutamide, glyburide, and glipizide.
- Effects or levels of this drug may be decreased by the tuberculosis drug rifampin.

Helpful hints:

- Have regular liver function tests while you're taking this drug. Liver damage is rare but serious.
- Take all of your medicine, even after you begin to feel better.
- Store the oral suspension at room temperature, and throw away any unused suspension after two weeks.

Flucytosine

Brand name: *Ancobon*

What this drug does for you:

This drug is used to treat serious fungal infections caused by specific yeast and bacteria.

Possible side effects of this drug:

- This drug commonly causes nausea, diarrhea, stomach pain, headache, fever, confusion, dizziness, and rash.
- Flucytosine may cause liver damage, with or without jaundice (yellow eyes and skin, dark urine, and whitish stools).
- Flucytosine may damage nerve tissues in your extremities. Symptoms include numbness or tingling in the hands or feet, lack of muscle coordination, and weakness.
- Flucytosine can lower the number of blood cells you have. If you don't have enough white blood cells, your immunity is down, and you can get a fever, sore throat, or pneumonia. If you are lacking red blood cells, you can become anemic, and that makes you tired and weak. Not having enough blood platelets makes you bruise easily and keeps your blood from clotting properly when you're injured. Be on the lookout for any of these symptoms of bone marrow depression.
- Rare side effects include dry mouth, loss of appetite, ulcer, low blood sugar and potassium levels, hallucinations, hearing loss, sensitivity of skin to light, hives, itching, chest pain, difficulty breathing, and heart attack.

Special warnings:

- If you have poor kidney function, you should take this drug with extreme caution.
- Blood levels of flucytosine should be monitored to prevent accumulation and toxicity.

Pregnancy and nursing mothers:

Category C. See page 9 for description of categories. Not known if drug is present in mother's milk.

Possible food and drug interactions:

- The herpes virus drug cytosine arabinoside may counteract the good effects of this drug.
- The antibiotic amphotericin B increases the action and toxicity of this drug.

Helpful hints:

- Your infection may not begin clearing up for weeks or months. Keep taking the drug as prescribed.
- If you take more than one capsule at once, you may want to take the capsules over a 15-minute period to help prevent stomach irritation.
- You should have regular blood, kidney, and liver tests while you're taking this drug.

Ketoconazole

Brand name: *Nizoral*

What this drug does for you:

This drug comes as a cream, shampoo, or tablets and is used to treat fungal infections including oral thrush and skin infections.

Possible side effects of this drug:

- This drug may cause nausea, itching, and stomach pain.
- Rare side effects include diarrhea, enlargement of breasts in men, impotence, decreased sperm counts, severe depression, sensitivity of skin to light, headache, dizziness, and sleepiness.
- Even though it is very rare, ketoconazole can lower the number of blood cells you have. If you don't have enough white blood cells, your immunity is down, and you can get a fever, sore throat, or pneumonia. If you are lacking red blood cells, you can become anemic, and that makes you tired and weak. Not having enough blood platelets makes you bruise easily and keeps your blood from clotting properly when you're injured. Be on the lookout for any of these symptoms of bone marrow depression.
- A very rare side effect is severe liver damage. Liver toxicity can be fatal. Contact your doctor if you have severe diarrhea, stomach pain, or fever or if you develop any symptoms of possible liver damage such as nausea, dark urine, pale stools, yellow eyes or skin, loss of appetite, or unusual fatigue.

Special warnings:

- Liver functions should be tested before treatment begins and should be carefully monitored during treatment, especially in people with a history of liver disease.
- This drug should be used with caution by men with prostate cancer.

Pregnancy and nursing mothers:

Category C. See page 9 for description of categories. Not known if drug is present in mother's milk. Do not nurse while taking this drug.

Possible food and drug interactions:

- Do not take ketoconazole with the allergy drug terfenadine because it may cause a dangerously rapid heartbeat.
- Taking this drug with the antihistamine astemizole may cause heartbeat irregularities.
- Antacids should be taken two hours after this drug because they reduce absorption.
- Effects or levels of this drug may be decreased by anticholinergics, histamine blockers, and the tuberculosis drug rifampin.
- This drug may increase levels or effects of corticosteroids, anticoagulants, and the immunosuppressant cyclosporine.
- If taken with the antifungal drug miconazole, this drug may cause very low blood sugar.

Helpful hints:

- You shouldn't drive a car or operate heavy machinery until you are sure the medicine isn't making you drowsy, dizzy, or less than alert.
- Take your medicine with food to help prevent nausea. Nausea should go away after you've been taking the drug for a while.
- Keep taking your medicine, even after you get better. The infection may return if you stop your medicine too early.
- This drug may make your skin extra-sensitive to sunlight, so protect your skin if you'll be outdoors in sunny weather.
- You may see improvement quickly, but continue to treat jock itch and ringworm for two weeks so that the fungus won't come back.

MALARIA DRUGS

Chloroquine

Brand name: *Aralen*

What this drug does for you:

This drug is used to treat severe attacks of malaria and amebic infections.

Possible side effects of this drug:

- This drug may cause ringing in the ears, skin problems, itching, stomach cramps, nausea, diarrhea, loss of appetite, headache, and psychotic episodes.
- This drug may cause irreversible damage to the retina of the eye. See your doctor immediately if any vision changes occur.
- Rare side effects include low blood pressure, hearing loss, and convulsions. If you feel a sense of fullness in your ears or have ringing in your ears, tell your doctor immediately. Those sensations could indicate nerve damage that could lead to hearing loss.

- Even though it is very rare, chloroquine can lower the number of blood cells you have. If you don't have enough white blood cells, your immunity is down, and you can get a fever, sore throat, or pneumonia. If you are lacking red blood cells, you can become anemic, and that makes you tired and weak. Not having enough blood platelets makes you bruise easily and keeps your blood from clotting properly when you're injured. Be on the lookout for any of these symptoms of bone marrow depression.

Special warnings:
- People with psoriasis, liver disease, the metabolic disease called porphyria, alcoholism, or G6PD deficiency should use chloroquine with caution.

Pregnancy and nursing mothers:
Category C. See page 9 for description of categories. New mothers who want to breast-feed should not take chloroquine. Chloroquine may cause serious adverse reactions in nursing infants.

Helpful hints:
- This drug may make your skin extra-sensitive to sunlight, so protect your skin if you'll be outdoors in sunny weather.
- To help you remember to take your medicine, take it with a meal on the same day each week.

Hydroxychloroquine

Brand name: *Plaquenil Sulfate*

What this drug does for you:
This drug is used to treat severe attacks of malaria, rheumatoid arthritis, and lupus.

Possible side effects of this drug:
- This drug may cause ringing in the ears, skin problems, itching, stomach cramps, nausea, diarrhea, loss of appetite, headache, and psychotic episodes.
- This drug may cause irreversible damage to the retina of the eye. See your doctor immediately if any vision changes occur. Eye exams should be done regularly.
- Rare side effects include low blood pressure, hearing loss, and convulsions. If you feel a sense of fullness in your ears or have ringing in your ears, tell your doctor immediately. Those sensations could indicate nerve damage that could lead to hearing loss.
- Even though it is very rare, hydroxychloroquine can lower the number of blood cells you have. If you don't have enough white blood cells, your immunity is down, and you can get a fever, sore throat, or pneumonia. If you are lacking red blood cells, you can become anemic, and that makes you tired and weak. Not having enough blood platelets makes you bruise easily and keeps your blood from clotting properly when you're injured. Be on the lookout for any of these symptoms of bone marrow depression.

Special warnings:

- This drug may worsen the skin disease psoriasis or the metabolic disorder porphyria.
- People with liver disease, alcoholism, or G6PD deficiency should use this drug with caution.

Pregnancy and nursing mothers:

Category C. See page 9 for description of categories.

Helpful hints:

- It may take several weeks before you get any relief from your rheumatoid arthritis symptoms. If you don't improve in six months, you're doctor will probably stop your drug treatment.
- If this drug upsets your stomach, take it with food.

Pyrimethamine

Brand name: *Daraprim*

What this drug does for you:

This drug is used to treat and control malaria.

Possible side effects of this drug:

- Pyrimethamine may cause loss of appetite, vomiting, and tongue inflammation.
- Pyrimethamine can lower the number of blood cells you have. If you don't have enough white blood cells, your immunity is down, and you can get a fever, sore throat, or pneumonia. If you are lacking red blood cells, you can become anemic, and that makes you tired and weak. Not having enough blood platelets makes you bruise easily and keeps your blood from clotting properly when you're injured. Be on the lookout for any of these symptoms of bone marrow depression.
- Rare side effects include headache, dry mouth or throat, diarrhea, fever, abnormal skin pigmentation, skin eruptions, insomnia, lightheadedness, seizures, and depression. If skin rash occurs, stop taking this drug and contact your doctor immediately.

Special warnings:

- Alcoholics, people who are on folate therapy, or people who have poor liver or kidney functions should use pyrimethamine with caution.

Pregnancy and nursing mothers:

Category C. See page 9 for description of categories. Drug is present in mother's milk.

Possible food and drug interactions:

- If taken with sulfonamides, this drug may increase bone marrow suppression.
- This drug may cause liver toxicity if taken with the anti-anxiety drug lorazepam.

Helpful hint:
- Take with food to reduce vomiting or loss of appetite.

Quinacrine

Brand name: *Atabrine HCl*

What this drug does for you:
This drug is used to treat malaria, giardiasis (protozoa), and cestodiasis (tapeworm).

Possible side effects of this drug:
- Quinacrine may cause yellow discoloration of skin or urine, nausea, diarrhea, stomach cramps, loss of appetite, headache, dizziness, skin eruptions, and nightmares. Contact your doctor if any vision disturbances develop.
- This drug may cause mood changes and temporary psychosis.

Special warnings:
- The skin disease psoriasis and the metabolic disease porphyria may worsen.
- This drug should be used with caution by people over 60.
- People with liver disease, alcoholism, or G6PD deficiency, as well as those with a psychosis, should use with extreme caution.

Pregnancy and nursing mothers:
Do not take this drug to treat malaria during pregnancy unless absolutely necessary. Do not take this drug to treat giardiasis or cestodiasis during pregnancy. You should wait until after delivery.

Possible food and drug interaction:
- Do not take with the malaria drug primaquine because this drug increases primaquine's toxicity.

Helpful hint:
- Take your medicine after a meal with a full glass of liquid.

TUBERCULOSIS DRUGS

Ethambutol

Brand name: *Myambutol*

What this drug does for you:
This drug is used to treat pulmonary tuberculosis in combination with other antituberculous drugs. Ethambutol prevents growth of the bacteria that causes tuberculosis.

Possible side effects of this drug:
- Ethambutol may cause nausea, stomach upset or pain, loss of appetite, visual disturbances, hallucinations, disorientation, dizziness, confusion,

headache, fever, numbness and tingling in the hands and feet, joint pain, low number of blood platelets, abnormal liver function, itching, dermatitis, and gout.

Special warnings:

- People with poor kidney function may need smaller doses. Kidney and liver functions and blood tests should be periodically checked if you take this drug for a long time.
- This drug may cause vision problems which can be irreversible in some cases. Eye exams should be done regularly. Use with extreme caution if you have cataracts, optic neuritis, disorder of the retina of the eye caused by diabetes, or recurring eye inflammation. These conditions make it more difficult to determine changes in vision. Report any changes in vision in one or both eyes to your doctor.

Pregnancy and nursing mothers:

Not known if safe to use while you are pregnant. Not known if safe to use while you are breast-feeding.

Possible food and drug interaction:

- Antacids may delay and reduce absorption of this drug.

Helpful hints:

- You shouldn't drive a car or operate heavy machinery until you are sure the medicine isn't making you dizzy or less than alert.
- If you miss a dose, take it as soon as possible. If several hours have passed or it is nearing time for the next dose, don't try to catch up by doubling up your dose unless your doctor tells you to.

Isoniazid

Brand name: *Nydrazid* **(Generic available)**

What this drug does for you:

Isoniazid treats all forms of tuberculosis.

Possible side effects of this drug:

- This drug may cause jaundice, hepatitis, nausea, upset stomach, fever, rashes, high blood sugar, enlargement of breasts in men, inflammation of blood vessels or lymph glands, lupus-like syndrome, and nutritional deficiency of some forms of vitamin B, calcium, and phosphorus.
- In large doses, isoniazid may damage nerve tissues in your extremities. Symptoms include numbness or tingling in the hands or feet, lack of muscle coordination, and weakness.
- Isoniazid can lower the number of blood cells you have. If you don't have enough white blood cells, your immunity is down, and you can get a fever, sore throat, or pneumonia. If you are lacking red blood cells, you can become anemic, and that makes you tired and weak. Not having enough blood platelets makes you bruise easily and keeps your blood from clotting properly when you're injured. Be on the lookout for any of

these symptoms of bone marrow depression.

- Rare side effects include poor memory, convulsions, toxic psychosis, and diseases of the optic nerve of the eye.

Special warnings:

- This drug should not be used by people who have had any kind of severe reaction to isoniazid, including liver damage.
- Alcoholics and diabetics may need vitamin B supplements.
- Hepatitis is a rare but sometimes fatal side effect. Call your doctor if you experience weakness, loss of appetite, or vomiting. These symptoms may be signs of hepatitis.
- If you have chronic liver disease or poor kidney function, you should use this drug with caution.

Pregnancy and nursing mothers:

Not known if safe to use in pregnancy. Drug is present in mother's milk.

Possible food and drug interactions:

- This drug may increase the effects of the seizure drug phenytoin.
- Avoid alcohol while taking this drug. Alcohol increases the risk of liver damage from isoniazid.
- Taking this drug with large doses of acetaminophen increases your risk of liver damage.

Helpful hints:

- You can take your medicine with food to help prevent stomach irritation.
- Ask your doctor if you need to take vitamin B6 supplements.
- If you miss a dose, take it as soon as possible. If several hours have passed or it is nearing time for the next dose, don't try to catch up by doubling up your dose unless your doctor tells you to.

Pyrazinamide

Brand name: *None available* **(Generic available)**

What this drug does for you:

This drug is used to treat active tuberculosis.

Possible side effects of this drug:

- This drug may cause nausea, loss of appetite, joint and muscle pain, gout, painful or difficult urination, liver toxicity, anemia and other blood disorders, and allergic reactions including rash, hives, and itching.
- Rare side effects include acne, sensitivity to light, fever, porphyria, and kidney inflammation.
- Contact your doctor if you develop nausea, vomiting, loss of appetite, darkened urine, yellowish discoloration of eyes and skin, pain or swelling of joints, or fever.

Special warnings:

- Do not use pyrazinamide if you have gout or severe liver damage.
- If you have mild liver disease or diabetes, you should use this drug with

caution. Liver functions should be closely monitored.

Pregnancy and nursing mothers:

Category C. See page 9 for description of categories. Drug is present in mother's milk.

Possible food and drug interaction:

- This drug may interfere with certain urine tests.

Helpful hints:

- Your uric acid levels should be checked regularly while you are taking this drug. High uric acid levels can cause gout. Your doctor may need to take you off this drug if you develop signs of gouty arthritis.
- This drug may make your skin extra-sensitive to sunlight, so protect your skin if you'll be outdoors in sunny weather.
- If you miss a dose, take it as soon as possible. If several hours have passed or it is nearing time for the next dose, don't try to catch up by doubling up your dose unless your doctor tells you to.

Rifampin

Brand names: *Rifadin, Rimactane*

What this drug does for you:

This drug is used to treat all forms of tuberculosis and certain other bacterial infections.

Possible side effects of this drug:

- This drug may cause dizziness, headache, drowsiness, lack of coordination, visual abnormalities, weakness, confusion, menstrual abnormalities, nausea, heartburn, gas, stomach cramps, flushing, itching, rash, sore mouth or tongue, and flu-like symptoms.
- Rare side effects include liver damage and kidney failure. Watch yourself for signs of liver damage such as fatigue, loss of appetite, yellow skin and eyes, and dark urine.
- Even though it is rare, rifampin can lower the number of blood cells you have. If you don't have enough white blood cells, your immunity is down, and you can get a fever, sore throat, or pneumonia. If you are lacking red blood cells, you can become anemic, and that makes you tired and weak. Not having enough blood platelets makes you bruise easily and keeps your blood from clotting properly when you're injured. Be on the lookout for any of these symptoms of bone marrow depression.

Special warnings:

- People with liver disease should use this drug with caution. Liver functions should be closely monitored.
- Blood counts should be done before and throughout treatment.
- The metabolic disease porphyria may be worsened by this drug.
- This drug may discolor urine, stools, sweat, saliva, and tears red-orange. Soft contact lenses may be permanently stained.

Pregnancy and nursing mothers:

Category C. See page 9 for description of categories. Not known if drug is present in mother's milk.

Possible food and drug interactions:

- This drug may decrease levels or effects of the following drugs: anticoagulants, anticonvulsants, barbiturates, beta-blockers, corticosteroids, birth control pills, the immunosuppressant cyclosporine, diabetic drugs, the anti-anxiety drug diazepam, the heartbeat regulator quinidine, the antifungal drug ketoconazole, and the asthma drug theophylline.
- Effects of this drug may be increased by the gout drug probenecid.
- Avoid alcoholic beverages while taking this drug. The combination could cause liver damage.

Helpful hint:

- Preferably, take this drug on an empty stomach — at least one hour before or two hours after meals. If the drug irritates your stomach, you can take it with food.
- If you miss a dose, take it as soon as possible. If several hours have passed or it is nearing time for the next dose, don't try to catch up by doubling up your dose unless your doctor tells you to.

Natural Alternatives 🍎

BRONCHITIS (ACUTE)

- ◀ Chills
- ◀ Persistent coughing
- ◀ Fever
- ◀ Sore chest

Best ways to beat bronchitis

With bronchitis, the bark is almost always worse than the bite. You'll probably sound worse than you feel, but you'll still want relief. Here's how to heal your inflamed bronchial tubes fast and quiet a cough that just won't quit.

Get plenty of rest. The illness is usually short-lived — if you get enough rest.

Eat nutritiously. This is not the time to give in to cravings for junk food and empty calories. Your body needs nutrition ammunition to get rid of the infection.

Drink plenty of liquids. Drinking lots of fruit juice, tea, and water will help reduce the amount of mucus in your lungs.

Don't smoke. And don't let anyone smoke around you.

Use disposable tissues instead of handkerchiefs. You don't want to re-infect yourself with a germy handkerchief. Also, wash your hands frequently.

Try a vaporizer. Breathing warm, steamy air from a vaporizer should give you some relief.

Take care of your lungs. If you have a cold and don't want it to become bronchitis, be sure to take good care of yourself. Avoid dust, fumes, and extremely cold air, culprits which irritate your bronchial tubes. If you exercise in cold air, wear a face mask to warm the air you're breathing, and don't sleep in a very cold room.

Source —
Taber's Cyclopedic Medical Dictionary, F.A. Davis Company, Philadelphia, Pa., 1989

EAR INFECTIONS

◀ Discharge of pus from the ears   ◀ Fever
◀ Muffled hearing   ◀ Pain in the ear

Natural help for ear infections

Starting at age 3 months, many children are constantly troubled with earaches. Ear infections result in countless trips to the doctor and endless rounds of antibiotic prescriptions. Adults can get ear infections too.

There are only a few common-sense methods to fight ear infections naturally:

Strengthen the immune system. Plenty of rest, nutritious foods, and low stress are the keys to a strong immune system.

Take your vitamins. Be sure to get enough vitamin C and iron. Buy a good multivitamin plus iron, either for children or adults.

Restrict sugar. Eating sugar suppresses your body's production of infection-fighting antibodies.

Avoid cigarette smoke. Don't smoke, and don't let children be around smokers.

As grueling as it is to live with a child's marathon ear infections, the time will eventually pass. Children usually grow out of this stage at about age 3. Adult ear infections are rare and short-lived.

Source —
The Doctor's Complete Guide to Vitamins and Minerals, Dell Publishing, New York, 1994

GENERAL INFECTIONS

◀ Breathing difficulties   ◀ Fever
◀ Headache   ◀ Inflammation
◀ Itching   ◀ Pain
◀ Redness and swelling   ◀ Stomach problems

Natural ways to fight infection

The French philosopher Voltaire said, "The art of medicine consists of amusing the patient while nature cures the disease." This is more or less true for some infections, but not for others. If the infection is viral, you do have to treat the symptoms and wait it out. If it's bacterial, you'll probably need antibiotics to knock it out.

Your body does its best to fight off all kinds of infections. Here are some natural ways to build your body's defense system:

Boost your natural immune response with vitamin C. Here's another sound idea from mother's lips we didn't have to learn in school: Drink all your juice every day. Getting a good daily supply of vitamin C from orange juice really will help fight colds and flu.

Recently, a team of scientists at Arizona State University wanted to find out just how good vitamin C was at fighting off infection. They found that when the body is under stress (whether emotional or physical), it creates more of a chemical known as histamine.

Although small amounts of excess histamine are necessary to help the body cope with stress, too much histamine can be a kind of poison to the body. It can interfere with the body's natural immune responses that fight off infections and illnesses.

Scientists think that vitamin C might help get rid of the excess histamine and, therefore, help protect the body's natural immune defenses. The Arizona researchers discovered that taking 1,000 to 2,000 milligrams of vitamin C each day can lower the amount of histamine in the blood anywhere from 20 to 40 percent.

Vitamin C can't keep a determined cold or flu bug away, but it can make colds and serious respiratory infections less severe and last a shorter time.

Use garlic as a natural antibiotic. Garlic actually fights off some infections that modern antibiotics can't kill. In a recent study at Boston City Hospital, researchers found that an extract of fresh garlic cloves killed or slowed the growth of more than a dozen common bacteria.

If you feel like you're going to catch a cold or the flu, chow down on a clove or two of garlic. You may be able to catch the infection in its very early stage and not even get sick.

Raw garlic seems to fight infections better than cooked garlic, but cooked garlic is good for you too. (In fact, cooked garlic may be better than raw at protecting against heart disease.)

If you're bothered by garlic's strong odor, try garlic supplement tablets with an enteric coating. This coating prevents the garlic from dissolving until it reaches the intestines. These supplements tend to be more odor-free and effective than other types.

The many different brands of garlic supplements available vary widely in effectiveness. Kwai is one brand that has produced positive results in several clinical trials.

Don't smoke. Smoking lowers your resistance to infection. It introduces toxins into a body already trying to fight off infection and lowers the amount of vitamin C in your body.

Exercise, but moderately. If you are fighting an infection, it's OK to continue your exercise program, but don't push yourself too hard. Moderate exer-

Don't take antibiotics
unless you really need them

Pinpointing the culprit behind an infection is vitally important. Bacterial infections can be effectively treated with antibiotics; viral infections can't.

In the past, doctors would often prescribe antibiotics without knowing what type of infection was causing the problem. But we can't afford to take that approach anymore.

Antibiotics can knock out an infection without killing all the bacteria. The surviving bacteria breed offspring that are "resistant" to the antibiotic, which means the antibiotic isn't effective against them anymore. If you try a new antibiotic, the bacteria can become resistant to it too. The next time you get sinusitis or some other infection, it will be even harder to get rid of.

Antibiotics also kill beneficial bacteria that control the growth of yeast. If too much yeast grows, you can have yeast infections in your mouth, vagina, or elsewhere. This weakens your immune system and opens the door to infections that keep coming back.

The powerful new antibiotic drugs, Ceclor, Cefzil, and Suprax, kill a wide range of bacteria, which can lead to even more bacterial resistance. People infected with drug-resistant bacteria are more likely to need hospitalization, stay longer at the hospital, and die.

Today, public health officials are urging doctors to stop prescribing these powerful new antibiotics for the treatment of sinusitis. When your doctor prescribes antibiotics to you, ask plenty of questions to make sure you really need them.

Sources —
> *Journal of the American Academy of Physician Assistants* (6,3:228)
> *The American Medical Association Home Medical Encyclopedia*, Random House, New York, 1989

cise seems to boost your immune system. Exercise that's too strenuous has the opposite effect. Of course, if you are weak, dizzy, or have a fever, don't exercise until you are feeling better.

Stay away from sugary foods. Some studies show that sugar represses the immune system, so your body can't fight infections as effectively. Eat fresh fruits and vegetables and whole grains to give your body the best nutrition defense.

Revive while you sleep. Get plenty of rest. Robert Ludlum's super-spy characters tend to say, "Sleep is a weapon." Research has shown that it's true. A recent study showed that the activity of infection-fighting cells dropped by 30 percent after just one night of insomnia. When the study participants caught up on their sleep, the cell activity levels bounced right back.

Sources —
Encyclopedia of Natural Healing, Prima Publishing, Rocklin, Calif., 1991
Food Safety Notebook (4,9:85)
Food — Your Miracle Medicine: How Food Can Prevent and Cure Over 100 Symptoms and Problems, HarperCollins Publishers, New York, 1993
Heinerman's Encyclopedia of Fruits, Vegetables and *Herbs,* Parker Publishing, West Nyack, N.Y., 1988
Herbal Medicine, Beaconsfield Publishers, Beaconsfield, England, 1991
HerbalGram (30:11)
Journal of the American Dietetic Association (92,8:988)
Nutrition Research Newsletter (14,1:10)
The Honest Herbal by Varro E. Tyler, PhD, The Haworth Press, Binghamton, N.Y., 1993

INFLUENZA (FLU)

◀ Chills   ◀ Cough
◀ Fatigue   ◀ Fever
◀ Headache   ◀ Muscle aches
◀ Runny nose   ◀ Sore throat

What to do to fight the flu

Influenza or the "flu" got its name from the Italian word for influence. Long age, people thought that it was caused by the "influence of the stars and planets." Today, while influenza is usually not life-threatening, it can definitely influence your lifestyle temporarily.

Influenza is a viral infection of the nose, throat, and lungs. People often confuse it with the common cold. However, the flu causes a fever, while a cold doesn't.

The flu can be dangerous for older people, so people over 65 should get a flu shot every year. Otherwise, to get through the flu:

Rest. Get a few days of bed rest in a warm, well-ventilated room. Don't think that you can work right through it. Besides, if you go out in public, you'll expose others to the virus.

Take aspirin. Take aspirin or other pain relievers for the aches and fever. However, don't give aspirin to anyone under age 21. It can increase their risk of Reye's syndrome, a life-threatening condition involving the brain and liver. Use acetaminophen instead.

Drink fluids. Drink plenty of water, fruit juice, and other liquids. If the fever lasts for more than a few days, call your doctor.

Sources —
Age Page, What to Do About the Flu, National Institute of Health, 1994
The American Medical Association Encyclopedia of Medicine, Random House, 1989

LARYNGITIS

◀ Hoarseness
◀ Inability to speak in a normal tone
◀ Sore throat

When you speak in a squeak

For years, doctors have recommended gargling to treat the old silencer, laryngitis. But gargling is not effective, says UCLA otolaryngologist, Dr. Robert J. Feder. Instead, he recommends the following home remedies:

Drink room-temperature water, instead of cold or ice water, to keep your throat moist.

Don't whisper. Talk in a normal voice. Whispering strains the vocal cords as much as shouting. If you can't talk in a normal voice, don't talk at all.

Use a steam vaporizer for five minutes every few hours to moisten the throat.

Avoid throat lozenges with mint or menthol, which dry your throat tissues. Use flavors such as honey, wild cherry, or black currant.

Don't clear your throat. It may seem to help, but it actually irritates throat tissues.

When you can't voice your opinions, don't panic. Laryngitis is usually short-lived. Follow these tips and you'll be speaking up before you know it.

Source —
Nutrition Health Review (56,10:1)

SHINGLES

◀ Fever and fatigue
◀ Line of pain, itching, or burning along one side of your body
◀ Painful line of blisters

When chickenpox virus strikes back

While it's true that most people who have had chickenpox won't break out in that itchy rash again, the virus that causes chickenpox can lie dormant in your nerves for years until something triggers it to become active again. The result is far more serious than a little fever and itching; it's an illness known as shingles.

About one in five people who have had chickenpox will develop shingles. You're at risk if you're over 50 or if your immune system is down because of an illness, recent surgery, or stress.

Don't neglect this medical emergency. If you have the symptoms of shingles, you should see a doctor immediately. If not treated quickly, shingles can do permanent damage to your nerves and cause intense pain that may never go away. It can cause permanent scarring, and it may even damage your eyes.

> ## What's your temperature?
> Few people actually have a body temperature of 98.6 degrees. "Normal" for you may be anywhere between 96 and 100.8 degrees. It's also normal to have a higher temperature in the afternoon than in the morning.
>
> **Source —**
> *The Journal of the American Medical Association* (268,12:1578)

The receptionist who schedules your doctor's appointments may have no idea that your blisters need immediate treatment. Don't let her put off your appointment for later in the week. Several prescription drugs can fight the virus that causes shingles, but you must start taking the drugs within 72 hours after the blisters form to get the best results.

While shingles is not an illness you can care for with home remedies alone, you can relieve your pain while you wait for the antiviral drugs to run their course. Here's what to do:

Cool off with a compress. Compresses made of towels moistened with water can help relieve the pain.

Get some rest. You may want to stay in bed at first. Stretching skin that's blistered, even with the smallest movements, can cause intense pain.

Mix crushed aspirin with body lotion for a pain-relieving cream. Crush one 325-milligram aspirin tablet and mix with 2 tablespoons of lotion, such as Vaseline Intensive Care. Rub it on the affected area three or four times a day.

The skin absorbs the aspirin quickly, so you won't have to wait long for relief. Applying the lotion may be quite painful, but the relief will be worth it.

Get pepper cream relief. Once the blisters have healed, a nonprescription capsaicin cream such as Zostrix may work wonders to relieve your pain. The active ingredient in this skin cream, capsaicin, comes from red chili peppers.

It works by deadening nerves in the area you rub it on, but it may cause a slight burning or tingling when you first use it. Make sure you see capsaicin in the list of ingredients. Don't be confused by drugs that have similar names, like capsicum or capsicum oleoresin.

Keep infection away with antibiotic cream. Rub-on antibiotic creams, available at your local pharmacy, can help prevent blisters from becoming infected.

Don't spread the virus. Keep in mind that if you have shingles, you can spread the virus to others and cause chickenpox. You should be especially careful around small children who have not had chickenpox.

The good news is that, like chickenpox, you should only get shingles once. Try to take comfort in the thought that you'll never have to suffer with shingles again.

Sources —
Emergency Medicine (21,3:35)
Medical Tribune (31,2:9)
Medical Tribune for the Family Physician (35,19:2)
U.S. Pharmacist (18,8:20)

SINUS INFECTIONS

◄ Creamy yellow or green
  discharge from your nose
◄ Loss of sense of smell
◄ Pain and pressure in your face, especially
  between or around your eyes and nose

◄ Fever
◄ Little relief from decongestants
  and antihistamines
◄ Pain in your upper teeth
◄ Stuffy, aching nose

Stop the sinusitis cycle

You have all the classic symptoms of sinusitis: a stuffy nose, painful sinuses, postnasal drip. Your first impulse is to visit your doctor and insist that he prescribe an antibiotic so you can get some relief.

If you don't have an infection and your doctor writes that prescription, he may be contributing to serious consequences later. Your body could begin to harbor bacteria that are resistant to antibiotics. When you really get sick, you could be in trouble.

So what's the answer when you're suffering from sinusitis? For general relief from sinus congestion, try home remedies and an over-the-counter decongestant.

If your symptoms continue and the nasal discharge turns greenish-yellow, you may have a sinus infection. Your doctor will probably treat your sinusitis with antibiotics. Your best bet is one of the older, less expensive antibiotics such as Amoxil or Augmentin.

If you're prescribed an antibiotic, don't stop taking it when your symptoms disappear. Take every pill according to your doctor's directions.

Tricks to treating sinus problems

Sinusitis may go away in time. Otherwise, at best, it produces discomfort, at worst, serious medical consequences. If your sinusitis isn't too severe, you can treat yourself with some home remedies and over-the-counter medicines.

Your tongue's healing powers

Did you know that your tongue contains a natural antibiotic?

Your instinct to pop a cut finger in your mouth may have a basis in scientific fact. Apparently, all the moist surfaces of your body respond to injuries by producing infection-fighting peptides.

You've probably seen dogs and cats lick their own wounds. They may be doing more than cleaning them; they may be putting on some antibiotic too.

Source —
Science News (147,11:166)

Drink lots of fluids. Drinking fluids will moisten and thin your mucus and help your sinuses drain.

Vaporize your air. Vaporizers will help your sinuses drain too. Try adding menthol or eucalyptus preparations to the water.

Chew horseradish root or slurp soups made with garlic. Any hot and spicy herb or food will help open your nasal passages.

Sleep with your head up. Put blocks under the head of your bed or use pillows to keep your head elevated. This will help keep mucus from draining back into your sinuses. You don't want the mucus to sit in your sinuses and become infected.

Find out what's triggering your allergies. Allergies may be at the root of your nasal and sinus inflammation, especially if you also have itchy eyes. You may be able to get rid of your sinusitis by getting your allergies under control. See the Breathing Problems chapter for more information.

Get over-the-counter relief. You should be able to get relief from some type of over-the-counter drug. It's best to buy single ingredient products rather than combination products.

That way you can stop taking the decongestant, the cough medicine, or the aspirin one by one as the symptoms disappear. You will avoid taking too many medicines and cut down on unwanted side effects.

Antihistamines block the effect of histamines on your nose. While antihistamines reduce itching and sneezing, they may not work well for swelling sinuses and a dripping or stuffy nose.

Decongestants may be taken by mouth or as nasal sprays or drops. They reduce the swelling that clogs your airways. Nasal sprays or nose drops work quickly, can last up to 12 hours, and are quite safe to use for up to three days. If you use them for longer than three days, though, you risk a rebound effect harder to remedy than the original stuffiness. People with high blood pressure, heart disease, diabetes, or hyperthyroidism should not use nasal decongestants without the advice of their doctors.

The longer your sinusitis lasts, the less effective over-the-counter drugs become. If you've developed a drug tolerance to the nasal decongestants and antihistamines, simply switching to products with different ingredients from time to time may work. But you may have chronic sinusitis that needs more aggressive treatment.

You may need antibiotics. Have you cancelled plans because of your sinusitis? Do you have to take naps or miss work regularly? Do over-the-counter drugs do little for you? Do you have frequent colds or stubborn earaches?

You probably have a sinus infection that needs antibiotic treatment. Antibiotics are used to kill the bacteria that cause infection

Know when you need surgery. Very few cases of sinusitis require surgical treatment. Yet when sinus trouble never ends, you may need surgery, not just to relieve discomfort but to protect against serious consequences. Polyps or cysts that hold mucus can grow in your sinuses, and they can be cancerous or simply grow too large.

With so many tools at hand, there seems no reason now for anyone to be resigned to a lifetime of sinus discomfort.

Sources —
Consumer Reports (60,7:492)
FDA Consumer (26,8:20)
Health & Healing (3,10:6)
Journal of the American Academy of Physician Assistants (6,3:228)
Postgraduate Medicine (91,5:281)
The American Medical Association Home Medical Encyclopedia, Random House, New York, 1989
The Journal of the American Medical Association (273,3:214)

> Please check with your doctor for approval before taking or discontinuing any prescription drug or using a natural healing alternative.

MENTAL ILLNESS AND SLEEPING PROBLEMS

Prescription Drugs

Natural Alternatives

Prescription Drugs

ANTI-ANXIETY DRUGS

Alprazolam

Brand name: *Xanax* **(Generic available)**

What this drug does for you:

This benzodiazepine treats anxiety, anxiety associated with depression, and panic disorder by slowing down your nervous system.

Possible side effects of this drug:

- Usually, side effects from alprazolam disappear after you've been taking the drug for a while. Drowsiness and lightheadedness are by far the most common side effects.
- You may also experience headache, confusion, insomnia, low blood pressure, difficulty urinating, dry mouth, constipation, diarrhea, nausea, irritability, memory impairment, trouble speaking clearly, decreased sex drive, and increased or decreased appetite.

Special warnings:

- People with some kinds of glaucoma shouldn't use this drug.
- You can become dependent on alprazolam, especially if you take more than 4 mg per day for longer than eight to 12 weeks. To avoid seizures and other less severe withdrawal symptoms, such as heightened senses, muscle cramps, diarrhea, and blurred vision, you should quit taking the drug gradually under your doctor's supervision. Don't stop abruptly, and don't increase or decrease your dosage without your doctor's approval.
- People with poor liver, kidney, or lung functions and obese people should use alprazolam cautiously. The drug may stay in your body longer and increase your risk of side effects.
- You should have regular blood and urine tests if you are taking alprazolam for a long time.

Pregnancy and nursing mothers:

Category D. See page 9 for description of categories. If mother has taken drug during pregnancy, newborns may go through withdrawal. Drug is present in mother's milk.

Possible food and drug interactions:

- If you take alprazolam along with any drug that depresses your nervous system, such as other tranquilizers, alcohol, antihistamines, or muscle relaxants, the combination may dangerously depress your nervous system.
- Alprazolam may increase levels of the antidepressants imipramine and desipramine in your body.
- Effects of this drug may be increased by the ulcer drug cimetidine and by birth control pills.

Helpful hints:

- Don't drive a car or operate heavy machinery until you see how the medicine affects you.
- The usual adult starting dosage for anxiety is 0.25 to 0.5 mg three times a day.
- The average adult dosage for panic disorder is 5 to 6 mg daily.

Buspirone

Brand name: *BuSpar*

What this drug does for you:
Buspirone treats anxiety, probably by affecting brain chemicals such as serotonin.

It is one of the safest anti-anxiety drugs because you aren't likely to become addicted to it. It also doesn't make you as sedated and drowsy as most of the other anti-anxiety drugs.

Possible side effects of this drug:
- The most common side effects are dizziness, nausea, headache, nervousness, lightheadedness, excitement, insomnia, and fatigue.
- Other side effects reported by at least one in every 100 people taking buspirone are chest pain, disturbed dreams, ringing in the ears, sore throat, and nasal congestion.

Special warning:
- If you are getting off a benzodiazepine drug or another sedative drug in order to begin taking buspirone, make sure you withdraw slowly from your previous drug. Buspirone will not help prevent withdrawal symptoms from other drugs for anxiety.

Pregnancy and nursing mothers:
Category B. See page 9 for description of categories. Drug is present in mother's milk. You should avoid this drug while nursing if possible.

Possible food and drug interactions:
- It's best not to take this drug with antidepressant drugs called monoamine oxidase (MAO) inhibitors. The combination may cause high blood pressure.
- Studies haven't shown an interaction between alcohol and buspirone, but it's wise to avoid alcohol while taking this drug.
- Researchers have not studied the effects of taking buspirone along with other drugs for mental disorders, so you and your doctor should approach any combination cautiously. Buspirone has been shown to increase levels of the antipsychotic haloperidol.

Helpful hints:
- The usual starting dosage for adults is 5 mg three times a day. Most people eventually begin taking 20 to 30 mg per day. The maximum daily dosage is 60 mg.
- Even though buspirone isn't supposed to be sedating, you should still avoid driving a car or operating any dangerous machinery until you see how the drug will affect you.

Chlordiazepoxide

Brand names: *Librium, Libritabs*

What this drug does for you:
This benzodiazepine treats anxiety and alcohol withdrawal by slowing down your nervous system. It acts as a sedative, stimulates your appetite, and works as a mild pain reliever. You can take chlordiazepoxide capsules, tablets, or shots.

Possible side effects of this drug:
- Drowsiness, confusion, and lack of coordination are the most common side effects.
- Rare side effects are fainting, skin eruptions, swelling, minor menstrual irregularities, nausea, constipation, and decreased or increased sex drive.

Special warnings:
- You can become dependent on chlordiazepoxide. To avoid seizures and other less severe withdrawal symptoms, such as heightened senses, muscle cramps, diarrhea, and blurred vision, you should quit taking the drug gradually under your doctor's supervision. Don't stop abruptly, and don't increase or decrease your dosage without your doctor's approval.
- People with poor liver, kidney, or lung functions and obese people should use chlordiazepoxide cautiously. The drug may stay in your body longer and increase your risk of side effects.
- People with a group of disorders called porphyria should use chlordiazepoxide cautiously.
- You should have regular blood and urine tests if you are taking chlordiazepoxide for a long time.

Pregnancy and nursing mothers:
This drug may cause birth defects if used during pregnancy. Drug is present in mother's milk.

Possible food and drug interactions:
- If you take chlordiazepoxide along with any drug that depresses your nervous system, such as other tranquilizers, alcohol, antihistamines, or muscle relaxers, the combination may dangerously depress your nervous system.
- You shouldn't take chlordiazepoxide when you are taking other drugs for mental disorders, especially monoamine oxidase (MAO) inhibitors and phenothiazines.
- Effects of this drug may be increased by the ulcer drug cimetidine and by birth control pills.

Helpful hints:
- Don't drive a car or operate heavy machinery until you see how the medicine affects you.
- The usual adult dosage depends on how severe your anxiety is. It ranges

from 5 mg to 25 mg, three or four times daily.
- Older people should probably take a low dosage (5 mg, two to four times daily) to reduce the chances of becoming oversedated.

Clorazepate

Brand names: *Tranxene-SD, Tranxene-SD Half Strength, Tranxene T-TAB, Gen-Xene* **(Generic available)**

What this drug does for you:
This benzodiazepine treats anxiety, helps manage seizures, and treats alcohol withdrawal by slowing down your nervous system. It acts as a sedative, stimulates your appetite, and works as a mild pain reliever.

Possible side effects of this drug:
- Drowsiness is the most common side effect.
- Less common side effects are dizziness, stomach problems, nervousness, blurred vision, headache, and confusion.
- Rare side effects are insomnia, skin rashes, fatigue, urination problems, irritability, double vision, depression, tremor (shakiness), and slurred speech.

Special warnings:
- People with some kinds of glaucoma shouldn't use this drug.
- You can become dependent on clorazepate. To avoid seizures and other less severe withdrawal symptoms, such as heightened senses, muscle cramps, diarrhea, and blurred vision, you should quit taking the drug gradually under your doctor's supervision. Don't stop abruptly, and don't increase or decrease your dosage without your doctor's approval.
- People with poor liver, kidney, or lung functions should use clorazepate cautiously. The drug may stay in your body longer and increase your risk of side effects.
- You should have regular blood and urine tests if you are taking clorazepate for a long time.

Pregnancy and nursing mothers:
This drug may cause birth defects if used during pregnancy. Drug is present in mother's milk.

Possible food and drug interactions:
- If you take clorazepate along with any drug that depresses your nervous system, such as other tranquilizers, alcohol, antihistamines, or muscle relaxers, the combination may dangerously depress your nervous system.
- If possible, you shouldn't take clorazepate when you are taking other drugs for mental disorders, especially monoamine oxidase (MAO) inhibitors and phenothiazines.

Helpful hints:
- Don't drive a car or operate heavy machinery until you see how the medicine affects you.

- The usual adult dosage is 15 to 60 mg a day.
- Older people should begin with a low dosage to reduce the chances of becoming oversedated.

Diazepam

Brand names: *Valium, Valrelease* **(Generic available)**

What this drug does for you:

This benzodiazepine treats anxiety, relieves muscle spasms, helps manage seizures, and treats alcohol withdrawal by slowing down your nervous system. It acts as a sedative, stimulates your appetite, and works as a mild pain reliever.

Possible side effects of this drug:

- Drowsiness, fatigue, and lack of coordination are by far the most common side effects.
- Less common side effects are confusion, depression, slurred speech, headache, fainting, tremor (shakiness), dizziness, constipation, nausea, urinary problems, changes in sex drive, heart problems, blurred vision, skin rash, and hives.

Special warnings:

- People with some kinds of glaucoma shouldn't use this drug.
- You can become dependent on diazepam. To avoid seizures and other less severe withdrawal symptoms, such as heightened senses, muscle cramps, diarrhea, and blurred vision, you should quit taking the drug gradually under your doctor's supervision. Don't stop abruptly, and don't increase or decrease your dosage without your doctor's approval.
- People with poor liver, kidney, or lung functions should use diazepam cautiously. The drug may stay in your body longer and increase your risk of side effects.
- You should have regular blood and urine tests if you are taking diazepam for a long time.

Pregnancy and nursing mothers:

This drug may cause birth defects if used during pregnancy. Drug is present in mother's milk.

Possible food and drug interactions:

- If you take diazepam along with any drug that depresses your nervous system, such as other tranquilizers, alcohol, antihistamines, or muscle relaxers, the combination may dangerously depress your nervous system.
- You shouldn't take diazepam when you are taking other drugs for mental disorders, especially monoamine oxidase (MAO) inhibitors and phenothiazines.
- Effects of this drug may be increased by the ulcer drug cimetidine.

Helpful hints:

- Don't drive a car or operate heavy machinery until you see how the med-

icine affects you.
- The usual adult dose is 2 mg to 10 mg, two to four times daily.
- Older people should begin with a low dose (2 mg to 2 1/2 mg, once or twice daily) to reduce the chances of becoming oversedated.

Hydroxyzine

Brand names: *Atarax, Vistaril* **(Generic available)**

What this drug does for you:
This drug is used to relieve anxiety and tension, to relieve itching caused by allergies, and as a sedative before surgery. Hydroxyzine is an antihistamine that suppresses the nervous system. It also relieves nausea, relaxes your muscles, and works as a bronchodilator and a pain reliever.

You should notice the effects of any form of this drug (tablets, capsules, or syrup) within 15 to 30 minutes.

Possible side effects of this drug:
- Dry mouth and drowsiness are common side effects, but they tend to go away after you've been taking the drug for a while.
- Rarely, large doses of the drug can cause convulsions or tremors.

Special warnings:
- Check with your doctor before taking hydroxyzine if you have an enlarged prostate, urination problems, glaucoma, or heart rhythm problems.

Pregnancy and nursing mothers:
This drug may cause birth defects if you use it while you're pregnant. It is not known whether this drug is present in mother's milk.

Possible food and drug interactions:
- Hydroxyzine may increase the action of drugs that depress the nervous system, such as meperidine, barbiturates, narcotics, and non-narcotic pain relievers. These drugs are sometimes used together before surgery.
- When you're taking hydroxyzine, avoid alcohol and other depressants such as tranquilizers and sleeping pills.

Helpful hints:
- Don't drive a car or operate heavy machinery until you see how the medicine affects you.
- The usual adult dosage for anxiety is 50 to 100 mg four times a day.
- For itching, the usual adult dosage is 25 mg three or four times a day.

Lorazepam

Brand name: *Ativan* **(Generic available)**

What this drug does for you:
This benzodiazepine treats anxiety and anxiety associated with depression by slowing down your nervous system.

Possible side effects of this drug:

- Usually, side effects from lorazepam disappear after you've been taking the drug for a while. Drowsiness and dizziness are the most common side effects.
- You may also experience weakness, unsteadiness, depression, nausea, change in appetite, headache, sleep disturbances, and skin problems.

Special warnings:

- People with some kinds of glaucoma shouldn't use this drug.
- You can become dependent on lorazepam. To avoid seizures and other less severe withdrawal symptoms, such as heightened senses, muscle cramps, diarrhea, and blurred vision, you should quit taking the drug gradually under your doctor's supervision. Don't stop abruptly, and don't increase or decrease your dosage without your doctor's approval.
- People with poor liver, kidney, or lung functions should use lorazepam cautiously. The drug may stay in your body longer and increase your risk of side effects.
- You should have regular blood and urine tests if you are taking lorazepam for a long time.

Pregnancy and nursing mothers:

You should not take this drug while you're pregnant. It is not known whether drug is present in mother's milk. However, since other benzodiazepine tranquilizers are present in mother's milk, lorazepam probably is too.

Possible food and drug interactions:

- If you take lorazepam along with any drug that depresses your nervous system, such as other tranquilizers, alcohol, antihistamines, or muscle relaxers, the combination may dangerously depress your nervous system.

Helpful hints:

- Don't drive a car or operate heavy machinery until you see how the medicine affects you.
- The usual adult dosage is 2 to 6 mg a day. You usually take the largest dose at bedtime.

Meprobamate

Brand names: *Equanil, MB-TAB, Meprospan, Miltown*

What this drug does for you:

This drug relieves severe anxiety and nervousness.

Possible side effects of this drug:

- This drug may cause a headache, drowsiness, dizziness, excitement, visual disorders, lack of coordination, weakness, slurred speech, heart palpitations or an irregular heartbeat, low blood pressure, fainting, nausea, diarrhea, and a tingling or prickling feeling.
- If you have an allergic reaction to the drug, your symptoms could include itching, hives, rashes, swelling, fever, chills, urinary problems, skin dis-

orders, and wheezing.

Special warnings:

- Don't use this drug if you have the metabolic disease called porphyria.
- If you have liver or kidney problems, epilepsy, alcoholism, or a history of drug abuse, you should talk with your doctor about your condition before taking this drug.
- You can become dependent on meprobamate. To avoid seizures and other less severe withdrawal symptoms, such as heightened senses, muscle cramps, diarrhea, and blurred vision, you should quit taking the drug gradually under your doctor's supervision. Don't stop abruptly, and don't increase or decrease your dosage without your doctor's approval.

Pregnancy and nursing mothers:

You should not use this drug while you're pregnant. It can cause birth defects. Drug is present in mother's milk in very high amounts.

Possible food and drug interactions:

- If you take meprobamate along with any drug that depresses your nervous system, such as other tranquilizers, alcohol, antihistamines, or muscle relaxers, the combination may dangerously depress your nervous system.

Helpful hints:

- Don't drive a car or operate heavy machinery until you see how the medicine affects you.
- The usual adult daily dosage is 1200 mg to 1600 mg.

Oxazepam

Brand name: *Serax* **(Generic available)**

What this drug does for you:

This benzodiazepine treats anxiety, tension, agitation, irritability, and anxiety associated with depression by slowing down your nervous system. It also helps treat the symptoms of alcohol withdrawal.

Oxazepam is one of the safer benzodiazepine tranquilizers, mainly because it doesn't stay in your body as long as the others.

Possible side effects of this drug:

- Usually, side effects from oxazepam disappear after you've been taking the drug for a while. Drowsiness and lightheadedness are the most common side effects.
- Other side effects are dizziness, headache, fainting, and excitement.
- Rare side effects are skin rashes, nausea, swelling, slurred speech, shakiness, and a change in your sex drive.

Special warnings:

- People with some kinds of glaucoma shouldn't use this drug.
- You can become dependent on oxazepam, especially if you take more than 4 mg per day for longer than eight to 12 weeks. To avoid seizures

and other less severe withdrawal symptoms, such as heightened senses, muscle cramps, diarrhea, and blurred vision, you should quit taking the drug gradually under your doctor's supervision. Don't stop abruptly, and don't increase or decrease your dosage without your doctor's approval.

- Very rarely, oxazepam has caused low blood pressure. You should take this drug cautiously if a drop in blood pressure could cause heart trouble for you.
- You should have regular blood counts and liver-function tests while you're taking this drug.

Pregnancy and nursing mothers:

Taking this drug while you're pregnant may cause birth defects. Drug is present in mother's milk.

Possible food and drug interactions:

- If you take oxazepam along with any drug that depresses your nervous system, such as other tranquilizers, alcohol, antihistamines, or muscle relaxers, the combination may dangerously depress your nervous system.

Helpful hints:

- Don't drive a car or operate heavy machinery until you see how the medicine affects you.
- The usual adult dose for mild to moderate anxiety is 10 to 15 mg, three or four times a day.
- The usual adult dose for severe anxiety syndromes is 15 to 30 mg, three or four times daily.
- The usual starting dose for older adults with anxiety, tension, and agitation is 10 mg, three times daily.

ANTIDEPRESSANTS

Amitriptyline

Brand names: *Elavil, Endep* (Generic available)

What this drug does for you:

Amitriptyline treats the symptoms of depression. It is a tricyclic antidepressant with strong sedative effects. It increases the amount of serotonin or norepinephrine in your central nervous system.

Possible side effects of this drug:

- Amitriptyline is one of the most sedating tricyclic antidepressants. It will probably make you drowsy, at least for the first few weeks.
- Other common side effects are dizziness, dry mouth, headache, increased appetite, nausea, unpleasant taste, or a black-colored tongue. You could also have diarrhea, increased sweating, ringing in the ears, breast enlargement in males and females, hair loss, and sensitivity to light.

- More serious side effects are blurred vision, confusion, constipation, decreased sexual ability, difficulty in speaking or swallowing, eye pain, fainting, irregular heartbeat, hallucinations, shakiness, nervousness, shuffling walk, a mask-like face, loss of balance control, a change in blood sugar levels or blood pressure levels, hepatitis, jaundice, seizures, coma, heart attack, and stroke.
- If you suddenly quit taking this drug, you could have nausea, headache, and a general feeling of fatigue. If you gradually quit taking the drug, you may still experience irritability, restlessness, and dream and sleep disturbances.

Special warnings:
- You shouldn't use this drug when you are recovering from a heart attack.
- If you have a history of seizures, liver problems, urinary retention, thyroid problems, increased pressure in the eye, or heart problems, you should talk with your doctor about your condition before you take amitriptyline.
- When possible, you should quit taking amitriptyline several days before surgery.

Pregnancy and nursing mothers:
If possible, you should not take amitriptyline while you are pregnant. No good studies have been done, but some women taking amitriptyline have had babies with birth defects. Drug is present in mother's milk. You should not use this drug while you are nursing.

Possible food and drug interactions:
- You should never take amitriptyline while taking the antidepressants called monoamine oxidase (MAO) inhibitors. If you've been taking an MAO inhibitor, you should stay off it for two weeks before you begin taking amitriptyline. The combination can cause a high fever, convulsions, and death.
- Any of the type of antidepressants called selective serotonin reuptake inhibitors (fluoxetine, sertraline, and paroxetine) can cause amitriptyline to reach dangerously high levels in your body. If you are taking these antidepressants at the same time, your doctor should monitor you closely. You may need lower than normal doses of both drugs. You also should not quickly switch from fluoxetine to a tricyclic antidepressant like amitriptyline. You may need to wait five weeks for the fluoxetine to clear out of your body.
- Some blood-pressure-lowering drugs may not work as well if you also take amitriptyline.
- If you take amitriptyline along with any drug that depresses your nervous system, such as tranquilizers, alcohol, antihistamines, or muscle relaxers, the combination may dangerously depress your nervous system.
- Taking disulfiram, a drug that helps you overcome alcohol addiction, and amitriptyline at the same time can cause delirium.
- Your doctor should supervise you closely for side effects if you take

amitriptyline along with any anticholinergic drugs such as some anti-histamines and muscle relaxants or along with any sympathomimetic drugs such as some decongestants.

- Cimetidine, an ulcer drug, can increase the levels of amitriptyline in your body.
- Taking ethchlorvynol, a drug for insomnia, and amitriptyline at the same time can cause delirium.

Helpful hints:
- Don't drive a car or operate heavy machinery until you see how the medicine affects you. Drowsiness and dizziness usually go away after a few weeks.
- Be careful in hot weather. This drug could make you sweat less in high temperatures, so you're more likely to get a high fever or heatstroke.
- This drug is very likely to cause dry mouth and constipation, so you should drink plenty of fluids and eat a high-fiber diet.
- The usual starting dosage is 75 mg a day, taken in divided doses. Some people take 150 mg a day. The usual maintenance dosage is 50 to 100 mg a day. Since amitriptyline has a sedative effect, you may want to take the largest dose in the late afternoon or at bedtime.

Amoxapine

Brand name: *Asendin* **(Generic available)**

What this drug does for you:
Amoxapine treats the symptoms of depression and depression accompanied by anxiety. It is a tricyclic antidepressant with mild sedative effects. It increases the amount of serotonin or norepinephrine in your central nervous system.

Amoxapine works more quickly than some of the other tricyclic antidepressants — possibly within four to seven days and usually within two weeks.

Possible side effects of this drug:
- The most common reactions to amoxapine are drowsiness, dry mouth, constipation, and blurred vision.
- You may also experience anxiety, insomnia, shakiness, heart palpitations, confusion, excitement, nausea, dizziness, headache, fatigue, weakness, increased appetite, and increased sweating.
- Some people may get a skin rash or a fever when taking amoxapine. Usually, this allergic reaction happens in the first few days you're on the drug.
- A rare side effect of amoxapine is tardive dyskinesia, a disorder where certain muscles or muscle groups move slowly and uncontrollably. This side effect is dangerous because it may not go away when you quit taking the drug. Lip smacking, puffing of cheeks, or any uncontrolled movement is a sign of tardive dyskinesia.
- Another rare but dangerous side effect is neuroleptic malignant syndrome. Some signs of the syndrome are a high fever, rigid muscles, an

irregular or rapid heartbeat, and sweating.

Special warnings:

- You shouldn't use this drug when you are recovering from a heart attack.
- If you have a history of seizures, urinary retention, increased pressure in the eye, or heart problems, you should talk with your doctor about your condition before you take amoxapine.
- Use this drug with caution if you have heart disease, certain kinds of glaucoma (consult your doctor), or urinary retention.
- If you have a history of seizures or convulsions, you should use this drug with extreme caution.
- You shouldn't drive a car or operate heavy machinery until you are sure the medicine isn't making you drowsy or less than alert.

Pregnancy and nursing mothers:

Category C. See page 9 for description of categories. Drug is present in mother's milk.

Possible food and drug interactions:

- You should never take amoxapine while taking the antidepressants called monoamine oxidase (MAO) inhibitors. If you've been taking an MAO inhibitor, you should stay off it for two weeks before you begin taking amoxapine. The combination can cause a high fever, convulsions, and death.
- Any of the type of antidepressants called selective serotonin reuptake inhibitors (fluoxetine, sertraline, and paroxetine) can cause amoxapine to reach dangerously high levels in your body. If you are taking these antidepressants at the same time, your doctor should monitor you closely. You may need lower than normal doses of both drugs. You also should not quickly switch from fluoxetine to a tricyclic antidepressant like amoxapine. You may need to wait five weeks for the fluoxetine to clear out of your body.
- If you take amoxapine along with any drug that depresses your nervous system, such as tranquilizers, alcohol, antihistamines, or muscle relaxers, the combination may dangerously depress your nervous system.
- Your doctor should supervise you closely for side effects if you take amoxapine along with any anticholinergic drugs such as some antihistamines and muscle relaxants.
- Cimetidine, an ulcer drug, can increase the levels of amoxapine in your body.

Helpful hints:

- Don't drive a car or operate heavy machinery until you see how the medicine affects you. Drowsiness and dizziness usually go away after a few weeks.
- The usual adult dosage of amoxapine is 200 to 300 mg daily. Most people take a single dose at bedtime. If you take more than 300 mg a day, you shouldn't take it all at once.

Bupropion

Brand name: *Wellbutrin*

What this drug does for you:

Bupropion relieves the symptoms of depression. It increases the amount of serotonin, norepinephrine, and dopamine in your central nervous system. Unlike many of the other antidepressants, it does not have sedative effects.

Possible side effects of this drug:

- Many people experience dry mouth, headache, nausea, constipation, shakiness, agitation, anxiety, restlessness, and insomnia when they first begin taking bupropion.
- Weight loss is a common side effect of bupropion. If you can't afford to lose any weight, you may not want to begin taking bupropion.
- Rarer side effects are skin rash, dizziness, an irregular heartbeat, some menstrual complaints, sweating, and blurred vision.
- Bupropion is four times more likely to cause seizures than other antidepressants. Approximately three out of every 1,000 people taking 450 mg or less of bupropion a day experience a seizure. See the Helpful hints section for advice on reducing your risk.

Special warnings:

- People with a seizure disorder should not take bupropion.
- People who have had the eating disorders bulimia or anorexia nervosa have a higher risk of seizures if they take bupropion. You also have a higher risk of seizures if you have a history of head injury or a tumor of the central nervous system.
- You should use this drug cautiously when you are recovering from a heart attack or if your heart disease is unstable.
- People with liver or kidney damage probably need lower doses of bupropion and should be closely watched for any toxic effects.

Pregnancy and nursing mothers:

Category B. See page 9 for description of categories. You should not use this drug while you are nursing.

Possible food and drug interactions:

- People taking antipsychotics, other antidepressants, or people who have suddenly quit taking a benzodiazepine (a drug for anxiety) are at greater risk of seizures if they also take bupropion.
- You should never take bupropion while taking the antidepressants called monoamine oxidase (MAO) inhibitors. If you've been taking an MAO inhibitor, you should stay off it for two weeks before you begin taking bupropion.
- You shouldn't drink alcohol while you're taking bupropion because alcohol increases your risk of seizures.
- Drugs that affect liver function such as carbamazepine, cimetidine, phenobarbital, and phenytoin can increase or decrease the effectiveness of bupropion.

- If you take bupropion at the same time as levodopa, you may have more side effects.

Helpful hints:
- To reduce the risk of seizures, don't take more than 450 mg of bupropion a day. You should divide your dosage — never take more than 150 mg at one time. If you forget a dose, don't double up on your next dose. Also, if you and your doctor decide you need to increase your dosage, begin taking more medicine gradually.
- As with any drug that affects your central nervous system, you shouldn't drive a car or operate heavy machinery until you are sure the medicine isn't making you drowsy or less than alert.
- The usual adult dosage is 300 mg, taken three times a day.
- It's best to allow at least six hours between each dose.
- If you are having trouble sleeping, try not to take a dose right at bedtime.
- You may take bupropion for four weeks before you notice any improvement in your depression.

Clomipramine

Brand name: *Anafranil*

What this drug does for you:
Clomipramine is a tricyclic antidepressant used to treat obsessive-compulsive disorder (OCD). Obsessions are thoughts you have over and over again that interfere with your day-to-day life. Compulsions are meaningless actions you purposely perform again and again, such as counting things or washing your hands.

Possible side effects of this drug:
- Even though less than 1 percent of the people taking clomipramine have seizures, they are still the most significant risk of taking clomipramine.
- One very common side effect is sexual dysfunction in men. Forty-two percent of the men in one study were unable to ejaculate and 20 percent experienced impotence.
- Other common side effects are dry mouth, constipation, nausea, upset stomach, sleepiness, shakiness, twitching muscles, dizziness, nervousness, fatigue, sweating, urination problems, weight gain, and visual changes.
- You may experience some withdrawal symptoms (dizziness, nausea, sleep disturbances, irritability, etc.) if you stop taking the drug suddenly.

Special warnings:
- You shouldn't use this drug when you are recovering from a heart attack.
- You should use clomipramine cautiously if you have a history of seizures, alcoholism, or brain damage.
- You should quit taking clomipramine before surgery with general anes-

thetics if possible.
- If you have any of the following conditions, you should use clomipramine with caution: an overactive thyroid, increased pressure in the eye, urinary retention, poor liver function, or tumors of the adrenal medulla.

Pregnancy and nursing mothers:
Category C. See page 9 for description of categories. Drug is present in mother's milk. You should not use this drug while you are nursing.

Possible food and drug interactions:
- The antipsychotic drug haloperidol, the attention-deficit disorder drug methylphenidate, the ulcer drug cimetidine, and certain antidepressants such as fluoxetine may increase levels of clomipramine in your body.
- Clomipramine may increase levels of phenobarbital and the heart drugs warfarin and digoxin in your body.
- You should never take clomipramine while taking the antidepressants called monoamine oxidase (MAO) inhibitors. If you've been taking an MAO inhibitor, you should stay off it for two weeks before you begin taking clomipramine. The combination can cause a high fever, convulsions, and death.
- Smoking may reduce the effectiveness of clomipramine.
- People taking antipsychotics, other antidepressants, or people who have suddenly quit taking a benzodiazepine (a drug for anxiety) are at greater risk of seizures if they also take clomipramine.
- If you take clomipramine along with any drug that depresses your nervous system, such as tranquilizers, alcohol, antihistamines, or muscle relaxers, the combination may dangerously depress your nervous system.
- Some blood-pressure-lowering drugs may not work as well if you also take clomipramine.
- Your doctor should supervise you closely for side effects if you take clomipramine along with any anticholinergic drugs such as some antihistamines and muscle relaxants or along with any sympathomimetic drugs such as some decongestants.
- The seizure drug phenytoin and various barbiturates may decrease levels of clomipramine in your body.

Helpful hints:
- As with any drug that affects your central nervous system, you shouldn't drive a car or operate heavy machinery until you are sure the medicine isn't making you drowsy or less than alert.
- Take your medicine with meals so it won't upset your stomach.
- The usual starting adult dosage is 25 mg daily. Your doctor may gradually increase your dosage to a maximum of 250 mg daily. Eventually, you can take your total daily dose at bedtime so you won't be sleepy during the day.

Desipramine

Brand name: *Norpramin* **(Generic available)**

What this drug does for you:

Desipramine treats the symptoms of depression. It is a tricyclic antidepressant, and it increases the amount of serotonin and, especially, norepinephrine in your central nervous system.

You may see results in two to five days, but you usually don't get the full benefits until you've been taking the drug for two to three weeks.

Possible side effects of this drug:

- Common side effects are dizziness, drowsiness, dry mouth, headache, increased appetite, nausea, unpleasant taste, or a black-colored tongue. You could also have diarrhea, increased sweating, ringing in the ears, breast enlargement in males and females, hair loss, and sensitivity to light.
- More serious side effects are blurred vision, confusion, constipation, decreased sexual ability, difficulty in speaking or swallowing, eye pain, fainting, irregular heartbeat, hallucinations, shakiness, nervousness, shuffling walk, a mask-like face, loss of balance control, a change in blood sugar levels or blood pressure levels, hepatitis, jaundice, seizures, coma, heart attack, or stroke.
- If you suddenly quit taking this drug, you could have nausea, headache, and a general feeling of fatigue. If you gradually quit taking the drug, you may still experience irritability, restlessness, and dream and sleep disturbances.

Special warnings:

- You shouldn't take this drug when you are recovering from a heart attack.
- You should take this drug very cautiously if you have heart disease, urinary retention, glaucoma, thyroid disease, or a history of seizures.
- When possible, you should quit taking desipramine several days before surgery.

Pregnancy and nursing mothers:

Not known if it's safe to take this drug while pregnant. Not known if it's safe to take this drug while nursing.

Possible food and drug interactions:

- The ulcer drug cimetidine, the phenothiazine tranquilizers, and the heart drugs propafenone and flecainide can increase the levels of desipramine in your body.
- Cigarette smoking, barbiturates, and alcohol may decrease the effectiveness of this drug.
- You should never take desipramine while taking the antidepressants called monoamine oxidase (MAO) inhibitors. If you've been taking an MAO inhibitor, you should stay off it for two weeks before you begin taking desipramine. The combination can cause a high fever, convulsions,

and death.
- Some blood-pressure-lowering drugs may not work as well if you also take desipramine.
- If you take desipramine along with any drug that depresses your nervous system, such as tranquilizers, alcohol, antihistamines, or muscle relaxers, the combination may dangerously depress your nervous system.
- Your doctor should supervise you closely for side effects if you take desipramine along with any anticholinergic drugs such as some antihistamines and muscle relaxants or along with any sympathomimetic drugs such as some decongestants.
- Any of the type of antidepressants called selective serotonin reuptake inhibitors (fluoxetine, sertraline, and paroxetine) can cause desipramine to reach dangerously high levels in your body. If you are taking these antidepressants at the same time, your doctor should monitor you closely. You may need lower than normal doses of both drugs.

Helpful hints:
- As with any drug that affects your central nervous system, you shouldn't drive a car or operate heavy machinery until you are sure the medicine isn't making you drowsy or less than alert.
- The usual adult dose is 100 to 200 mg a day. You shouldn't take more than 300 mg a day.

Doxepin

Brand names: *Adapin, Sinequan, Zonalon* (Generic available)

What this drug does for you:
Doxepin treats the symptoms of depression and anxiety. It is a tricyclic antidepressant with strong sedative effects. It increases the amount of norepinephrine in your central nervous system.

Possible side effects of this drug:
- Doxepin will probably make you drowsy, at least for the first few weeks.
- Other common side effects are dizziness, dry mouth, headache, increased appetite, nausea, unpleasant taste, or a black-colored tongue. You could also have diarrhea, increased sweating, ringing in the ears, breast enlargement in males and females, hair loss, and sensitivity to light.
- More serious side effects are blurred vision, confusion, constipation, decreased sexual ability, difficulty in speaking or swallowing, eye pain, fainting, irregular heartbeat, hallucinations, shakiness, nervousness, shuffling walk, a mask-like face, loss of balance control, a change in blood sugar levels or blood pressure levels, hepatitis, jaundice, seizures, coma, heart attack, and stroke.
- If you suddenly quit taking this drug, you could have nausea, headache, and a general feeling of fatigue. If you gradually quit taking the drug, you may still experience irritability, restlessness, and dream and sleep

disturbances.

Special warning:
- People with glaucoma or urinary retention should not use doxepin.

Pregnancy and nursing mothers:
Not known if safe to use while pregnant. No test has been done with nursing mothers, but there has been one report of a nursing baby having drowsiness and sleep apnea (a disorder where you stop breathing for short periods of time while you sleep) when his mother was taking doxepin.

Possible food and drug interactions:
- Doxepin may be a good choice for people with high blood pressure, because it doesn't significantly affect the action of guanethidine and other similar blood-pressure-lowering drugs.
- Doxepin is sometimes given to alcoholics for depression and anxiety, but you should avoid alcohol while taking the drug. Your normal response to the alcohol could be dangerously increased.
- You should never take doxepin while taking the antidepressants called monoamine oxidase (MAO) inhibitors. If you've been taking an MAO inhibitor, you should stay off it for two weeks before you begin taking doxepin.
- The ulcer drug cimetidine, the phenothiazine tranquilizers, the heart drugs propafenone and flecainide, and any of the type of antidepressants called selective serotonin reuptake inhibitors (fluoxetine, sertraline, and paroxetine) can increase the levels of doxepin in your body. If you are taking doxepin and any of these other drugs at the same time, you may need lower than normal doses of both drugs.
- Your doctor should supervise you closely for side effects if you take doxepin along with any anticholinergic drugs such as some antihistamines and muscle relaxers.
- For diabetics, taking tolazamide and doxepin at the same time can cause severe hypoglycemia.

Helpful hints:
- Don't drive a car or operate heavy machinery until you see how the medicine affects you. Drowsiness and dizziness usually go away after a few weeks.
- The usual adult dose is 75 to 150 mg per day. You can take a dose of 150 mg or less at one time, usually at bedtime.
- You may need to take doxepin for two to three weeks before your depression is relieved.

Fluoxetine

Brand name: *Prozac*

What this drug does for you:
Fluoxetine treats the symptoms of depression and obsessive-compulsive disorder by increasing the amount of serotonin in your central nervous system.

Possible side effects of this drug:

- Anxiety, insomnia, and weight loss are three very common side effects of fluoxetine.
- Other common side effects are drowsiness, fatigue, tremor (shakiness), sweating, upset stomach, nausea, diarrhea, dizziness, and lightheadedness.
- You may also experience dry mouth, abnormal vision, decreased sex drive, and abnormal ejaculation.
- Tell your doctor if you develop a rash or hives while taking fluoxetine. You may have to stop taking the drug, because more serious reactions can accompany the rash.
- This drug has many other side effects, but they are rare. Check with your doctor if you have chills or fever, joint or muscle pain, trouble breathing, or any more serious problems.

Special warnings:

- Fluoxetine can stay in your body for up to five weeks after you stop taking it. You may need to wait five weeks before you take any drug that may interact with fluoxetine.
- You may need a lower than normal dosage of fluoxetine if you have liver or kidney disease. Your doctor should monitor you closely for side effects.
- Take this drug with caution if you have a history of seizures.
- For people with diabetes, fluoxetine can affect your blood sugar control.

Pregnancy and nursing mothers:

Category B. See page 9 for description of categories. Drug is present in mother's milk. You should not take fluoxetine while you are nursing.

Possible food and drug interactions:

- Taking fluoxetine while you are also taking other antidepressants can increase the levels of both drugs in your body.
- You should never take fluoxetine while taking the antidepressants called monoamine oxidase (MAO) inhibitors. If you've been taking an MAO inhibitor, you should stay off it for two weeks before you begin taking fluoxetine. You should stay off fluoxetine for five weeks before you begin taking an MAO inhibitor.
- If you are taking flecainide, vinblastine, carbamazepine, or any tricyclic antidepressant, you may need to decrease your dosage of the drug once you start taking fluoxetine. Consult your doctor.
- Tryptophan and paroxetine together can cause agitation, restlessness, and upset stomach. You may want to avoid foods high in tryptophan, such as meats, poultry, fish, liver, kidney, eggs, nuts, peanut butter, broad beans, and wheat germ.
- Fluoxetine may increase or decrease levels of the antipsychotic lithium, so lithium levels should be monitored while using this drug.
- Fluoxetine may cause diazepam to stay in your body longer than usual.
- Fluoxetine may increase levels of phenytoin in your body.
- Digoxin and coumadin may interact with fluoxetine.

Helpful hints:

- You can take fluoxetine with or without food.
- As with any drug that affects your central nervous system, you shouldn't drive a car or operate heavy machinery until you are sure the medicine isn't making you drowsy or less than alert.
- The usual starting dose for adults is 20 mg a day, taken in the morning. The maximum dose is 80 mg a day.

Imipramine

Brand name: *Tofranil* **(Generic available)**

What this drug does for you:

Imipramine treats the symptoms of depression. It is a tricyclic antidepressant with moderate sedative effects. It increases the amount of norepinephrine in your central nervous system.

Imipramine is also used to treat bed-wetting for children over 6.

Possible side effects of this drug:

- Imipramine is one of the most sedating tricyclic antidepressants. It will probably make you drowsy, at least for the first few weeks.
- Other common side effects are dizziness, dry mouth, headache, increased appetite, nausea, unpleasant taste, or a black-colored tongue. You could also have diarrhea, increased sweating, ringing in the ears, breast enlargement in males and females, hair loss, and sensitivity to light.
- More serious side effects are blurred vision, confusion, constipation, decreased sexual ability, difficulty in speaking or swallowing, eye pain, fainting, irregular heartbeat, hallucinations, shakiness, nervousness, shuffling walk, a mask-like face, loss of balance control, a change in blood sugar levels or blood pressure levels, hepatitis, jaundice, seizures, coma, heart attack, or stroke.
- If you suddenly quit taking this drug, you could have nausea, headache, and a general feeling of fatigue. If you gradually quit taking the drug, you may still experience irritability, restlessness, and dream and sleep disturbances.
- If you develop a fever and a sore throat while taking this drug, you need to have certain blood tests done. You may have to quit taking imipramine.

Special warnings:

- You shouldn't use this drug when you are recovering from a heart attack.
- If you have a history of seizures, liver or kidney problems, urinary retention, thyroid problems, increased pressure in the eye, or heart problems, you should talk with your doctor about your condition before you take imipramine. You may need to be carefully monitored by your doctor while you're taking imipramine.
- When possible, you should quit taking imipramine several days before surgery.

Pregnancy and nursing mothers:

If possible, you should not take imipramine while you are pregnant. No good studies have been done, but some women taking imipramine have had babies with birth defects. Drug is present in mother's milk. You should not use this drug while you are nursing.

Possible food and drug interactions:

- You should never take imipramine while taking the antidepressants called monoamine oxidase (MAO) inhibitors. If you've been taking an MAO inhibitor, you should stay off it for two weeks before you begin taking imipramine. The combination can cause a high fever, convulsions, and death.
- If you take imipramine along with any drug that depresses your nervous system, such as tranquilizers, alcohol, antihistamines, or muscle relaxers, the combination may dangerously depress your nervous system.
- Your doctor should supervise you closely for side effects if you take imipramine along with any anticholinergic drugs such as some antihistamines and muscle relaxants or along with any sympathomimetic drugs such as some decongestants.
- Cimetidine, an ulcer drug, methylphenidate, and fluoxetine can increase the levels of imipramine in your body.
- Some blood-pressure-lowering drugs, such as guanethidine and clonidine, may not work as well if you also take imipramine.
- Barbiturates and phenytoin can decrease levels of imipramine in your body.

Helpful hints:

- Don't drive a car or operate heavy machinery until you see how the medicine affects you. Drowsiness and dizziness usually go away after a few weeks.
- The usual starting dosage is 75 mg a day. The usual maintenance dosage is 50 to 150 mg a day. Since imipramine has a sedative effect, you may want to take the largest dose in the late afternoon or bedtime.
- You may take imipramine one to three weeks before you notice an improvement in your depression.
- Don't expose yourself to too much sunlight, because imipramine makes your skin extra-sensitive to sunlight.

Maprotiline

Brand name: *Ludiomil* (Generic available)

What this drug does for you:

Maprotiline treats the symptoms of depression and the anxiety that can accompany depression. It is a tetracyclic antidepressant that works by increasing the amount of norepinephrine in your central nervous system.

Possible side effects of this drug:

- Maprotiline basically has the same side effects as the tricyclic antidepressants. Drowsiness and dry mouth are the most common side effects. Also common are nervousness, anxiety, insomnia, agitation, dizziness, shakiness, constipation, blurred vision, nausea, weakness and fatigue, and headache.

- Rare side effects are impotence, a change in blood sugar level or blood pressure level, vomiting, diarrhea, difficulty swallowing, jaundice, sweating, flushing, rapid heartbeat, heart block, fainting, enlargement of breasts in men and women, nasal congestion, hair loss, numbness or tingling, ringing in the ears, hallucinations, delusions, lack of coordination, itching, rash, and sensitivity to light.

Special warnings:

- You shouldn't use this drug when you are recovering from a heart attack.
- If you have a history of seizures, liver problems, urinary retention, thyroid problems, increased pressure in the eye, or heart problems, you should talk with your doctor about your condition before you take maprotiline.
- When possible, you should quit taking maprotiline several days before surgery.

Pregnancy and nursing mothers:

Category B. See page 9 for description of categories. Drug is present in mother's milk.

Possible food and drug interactions:

- You should never take maprotiline while taking the antidepressants called monoamine oxidase (MAO) inhibitors. If you've been taking an MAO inhibitor, you should stay off it for two weeks before you begin taking maprotiline. The combination can cause a high fever, convulsions, and death.
- Taking maprotiline with phenothiazines (a type of tranquilizer) increases your risk of seizures.
- If you take maprotiline along with any drug that depresses your nervous system, such as tranquilizers, alcohol, antihistamines, or muscle relaxers, the combination may dangerously depress your nervous system.
- Your doctor should supervise you closely for side effects if you take maprotiline along with any anticholinergic drugs such as some antihistamines and muscle relaxants or along with any sympathomimetic drugs such as some decongestants.
- Some blood-pressure-lowering drugs such as guanethidine may not work as well if you also take maprotiline.
- Any of the type of antidepressants called selective serotonin reuptake inhibitors (fluoxetine, sertraline, and paroxetine) can cause maprotiline to reach dangerously high levels in your body. If you are taking these antidepressants at the same time, your doctor should monitor you closely. You may need lower than normal doses of both drugs.
- Cimetidine, an ulcer drug, can increase the levels of maprotiline in your body.
- The seizure drug phenytoin and various barbiturates may lower the lev-

els of maprotiline in your body.

Helpful hints:

- As with any drug that affects your central nervous system, you shouldn't drive a car or operate heavy machinery until you are sure the medicine isn't making you drowsy or less than alert.
- It usually takes two to three weeks of taking maprotiline before you notice any improvement in your depression.
- The usual starting dosage for adults in 75 mg a day. The maximum recommended dosage is 150 mg a day, although some severely depressed people take 225 mg a day.

Nortriptyline

Brand name: *Pamelor* **(Generic available)**

What this drug does for you:

Nortriptyline treats the symptoms of depression. It is a tricyclic antidepressant with mild sedative effects. It increases the amount of norepinephrine in your central nervous system.

Possible side effects of this drug:

- Common side effects are dizziness, drowsiness, dry mouth, headache, increased appetite, nausea, unpleasant taste, or a black-colored tongue. You could also have diarrhea, increased sweating, ringing in the ears, breast enlargement in males and females, hair loss, and sensitivity to light.
- More serious side effects are blurred vision, confusion, constipation, decreased sexual ability, difficulty in speaking or swallowing, eye pain, fainting, irregular heartbeat, hallucinations, shakiness, nervousness, shuffling walk, a mask-like face, loss of balance control, a change in blood sugar levels or blood pressure levels, hepatitis, jaundice, seizures, coma, heart attack, or stroke.
- If you suddenly quit taking this drug, you could have nausea, headache, and a general feeling of fatigue. If you gradually quit taking the drug, you may still experience irritability, restlessness, and dream and sleep disturbances.

Special warnings:

- You shouldn't use this drug when you are recovering from a heart attack.
- If you have a history of seizures, liver problems, urinary retention, thyroid problems, increased pressure in the eye, or heart problems, you should talk with your doctor about your condition before you take nortriptyline.
- When possible, you should quit taking nortriptyline several days before surgery.

Pregnancy and nursing mothers:

Not known if drug is safe to use while pregnant. Not known if drug is safe to use while nursing.

Possible food and drug interactions:

- You should never take nortriptyline while taking the antidepressants called monoamine oxidase (MAO) inhibitors. If you've been taking an MAO inhibitor, you should stay off it for two weeks before you begin taking nortriptyline. The combination can cause a high fever, convulsions, and death.
- Any of the type of antidepressants called selective serotonin reuptake inhibitors (fluoxetine, sertraline, and paroxetine) can cause nortriptyline to reach dangerously high levels in your body. If you are taking these antidepressants at the same time, your doctor should monitor you closely. You may need lower than normal doses of both drugs. You also should not quickly switch from fluoxetine to a tricyclic antidepressant like nortriptyline. You may need to wait five weeks for the fluoxetine to clear out of your body.
- Some blood-pressure-lowering drugs may not work as well if you also take nortriptyline.
- If you take nortriptyline along with any drug that depresses your nervous system, such as tranquilizers, alcohol, antihistamines, or muscle relaxants, the combination may dangerously depress your nervous system.
- Your doctor should supervise you closely for side effects if you take nortriptyline along with any anticholinergic drugs such as some antihistamines and muscle relaxants or along with any sympathomimetic drugs such as some decongestants.
- Cimetidine, an ulcer drug, can increase the levels of nortriptyline in your body.
- Taking quinidine and nortriptyline at the same time can increase the levels of nortriptyline in your body.
- Taking reserpine and nortriptyline at the same time can cause a "stimulating" effect for some depressed people.
- For diabetics taking chlorpropamide, taking nortriptyline can cause hypoglycemia.

Helpful hints:

- As with any drug that affects your central nervous system, you shouldn't drive a car or operate heavy machinery until you are sure the medicine isn't making you drowsy or less than alert.
- The usual adult dose is 25 mg three or four times daily. You can take capsules or liquid.

Paroxetine

Brand name: *Paxil*

What this drug does for you:

Paroxetine treats the symptoms of depression by increasing the amount of serotonin in your central nervous system. Like fluoxetine, sertraline, and venlafaxine, paroxetine is a selective serotonin reuptake inhibitor.

Possible side effects of this drug:

- The most common side effects of paroxetine are weakness, sweating, nausea, decreased appetite, sleepiness, dizziness, insomnia, shakiness, and nervousness. Around 10 to 13 percent of men have trouble with delayed ejaculation and other sexual problems. After taking paroxetine for four to six weeks, some side effects should go away, especially nausea and dizziness.
- Much rarer side effects are heart palpitations, low blood pressure when you stand up, dry mouth, rash, constipation, diarrhea, gas, lump or tightness in your throat, increased appetite, achy muscles, decreased sex drive, blurred vision, a strange taste in your mouth, and frequent or difficult urination.

Special warnings:

- You may need a lower than normal dosage of paroxetine if you have liver or kidney disease. Your doctor should monitor you closely for side effects.
- Take this drug with caution if you have a history of seizures.

Pregnancy and nursing mothers:

Category B. See page 9 for description of categories. Drug is present in mother's milk.

Possible food and drug interactions:

- You should never take paroxetine while taking the antidepressants called monoamine oxidase (MAO) inhibitors. If you've been taking an MAO inhibitor, you should stay off it for two weeks before you begin taking paroxetine. You should stay off paroxetine for at least two weeks before you begin taking an MAO inhibitor.
- You shouldn't drink alcohol while taking paroxetine.
- Tryptophan and paroxetine together can cause agitation, restlessness, and upset stomach. You may want to avoid foods high in tryptophan, such as meats, poultry, fish, liver, kidney, eggs, nuts, peanut butter, broad beans, and wheat germ.
- Paroxetine may cause increased bleeding if you take it while you are taking warfarin.
- The ulcer drug cimetidine may increase levels or effects of paroxetine.
- The sedative phenobarbital may lower levels of paroxetine in your body.
- Phenytoin and paroxetine may interact.
- If you are taking phenothiazines, quinidine, certain antiarrhythmics such as propafenone, flecainide, and encainide, or any antidepressant, you may need to decrease your dosage of the drug once you start taking paroxetine. You may also need a lower than normal dosage of paroxetine. Consult your doctor.

Helpful hints:

- As with any drug that affects your central nervous system, you shouldn't drive a car or operate heavy machinery until you are sure the medicine isn't making you drowsy or less than alert.
- Most people notice an improvement in their depression after one to four weeks on paroxetine.

- The usual starting dose for adults is 20 mg a day, taken in the morning. The maximum dose is 50 mg a day.

Phenelzine

Brand name: *Nardil*

What this drug does for you:

Phenelzine is a monoamine oxidase (MAO) inhibitor. It treats depression, usually mixed with anxiety, phobias, or hypochondria.

Most people take phenelzine because they have been unable to get relief from other medicines. MAO inhibitors have many potentially serious side effects and many dangerous interactions with foods and other drugs.

Possible side effects of this drug:

- The most serious reaction to phenelzine is severe high blood pressure. It can be deadly. You should have your blood pressure checked often, and you should immediately tell your doctor about any heart palpitations or frequent headaches you have. Other symptoms of unusually high blood pressure are severe chest pain, enlarged pupils, increased sensitivity of eyes to light, increased sweating, nausea, and stiff or sore neck.
- You should also tell your doctor if you have dizziness or lightheadedness when you get up from a lying or sitting position.
- Most side effects of MAO inhibitors are not very severe, and they tend to go away after you've been taking the drug for a while. You may experience drowsiness, headache, tremors, twitching, dizziness, dry mouth, constipation, stomach problems, weight gain, rash, sweating, blurred vision, nervous jitters, difficulty urinating, prickling or tingling in hands or feet, fluid retention, glaucoma, and sexual disturbances such as difficulty ejaculating.

Special warnings:

- This drug should not be used by people with poor liver function, heart failure, or a tumor that produces adrenaline (pheochromocytoma)
- You should quit taking phenelzine 10 days before having surgery that requires anesthesia.
- For diabetics, phenelzine may cause hypoglycemia.

Pregnancy and nursing mothers:

Category C. See page 9 for description of categories. Not known if drug is present in mother's milk. You shouldn't take this drug while nursing.

Possible food and drug interactions:

- Taking any of the following drugs while taking MAO inhibitors can cause extremely high blood pressure: buspirone, epinephrine, norepinephrine, amphetamines, methylphenidate, phenylalanine, dopamine, methyldopa, tryptophan, and tyrosine.
- You can have extremely high blood pressure when you eat any foods high in tyramine or dopamine while taking MAO inhibitors: yogurt, aged cheese, liver, avocados, bananas, broad beans, sauerkraut, wine, beer,

and pickled, dried, or smoked meats, fish or vegetables (including salami and pepperoni). You should also avoid large amounts of caffeine and chocolate.

- Foods high in tryptophan can cause confusion, delirium, and agitation: meats, poultry, fish, liver, kidney, eggs, nuts, peanut butter, broad beans, and wheat germ.
- Over-the-counter medicines you should avoid while taking phenelzine include:

  > Cough and cold preparations (including any containing dextromethorphan)
  > Nasal decongestants (tablets, drops, or sprays)
  > Hay-fever medications
  > Sinus medications
  > Asthma inhalers
  > Weight-reducing medicines or appetite-controlling medicines
  > "Pep" pills
  > L-tryptophan-containing medicines

- Phenelzine may dangerously increase the effects of depressants and sedatives, including alcohol.
- Taking phenelzine with meperidine (Demerol) may cause high fever, seizures, and coma.
- Taking phenelzine with other antidepressants could cause a negative drug interaction. In fact, you should wait at least 10 days after you quit taking phenelzine before you begin taking another antidepressant or the anti-anxiety buspirone. You should wait 14 days before you begin taking bupropion.
- After taking the antidepressant fluoxetine, you should wait five weeks before you begin taking phenelzine.
- You should not take phenelzine while taking guanethidine. If you take other high blood pressure drugs, such as thiazide diuretics and beta blockers, you should take phenelzine cautiously.

Helpful hints:
- The usual starting dose for adults is 15 mg three times a day. Your doctor may increase your dosage at first, then slowly reduce your dosage until you take just 15 mg once a day or every other day.
- You may not notice any improvement in your depression until you've been taking phenelzine for four weeks.

Protriptyline

Brand name: *Vivactil*

What this drug does for you:
Protriptyline treats the symptoms of depression. It is a nonsedating tricyclic antidepressant, and it works particularly well for depressed people who are withdrawn and lack energy.

Possible side effects of this drug:

- Protriptyline has the same basic side effects as the other tricyclic antidepressants. It isn't sedating, and it's more likely to make you agitated and anxious. It also is more likely to produce some heart-related side effects such as a rapid heartbeat and low blood pressure.
- Common side effects of tricyclic antidepressants are dizziness, drowsiness, dry mouth, headache, increased appetite, nausea, unpleasant taste, or a black-colored tongue. You could also have diarrhea, increased sweating, ringing in the ears, breast enlargement in males and females, hair loss, and sensitivity to light.
- More serious side effects are blurred vision, confusion, constipation, decreased sexual ability, difficulty in speaking or swallowing, eye pain, fainting, irregular heartbeat, hallucinations, shakiness, nervousness, shuffling walk, a mask-like face, loss of balance control, a change in blood sugar levels or blood pressure levels, hepatitis, jaundice, seizures, coma, heart attack, or stroke.
- If you suddenly quit taking this drug, you could have nausea, headache, and a general feeling of fatigue. If you gradually quit taking the drug, you may still experience irritability, restlessness, and dream and sleep disturbances.

Special warnings:

- You shouldn't take this drug when you are recovering from a heart attack.
- You should take this drug very cautiously if you have heart disease, urinary retention, glaucoma, thyroid disease, or a history of seizures.
- When possible, you should quit taking protriptyline several days before surgery.

Pregnancy and nursing mothers:

Not known if it's safe to take this drug while pregnant. Not known if it's safe to take this drug while nursing.

Possible food and drug interactions:

- You should never take protriptyline while taking the antidepressants called monoamine oxidase (MAO) inhibitors. If you've been taking an MAO inhibitor, you should stay off it for two weeks before you begin taking protriptyline. The combination can cause a high fever, convulsions, and death.
- Some blood-pressure-lowering drugs such as guanethidine may not work as well if you also take protriptyline.
- If you take protriptyline along with any drug that depresses your nervous system, such as tranquilizers, alcohol, antihistamines, or muscle relaxants, the combination may dangerously depress your nervous system.
- Your doctor should supervise you closely for side effects if you take protriptyline along with any anticholinergic drugs such as some antihistamines and muscle relaxants or along with any sympathomimetic drugs such as some decongestants.

- The ulcer drug cimetidine can increase the levels of protriptyline in your body.

Helpful hints:

- As with any drug that affects your central nervous system, you shouldn't drive a car or operate heavy machinery until you are sure the medicine isn't making you drowsy or less than alert.
- Be careful in hot weather. This drug could make you sweat less in high temperatures, so you're more likely to get a high fever or heatstroke.
- This drug is very likely to cause dry mouth and constipation, so you should drink plenty of fluids and eat a high-fiber diet.
- The usual adult dosage is 15 to 40 mg a day divided into three or four doses.
- Protriptyline may cause insomnia, so try not to take the medicine late in the day.

Sertraline

Brand name: *Zoloft*

What this drug does for you:

Sertraline treats the symptoms of depression by increasing the amount of serotonin in your central nervous system. Like fluoxetine, paroxetine, and venlafaxine, sertraline is a selective serotonin reuptake inhibitor.

Possible side effects of this drug:

- The most common side effects of sertraline are nausea, diarrhea and stomachache, tremor (shakiness), dizziness, insomnia, sleepiness, increased sweating, dry mouth, decreased appetite, and sexual problems for men (mainly a delay in ejaculation).
- Much rarer side effects are heart palpitations, low blood pressure when you stand up, confusion, rash, constipation, gas, increased appetite, achy muscles, hot flushes, fever, agitation, blurred vision, a strange taste in your mouth, and frequent or difficult urination.

Special warnings:

- You may need a lower than normal dosage of sertraline if you have liver or kidney disease. Your doctor should monitor you closely for side effects.
- Take this drug with caution if you have a history of seizures.

Pregnancy and nursing mothers:

Category B. See page 9 for description of categories. Not known if drug is present in mother's milk.

Possible food and drug interactions:

- You should never take sertraline while taking the antidepressants called monoamine oxidase (MAO) inhibitors. If you've been taking an MAO inhibitor, you should stay off it for two weeks before you begin taking sertraline. You should stay off sertraline for at least two weeks before you begin taking an MAO inhibitor.
- Although lab experiments haven't shown an interaction between alcohol

and sertraline, you shouldn't drink alcohol while taking this drug.
- Sertraline may cause increased bleeding if you take it while you are taking warfarin. Sertraline may affect levels of warfarin and digitoxin in your body, and vice versa.
- The ulcer drug cimetidine may increase levels or effects of sertraline.
- If you take lithium, your lithium levels should be closely monitored after you begin taking sertraline.

Helpful hints:
- As with any drug that affects your central nervous system, you shouldn't drive a car or operate heavy machinery until you are sure the medicine isn't making you drowsy or less than alert.
- The usual starting dose for adults is 50 mg once a day. The maximum dose is 200 mg a day. You can take your medication in the morning or the evening.

Trazodone

Brand name: *Desyrel* **(Generic available)**

What this drug does for you:
Trazodone treats depression, possibly by increasing the amount of serotonin in the central nervous system.

Possible side effects of this drug:
- The most common side effects are dizziness, drowsiness, dry mouth, and nausea.
- One of the worst side effects of trazodone is painful, prolonged penile erections. You should let your doctor know immediately if you experience this reaction. You may need drugs or surgery to correct the condition.
- Other side effects experienced by more than 1 percent of people taking trazodone are swelling, blurred vision, constipation, high or low blood pressure, confusion, headache, insomnia, achy muscles, lack of coordination, shakiness, tired and itchy eyes, sinus congestion, ringing in the ears, and weight gain.

Special warnings:
- You shouldn't take trazodone when you are recovering from a heart attack. If you have heart disease, you should take the drug very cautiously. It can cause an irregular heartbeat.
- You should quit taking trazodone for as long as possible before surgery with general anesthesia.

Pregnancy and nursing mothers:
Category C. See page 9 for description of categories. Drug is probably present in mother's milk. (Lab experiments have shown that it's present in rat's milk.)

Possible food and drug interactions:
- Since trazodone can cause low blood pressure, you may need a lower

dose of your blood-pressure-lowering drug.

- If you take trazodone along with any drug that depresses your nervous system, such as tranquilizers, alcohol, antihistamines, or muscle relaxers, the combination may dangerously depress your nervous system.
- Trazodone may increase levels of the heart drug digoxin and the seizure drug phenytoin.
- Your doctor should monitor you carefully for side effects if you will be taking monoamine oxidase (MAO) inhibitors and trazodone at the same time.
- Trazodone may cause increased bleeding if you take it while you are taking warfarin.

Helpful hints:

- Take trazodone after you eat a meal or a snack. You will absorb the drug better, and you are less likely to feel dizzy and lightheaded.
- This drug does cause drowsiness, so you may want to take your largest dose at bedtime.
- As with any drug that affects your central nervous system, you shouldn't drive a car or operate heavy machinery until you see how the medicine affects you.
- You may experience some relief from your depression right away, but it can take up to four weeks for you to notice any improvement.
- The usual starting dose for adults is 150 mg a day. The maximum dose is 400 mg a day.

ANTIPSYCHOTICS

Fluphenazine

Brand name: *Prolixin*

What this drug does for you:

This phenothiazine is used to treat symptoms of various mental illnesses, such as schizophrenia and mania. It is a tranquilizer.

Possible side effects of this drug:

- All antipsychotics commonly cause sleepiness, dry mouth, urine retention, confusion, and low blood pressure. These side effects are less common with fluphenazine than with some of the other phenothiazines.
- Some of the less common side effects of fluphenazine are restlessness, excitement, bizarre dreams, nausea, loss of appetite, sweating, headache, constipation, frequent urination, blurred vision, rapid heartbeat, nasal congestion, swelling, enlargement of breasts in men, impotence, increased sex drive in women, and skin disorders including a sensitivity to light.
- With any antipsychotic you take, you risk nerve problems as a rare side effect. These problems include tardive dyskinesia (out-of-control movements of the lips, tongue, fingers, toes, or other muscle groups), drug-

induced parkinsonism (difficulty speaking or swallowing, loss of balance, muscle spasms, stiff arms or legs, trembling, and shaking), restless leg syndrome, and weak or tired muscles. Very rarely, these problems remain even after you quit taking the drug. These nerve problems are more common with fluphenazine than with some of the other phenothiazines. Catching the nerve disorders quickly is important, so be sure to let your doctor know immediately if you notice any of these symptoms.

Special warnings:

- People with brain damage, severely depressed people, and people taking large doses of hypnotics shouldn't take fluphenazine.
- You should take this drug very cautiously if you have a history of epilepsy, heart disease, or liver disease. You should also be careful with this drug if you work in extreme heat or around phosphorus insecticides.

Pregnancy and nursing mothers:

Not known if safe to use while pregnant. Not known if safe to use while nursing.

Possible food and drug interactions:

- If you take any phenothiazine along with a drug that depresses your nervous system, such as other tranquilizers, alcohol, antihistamines, or muscle relaxers, the combination may dangerously depress your nervous system.
- This drug may increase the effects of atropine.

Helpful hints:

- As with any drug that affects your central nervous system, you shouldn't drive a car or operate heavy machinery until you are sure the medicine isn't making you drowsy or less than alert.
- This drug can cause pregnancy test results to be unreliable.
- The usual starting dosage for adults is 2.5 to 10 mg a day. You should take your doses six to eight hours apart. The usual maintenance dosage is 1 or 5 mg a day.
- The oral concentrate form should be added to water, tomato or fruit juice (except apple), milk, or caffeine-free soft drinks just before you take it. You should not mix the medicine with caffeinated drinks, drinks with tannins (for example: tea, coffee, and red wines), or apple juice.
- Gently shake the elixir form before you use it. If the medicine does not become clear when you shake it, you shouldn't use it.
- Don't quit taking this drug suddenly. If you do, you may experience stomach pain, nausea, dizziness, and shakiness.

Haloperidol

Brand name: *Haldol* (Generic available)

What this drug does for you:

This tranquilizer treats schizophrenia and other mental illnesses, severe hyperactivity and other behavior problems in children, and the tics and offensive language of Tourette's syndrome.

Possible side effects of this drug:

- All antipsychotics commonly cause sleepiness, dry mouth, urine retention, blurred vision, confusion, and low blood pressure. These side effects are less common with haloperidol than with some of the other phenothiazines.
- Some of the less common side effects of haloperidol are restlessness, excitement, bizarre dreams, nausea, loss of appetite, sweating, headache, constipation, frequent urination, rapid heartbeat, nasal congestion, swelling, enlargement of breasts in men or lactation (secreting milk) in women, impotence, increased sex drive, menstrual irregularities, damage to your liver, and skin disorders including a sensitivity to light.
- With any antipsychotic you take, you risk nerve problems as a rare side effect. These problems include tardive dyskinesia (out-of-control movements of the lips, tongue, fingers, toes, or other muscle groups), drug-induced parkinsonism (difficulty speaking or swallowing, loss of balance, muscle spasms, stiff arms or legs, trembling, and shaking), restless leg syndrome, and weak or tired muscles. Very rarely, these problems remain even after you quit taking the drug. Catching the nerve disorders quickly is important, so be sure to let your doctor know immediately if you notice any of these symptoms.

Special warnings:

- People with Parkinson's disease should not use this drug.
- People with a history of heart problems or seizures or people who take anticoagulants (such as phenindione) should take this drug with extreme caution.

Pregnancy and nursing mothers:

This drug may cause birth defects. You shouldn't use it while pregnant. You should not breast-feed while taking this drug.

Possible food and drug interactions:

- Taking haloperidol with lithium may cause toxic effects on the brain and nervous system. Your doctor should monitor you closely.
- If you take haloperidol along with a drug that depresses your nervous system, such as other tranquilizers, alcohol, antihistamines, or muscle relaxers, the combination may dangerously depress your nervous system. Alcohol and haloperidol combined can also cause very low blood pressure.
- You should be very careful when taking haloperidol and an antiparkinson drug at the same time.

Helpful hints:

- As with any drug that affects your central nervous system, you shouldn't drive a car or operate heavy machinery until you are sure the medicine isn't making you drowsy or less than alert.

- Make sure you get plenty to drink even if you don't feel thirsty. Some people who take this drug get dehydrated and sick.
- Don't quit taking this drug suddenly. If you do, you may experience stomach pain, nausea, dizziness, and shakiness.
- How much of this drug you take will depend on many factors, including the severity of your symptoms and your age. The starting dosage for adults can range from 0.5 mg twice a day to 5 mg three times a day.

Lithium

Brand names: *Eskalith, Lithium Carbonate, Lithonate, Lithotabs*

What this drug does for you:

Lithium treats the manic stages of manic depression, the condition in which your mood swings dramatically from very depressed to very excited, agitated, talkative, and aggressive.

Possible side effects of this drug:

- Lithium can be toxic at low doses. You should watch for early symptoms such as tremors, lack of coordination, diarrhea, weakness, vomiting, and drowsiness. If you have these symptoms, don't take your next dose of lithium and call your doctor immediately. Later symptoms of toxicity are blurred vision, dizziness, and convulsions.
- You may experience shaky hands, frequent urination, thirstiness, nausea, and a general discomfort when you first begin taking lithium. These side effects should go away after you've been taking the drug for a while. If they don't go away, you may need a lower dosage.
- Less common side effects are blackouts, slurred speech, loss of bladder control, irregular heartbeat, low blood pressure, weight loss or gain, swelling, hair loss, dry skin, dry mouth, and dehydration.

Special warning:

- Use this drug with extreme caution if you have cardiovascular disease, kidney disease, dehydration, or low sodium levels, or if you take diuretics.

Pregnancy and nursing mothers:

Category D. See page 9 for a description of the categories. Lithium can cause birth defects and should not be used while you are pregnant. Drug is present in mother's milk. You should not use this drug while you are nursing.

Possible food and drug interactions:

- Taking lithium and the antipsychotic haloperidol at the same time may cause toxicity and brain damage. If you take lithium along with any antipsychotic, you and your doctor should watch closely for side effects, such as shakiness, weakness, fever, and confusion.
- Lithium may increase the effects of neuromuscular blockers such as metocurine iodide.
- Nonsteroidal anti-inflammatories (NSAIDs), such as indomethacin and piroxicam, can increase lithium levels.
- Diuretics, calcium channel blockers, and ACE inhibitors such as capto-

pril can increase lithium levels in your body. That increases your risk of lithium toxicity.
- The following may decrease the effects of lithium: acetazolamide, caffeine, and sodium bicarbonate.
- Taking carbamazepine and lithium at the same time can cause toxic side effects.
- Fluoxetine can increase or decrease your lithium levels.

Helpful hints:
- As with any drug that affects your central nervous system, you shouldn't drive a car or operate heavy machinery until you are sure the medicine isn't making you drowsy or less than alert.
- Make sure you drink plenty of fluids and eat a balanced diet that includes salt. If you sweat a lot or have diarrhea, you need extra fluids, and you may need salt supplements.
- For acute mania, the usual adult dosage is 600 mg three times a day. For long-term control, the usual adult dosage is 300 mg three or four times a day.

Molindone

Brand name: *Moban*

What this drug does for you:
This drug is a strong tranquilizer used to treat schizophrenia and aggressive or bizarre behavior. It works as a tranquilizer without causing muscle relaxation or lack of coordination.

Possible side effects of this drug:
- The most common side effect, drowsiness, usually goes away after you've been taking the drug for a while.
- Other side effects are depression, blurred vision, rapid heartbeat, nausea, dry mouth, difficult urination, constipation, changes in menstrual periods, swelling of breasts, increased sex drive, and skin rash.
- With any antipsychotic you take, you risk nerve problems as a rare side effect. These problems include tardive dyskinesia (out-of-control movements of the lips, tongue, fingers, toes, or other muscle groups), drug-induced parkinsonism (difficulty speaking or swallowing, loss of balance, muscle spasms, stiff arms or legs, trembling, and shaking), restless leg syndrome, and weak or tired muscles. Very rarely, these problems remain even after you quit taking the drug. Catching the nerve disorders quickly is important, so be sure to let your doctor know immediately if you notice any of these symptoms.

Special warnings:
- This drug should not be used by people who are already heavily sedated.
- This drug contains sulfites. Some people with asthma are sensitive to sulfites.

Pregnancy and nursing mothers:

Not known if drug is safe to use while pregnant. Animal studies haven't shown an increased risk of birth defects. Not known if drug is safe to use while nursing.

Possible food and drug interactions:

- Don't use alcohol or other depressants while taking this drug.
- The molindone tablets contain calcium sulfate, which can decrease the absorption of phenytoin and tetracycline.

Helpful hints:

- As with any drug that affects your central nervous system, you shouldn't drive a car or operate heavy machinery until you are sure the medicine isn't making you drowsy or less than alert. Drowsiness will usually go away after you've been taking the drug for a while.
- The usual starting dosage for adults is 50 to 75 mg a day. The maintenance dosage can range from 15 mg a day to 225 mg a day, depending on the severity of your symptoms.

Perphenazine

Brand name: *Trilafon* (Generic available)

What this drug does for you:

Perphenazine tablets, concentrate, or injections treat mental illnesses and control severe nausea and vomiting. Perphenazine is a phenothiazine-type tranquilizer.

Possible side effects of this drug:

- All antipsychotics commonly cause sleepiness, dry mouth, urine retention, confusion, and low blood pressure. These side effects are less common with perphenazine than with some of the other phenothiazines.
- Some of the less common side effects of perphenazine are restlessness, excitement, bizarre dreams, nausea, loss of appetite, sweating, headache, constipation, frequent urination, blurred vision, rapid heartbeat, nasal congestion, swelling, enlargement of breasts in men, impotence, increased sex drive in women, and skin disorders including a sensitivity to light.
- With any antipsychotic you take, you risk nerve problems as a rare side effect. These problems include tardive dyskinesia (out-of-control movements of the lips, tongue, fingers, toes, or other muscle groups), drug-induced parkinsonism (difficulty speaking or swallowing, loss of balance, muscle spasms, stiff arms or legs, trembling, and shaking), restless leg syndrome, and weak or tired muscles. Very rarely, these problems remain even after you quit taking the drug. These nerve problems are more common with perphenazine than with some of the other phenothiazines. Catching the nerve disorders quickly is important, so be sure to let your doctor know immediately if you notice any of these symptoms.
- If your body temperature goes up, that may be a signal that you can't tol-

erate this drug.

Special warnings:
- Use this drug cautiously if you have a history of seizures, poor kidney function, lung infections, asthma, or emphysema.
- You should also be careful with this drug if you work in extreme heat or around phosphorus insecticides.

Pregnancy and nursing mothers:
Not known if safe to use this drug while you're pregnant. Not known if safe to use this drug while you're nursing.

Possible food and drug interactions:
- You can't use perphenazine along with large amounts of any drug that depresses your nervous system, such as other tranquilizers, alcohol, antihistamines, pain relievers, or muscle relaxers. The combination may dangerously depress your nervous system. If you are taking any of these depressants at the same time, you'll probably need a lower than normal dosage of each drug. Alcohol combined with perphenazine could also cause extremely low blood pressure.
- Perphenazine may increase the effects of atropine.

Helpful hints:
- As with any drug that affects your central nervous system, you shouldn't drive a car or operate heavy machinery until you are sure the medicine isn't making you drowsy or less than alert. Drowsiness will usually go away after you've been taking the drug for a while.
- Your blood counts and liver and kidney functions should be checked regularly while you're taking this drug.
- For mental illness that isn't too severe, the usual starting dosage for adults is 4 to 8 mg three times a day.
- For severe nausea and vomiting, the usual adult dosage is 8 to 16 mg two to four times a day. Don't take more than 64 mg a day.
- Don't quit taking this drug suddenly. If you do, you may experience stomach pain, nausea, dizziness, and shakiness.
- The concentrate form is best taken in liquids such as orange, grapefruit, tomato, pineapple, apricot, or prune juice, carbonated orange drink, homogenized milk, or water. Don't use caffeinated drinks including tea, or apple juice.

Thioridazine Hydrochloride

Brand name: *Mellaril* **(Generic available)**

What this drug does for you:
This phenothiazine is used to treat depression, anxiety, sleep disturbances, and fears. It also treats severe hyperactivity and other behavior problems in children. Thioridazine is a tranquilizer.

Possible side effects of this drug:
- All antipsychotics commonly cause sleepiness, dry mouth, urine reten-

tion, confusion, and low blood pressure when you stand up. These side effects are more common with thioridazine than with some of the other phenothiazines, but they should go away after you've been taking the drug for a while.

- Some of the less common side effects of thioridazine are restlessness, excitement, bizarre dreams, nausea, diarrhea, stuffy nose, headache, constipation, blurred vision and other vision changes, rapid heartbeat, changes in the menstrual period, swelling of breasts, difficult ejaculation, skin disorders including a sensitivity to light, and blood disorders.
- With any antipsychotic you take, you risk nerve problems as a rare side effect. These problems include tardive dyskinesia (out-of-control movements of the lips, tongue, fingers, toes, or other muscle groups), drug-induced parkinsonism (difficulty speaking or swallowing, loss of balance, muscle spasms, stiff arms or legs, trembling, and shaking), restless leg syndrome, and weak or tired muscles. Very rarely, these problems remain even after you quit taking the drug. These nerve problems are less common with thioridazine than with some of the other phenothiazines. Catching the nerve disorders quickly is important, so be sure to let your doctor know immediately if you notice any of these symptoms.

Special warning:
- You should take this drug very cautiously if you have heart disease with blood pressure problems. You should also be careful with this drug if you work in extreme heat or around phosphorus insecticides.

Pregnancy and nursing mothers:
  Use in pregnancy and nursing only if the potential benefits to the mother outweigh the risks to the baby.

Possible food and drug interactions:
- If you take any phenothiazine along with a drug that depresses your nervous system, such as other tranquilizers, alcohol, antihistamines, or muscle relaxers, the combination may dangerously depress your nervous system.
- This drug may increase the effects of atropine.
- Levels of thioridazine may be increased by the beta-blockers propranolol and pindolol.

Helpful hints:
- As with any drug that affects your central nervous system, you shouldn't drive a car or operate heavy machinery until you are sure the medicine isn't making you drowsy or less than alert.
- For depressed, fearful, or anxious adults, the dosage ranges from 20 mg a day to 200 mg a day. People with severe mental illness can be prescribed up to 800 mg a day.
- Add the concentrate form to water or juice (not apple juice) just before you drink it.
- Don't quit taking this drug suddenly. If you do, you may experience stomach pain, nausea, headache, insomnia, dizziness, and shakiness.

Thiothixene

Brand name: *Navane* (Generic available)

What this drug does for you:

Thiothixene is a tranquilizer used to treat mental illness, such as loss of contact with reality and personality disorders. Thiothixene is similar to some of the phenothiazines.

Possible side effects of this drug:

- All antipsychotics commonly cause sleepiness, dry mouth, urine retention, and confusion. These side effects are less common with thiothixene than with some of the other antipsychotics. The drowsiness should go away after you've been taking the drug for a while. Thiothixene also commonly causes low blood pressure.
- Some of the less common side effects of thiothixene are restlessness, excitement, insomnia, breast enlargement, changes in menstrual period, changes in blood sugar, blurred vision and other vision changes, stuffy nose, sweating, constipation, impotence, fever, weight loss, nausea, diarrhea, weakness, increase in appetite and weight, blood disorders, liver damage, and skin disorders including a sensitivity to light.
- With any antipsychotic you take, you risk nerve problems as a rare side effect. These problems include tardive dyskinesia (out-of-control movements of the lips, tongue, fingers, toes, or other muscle groups), drug-induced parkinsonism (difficulty speaking or swallowing, loss of balance, muscle spasms, stiff arms or legs, trembling, and shaking), restless leg syndrome, and weak or tired muscles. Very rarely, these problems remain even after you quit taking the drug. These nerve problems are more common with thiothixene than with some of the other phenothiazines. Catching the nerve disorders quickly is important, so be sure to let your doctor know immediately if you notice any of these symptoms.

Special warnings:

- You should not take this drug if you have circulatory collapse, if your central nervous system is depressed for any reason, or if you have certain kinds of blood disorders.
- You should take this drug very cautiously if you have heart disease, a history of seizures, or if you work in extreme heat.

Pregnancy and nursing mothers:

Not known if safe to use while pregnant. Animal studies have not shown an increased risk of birth defects. Not known if safe to use while nursing.

Possible food and drug interactions:

- If you take any phenothiazine along with a drug that depresses your nervous system, such as other tranquilizers, alcohol, antihistamines, or muscle relaxers, the combination may dangerously depress your nervous system and cause very low blood pressure.
- This drug may increase the effects of atropine.

Helpful hints:

- As with any drug that affects your central nervous system, you shouldn't drive a car or operate heavy machinery until you are sure the medicine isn't making you drowsy or less than alert.
- This drug can cause pregnancy test results to be unreliable.
- The usual starting dose for adults ranges from 2 mg three times a day to 5 mg twice daily. Later, your doctor may increase your dosage to 15 to 60 mg a day.
- This drug may make your skin extra-sensitive to sunlight, so protect your skin if you'll be outdoors in sunny weather.

Trifluoperazine

Brand name: *Stelazine*

What this drug does for you:

This phenothiazine is used to treat mental illnesses, such as loss of contact with reality and personality disorders. Trifluoperazine can also be used to treat anxiety. It is a tranquilizer.

Possible side effects of this drug:

- All antipsychotics commonly cause sleepiness, dry mouth, urine retention, confusion, and low blood pressure. These side effects are less common with trifluoperazine than with some of the other phenothiazines. The drowsiness should go away after you've been taking the drug for a while. Trifluoperazine also commonly causes low blood pressure.
- Some of the less common side effects of trifluoperazine are restlessness, excitement, bizarre dreams, nausea, loss of appetite, sweating, headache, constipation, frequent urination, blurred vision, rapid heartbeat, nasal congestion, swelling, enlargement of breasts in men, impotence, increased sex drive in women, and skin disorders including a sensitivity to light.
- With any antipsychotic you take, you risk nerve problems as a rare side effect. These problems include tardive dyskinesia (out-of-control movements of the lips, tongue, fingers, toes, or other muscle groups), drug-induced parkinsonism (difficulty speaking or swallowing, loss of balance, muscle spasms, stiff arms or legs, trembling, and shaking), restless leg syndrome, and weak or tired muscles. Very rarely, these problems remain even after you quit taking the drug. These nerve problems are more common with trifluoperazine than with some of the other antipsychotics. Catching the nerve disorders quickly is important, so be sure to let your doctor know immediately if you notice any of these symptoms.
- If you get a sore throat or other signs of an infection while you're taking this drug, let your doctor know. Trifluoperazine can lower your immunity.
- If you get a fever and flu-like symptoms, the drug may be damaging your liver.

Special warnings:
- People who have depressed central nervous systems, some blood disorders, bone marrow depression, or liver damage shouldn't take trifluoperazine.
- This drug contains sulfites. Some people with asthma are sensitive to sulfites.
- You should take this drug very cautiously if you have a history of epilepsy, heart disease, glaucoma, or liver disease.
- You should also be careful with this drug if you work in extreme heat.

Pregnancy and nursing mothers:
It may not be safe to take this drug while you are pregnant. Drug is present in mother's milk.

Possible food and drug interactions:
- If you take any phenothiazine along with a drug that depresses your nervous system, such as other tranquilizers, alcohol, antihistamines, or muscle relaxers, the combination may dangerously depress your nervous system.
- Trifluoperazine may decrease the effects of anticoagulants and blood pressure drugs such as guanethidine.
- Taking trifluoperazine and propranolol at the same time can increase the levels of both drugs.
- If you take trifluoperazine with thiazide diuretics, you may have very low blood pressure.
- Trifluoperazine may increase levels of the anticonvulsant phenytoin, possibly to toxic levels.

Helpful hints:
- As with any drug that affects your central nervous system, you shouldn't drive a car or operate heavy machinery until you are sure the medicine isn't making you drowsy or less than alert.
- This drug can cause pregnancy test results to be unreliable.
- For nonpsychotic anxiety, the usual starting dosage for adults is 1 or 2 mg twice daily. You shouldn't take more than 6 mg per day, and you shouldn't take the drug for longer than 12 weeks.
- For psychotic disorders, most people start with 2 to 5 mg twice a day and go up to 15 to 20 mg daily.
- The oral concentrate form should be added to 2 or more ounces of liquid just before you take it. You can use tomato or fruit juice, milk, carbonated beverages, coffee, tea, or water. You can also take your medicine in soft foods such as soup or pudding.

DRUGS FOR INSOMNIA

Butabarbital Sodium

Brand name: *Butisol Sodium* **(Generic available)**

What this drug does for you:
This barbiturate is used to promote sleep and to relieve anxiety and tension. Butabarbital is an "intermediate" barbiturate — it usually begins working in 45 minutes to an hour, and lasts about six to eight hours.

Possible side effects of this drug:
- The most common side effect is daytime sleepiness.
- Rarer side effects are agitation, confusion, nightmares, nervousness, dizziness, very slow breathing, low blood pressure, nausea, headache, skin rash, and fever.

Special warnings:
- You can become addicted to this drug. You must not increase your dose without talking to your doctor. Some symptoms of intoxication with barbiturates are walking unsteadily, slurred speech, confusion, and irritability.
- You should withdraw from butabarbital slowly (for example, decrease the dose from three to two doses a day for one week). If you quit taking the drug quickly, you may have nightmares, insomnia, anxiety, dizziness, and nausea. If you're addicted to the drug and you quit taking it suddenly, you may have delirium, convulsions, and death.
- People with a group of disorders called porphyria should not use barbiturates.

Pregnancy and nursing mothers:
Category D. See page 9 for description of categories. You must not use this drug while you're pregnant. Drug is present in mother's milk.

Possible food and drug interactions:
- If you take butabarbital sodium along with a drug that depresses your nervous system, such as tranquilizers, alcohol, antihistamines, or muscle relaxers, the combination may dangerously depress your nervous system.
- Butabarbital sodium may increase the effects of corticosteroids.
- This drug may decrease the effectiveness of anti-clotting drugs like warfarin, the anti-fungal drug griseofulvin, birth control pills, and doxycycline.
- Butabarbital sodium may increase the effects of phenytoin.
- Sodium valproate, valproic acid, and monoamine oxidase (MAO) inhibitors may increase the depressant effects of butabarbital sodium.

Helpful hints:
- Butabarbital loses its ability to promote sleep after two weeks of taking it regularly.

- You shouldn't drive a car or operate heavy machinery until you are sure the medicine isn't making you drowsy or less than alert.
- You should have regular blood, liver, and kidney tests if you take this drug for a long time.
- If you take birth control pills, you should use another type of contraception while you're taking butabarbital sodium.
- The usual adult dosage for a daytime sedative is 15 to 30 mg, three or four times daily. As a bedtime hypnotic, the usual adult dosage is 50 to 100 mg.

Flurazepam

Brand name: *Dalmane* (Generic available)

What this drug does for you:
Flurazepam is a hypnotic drug used to treat insomnia. It is a benzodiazepine. Some drugs for insomnia stop working after you take them for two weeks, but flurazepam works for at least 28 nights in a row. Flurazepam is cleared out of the body more slowly than some of the other benzodiazepines, so it is more likely to accumulate and cause daytime sleepiness and certain other side effects.

Possible side effects of this drug:
- The most common side effects, especially in older people, are dizziness, drowsiness, light-headedness, and lack of coordination.
- Other side effects are headache, heartburn, upset stomach, nausea, diarrhea, constipation, nervousness, talkativeness, irritability, heart palpitations, chest pain, joint pain, and urinary problems.
- Rare side effects are sweating, flushing, difficulty focusing, blurred vision, low blood pressure, shortness of breath, skin rash, dry mouth, bitter taste, slurred speech, confusion, restlessness, and hallucinations.
- Some people have memory loss for several hours after taking a benzodiazepine. Make sure you'll be able to get a full night's sleep after taking your medicine.
- Benzodiazepines cause some people's behavior to change. For instance, you may become more aggressive and agitated.

Special warnings:
- You can become dependent on flurazepam. To avoid seizures and other less severe withdrawal symptoms, such as heightened senses, muscle cramps, diarrhea, and blurred vision, you should quit taking the drug gradually under your doctor's supervision. Don't stop abruptly, and don't increase or decrease your dosage without your doctor's approval.
- People with poor liver, kidney, or lung functions should use flurazepam cautiously. The drug may stay in your body longer and increase your risk of side effects.

Pregnancy and nursing mothers:
This drug may cause birth defects. You should not take it while you are preg-

nant.

Possible food and drug interaction:
- If you take flurazepam along with a drug that depresses your nervous system, such as tranquilizers, alcohol, antihistamines, or muscle relaxants, the combination may dangerously depress your nervous system.

Helpful hints:
- You shouldn't drive a car or operate heavy machinery until you are sure the medicine isn't making you drowsy or less than alert. Be careful the day after you've taken flurazepam, as well as the night you take it.
- The usual adult dose is 30 mg at bedtime. Some people just need 15 mg.
- You may have trouble sleeping for the first couple of nights after you stop taking this drug.

Phenobarbital

Brand name: *Solfoton* (Generic available)

What this drug does for you:
This strong barbiturate is used to promote sleep and to relieve anxiety and tension. Phenobarbital is a long-acting barbiturate — it takes one hour or longer to begin working and lasts about 10 to 12 hours.

Possible side effects of this drug:
- The most common side effect is daytime sleepiness.
- Rarer side effects are agitation, confusion, nightmares, nervousness, dizziness, very slow breathing, low blood pressure, nausea, headache, skin rash, and fever.

Special warnings:
- You can become addicted to this drug. You must not increase your dose without talking to your doctor. Some symptoms of intoxication with barbiturates are walking unsteadily, slurred speech, confusion, and irritability.
- You should withdraw from phenobarbital slowly (for example, decrease the dose from three to two doses a day for one week). If you quit taking the drug quickly, you may have nightmares, insomnia, anxiety, dizziness, and nausea. If you're addicted to the drug and you quit taking it suddenly, delirium, convulsions, and death may result.
- People with a group of disorders called porphyria should not use barbiturates.

Pregnancy and nursing mothers:
Category D. See page 9 for description of categories. You must not use this drug while you're pregnant. Drug is present in mother's milk.

Possible food and drug interactions:
- If you take phenobarbital along with a drug that depresses your nervous system, such as tranquilizers, alcohol, antihistamines, or muscle relaxers, the combination may dangerously depress your nervous system.

- Phenobarbital may increase the effects of corticosteroids.
- This drug may decrease the effectiveness of anti-clotting drugs like warfarin, the anti-fungal drug griseofulvin, birth control pills, and doxycycline.
- Phenobarbital may increase the effects of phenytoin.
- Sodium valproate, valproic acid, and monoamine oxidase (MAO) inhibitors may increase the depressant effects of phenobarbital.

Helpful hints:
- Phenobarbital loses its ability to promote sleep after two weeks of taking it regularly.
- You shouldn't drive a car or operate heavy machinery until you are sure the medicine isn't making you drowsy or less than alert.
- You should have regular blood, liver, and kidney tests if you take this drug for a long time.
- If you take birth control pills, you should use another type of contraception while you're taking phenobarbital.
- The usual dose for adults with insomnia is 100 mg at bedtime.

Quazepam

Brand name: *Doral*

What this drug does for you:
Quazepam is a hypnotic drug used to treat insomnia. It is a benzodiazepine. Some drugs for insomnia stop working after you take them for two weeks, but quazepam works for at least 28 nights in a row. Quazepam is cleared out of the body more slowly than some of the other benzodiazepines, so it is more likely to accumulate and cause daytime sleepiness and certain other side effects.

Possible side effects of this drug:
- The most common side effects, especially in older people, are daytime drowsiness and headache. Daytime sleepiness may last for several days after you quit taking the drug. Also common are fatigue, dizziness, dry mouth, and upset stomach.
- Other side effects are weakness, confusion, lack of coordination, shakiness, depression, nervousness, irritability, impotence, decreased sex drive, nightmares, blurred vision and other vision disturbances, loss of bladder control or difficulty urinating, heart palpitations, nausea, constipation, diarrhea, slurred speech, and menstrual irregularities.
- Some people have memory loss for several hours after taking a benzodiazepine. Make sure you'll be able to get a full night's sleep after taking your medicine.
- Benzodiazepines cause some people's behavior to change. For instance, you may become more aggressive and agitated.

Special warnings:
- You can become dependent on quazepam. To avoid seizures and other

less severe withdrawal symptoms, such as heightened senses, muscle cramps, diarrhea, and blurred vision, you should quit taking the drug gradually under your doctor's supervision. Don't stop abruptly, and don't increase or decrease your dosage without your doctor's approval.

- People with poor liver, kidney, or lung function should use quazepam cautiously. The drug may stay in your body longer and increase your risk of side effects.

Pregnancy and nursing mothers:

Category X. See page 9 for a description of categories. This drug may cause birth defects. You should not take it while you are pregnant.

Possible food and drug interactions:

- If you take quazepam along with a drug that depresses your nervous system, such as tranquilizers, alcohol, antihistamines, or muscle relaxants, the combination may dangerously depress your nervous system.

Helpful hints:

- You shouldn't drive a car or operate heavy machinery until you are sure the medicine isn't making you drowsy or less than alert. Be careful the day after you've taken quazepam, as well as the night you take it.
- The usual starting dose for adults is 15 mg at bedtime. Some people just need 7.5 mg.
- You may have trouble sleeping for the first couple of nights after you stop taking this drug.

Secobarbital

Brand name: *Seconal Sodium* (Generic available)

What this drug does for you:

This barbiturate is used to promote sleep and to relieve anxiety and tension. Secobarbital is a short-acting barbiturate — it begins working in 10 to 15 minutes and lasts about three to four hours.

Possible side effects of this drug:

- The most common side effect is daytime sleepiness.
- Some rarer side effects are agitation, confusion, nightmares, nervousness, dizziness, very slow breathing, low blood pressure, nausea, constipation, headache, skin rash, and fever.

Special warnings:

- You can become addicted to this drug. You must not increase your dose without talking to your doctor. Some symptoms of intoxication with barbiturates are walking unsteadily, slurred speech, confusion, and irritability.
- You should withdraw from secobarbital slowly (for example, decrease the dose from three to two doses a day for one week). If you quit taking the drug quickly, you may have nightmares, insomnia, anxiety, dizziness, and nausea. If you're addicted to the drug and you quit taking it suddenly, delirium, convulsions, and death may result.

- People with a group of disorders called porphyria should not use barbiturates.

Pregnancy and nursing mothers:

Category D. See page 9 for description of categories. You must not use this drug while you're pregnant. Drug is present in mother's milk.

Possible food and drug interactions:

- If you take secobarbital along with a drug that depresses your nervous system, such as tranquilizers, alcohol, antihistamines, or muscle relaxants, the combination may dangerously depress your nervous system.
- Secobarbital may increase the effects of corticosteroids.
- This drug may decrease the effectiveness of anti-clotting drugs like warfarin, the anti-fungal drug griseofulvin, birth control pills, and doxycycline.
- Secobarbital may increase the effects of phenytoin.
- Sodium valproate, valproic acid, and monoamine oxidase (MAO) inhibitors may increase the depressant effects of secobarbital.

Helpful hints:

- Secobarbital loses its ability to promote sleep after two weeks of taking it regularly.
- You shouldn't drive a car or operate heavy machinery until you are sure the medicine isn't making you drowsy or less than alert.
- You should have regular blood, liver, and kidney tests if you take this drug for a long time.
- If you take birth control pills, you should use another type of contraception while you're taking secobarbital.
- The usual dose for adults with insomnia is 100 mg at bedtime.

Temazepam

Brand name: *Restoril* **(Generic available)**

What this drug does for you:

Temazepam is a hypnotic drug used to treat insomnia. It is a benzodiazepine. Temazepam seems to cause less daytime sleepiness than some of the longer-acting benzodiazepines.

Possible side effects of this drug:

- The most common side effect, especially in older people, is daytime drowsiness. Daytime sleepiness may last for several days after you quit taking the drug. Other side effects are fatigue, headache, nervousness, dizziness, nightmares, weakness, blurred vision, dry mouth, diarrhea, and upset stomach.
- Rare side effects are shakiness, backache, burning eyes, memory loss, hallucinations, and restlessness.
- Some people have memory loss for several hours after taking a benzodiazepine. Make sure you'll be able to get a full night's sleep after taking your medicine.

- Benzodiazepines cause some people's behavior to change. For instance, you may become more aggressive and agitated.

Special warnings:

- You can become dependent on temazepam. To avoid seizures and other less severe withdrawal symptoms, such as heightened senses, muscle cramps, diarrhea, and blurred vision, you should quit taking the drug gradually under your doctor's supervision. Don't stop abruptly, and don't increase or decrease your dosage without your doctor's approval.
- People with poor liver, kidney, or lung function should use temazepam cautiously. The drug may stay in your body longer and increase your risk of side effects.

Pregnancy and nursing mothers:

Category X. See page 9 for a description of categories. This drug may cause birth defects. You should not take it while you are pregnant.

Possible food and drug interaction:

- If you take temazepam along with a drug that depresses your nervous system, such as tranquilizers, alcohol, antihistamines, or muscle relaxants, the combination may dangerously depress your nervous system. Never drink alcohol while taking any benzodiazepine.

Helpful hints:

- You shouldn't drive a car or operate heavy machinery until you are sure the medicine isn't making you drowsy or less than alert. Be careful the day after you've taken temazepam, as well as the night you take it.
- The usual starting dose for adults is 15 mg at bedtime. Some people just need 7.5 mg.
- Take temazepam at least 30 minutes before bedtime.
- You may have trouble sleeping for the first couple of nights after you stop taking this drug.
- It's best not to take hypnotics for more than seven to 10 days.

Triazolam

Brand name: *Halcion* (Generic available)

What this drug does for you:

Triazolam is a hypnotic drug used to treat insomnia. It is a short-acting benzodiazepine. Since it is short-acting, it is more likely than some of the other benzodiazepines to cause rebound insomnia (increased sleeping problems, especially during the last third of the night) and anxiety or nervousness during the day.

Possible side effects of this drug:

- The most common side effects, especially in older people, are daytime drowsiness, dizziness, and lightheadedness. Also common are nervousness, headache, lack of coordination, and nausea.
- Other side effects are weakness, confusion, shakiness, depression, irri-

tability, impotence, decreased sex drive, nightmares, blurred vision and other vision disturbances, loss of bladder control or difficulty urinating, heart palpitations, nausea, constipation, diarrhea, slurred speech, and menstrual irregularities.

● Some people have memory loss for several hours after taking a benzodiazepine. Make sure you'll be able to get a full night's sleep after taking your medicine.

● Benzodiazepines cause some people's behavior to change. For instance, you may become more aggressive and agitated.

Special warnings:

● You can become dependent on triazolam. To avoid seizures and other less severe withdrawal symptoms, such as heightened senses, muscle cramps, diarrhea, and blurred vision, you should quit taking the drug gradually under your doctor's supervision. Don't stop abruptly, and don't increase or decrease your dosage without your doctor's approval.

● People with poor liver, kidney, or lung function should use triazolam cautiously. The drug may stay in your body longer and increase your risk of side effects.

Pregnancy and nursing mothers:

Category X. See page 9 for a description of categories. This drug may cause birth defects. You should not take it while you are pregnant. Triazolam is present in mother's milk. Nursing mothers should not take triazolam.

Possible food and drug interaction:

● If you take triazolam along with a drug that depresses your nervous system, such as tranquilizers, alcohol, antihistamines, or muscle relaxants, the combination may dangerously depress your nervous system.

Helpful hints:

● You shouldn't drive a car or operate heavy machinery until you are sure the medicine isn't making you drowsy or less than alert. Be careful the day after you've taken triazolam, as well as the night you take it.

● The usual starting dose for adults is 15 mg at bedtime. Some people just need 7.5 mg.

● You may have trouble sleeping for the first couple of nights after you stop taking this drug.

● It's best not to take hypnotics for more than seven to 10 days.

Zolpidem Tartrate

Brand name: *Ambien*

What this drug does for you:

Zolpidem is a short-acting hypnotic drug used to treat insomnia. Since it is short-acting, it is more likely than some of the other hypnotics to cause rebound insomnia (increased sleeping problems, especially during the last third of the night) and anxiety or nervousness during the day. It is less likely to cause daytime sleepiness.

Possible side effects of this drug:

- The most common side effects, especially in older people, are daytime drowsiness, dizziness, headache, diarrhea, and nausea.
- Other side effects are dry mouth, allergy, back pain, chest pain, heart palpitations, lightheadedness, depression, abnormal dreams, anxiety, constipation, sinusitis, and rash.
- Although it's rare with zolpidem, some people have memory loss for several hours after taking a hypnotic. Make sure you'll be able to get a full night's sleep after taking your medicine.
- Hypnotics like zolpidem cause some people's behavior to change. For instance, you may become more aggressive and agitated.

Special warnings:

- You can become dependent on zolpidem. To avoid seizures and other less severe withdrawal symptoms, such as heightened senses, muscle cramps, diarrhea, and blurred vision, you should quit taking the drug gradually under your doctor's supervision. Don't stop abruptly, and don't increase or decrease your dosage without your doctor's approval.
- People with poor liver, kidney, or lung function should use zolpidem cautiously. The drug may stay in your body longer and increase your risk of side effects.

Pregnancy and nursing mothers:

Category B. See page 9 for a description of categories. Zolpidem is present in mother's milk. Nursing mothers should not take zolpidem.

Possible food and drug interactions:

- If you take zolpidem along with a drug that depresses your nervous system, such as tranquilizers, alcohol, antihistamines, or muscle relaxants, the combination may dangerously depress your nervous system. Never drink alcohol while taking sleeping medicines.

Helpful hints:

- You will absorb zolpidem more slowly (and fall asleep more slowly) if you take it with or immediately after a meal. Take it without food to fall asleep faster.
- You shouldn't drive a car or operate heavy machinery until you are sure the medicine isn't making you drowsy or less than alert. Be careful the day after you've taken zolpidem, as well as the night you take it.
- The usual dose for adults is 10 mg at bedtime.
- It's best not to take hypnotics for more than seven to 10 days.
- You may have trouble sleeping the first night or two after you stop taking zolpidem. This rebound insomnia will go away.

Natural Alternatives

ANXIETY

- ◀ Blurred vision
- ◀ Difficulty breathing, shortness of breath
- ◀ Dry mouth
- ◀ Fidgeting
- ◀ Irritability
- ◀ Poor memory or concentration
- ◀ Ringing in the ears
- ◀ Sweaty or clammy skin
- ◀ Chest pain
- ◀ Dizziness
- ◀ Eyelid twitching
- ◀ Headache
- ◀ Muscle aches
- ◀ Rapid, pounding heartbeat
- ◀ Stomach pain, nausea, vomiting

Fight your fears the natural way

Are your worry dolls getting overworked? Does the thought of an eight-legged creature send you fleeing for the nearest chair? Well then, count yourself as one of the millions of people who experience anxiety.

Before you scramble for the closest psychiatrist's couch and examine your feelings toward your parents, realize that anxiety is a natural response that comes in several degrees, many of which are considered healthy.

Anxiety is part of your natural protective fight-or-flight response. It motivates you to high performance such as studying hard for a big test or meeting a deadline. It is when the fear, or trying to avoid the fear, begins to take over your daily life that you need to take action. If anxiety is driving you relentlessly and recklessly down the road of life, you need to kick fear out of the driver's seat and take control. Here's what to do:

Cut down on the caffeine. Chasing your fears away may be as simple as limiting your intake of coffee, sodas, and other caffeinated products. These drinks can cause physical reactions, such as a rapid heartbeat, that make your body think it's having an anxiety attack.

Get a physical. Before you start sizing straight jackets, get a physical exam. Many physical symptoms of anxiety are caused by other medical problems such as anemia, diabetes, or heart problems. Even prescription drugs like asthma inhalers, diet pills, and decongestants can cause anxiety-like symptoms.

Then get physical. Once your doctor has ruled out potential medical problems, and he's OK'd a regular exercise program, get with it! Exercise is a good way to work out anxious thoughts. And the physical response to exercise is a rush of endorphins, chemicals produced in the brain that actually make you feel better

Take a second look. Most people with anxiety disorders have false views of the situation and their emotions. Through therapy, you can learn to re-examine anxious thinking and find new ways of viewing the environment.

Belief system therapy (often called cognitive therapy by psychologists) has been the clear champion over other forms of therapy. In belief system therapy, you examine beliefs which may be causing your anxiety and work on replacing these beliefs with healthier ones.

Face your fears. "The only thing we have to fear is fear itself." President Franklin Delano Roosevelt's wise words may have inspired a country, but they do little to allay the fears of someone having an anxiety attack. But FDR was right, fear is what causes your discomfort.

And avoiding your fears will only make them worse. Work on gradually placing yourself in the harmless situations that cause you needless anxiety. Use relaxation techniques, such as breathing deeply and slowly, to keep yourself calm.

Relax. Working your way from the top of your head to the tips your toes, tense and relax each group of muscles. Practice this technique on a regular basis, and you'll find your tension level reduced during everyday activities.

Don't bottle it up. Liquid courage doesn't last long. Alcohol and drugs may temporarily numb your worries, but they only mask the anxiety and can lead to more serious problems. One-third of people with anxiety disorders abuse alcohol and drugs.

Don't depend on prescribed drugs. A short-term dose of prescribed drugs may help you through some rough times, especially in the beginning of therapy. But you and your doctor must work on helping you cope without drugs.

Widely prescribed drugs like benzodiazepines can have serious side effects, and users often experience withdrawal symptoms. Since medicine does not help you learn to deal with your anxieties, you're likely to be no better, and in some cases you may be worse, than you were before you started taking the drugs.

Set aside a specific worry time. Pick a place and a time for worrying — about a half hour should be plenty. Quickly jot down random worries as they occur, then immediately push them out of your head until you reach the place and time you've set aside for worry. During the half hour you've set aside, review all your worries and write down as many solutions as you can think of. At the end of your session, choose a solution and commit to trying it out.

Although anxiety may feel like a crippling disease, it is not only controllable but reversible. The first steps are to admit your fear and not be ashamed. Instead of denying the feelings, look for what is causing your anxiety. Don't be afraid to seek professional counseling if you need help. Once you have discovered your fear, use the natural techniques listed above to help you throw away your worry dolls and begin to relax.

Sources —
   American Family Physician (49,1:161 and 50,8:1745)
   British Medical Review (1309,6950:321)
   Consultant (35,4:473)
   Psychology Today (27,3:34)

Repressed emotions raise cholesterol

You know that high cholesterol is bad for you, so you take steps to keep it low. You watch what you eat, you exercise regularly ... but do you check your emotions? A study at Miriam Hospital found that holding in your feelings can be just as bad as eating that jelly doughnut. Dr. Raymond Niaura studied young men and women for a connection between cholesterol levels, personalities, and anxiety. Although the study showed no difference for women, the cholesterol levels for men differed according to how they dealt with anxiety.

Men with low cholesterol levels were honest about their emotions, including anxiety. Men who denied their negative emotions averaged cholesterol levels of 200 mg/dl — 40 points higher than the levels of the men who admitted feeling anxious. Anxiety is a natural protective response. When it is triggered, your body transports fat out of storage and into the blood. Men who repress anxiety actually have a more intense response and get more harmful fat into the bloodstream, raising cholesterol levels.

So while cutting back on some things, like smoking and ice cream, can lower your cholesterol, saying no to your emotions could do harm. Admitting your anxiety could open up a whole new avenue to health.

Source —
Psychology Today (89, 23:24)

DEPRESSION

◄ Difficulty concentrating or staying awake
◄ Feeling guilty or worthless
◄ General aches and pains
◄ Headache
◄ Lack of interest in hobbies, sports, or sex
◄ Sleep too much or can't fall asleep
◄ Weight gain or loss
◄ Digestive difficulties
◄ Feeling hopeless and worried all the time
◄ Increased or decreased appetite
◄ No energy
◄ Restless
◄ Thoughts of death and suicide

It's more than the blues

It's perfectly normal to feel sad sometimes, especially when sad things happen in your life. And it may take a while to feel better. But if you can't shake these bad feelings for weeks and months, or if you have these feelings when nothing bad has happened to you, you may be suffering from clinical depression, and you probably need to get some help. Depression is a medical disorder, like heart disease or diabetes, and it can affect both your behavior and your physical health.

Once you're working with a doctor to help you conquer your depression, there are some natural things you can do to make yourself feel better.

Make sure your doctor knows about all the medicine you're taking. Depression has been linked to beta blockers, drugs widely prescribed for high blood pressure. Researchers now say beta blockers may only cause depression in a few people, but many other prescription drugs list depression as a side effect. If you suspect a drug is behind your blues, discuss alternatives with your doctor — like discontinuing the drug, changing your dosage, or switching to a drug less likely to cause depression.

Skip the guilt trip. Depression affects people of all income levels, races, and religions. You can't make it go away by just "cheering up" or "toughing it out" because clinical depression is an illness.

Lend a helping hand. This suggestion seems to work especially well for older people. Try helping out in informal ways, such as caring for children, cooking, or shopping. You'll feel useful and have a sense of being in control, a good weapon against depression.

Move your body to heal your mind. When you feel down, your natural instinct may be to retreat and be alone, watch a lot of television, and snack uncontrollably. But that strategy rarely helps. A recent study of over 400 people concluded that the top way to stop mild depression was exercise.

According to the Canadian Fitness and Lifestyle Research Institute, evidence is mounting that exercise can actually prevent depression, as well as help people already experiencing mild to moderate symptoms. Exercise even helps those with severe emotional illness, when used in combination with other treatments. The Canadian researchers noted that depressed people often show marked improvement after two to six months of regular exercise.

How can moving your body heal your mind? No one knows for sure, but scientists suspect that the brain counters the stimulus of exercising your muscles by releasing endorphins that cause pleasurable sensations and elevate mood.

Get busy. It may sound too simple, but working on a hobby that brings you pleasure may help your depression. The same is true for tackling chores you've been putting off. You'll enjoy a real sense of accomplishment and purpose.

Try problem-solving treatment. A British study published in 1995 explains an interesting new method of psychotherapy called problem-solving treatment. The basic idea is that emotional problems are caused by problems in living, and sometimes a person is completely overwhelmed. Dealing effectively with the problems can help the symptoms improve. A therapist or other trained doctor helps the depressed person identify and map out a plan to deal with his problems one at a time. This treatment for depression has been found to be very successful, as well as cost-effective, and it doesn't involve any drugs

---

Some depression drugs lead to bad breath

Some prescription drugs, such as antidepressants or medication for angina, can cause your breath to smell bad. Many of these drugs cause dry mouth, which can lead to bad breath. You can defeat the effects of these drugs by drinking more water.

Sources —
British Medical Journal (6923,308:217)
Dental Update (20,2:57)

or long-term treatment.

For more information, see *How to solve a problem in six easy steps* later in this chapter.

Soothe your soul with music. "Music alone with sudden charms can bind the wand'ring sense, and calme the troubled mind," wrote 17th century dramatist William Congreve.

Twentieth century scientists say that's more than a poetic idea. In fact, when researchers asked over 500 adults what worked best to overcome a bad mood, listening to music was high on the list, topped only by exercise.

A recent study of 30 depressed elderly adults aged 61 to 86 concluded that music can lift depression. Research subjects were divided into two groups. One received no treatment while the other relaxed by listening to music. The untreated group didn't get better, but those who used music as part of their therapy soon had improved moods and higher self-esteem.

Let in the light. Another way to help rid yourself of depression is to check into the possibility of light therapy. If your blues seem linked to the dark, bleak days of autumn and winter, you may have a form of depression known as SAD (Seasonal Affective Disorder).

According to the U.S. Department of Health and Human Services, mild or moderate seasonal depression due to a lack of natural light can be successfully treated using a special bright light bulb. It "tricks" the body into thinking you've experienced a few extra hours of daylight each day.

To find out if you are a candidate for light therapy, talk to your doctor.

Be good to yourself. Perhaps the best way to help yourself feel better when you are down is simply to be good to yourself. Try not to see life only in terms of black and white, and don't expect yourself or others to be perfect.

And don't hesitate to seek professional counseling if you need help. Ask your doctor or local mental health center for a referral. You may also want to ask them to put you in touch with a local support group so you can learn how other people are handling their depression.

Most of all, remember that your depression didn't develop overnight, and it won't disappear magically in a split second either. But with the right help — including doing everything you can to help yourself feel better — you will win the battle of the blues.

Eat right to fight depression

What you eat can have a huge effect on your health. A lack of calcium may result in bone-weakening osteoporosis, for example, and a high-fat diet increases your risk of heart disease. But it's not so well-known that what you eat can also affect your mood. Consuming the wrong foods can contribute to depression, while making some specific diet changes may boost your mood back to the sunny side.

Crush comfort-food cravings! It's perfectly normal to turn to food for comfort occasionally, and munching on a chocolate chip cookie every now and then when you are blue is relatively harmless.

But for people who have a serious problem with depression, using sweets as a kind of "self-medication" can start a dangerous cycle of not only overeating, but also eating foods that actually make depression worse.

Don't crash down from a sugar "high." Eating sugar makes you feel better for a while, but then you may feel worse — until you eat more sugar.

Researchers suspect that sugar causes your body to release endorphins — the same brain chemicals that blunt pain, elevate mood, and produce a "runner's high."

A sugar-triggered endorphin rush, however, unlike one produced by exercise, soon disappears. And endorphin levels drop even lower than before you had that candy bar or cola. In one study, even people who were not depressed felt better when they stopped eating sugar. If you decide to eliminate sugar from your diet to help your mood, remember to check labels. It's a "hidden" ingredient in many products — including flavored yogurt, catsup, cereals, fruit drinks, and granola bars.

All those empty calories are another reason to forget about eating sweets. You may end up lacking important nutrients, including calcium, magnesium, and selenium, and that can contribute to lethargy and depression.

Also, caffeine can make a normal drop in blood sugar seem worse, so eliminating or reducing consumption of coffee and caffeine-containing colas may help improve mood swings as well.

Lift your mood with complex carbos. So how can you eliminate sugar and still get its mood-lifting benefits? Sugar, refined flour, and other refined starch products are simple carbohydrates. Complex carbohydrates, like whole-grain breads and cereals, are a better choice. Researchers at the University of South Alabama studied the effects of simple versus complex carbohydrates. Both stimulate the production of serotonin, a brain chemical that helps elevate mood. The mood-lifting effects of the complex carbohydrates lasted much longer.

Another reason to fill up on complex carbohydrates is that you'll increase your body's supply of tryptophan, an amino acid that can help banish depression. A few years ago, the U.S. Food and Drug Administration (FDA) pulled supplements containing tryptophan off U.S. store shelves when contaminated batches of the pills were found to be the cause of a painful muscular disorder.

But you can increase your body's supply of the amino acid naturally, without any supplements, by eating more complex carbohydrates like oatmeal, brown rice, and whole-wheat muffins.

Perk up with protein. Not everyone responds with a sunnier disposition after trying a diet that relies heavily on complex carbohydrates, however. Some people feel better when they eat more protein.

If high-carbo eating doesn't improve your mood, try a lean turkey sandwich and some low-fat milk. The reason? Researchers theorize that the amino acid tyrosine, found in abundance in milk and poultry, increases the body's ability to use more of the mood-raising brain chemical norepinephrine. For some people, that change in diet is just what their particular body chemistry needs to banish fatigue and depression.

Don't wait too long to eat. Skipping meals not only robs you of needed vitamins and minerals but it can make a bad mood worse by causing blood sugar

How to solve a problem in six easy steps

Too many people go round the mulberry bush of worry and frustration when confronted with a problem. One common reason for this is that people are searching for the "perfect" solution. The truth is, perfect solutions don't exist. There is only the solution that's best suited to your time and place. Just knowing you don't have to make a perfect decision should take a load off your mind. So will this six-step system for solving a problem.

Step 1) Identify the problem. You may have more than one problem that needs solving, but you should work through each problem separately.

Step 2) Make a list of all possible answers, no matter how ridiculous or outrageous they seem.

Step 3) Choose the solution which seems best. If two solutions are very close and you can't decide, toss a coin. You can try one and if it doesn't work, try the other one.

Step 4) Take action.

Step 5) Re-evaluate. Ask yourself: How are things going? Is the problem solved? If the problem is not solved, what additional action should I take to solve the problem?

Step 6) Repeat steps four and five until the problem is resolved.

Work through this process on paper. Sometimes you will come up with a really great solution but forget about it when the time comes to make your decision. This is because the brain tends to discard original ideas and opt for old tried and true favorites or what seems more likely to work.

There. Now don't you feel better already?

Source —

Confessions of a Healer: The Truth from an Unconventional Family Doctor, MacMurray & Beck, Aspen, Colo., 1994

levels to drop. If you wait too long to eat, researchers have found, blood-sugar levels may not rise back to normal. And that can increase fatigue and depression.

Dieting can be a downer. One more way food can lead to the blues is that great American pastime — dieting. Not eating what you want or feeling guilty about eating fattening foods is no fun. Seriously overweight people have a higher than average risk of depression due to the stress of repeatedly going on diets.

Beat the blues with B vitamins. Studies have found that people who take in the least vitamin B12 are the most likely to suffer from depression and other mental problems, including memory loss and anxiety.

A deficiency of folic acid, another member of the B-complex family, has been linked to mood swings, anxiety, and depression. In fact, British scientists studying a group of people suffering from depression-related psychological problems found that over 30 percent of the research subjects had low levels of folic acid. When these people were given folic acid supplements, they improved dramatically.

You can get B6 and B12 in chicken, fish, pork, eggs, whole-wheat breads and cereals, dairy products, peanuts, and walnuts. Some foods rich in folic acid are broccoli, spinach, collards, oranges, lemons, grapefruit, beans, and whole-grain breads and cereals. Other foods may soon be fortified with folic acid to make sure everyone gets an ample supply of the vitamin. Check the labels on the food you buy to see if this important vitamin is included.

Don't forget vitamin C. A team of researchers from the Institute of Nutrition in Germany studied the effects of slight vitamin deficiencies on 1,082 otherwise healthy young men (ages 17 to 29 years), and they found some encouraging results.

The men who were suffering from mild vitamin deficiencies experienced more depression, nervousness, irritability, anxiety, fear, and even poorer memory and concentration skills. The good news, however, is that these same men seemed to benefit from vitamin supplements. Taking vitamin C supplements led to decreased nervousness, less depression, and improved emotional stability.

A healthy diet should provide almost all of your nutritional needs without having to take extra supplements. Some natural sources of vitamin C are green and red peppers, collard greens, broccoli, tomatoes, potatoes, spinach, strawberries, oranges, and other citrus fruits.

Sources —

Annals of Internal Medicine (117,10:820)

Annals of the New York Academy of Sciences (669:352)

Answers to Your Questions About Clinical Depression, National Mental Health Association, 1021 Prince Street, Alexandria, Va. 22314–2971

Archives of Internal Medicine (152,2:381)

British Medical Journal (306,6878:655; 308,6926:446; 308,6940:1328 and 310,6977:441)

Depression in Primary Care: Detection, Diagnosis, and Treatment, U.S. Department of Health and Human Services, 2101 East Jefferson Street, Suite 501, Rockville, Md. 20852, 1993

Depression is a Treatable Illness: A Patient's Guide, U.S. Department of Health and Human Services, 2101 East Jefferson Street, Suite 501, Rockville, Md. 20852, 1993

Food and Mood: The Complete Guide to Eating Well and Feeling Your Best, Henry Holt and Co., New York, 1995

Journal of Gerontology (47,5:300)

Journal Watch (12,10:74)

Medical Abstracts (15,1:8)

Medical Tribune (34,14:16 and 35,6:18)

Medical World News (34,11:13)

Nutrition Research Newsletter (13,11/12:122)

Physician Assistant (17,1:62)

Postgraduate Medicine (91,1:255,261)

Science News (141,13:213; 144,5:79 and 144,17:263)

The Atlanta Journal/Constitution (June 24, 1993, W8; Nov. 10, 1994, K1)

The Canadian Medical Association Journal (151,8:1163)

The Lancet (341,8852:1087)

MENTAL ILLNESS

◀ Delusions
◀ Hallucinations
◀ Hearing voices in your head
◀ Out of touch with reality

◀ Episodes of manic joy and energy
   followed by deep depression
◀ Inability to interact with other
   people

Dealing with schizophrenia and manic depression

For people suffering from any type of psychosis, life is like being locked alone in a carnival fun house ... without the fun. You hear voices, have severe hallucinations and delusions, you see and hear people not there. Trapped, psychotics lose touch with reality and the world.

Two psychotic illnesses, bipolar disorder (also known as manic depression) and schizophrenia, open their doors in adolescence or early adulthood. Although they affect only a small part of the population, they are often lifetime illnesses.

Schizophrenia is sometimes described as a "split personality." Schizophrenics often withdraw into themselves and began existing in a mixed-up world of their imagination.

Manic depression is a pendulum behavior that runs the range of emotion. In the manic mode a person has extreme irritability, increased energy, rapid talking, and overwhelming racing thoughts. Eventually depression takes over and feelings of hopelessness and guilt consume the person.

Although scientists are not sure what causes mental illness, many believe that it's due to abnormal brain functions. A new type of brain scanning, PET, may help solve the mystery.

For now, the primary treatment for people suffering from psychotic illness is medication and therapy. Since psychosis is difficult for the family as well as those affected, family therapy and support groups are often recommended.

People suffering from psychosis can lead normal, productive lives. With support from their family and professionals, they can shut the doors of the carnival fun house and enjoy the sounds and sights of life.

Sources —

Bipolar Disorder, National Institute of Mental Health, 1993

Cecil Textbook of Medicine, Harcourt Brace Jovanovich, Philadelphia, Pa., 1992

The American Medical Association Encyclopedia of Medicine, Random House, New York, 1989

OBSESSIVE-COMPULSIVE DISORDER

◄ Always dieting
◄ Buying and storing more food or other items than you can use
◄ Continually exercising and striving to be fit
◄ Counting anything and everything
◄ Fear of violence by yourself or others
◄ Spending hours cleaning or washing
◄ Workaholism

◄ Brooding over a word, phrase, or unanswerable problem
◄ Constantly checking and rechecking things
◄ Driving need to perform all tasks perfectly
◄ Strong fear of germs and dirt

When obsession takes over

You're positive that you turned the iron off and even unplugged it before you came to work this morning, but now you're beginning to have doubts. You visualize the iron burning through the board and flames igniting in the laundry room. You see the fire spreading through your house, engulfing the carpet, the furniture, the curtains. You imagine arriving home to find your house burned to the ground.

Even though you consciously know that this fantasy is ridiculous, you can't get your mind off it. At lunchtime, you drive home to be sure the iron is turned off. Back at work, the feeling of dread stays with you all afternoon, and you can't stop thinking about that iron. Finally, you become so upset by the imagined situation that you leave work early to go home and check again to see if your house is still there.

If this is just an isolated incident, you are probably having a stressful week or are really subconsciously worried about something else. But if this kind of thing happens frequently, you may have Obsessive-Compulsive Disorder.

Understand obsessions and compulsions. An obsession consists of frightening and insistent thoughts, such as fear that something horrible will happen or bizarre sexual fantasies. (One OCD sufferer's wife had trouble getting the laundry done because her husband kept opening the washing machine to make sure the cat wasn't inside.)

A compulsion consists of repetitive acts, such as counting one's steps or repeating the same words or washing the same foot over and over. Obsessions and compulsions go together. The obsessive fears lead to anxiety, and the anxiety is relieved by the compulsive actions. So it makes sense that compulsions naturally follow obsessions.

Know when your need for order is out of control. OCD seems to be related to a need for orderliness and perfectionism.

Just because you like to keep things neat and orderly or you double-check doors or stove burners doesn't mean you have OCD. But if your neat habits or your tendency to check things begins to take more than an hour a day or if it interferes with your normal daily routine, you should talk with your doctor.

Get your hands dirty. Several natural methods have helped some people with OCD. One is behavioral therapy. It calls for you to write down all of your symptoms and face them honestly. Then you must take action against them.

For instance, if you are a compulsive hand washer, dirty your hands. Then look at them and don't wash them for a specified time. Many people find it helpful to work through these behavioral changes with a qualified therapist.

Get it out of your system. Another behavioral method is to deliberately perform your compulsive acts until you can't stand it anymore. For example, if you check the stove burners 25 times, force yourself to check them 200 times. When you are thoroughly sick of doing it, you may gain some insight into your behavior.

Involve your family. Families who receive therapy learn how to help an obsessive-compulsive break free of this disorder. Therapists teach family members how to offer understanding and how to stop supporting the sufferer in obsessive-compulsive behavior patterns.

Control stress. Symptoms of obsessive-compulsive disorder are likely to recur if you don't manage your stress well.

OCD is more widespread than people once thought. Most sufferers keep their condition secret out of shame. But more and more people are coming forward. Estimates of the number of people with OCD in the United States range from 4 million to 5 million. It strikes men, women, and all ethnic groups equally. It can start at any age, including early childhood, but age 18 to 20 is the most common time.

If you think you or a family member has OCD, consult your doctor. Before choosing a therapist, make sure he has worked with obsessive-compulsives. For additional information, call the Obsessive-Compulsive Foundation National Headquarters at 203-878-5669.

Sources —

American Family Physician (49,5:1129, 1142)
American Journal of Psychiatry (150,3:460)
Bioscience (42,6:257)
FDA Consumer (26,4:6)
Health (8,5:78)
The American Medical Association Encyclopedia of Medicine, Random House, New York, 1989
The Boy Who Couldn't Stop Washing, E.P., Dutton, New York, 1989
The Good News About Panic, Anxiety & Phobias, Villard Books, New York, 1989
The Journal of the American Board of Family Practice (6,5:507)
The Wall Street Journal (April 25, 1994, A1)

PANIC DISORDER

- ◀ Chest pains
- ◀ Difficulty breathing
- ◀ Fast, shallow breathing
- ◀ Fear of going crazy
- ◀ Feeling faint
- ◀ Feeling that everything is unreal
- ◀ Pins and needles sensations
- ◀ Sweating
- ◀ Choking
- ◀ Dizziness
- ◀ Fear of doing something uncontrolled or embarrassing during an attack
- ◀ Nausea, stomach pain
- ◀ Rapid heartbeat
- ◀ Trembling

Stop the panic

According to Greek mythology, panic comes from Pan, the god of shepherds and their flocks, hunters, forests, and wildlife. Long ago, people passing through lonely wilderness areas associated the scary night sounds with Pan, and they experienced a new level of fear — "pan"ic. Panic may be Pan's legacy, but if you've ever been in the suffocating grip of a panic attack, you know that panic is one legacy you'd just as soon leave behind. Panic causes uncomfortable physical symptoms, and the fear of future attacks drains your life of joy and pleasure.

You're not alone. Panic attacks and anxiety disorders are among the most common problems treated by mental health professionals. About one in every 10 people has had a panic attack.

When panic attacks or the fear of having them becomes so frequent or severe that you can't function properly, it's diagnosed as a panic disorder. Between 4 and 6 percent of the general population suffer from panic disorder.

"It's common to have a panic attack when you're under tremendous stress," said Dr. Cynthia Last, director of the Anxiety Treatment Center at Nova Southeastern University in Davie, Florida. "It's the fear about the attacks that tends to make them keep coming, so it's kind of a vicious circle."

Stressed out! Basically, a panic attack is one reaction a person's body can have to stress, and there is a strong genetic link, Last said. You also can have a panic attack as a result of other mental health problems, such as post-traumatic stress disorder, obsessive-compulsive disorder, or a phobia.

"Any major life change, good or bad, can bring on an attack," she said. "There seems to be a link between hormonal and endocrinologic changes too. We see panic in women who have had babies or are going through menopause."

Panic attacks come in two varieties — the kind that is linked to the circumstance, like the person who has a panic attack every time he gets in an elevator or flies on an airplane, and the kind that seems to come out of the blue and is unrelated to the immediate situation.

It can take some time to figure out what triggers the second kind, but it's linked to something stressful, Last said.

You can be cured. "It's definitely a treatable disorder," said Dr. Thomas Mellman, director of the anxiety disorder and post-traumatic stress disorders program at the University of Miami. "Treatment can be several things. Sometimes it's a relatively straightforward debriefing. For others, it's just the passage of time or supportive interaction with others. Those all can help. But like any other problem, the longer it's established the more difficult it is to intervene."

Exercise, cut out caffeine, face your fears, and learn to relax. For more specifics, see the general anxiety article at the beginning of this chapter.

Think yourself out of a panic attack. Handle a panic attack with these four steps:

◁ Stay where you are. It may be tough, but try. It's very important to stay and face the situation.
◁ Breathe slowly and try to relax. Start at your head and work your way down through each part of the body, tensing and relaxing muscles.
◁ Visualize a pleasant experience or place.
◁ Think to yourself that the feeling is uncomfortable, but it's not dangerous and it will pass.

Sources —
Dr. Cynthia Last, director, Anxiety Treatment Center at Nova Southeastern University, Davie, Fla.
Dr. Thomas Mellman, director of the anxiety disorders and post-traumatic stress disorders program at the University of Miami, Fla.

SLEEPING PROBLEMS

◀ Can't go to sleep
◀ Fitful, restless sleep
◀ Waking frequently during the night
◀ Chronic fatigue
◀ Tossing and turning in bed
◀ Waking too early in the morning

Rest for the weary

Seem like the sandman has a grudge against you?

If you're tired of counting sheep and still not getting sleep, here's how to out-smart the sandman and get the sound sleep you need.

Find out how much sleep you need. It varies with the individual, but if you're getting seven or eight hours a night, you're probably all right. If you're over 60, you might need only five or six hours. You can judge how much sleep you need by your sense of well-being. If you've had bouts of insomnia, you know how rotten you feel the next day: tired, less able to concentrate, and probably irritable.

Don't seek slumber through sleeping pills. Such medications may break the pattern of insomnia and help you sleep at first, but they can have all kinds of side effects including "hangovers," drowsiness, dizziness, uncontrollable mood swings, even diarrhea.

Prescription drugs can lead to dependence and also to "rebound insomnia." After a few weeks of use their effectiveness wears off and the sleeplessness comes back worse than before. It's far better to achieve sleep in more natural ways.

Seven steps to snore-free sleeping

If snoring, yours or someone else's, is keeping you awake at night, try the tips below:

◁ Sleep on your side. You're more likely to snore when you sleep on your back. To help keep yourself on your side during the night, sew a tennis ball into the back of your pajamas, or simply stuff a couple of tennis balls into a sock, and pin it to the back of your pajamas.

◁ Avoid thick pillows that cause your neck to bend forward. This pinches the airways, making snoring worse. However, if you elevate your entire upper body with pillows, that may help.

◁ Stop smoking. Smoking causes the tissues of the throat to swell, and the nicotine disturbs sleep patterns.

◁ Stay away from alcohol, sleeping pills, and tranquilizers at bedtime. These relax the muscles of your throat, making snoring more likely.

◁ Use a saline spray before you head for bed. You can either purchase a saline spray at your local drugstore or make your own by mixing a cup of lukewarm water, a half teaspoon of salt, and a pinch of baking soda. These sprays help to open nasal passages, so you're less likely to breathe through your mouth and snore.

◁ Consider using a humidifier in your bedroom. Low humidity can dry out mucous membranes, increasing irritation and adding to the snoring problem.

◁ Lose weight. Extra weight, especially in the neck area, can cause pressure on your throat, collapsing already narrow air passages.

Sources —
American Review of Respiratory Diseases (144,5:1130)
British Medical Journal (300,6739:1557)
Chest (99,6:1378 and 107,5:1283)
The Home Remedies Handbook, Publications International, Lincolnwood, Ill., 1993
The Wellness Encyclopedia, Houghton Mifflin, Boston, 1991

Root out hidden causes. The causes of insomnia are many: anxiety; poor diet; lack of exercise; use of alcohol, drugs, or caffeine; low blood sugar; indigestion; lack of calcium and magnesium; and food intolerance.

In many cases, the cause is unknown. If you have a specific physical problem that may be disturbing your sleep, such as low blood sugar, food intolerance, or sleep apnea (when you stop breathing for 10-second periods at least 30 times during the night), you should work with your doctor to correct it. Otherwise, to overcome insomnia — or even better, to prevent it — consider the following tips:

Set your biological clock with sunlight. Whenever possible, spend at least 15 minutes in bright early-morning sunlight. Exposure to sunlight between 7 a.m. and 9 a.m. helps set your biological clock to a 24-hour light/dark cycle. It gears your body to recognize night as the time to sleep.

Drink decaf at night. Don't drink coffee, tea, or anything else containing caffeine within six hours of bedtime. Some authorities advise eliminating caffeine altogether.

Soak in a warm bath before bed. A bath will relax your muscles and soothe your nerves.

Save the bedroom for sleep and sex. The bedroom is not appropriate for work or arguing. Let it be a sleep sanctuary, so that you only associate relaxation and rest with that room.

Get vigorous exercise on a regular basis. A recent study shows that exercise may be all older Americans need to fall asleep faster and sleep better.

Study participants, who were ages 50 to 76, had four workouts a week: two workouts of stretching, aerobics, and strength training, and two workouts of brisk walking.

After four months, the exercisers fell asleep faster and slept for an hour longer each night. Researchers aren't sure just why exercise helps so much, but they think it may be linked to stress reduction.

Go to bed at the same time every night. But only go to bed if you feel sleepy. If you don't, stay up and read or watch television till your eyelids get heavy.

Sweeten your dreams with a cup of honeyed herbal tea. Both chamomile and honey have sleep-inducing properties, so 30 or 40 minutes before bed drink a cup of chamomile tea with a spoonful of honey stirred in. (The honey also makes the tea taste better.)

Don't drink alcohol near bedtime. Alcohol may help you drop off, but it also may interfere with your normal sleep patterns and wake you up later.

Warm some milk. The old folk remedy, warm milk, works for some people, though scientists don't know why.

Don't look at the clock, and don't keep trying. If you can't get to sleep, get up, go to another room, read, listen to music, play solitaire. Or stay in bed and concentrate on being awake. Simply opening your eyes and looking at the shadows around the room often works. This technique, crazy as it sounds, relieves your mind from the anxiety of not being able to fall asleep, and you're soon snoozing soundly.

Consider melatonin. If none of these other natural methods are working for you, you may want to try melatonin supplements, which you can find in your local health food store or pharmacy.

Melatonin is a nocturnal hormone that tells your body when to sleep. Studies have found that older people who boost their melatonin levels can fall asleep just minutes after closing their eyes without the negative side effects of prescribed sleeping pills. They can also sleep 10 percent longer, which amounts to about 45 extra minutes of sleep for the average person.

Before you take melatonin, be sure to read the instructions on the package. If you're taking prescription medications, let your doctor know you're taking melatonin. Its interactions with some medications still aren't clear.

And keep in mind that the FDA hasn't yet approved the use of melatonin supplements. Therefore, the manufacture of melatonin is not regulated. Without FDA approval, you have no guarantee that the melatonin you buy will be consistently pure and safe.

Tell yourself it won't last. Comfort yourself with this thought: "I'm suffering now, but it won't last forever. In the next day or two, things will return to normal and I'll be sleeping peacefully again."

If these techniques don't work, and you have a stubborn case of insomnia that hangs on for weeks, better consult your doctor. But with luck and a little preparation you won't have to. Sweet dreams.

Sources —

Alternative Medicine, Future Medicine Publishing, Puyallup, Wash., 1993
FDA Consumer (23,8:13 and 28,7:14)
Food — Your Miracle Medicine, HarperCollins Publishers, New York, 1993
Journal Watch (14,5:38)
Prescription for Natural Healing, Avery Publishing, New York, 1990
The Atlanta Journal/Constitution (Nov. 21, 1994, C4)
The Journal of the American Medical Association (269,12:1548 and 273,1:6)
U.S. Pharmacist (18,5:47)

Drugs that cause insomnia

Insomnia affects about one-third of adult Americans at some time in their lives. For some of us, it's a frequent companion. Stress and anxiety are causes that you might suspect first, but there are a number of health problems that can claim insomnia as a symptom. Prescription and over-the-counter drugs used to treat these health problems can be a cause of insomnia too.

Some of the most common insomnia-causing drugs or drug ingredients are:

◁ Alcohol
◁ Antineoplastics
◁ Caffeine
◁ Diuretics
◁ Nicotine
◁ Phenytoin (Dilantin)
◁ Stimulants
◁ Theophylline
◁ Thyroid hormone

◁ Antihypertensives
◁ Beta-blockers
◁ Corticosteroids
◁ Levodopa
◁ Oral contraceptives
◁ Selective serotonin reuptake inhibitors and protriptyline (Vivactil)

If you are taking any of these prescription drugs or drugs containing these ingredients and you are suffering from insomnia, consult your doctor to see if your dosage might be modified to get rid of that particular side effect. If alcohol, caffeine, and nicotine are part of your lifestyle, try eliminating them and see if your insomnia improves.

Source —

American Family Physician (51,1:191)

MISCELLANEOUS DISORDERS

Prescription Drugs ℞

AIDS DRUGS

Didanosine

Brand name: *Videx*

What this drug does for you:
This antiviral drug is used to slow the growth of the human immunodeficiency virus (HIV). It is used to treat advanced HIV when zidovudine (AZT) hasn't been effective. The drug is available as tablets or a powder

Possible side effects of this drug:
- This drug may cause diarrhea, chills, fever, rash, itching, stomach pain, unusual weakness and tiredness, headache, nausea, and pneumonia. The buffered powder form often causes diarrhea.
- Rare side effects include shortness of breath, swelling of feet or lower legs, unusual bleeding and bruising, yellow skin and eyes, anxiety, difficulty sleeping, dry mouth and altered taste, yeast infection of the mouth, loss of hair, irritability, and restlessness.
- Pancreatitis is the major problem associated with this drug. Symptoms of pancreatitis may include nausea, vomiting, or stomach pain. If you develop any of these symptoms, call your doctor immediately. Pancreatitis can be fatal.
- A common side effect is peripheral neuropathy, damage to the nerves in the extremities. Some symptoms are pain, tingling or numbness in the hands or feet.

- Convulsions (seizures) and liver damage are also rare but serious side effects.
- This drug may cause an abnormal amount of uric acid in the blood.

Special warnings:
- People with liver or kidney problems may need a reduced dose.

Pregnancy and nursing mothers:
Category B. See page 9 for description of categories. Not known if drug is present in mother's milk.

Possible food and drug interactions:
- The buffered tablet and pediatric forms should not be taken at the same time as tetracycline antibiotics or antacids. These two forms should not be taken with quinolone antibiotics.
- If you are taking any other drugs that cause peripheral neuropathy or pancreatitis, you should take didanosine with caution.
- Avoid alcohol while taking didanosine.
- This drug may affect many laboratory tests including certain blood tests, liver enzymes, uric acid, and bilirubin.

Helpful hints:
- Take this drug on an empty stomach.
- The buffered powder should be mixed with water, not fruit juice or any other acidic beverage. Clean up any powder you spill with a damp cloth to avoid generating dust.
- Adults should take two tablets at each dose.

DRUGS TO TREAT ANEMIA/NUTRITION DEFICIENCIES

Ferrous Sulfate

Brand name: *Feosol, Fero-Folic, Iberet-Folic* (Generic available)

What this drug does for you:
This drug is used to treat iron-deficiency anemia and to prevent iron deficiency. Your body needs iron to make hemoglobin, a part of red blood cells. Hemoglobin allows red blood cells to carry oxygen throughout the body.

Possible side effects of this drug:
- This drug may cause constipation, nausea, and diarrhea. Some signs of an iron overdose are tiredness, vomiting, stomach pain, black and tarry stools, a weak and rapid pulse, and low blood pressure.

Special warnings:
- Discuss any plans for pregnancy with your doctor.
- Liquid forms may temporarily stain teeth.

Pregnancy and nursing mothers:
Check with your doctor before using this product if you are pregnant or

nursing.

Possible food and drug interaction:

- Iron may decrease the effectiveness of the antibiotic tetracycline. Don't take antibiotics within two hours of taking iron.
- Antacids may decrease levels or effects of this drug. Don't take antacids within two hours of taking iron.
- Certain foods such as eggs, milk, yogurt, whole-grain breads and cereals, coffee, and tea may decrease iron absorption.

Helpful hints:

- Take this drug on an empty stomach. However, if it causes an upset stomach, you can take it with or after food.
- Mix liquid formulas with water or juice and drink through a straw to help prevent stained teeth.
- Do not chew or crush sustained-release tablets or capsules.
- If you miss a dose, take it as soon as you remember. But if it is nearing time for your next dose, don't double up your doses (unless your doctor tells you to).

Potassium Chloride

Brand names: *K+8, K+10, K+Care, K-Dur, K-Lor, K-Lyte/C1, K-Norm, K-Tab, Kaon CL 10, Klor-Con, Klotrix, Micro-K, Micro-K LS, Rum-K, Slow-K, Ten-K* **(Generic available)**

What this drug does for you:

This drug is used to maintain the body's supply of potassium when you don't get enough through your diet or anytime potassium is depleted due to illness or drugs.

Possible side effects of this drug:

- This drug may cause nausea, vomiting, gas, diarrhea, upset stomach, and rash.
- The capsules and tablets can cause ulcers and bleeding in the stomach and intestines. If you have very dark stools, stomach pain, or vomiting, contact your doctor.

Special warnings:

- If you have poor kidney function or heart disease, you should use this drug with caution.
- Blood levels of potassium should be checked frequently.

Pregnancy and nursing mothers:

Category C. See page 9 for description of categories. Potassium supplements should have little effect on a mother's milk, but check with your doctor before you begin breast-feeding.

Possible food and drug interactions:

- This drug may lead to dangerously high levels of potassium if taken with ACE inhibitors or potassium-sparing diuretics.

Helpful hints:
- Swallow tablets whole. Don't crush or chew.
- Take this drug with a full glass of water or liquid.
- To avoid upset stomach, take this drug with food.

MISCELLANEOUS DRUGS

Azathioprine

Brand name: *Imuran*

What this drug does for you:
These tablets are used to help suppress the immune system and prevent rejection in kidney transplants. Azathioprine is also used to treat rheumatoid arthritis in people who don't respond to other drugs. Doctors prescribe this drug for other illnesses, too: ulcerative colitis, myasthenia gravis, Behcet's syndrome, and Crohn's disease.

Possible side effects of this drug:
- This drug may cause severe nausea and vomiting, fever, rash, diarrhea, muscular pain, and low blood pressure.
- Azathioprine can lower the number of blood cells you have. If you don't have enough white blood cells, your immunity is down, and you can get a fever, sore throat or pneumonia. If you are lacking red blood cells, you can become anemic, and that makes you tired and weak. Not having enough blood platelets makes you bruise easily and keeps your blood from clotting properly when you're injured. Be on the lookout for any of these symptoms of bone marrow depression.

Special warnings:
- You must try to avoid, and report immediately to your doctor, even mild infections such as colds, fever, sore throat, and general feelings of discomfort.
- Imuran can, in very rare cases, become toxic to the liver.
- It may take up to 12 weeks for the drug to become effective for rheumatoid arthritis.

Pregnancy and nursing mothers:
Category D. See page 9 for description of categories. Drug is present in mother's milk.

Possible food and drug interactions:
- Azathioprine may cause a drop in your white blood cell count if used with high blood pressure drugs called ACE inhibitors or with other drugs that lower the white blood cell count.
- Allopurinol, a drug used to treat gout, may increase the effects of azathioprine.

Helpful hints:
- If you miss a dose, take it as soon as you remember. But if it is nearing

time for your next dose, don't double up your doses (unless your doctor tells you to).
- Azathioprine may upset your stomach. Take it with food or milk.

Chlorhexidine Gluconate

Brand name: *Peridex*

What this drug does for you:
This antibacterial drug is used to treat gingivitis.

Possible side effects of this drug:
- This drug may cause a change in taste and an increase in plaque. It may also stain your teeth, fillings, and mouth.

Special warning:
- Have your teeth cleaned at least every six months.

Pregnancy and nursing mothers:
Category B. See page 9 for a description of categories. Check with your doctor if you are pregnant or planning to get pregnant. It is not known if accidentally swallowed drug is present in mother's milk.

Helpful hints:
- Use twice daily for 30 seconds after you brush your teeth.
- Don't eat or drink for several hours after using this drug.
- Don't swallow the oral rinse.

Cyclosporine

Brand name: *Sandimmune*

What this drug does for you:
This oral solution is used to suppress the immune system and protect against rejection in heart, bone marrow, liver, and kidney transplants. Doctors may prescribe this drug for other illnesses including Crohn's disease, severe psoriasis, aplastic anemia, multiple sclerosis, alopecia areata, pemphigus and pemphigoid, Behcet's disease, myasthenia gravis, and atopic dermatitis.

Possible side effects of this drug:
- Cyclosporine commonly causes kidney damage, high blood pressure, excessive hair growth, tremor, acne, enlarged gums, cramps, diarrhea, nausea, tingling, and convulsions. Two percent or less of the people taking this drug experience headache, allergic reactions, loss of appetite, confusion, conjunctivitis, swelling, fever, brittle fingernails, stomach pain, hearing loss, hiccups, high blood sugar, muscle pain, stomach ulcer, and ringing in the ears.
- Cyclosporine can lower the number of blood cells you have. If you don't have enough white blood cells, your immunity is down, and you can get a fever, sore throat or pneumonia. If you are lacking red blood cells, you

can become anemic, and that makes you tired and weak. Not having enough blood platelets makes you bruise easily and keeps your blood from clotting properly when you're injured. Be on the lookout for any of these symptoms of bone marrow depression.

- Rare side effects include anxiety, chest pain, constipation, depression, hair breaking, blood in the urine, joint pain, tiredness, mouth sores, heart attack, night sweats, inflammation of the pancreas, itching, difficulty swallowing, tingling, bleeding in the stomach, visual disturbances, weakness, and weight loss.

Special warnings:

- You should have your liver and kidney functions checked often while you take this drug.
- Don't take this drug if you are allergic to castor oil.
- This drug may increase your risk of skin cancer and cancer of the lymph system.

Pregnancy and nursing mothers:

Category C. See page 9 for description of categories. Drug is present in mother's milk.

Possible food and drug interactions:

- You should not take cyclosporine with other immunosuppressive drugs.
- Taking any of the following drugs while taking cyclosporine may increase your risk of kidney toxicity: gentamicin, tobramycin, vancomycin, cimetidine, ranitidine, diclofenac, amphotericin B, ketoconazole, melphalan, trimethoprim with sulfamethoxazole, and azapropazone.
- Drugs that decrease liver enzymes may increase levels of cyclosporine, and conversely, drugs that increase liver enzymes may decrease levels of cyclosporine.
- Taking any of the following drugs may increase levels of cyclosporine in your body: diltiazem, nicardipine, verapamil, ketoconazole, fluconazole, itraconazole, danazol, bromocriptine, metoclopramide, erythromycin, and methylprednisolone.
- Taking any of the following may decrease levels of cyclosporine in your body: rifampin, phenobarbital, phenytoin, and carbamazepine.

Helpful hints:

- Stir well and drink all at once. Don't allow it to stand.
- Oral solution may be mixed with orange juice, milk, or chocolate milk to improve the taste.
- Take at room temperature.
- Use a glass container when taking the solution.

Mesalamine

Brand names: *Asacol, Pentasa, Rowasa*

What this drug does for you:

This anti-inflammatory drug is used to treat certain types of ulcerative colitis, proctosigmoiditis, and proctitis. It reduces inflammation in the colon or rectum. Mesalamine is available as tablets, capsules, and rectal suppositories or suspension.

Possible side effects of this drug:

- This drug may cause weakness, stomach pain, headache, burping, nausea, diarrhea, fever, gas, sore throat, stuffy head and nose, muscle pain, dizziness, indigestion, constipation, swelling of the hands or feet, itching, rash, irregular menstrual periods, sweating, conjunctivitis, and cough.
- This drug may worsen colitis in some people. Contact your doctor if you develop rash, fever, stomach pain, cramping, bloody diarrhea, or headache.
- Very rarely, this drug has caused kidney damage.

Special warnings:

- Don't use this drug if you are allergic to aspirin.
- If you are allergic to sulfasalazine, you should use this drug with extreme caution.
- If you have poor liver or kidney functions or a history of kidney disease, you should use this drug with caution.

Pregnancy and nursing mothers:

Category B. See page 9 for description of categories. Drug is present in mother's milk.

Helpful hints:

- Tablets should be swallowed whole. If intact or partially intact tablets repeatedly appear in your stool, tell your doctor.
- You may not see improvement for up to three weeks. Usual treatment is one enema or two suppositories daily for three to six weeks.

Methylprednisolone

Brand name: *Depo-Medrol, Medrol, Solu-Medrol* **(Generic available)**

What this drug does for you:

This corticosteroid drug is used to treat or ease the symptoms of various disorders including the following: arthritis and related rheumatic diseases, endocrine disorders, lupus and other collagen diseases, allergic reactions, respiratory diseases, kidney disorders, skin diseases, blood disorders (various anemias), eye diseases, leukemia, colitis, enteritis, meningitis, and trichinosis. Methylprednisolone is available as tablets, injection, or retention enema.

Possible side effects of this drug:

- Most people will experience very few side effects if they take methyl-prednisolone for 10 days or less. Long-term use can cause many serious side effects including insomnia, inflammation of the pancreas, bloating, ulcers, increased pressure on the brain, headache, convulsions, dizzi-ness, sweating, slow healing of wounds, muscle weakness, fluid reten-tion, weakened bones, congestive heart failure, high blood pressure, worsening of diabetes, menstrual abnormalities, glaucoma, and cataracts.
- Methylprednisolone may cause or aggravate emotional or psychotic problems. Call your doctor if you experience any changes in mood.
- This drug may cause you to lose calcium and potassium and retain salt. You may need to restrict your salt intake and take potassium supple-ments.

Special warnings:

- People with fungal infections should not use this drug.
- Corticosteroid drugs may weaken your immune system and decrease your natural resistance to infections. Call your doctor immediately at the first sign of fever or infection.
- Don't get any vaccinations and take extra care to avoid exposure to peo-ple with chicken pox or measles. If you are exposed, let your doctor know right away.
- If you have high blood pressure, osteoporosis, diabetes, cirrhosis, under-active thyroid, myasthenia gravis (muscle weakness disease), poor kid-ney function, or diverticulitis, you should take this drug with caution.

Pregnancy and nursing mothers:

Not known if it's safe to take this drug while you are pregnant or nursing.

Possible food and drug interaction:

- Methylprednisolone may increase the risk of convulsions if taken with the antibiotic cyclosporin.

Helpful hint:

- Take with food to prevent upset stomach.
- If you've been taking high doses of methylprednisolone or you've been taking it for a long time, don't suddenly quit taking it. Withdrawing rapidly could cause nausea, fever, fainting and even be fatal.

Olsalazine

Brand name: *Dipentum*

What this drug does for you:

This drug is used to reduce the chance that ulcerative colitis will recur in people who cannot take sulfasalazine.

Possible side effects of this drug:

- This drug may cause nausea, diarrhea, stomach pain or cramps, loss of appetite, indigestion, bloating, inflammation of the mouth, itching, rash,

muscle or joint pain, headache, fatigue, depression, insomnia, and dizziness.
- This drug may worsen the symptoms of colitis. Colitis is inflammation of the colon, and symptoms include bloody diarrhea, stomach cramps, and fever.

Special warnings:
- Don't use this drug if you are allergic to salicylates.
- If you have kidney disease, you should use this drug with caution.

Pregnancy and nursing mothers:
Category C. See page 9 for description of categories. Not known if drug is present in mother's milk.

Possible food and drug interaction:
- Olsalazine may increase the effects of the anticoagulant warfarin.

Helpful hint:
- Take this drug with food in evenly divided doses.

Prednisolone Sodium Phosphate

Brand names: *Hydeltrasol, Pediapred*

What this drug does for you:
This drug is a corticosteroid. It is used to treat or ease the symptoms of various disorders including the following: allergic reactions, blood disorders such as anemia, collagen diseases such as lupus, endocrine system disorders, eye allergies and inflammatory conditions, fluid retention in diseases of the kidneys, intestinal diseases such as colitis, leukemia, multiple sclerosis, respiratory diseases such as tuberculosis, rheumatic diseases such as arthritis and bursitis, and skin diseases and eruptions.

Possible side effects of this drug:
- Most people will experience very few side effects if they take prednisolone for 10 days or less. Long-term use can cause many serious side effects including insomnia, fatigue, inflammation of the pancreas, bloating, ulcers, increased pressure on the brain, headache, convulsions, dizziness, sweating, slow healing of wounds, muscle weakness, fluid retention and swelling of the face, weakened bones, congestive heart failure, high blood pressure, worsening of diabetes, menstrual abnormalities, glaucoma, and cataracts.
- Prednisolone may cause or aggravate emotional or psychotic problems. Call your doctor if you experience any changes in mood.
- This drug may cause you to lose calcium and potassium and retain salt. You may need to restrict your salt intake and take potassium supplements.

Special warnings:
- People with fungal infections should not use this drug.
- Corticosteroid drugs may weaken your immune system and decrease your natural resistance to infections. Call your doctor immediately at

the first sign of fever or infection.

- Don't get any vaccinations and take extra care to avoid exposure to people with chicken pox or measles. If you are exposed, let your doctor know right away.
- If you have high blood pressure, osteoporosis, diabetes, cirrhosis, underactive thyroid, herpes simplex of the eye, myasthenia gravis (muscle weakness disease), poor kidney function, colitis, diverticulitis, or ulcer, you should take prednisolone with caution.

Pregnancy and nursing mothers:

Category C. See page 9 for description of categories. Drug is present in mother's milk.

Possible food and drug interaction:

- The effects of this drug may be increased by barbiturates.

Helpful hint:

- Take with food to prevent upset stomach.
- If you've been taking high doses of prednisolone or you've been taking it for a long time, don't suddenly quit taking it. Withdrawing rapidly could cause nausea, fever, fainting, and even be fatal.

Prednisone

Brand names: *Deltasone, Liquid Pred, Prednicen-M, Sterapred, Sterapred DS* (Generic available)

What this drug does for you:

This drug is a corticosteroid. It is used to treat or ease the symptoms of various disorders including the following: allergic reactions, blood disorders such as anemia, collagen diseases such as lupus, endocrine system disorders, eye allergies and inflammatory conditions, fluid retention in diseases of the kidneys, intestinal diseases such as colitis, leukemia, multiple sclerosis, respiratory diseases such as tuberculosis, rheumatic diseases such as arthritis and bursitis, and skin diseases and eruptions.

Possible side effects of this drug:

- Most people will experience very few side effects if they take prednisone for 10 days or less. Long-term use can cause many serious side effects including insomnia, fatigue, inflammation of the pancreas, bloating, ulcers, increased pressure on the brain, headache, convulsions, dizziness, sweating, slow healing of wounds, muscle weakness, fluid retention and swelling of the face, weakened bones, congestive heart failure, high blood pressure, worsening of diabetes, menstrual abnormalities, glaucoma, and cataracts.
- Prednisone may cause or aggravate emotional or psychotic problems. Call your doctor if you experience any changes in mood.
- This drug may cause you to lose calcium and potassium and retain salt. You may need to restrict your salt intake and take potassium supplements.

Special warnings:

- People with fungal infections should not use this drug.
- Corticosteroid drugs may weaken your immune system and decrease your natural resistance to infections. Call your doctor immediately at the first sign of fever or infection.
- Don't get any vaccinations and take extra care to avoid exposure to people with chicken pox or measles. If you are exposed, let your doctor know right away.
- If you have high blood pressure, osteoporosis, diabetes, cirrhosis, underactive thyroid, herpes simplex of the eye, myasthenia gravis (muscle weakness disease), poor kidney function, colitis, diverticulitis, or ulcer, you should take prednisone with caution.

Pregnancy and nursing mothers:

Not known if it's safe to take this drug while you are pregnant or nursing.

Possible food and drug interaction:

- The effects of this drug may be increased by barbiturates.

Helpful hint:

- Take with food to prevent upset stomach.
- If you've been taking high doses of prednisone or you've been taking it for a long time, don't suddenly quit taking it. Withdrawing rapidly could cause nausea, fever, fainting and even be fatal.

Sulfasalazine

Brand name: *Azulfidine* **(Generic available)**

What this drug does for you:

This anti-inflammatory drug is used to treat ulcerative colitis.

Possible side effects of this drug:

- Sulfasalazine may cause nausea, vomiting, headache, loss of appetite, upset stomach, infertility in men, itching, rash, hives, and fever.
- Rare side effects include allergic reactions, difficulty urinating, kidney stones or poor kidney function, mental depression, hallucinations, ringing in the ears, drowsiness, inflammation of the pancreas, hepatitis, and skin discoloration.
- Even though it is very rare, sulfasalazine can lower the number of blood cells you have. If you don't have enough white blood cells, your immunity is down, and you can get a fever, sore throat or pneumonia. If you are lacking red blood cells, you can become anemic, and that makes you tired and weak. Not having enough blood platelets makes you bruise easily and keeps your blood from clotting properly when you're injured. Be on the lookout for any of these symptoms of bone marrow depression.

Special warnings:

- This drug should not be used by people with the metabolic disease porphyria or by people with obstructions of the intestines or urinary tract.
- People with poor liver or kidney functions, asthma, blood diseases, or

G6PD deficiency should use with caution. This drug may cause destruction of red blood cells in people with G6PD deficiency.

- Blood and urine should be tested regularly throughout treatment.

Pregnancy and nursing mothers:
Category B. See page 9 for description of categories. Drug is present in mother's milk.

Possible food and drug interaction:
- Sulfasalazine may decrease levels of folic acid and the heart drug digoxin.

Helpful hints:
- Take this drug with food or milk to avoid upset stomach.
- Don't stop taking this drug because you feel better. Take the full course of treatment.
- Avoid prolonged exposure to the sun and wear a sunscreen and protective clothing.
- Shake oral suspension well before opening.
- Drink extra fluids while you're taking sulfasalazine to help prevent kidney stones.

Yohimbine

Brand names: *Aphrodyne, Erex, Yocon, Yohimex, Yovital* **(Generic available)**

What this drug does for you:
This drug is used to treat certain forms of impotence and male sexual dysfunction. Occasionally doctors prescribe yohimbine to dilate the pupil or to treat low blood pressure and dizziness when you change positions.

Possible side effects of this drug:
- Yohimbine may cause increased blood pressure, nervousness, irritability, excitement, rapid heart rate, headache, dizziness, tremor, increased activity, and flushing.

Special warnings:
- This drug should not be used by people with kidney disease, heart disease, or people with a history of stomach or intestinal ulcers.
- This drug is not recommended for use by women, children, the elderly, or people being treated for psychiatric disorders.

Pregnancy and nursing mothers:
Don't take this drug during pregnancy or while you are nursing.

Possible food and drug interactions:
- Don't take this drug with antidepressants or other mood-altering drugs.

DRUGS FOR PAGET'S DISEASE/BONE LOSS

Calcitonin-Salmon

Brand names: *Calcimar, Miacalcin*

What this drug does for you:
This hormone is used to treat the symptoms of Paget's disease, to decrease bone loss, and to decrease calcium levels in the blood.

Possible side effects of this drug:
- Calcitonin may cause nausea, vomiting, inflammation at the point of injection, flushing, rash, need to urinate at night, itching of earlobes, fever, eye pain, poor appetite, stomach pain, swelling of the feet, and a salty taste in the mouth. The nausea and vomiting tend to go away after you've been taking the drug for a while.

Special warnings:
- Don't use this drug if you are allergic to synthetic calcitonin. A severe shock reaction can result.
- This drug may cause a shortage of calcium in the blood.

Pregnancy and nursing mothers:
Category C. See page 9 for description of categories. Not known if drug is present in mother's milk.

Helpful hint:
- Store this drug in the refrigerator.
- Giving the injection at bedtime may help prevent some of the nausea and flushing.

Etidronate

Brand name: *Didronel*

What this drug does for you:
This hormone is used to treat the symptoms of bone loss in Paget's disease and to aid in proper bone healing after hip replacement surgery.

Possible side effects of this drug:
- Side effects of etidronate may include nausea, diarrhea, bone pain, brittle bones, mouth ulcers, rash, hives, itching, fluid retention, memory loss, confusion, and mental depression.

Special warnings:
- People with kidney disease should take etidronate with caution.
- People being treated for hypercalcemia should have their kidney functions carefully monitored.
- Taking high doses of etidronate or taking it for a long time may increase the risk of fractures. If you experience a fracture, your doctor may stop your drug treatment for a while.

Pregnancy and nursing mothers:
Category C. See page 9 for description of categories. Not known if drug is present in mother's milk.

Possible food and drug interactions:
- Levels of etidronate may be decreased by vitamin and mineral supplements, food (especially milk and other dairy products), and antacids that contain calcium, iron, magnesium, or aluminum.

Helpful hints:
- Take this drug two hours before meals, especially before eating foods high in calcium such as milk or other dairy products.
- Avoid taking vitamin and mineral supplements or antacids high in calcium, iron, magnesium, or aluminum within two hours of taking this drug.

Natural Alternatives

AIDS

◀ Depression
◀ Nausea
◀ Vomiting

◀ Diarrhea
◀ Susceptibility to infection
◀ Weight loss

The nutrition factor in AIDS treatment

As research has shown, there's nothing simple about the cause or progression of AIDS. And unfortunately, there are no simple treatments. However, specialists say the best way to manage symptoms is to take a variety of approaches. That means nutritional support and behavioral therapy along with prescription medication.

When you get HIV, one of the first things to suffer is your ability to digest and absorb food. This, in turn, can lead to weight loss, depression, muscle deterioration, organ damage, and inability to handle medication. Malnutrition and the action of the virus then become intertwined in a vicious cycle.

Fortunately, there are some very helpful things you can do for yourself to maintain good nutrition and fight the disease. Here are some of the recommendations from AIDS-treatment specialists.

Start with the right attitude about food. Emotions often influence your reactions to food, and sticking with a nutritious diet is easier if you can get some enjoyment from eating. Make meals a pleasant social activity. If you have the opportunity, eat with friends or family.

Begin eating with a healthy approach. Depression or substance abuse are often serious roadblocks to good nutrition. If these problems are keeping you from eating right, get professional help.

Plan ahead for convenience. Skipping meals or eating poorly can become problems if you're tired or feeling ill. That's why it's so important to make sure you have easy access to interesting, nutritious foods that require little preparation. Keep a ready supply of frozen or canned foods that can be made into meals.

Cook meals ahead and freeze them. On days when you feel up to shopping and cooking, prepare foods in quantity and freeze them for later use.

Take advantage of restaurant delivery and deli foods. Try your grocer's deli for a variety of already cooked foods. Or, use restaurant delivery services, checking carefully that foods are nutritious and handled safely.

Inquire locally about food services for people with HIV. In some communities, special organizations provide home-delivered meals geared to meet the needs of people with AIDS.

Get the most out of your meals. When you don't feel like eating much, you've got to make every bite count. And that means selecting meals that are balanced and nutrient-rich. Keep your diet low in fat. Filling up on high-fat foods may keep on the pounds, but you may be missing out on nutrients you need.

Carefully select foods and supplements for vitamin and mineral content. Vitamin and mineral depletion can be a serious problem for many people with AIDS. And research has found that even in the early stages of HIV, the Recommended Dietary Allowances (RDAs) may be insufficient. People often need additional zinc, vitamins B6 and B12, and antioxidant nutrients, including vitamins E and C. So choose your foods for their vitamin content and take supplements according to your doctor's instructions. But be careful. Unmonitored megadosing with vitamins and minerals (more than 10 times the RDA) can cause toxic reactions, interfere with drug actions, and increase the likelihood of infection.

Try liquid nutritional supplements if eating balanced meals is difficult. Groceries and drug stores today offer a variety of nutrition supplements that can be easily swallowed and are high-calorie and nutrient-dense.

Make your meals appealing. When you lose your sense of taste, food becomes boring. That's when it helps to try out new spices, textures, and flavors that could stimulate your taste buds.
   ◁ Marinate foods in onion- or garlic-based dressings. Onions and garlic in marinades will add flavor without adding overwhelming odor.
   ◁ Try new foods that are sour, spicy, or sweet tasting. If your customary foods are no longer interesting, experiment with different regional or ethnic flavorings.

Make food safety a priority. With your immune system under assault, the last thing you need is a case of food poisoning or a toxic chemical reaction. Make sure you or anyone handling your food strictly follows food safety recommendations such as these:
   ◁ Wash all fruits and vegetables. Preservative and insecticide reactions can be especially hard on your body .
   ◁ Cook all meats and fish thoroughly. Never eat raw seafood or raw eggs.
   ◁ Store and cook foods at recommended temperatures. Do not leave foods

that need refrigeration at room temperature, even to thaw.

Fight nausea with small meals. During periods of nausea, try eating small meals every few hours. When you're better, eat as much as you can. Stay away from cooking odors or strong-smelling foods. Try dry, saltier products in the morning. And replace fatty or very sweet foods with clear beverages or soups.

When mouth sores are a problem, avoid acidic, spicy or crunchy foods. Oranges, grapefruits, salty or spicy foods, and rough-textured products will aggravate mouth sores. Soak crisp or dry foods in liquid and always keep food temperatures mild.

For swallowing difficulties, replace kernel-type foods with smooth-texture products. Forget the nuts, rice, and popcorn. Smooth-texture foods like mashed fruits or vegetables work best.

Increase fluids, avoid fiber, and replace lost nutrients during bouts of diarrhea. Water, plus liquids with high nutrient value, such as broth and fruit juices, helps offset dehydration and nutrient loss. To keep from worsening the problem, avoid high-fiber fruits and grains, caffeine, lactose in dairy products, sweets, and fatty foods.

The role that nutrition plays in combating AIDS is just beginning to be understood. Some researchers even suggest that nutrition management could be an important factor in slowing the progress of AIDS. With the help of your doctor or an approved AIDS nutrition specialist, you can develop a diet plan to meet your needs and help you stay as healthy as possible.

Sources —
AIDS Alert (5,11:209)
AIDS Weekly (April 11, 1994)
American Journal of Psychiatry (150,11:1679)
FDA Consumer (29,3:16)
Journal of the American Dietetic Association (91,4:476 and 94,9:1018)

GINGIVITIS

◀ Bad breath　　　　　　　　◀ Bleeding gums
◀ Swollen gums　　　　　　　◀ Tender gums

Holding on to healthy teeth

Years ago, a severe case of gingivitis would have doomed you to a toothless smile for the rest of your life. From red gums to tooth loss, it was an accepted fate. Fortunately, times and dental practices have changed. Now that grim prognosis is about as realistic as the tooth fairy.

Today, your dentist has a choice of effective new drugs and surgical procedures that can slow or even reverse your gum disease. In addition, there's a lot you can do to fight the problem at home. Here are some easy, inexpensive do-it-yourself treatments recommended by dental experts.

Strengthen your teeth and gums with a proper diet. Healthy teeth and gums depend on good nutrition. Since vitamin deficiencies often contribute to gum problems, make sure you're getting a balanced, nutritionally sound diet. If that's difficult, consider vitamin supplements. Also, avoid problem foods. Sugary snacks and drinks increase the sticky residue on teeth and gums, promoting gum-decaying bacteria growth.

Don't smoke. Smoking has been shown to increase your risk for gum disease, possibly as much as five times the rate for nonsmokers.

Follow an oral hygiene program that controls plaque. Plaque is your real enemy in the battle against gingivitis. Whenever you eat or drink, a bacteria-laden residue called "plaque" develops in your mouth, clinging to all surfaces. Unless that film is removed, the bacteria will attack your teeth and gums, causing decay and inflammation. Professional dental checkups and cleanings are essential in plaque control. But your first line of defense must be a good, at-home dental routine designed to stop plaque before it leads to gum disease.

Plaque-fighting techniques

Do you brush after meals, floss daily and use mouthwash? If you're already doing these things but still have gingivitis, you may have to make some changes in your approach. Scientific studies show that how you brush and which products you use make a big difference in fighting plaque.

Start with the right toothbrush, and use it the right way. Correctly removing particles from between teeth and gums is your first step. Brush with a gentle circular motion along gum lines, holding the toothbrush at a 45-degree angle. And avoid gum damage by using a soft toothbrush.

Remove plaque from between teeth with floss. Floss daily. Gently guide the waxed or unwaxed floss between your teeth with index fingers or thumbs, using a sawing motion at the gum line and curving around each tooth to cover the side surfaces.

Finally, rinse with an approved anti-plaque mouthwash. With new developments in the field of plaque-reducing mouthrinses, you now have a greater choice of products recommended by the American Dental Association.

From the first-generation list of mouthrinses, Listerine and its generics have proven to be effective with a 25-percent reduction in plaque. After brushing, wash your mouth for 30 seconds, then refrain from eating or drinking for 30 minutes.

By using these easy-to-follow, convenient tips in conjunction with your dentist's prescribed treatment, you can hold on to your beautiful smile for years.

Sources —

Diabetes in the News (13,2:26)

Complete Guide to Symptoms, Illness and Surgery, The Putnam Berkeley Group, New York, 1995

Medical Update (17,7:3)

USA Today (122,2579:3)

U.S. Pharmacist (20,5:30)

What you need to Know About Periodontal Diseases, National Institute of Dental Research, P.O. Box 54793, Washington, D.C. 20032

IMPOTENCE

◄ Inability to achieve an erection of the penis
◄ Inability to maintain an erection

Put impotence to bed

Most men at one time or another are unable to raise or maintain an erection. Usually, the problem is just temporary. Impotence can be caused by illness, injury, stress, fatigue, emotional upset, or too much alcohol. Look below for three contributing factors you might not have thought of, and for some helpful exercises to overcome long-term impotence.

Smoking isn't sexy. Despite what television shows and slick magazine ads might make you believe, smoking isn't sexy. In fact, it's not only a nasty habit, it can make your sex life stink.

A recent study of 4,462 male Vietnam veterans showed that smokers have a 50-percent higher risk of impotence than nonsmokers and past smokers. Around 2 percent of nonsmokers and past smokers were impotent, and almost 4 percent of current smokers were impotent.

Smoking contributes to blockages in the arteries that lead to the penis. Without adequate blood flow, your penis can't maintain an erection. The solution to this problem is simple: Don't smoke.

High-fat food can foul up sex. A new study has found that men with high cholesterol are twice as likely to be impotent as men whose cholesterol levels are normal or low.

Researchers recorded cholesterol levels of 3,250 healthy men between the ages of 25 and 83. Men with total cholesterol higher than 240 mg/dl were twice as likely to have trouble achieving or maintaining an erection than men whose cholesterol levels were below 180 mg/dl. Men who had low levels of HDL (good cholesterol) were also twice as likely to suffer from impotence.

The same high-fat diet that narrows arteries and blocks blood flow to your heart also narrows the arteries that carry blood to your penis. Blood has to be able to get to your penis in order for you to achieve and maintain an erection.

Avoid romance-robbing drugs. Certain over-the-counter and prescription drugs can significantly decrease your interest in sex, causing impotence. Side effects can appear after only a few weeks or develop after you've been taking a drug for years.

Drugs that often inhibit sexual desire include antihistamines, antidepressants, antipsychotics, beta blockers, decongestants, and tranquilizers. Even if you suspect a drug is interfering with your love life, don't stop taking it until you talk with your doctor. Abruptly discontinuing certain medicines can be a deadly decision.

Your doctor can help you find a safe alternative. And the next time you get a new prescription, ask about the effects it could have on your sex life.

Try pelvic exercises. You may be able to exercise your way back to full sexual capacity. Recently, a team of Belgian urologists treated 150 men who suffered from impotence. Some men had operations and others did special pelvic muscle exercises, called Kegels. The exercises are contractions of the pelvic floor muscles — something pregnant women have been doing for years to help with childbirth.

One year after treatment, 58 percent of the men who performed the Kegel exercises were completely cured or were so satisfied with their improvement that they did not opt for surgery.

Some skeptical doctors say that the pelvic muscles don't have any influence on the blood flow to the penis. They say the men in the study improved because of the beneficial psychological effects of the therapy. At any rate, if you are suffering from a mild case of impotence, Kegels just might do the trick.

Kegel exercises

1) Identify the pelvic muscles that need exercising. You can do this by stopping and starting the flow of urine several times when using the bathroom.
2) Tighten the muscles a little at the time. Contract muscles slowly, hold for a count of 10, and relax the muscles slowly.
3) Repeat these exercises for the anal pelvic muscles. To find these muscles, imagine you're trying to hold back a bowel movement, without tensing your leg, stomach or buttock muscles.
4) Then practice tightening all pelvic muscles together, moving from back to front.
5) Start with five repetitions of each exercise three to five times a day. Gradually work up to 20 or 30 repetitions at once.

You will find that you can perform your Kegels just about anywhere and anytime. Chances are good that "pumping it up" with these pelvic exercises will have you back in top shape in no time.

Sources —

Before You Call the Doctor, Random-Ballantine, New York, 1992
British Journal of Urology (71,1:52)
Complete Guide to Symptoms, Illness & Surgery, The Putnam Berkeley Group, New York, 1995
Medical Tribune (34,5:19;36,1:17; and 36,2:5)
National Opinion Research Center (NORC), *General Society Survey*, 1993
Obstetrics and Gynecology (81,2:283)

PAIN AND ARTHRITIS

Prescription Drugs

Natural Alternatives

Prescription Drugs ℞

GOUT DRUGS

Allopurinol

Brand name: *Zyloprim* **(Generic available)**

What this drug does for you:

Allopurinol treats gout, an arthritis condition caused by too much uric acid in the blood, by reducing the amount of uric acid your body produces.

Possible side effects of this drug:

- The most common reaction to allopurinol is a severe gout attack after you begin taking the drug. Also common is a skin rash. Let your doctor know immediately if you have a skin rash, because you may have a dangerous

allergy to the drug. The rash may be accompanied by fever, chills, and joint and muscle pain.
- Other side effects include nausea, diarrhea, headache, and jaundice.
- Some rare possible side effects are boils, heart problems, asthma, infertility in men, intestinal bleeding, dizziness, asthma, and cataracts.
- Let your doctor know if you experience painful urination, blood in the urine, eye irritation, or swelling of the lips and mouth.
- Even though it is very rare, allopurinol can lower the number of blood cells you have. If you don't have enough white blood cells, your immunity is down, and you can get a fever, sore throat, or pneumonia. If you are lacking red blood cells, you can become anemic, and that makes you tired and weak. Not having enough blood platelets makes you bruise easily and keeps your blood from clotting properly when you're injured. Be on the lookout for any of these symptoms of bone marrow depression.

Special warning:
- People with preexisting kidney disease, liver disease, or high blood pressure should be carefully monitored.

Pregnancy and nursing mothers:
Category C. See page 9 for description of categories. Drug is present in mother's milk.

Possible food and drug interactions:
- Allopurinol may increase the effects of the anticoagulant dicumarol and the immunosuppressant azathioprine.
- Allopurinol may cause skin rash when taken at the same time as the antibiotics amoxicillin and ampicillin.
- Don't take allopurinol with high doses of vitamin C as it may cause kidney stones.

Helpful hints:
- This drug may upset your stomach less if you take it with food.
- While you're taking this drug, drink 10 to 12 glasses of fluid per day to help prevent kidney stones.
- If you forget to take a dose of your medicine, you don't need to double your dose at the next scheduled time.
- You may not notice any improvement in your gout for two to six weeks. Don't get discouraged and quit taking your medicine.
- You shouldn't drive a car or operate heavy machinery until you are sure the medicine isn't making you drowsy or less than alert.

Probenecid

Brand name: *Benemid* **(Generic available)**

What this drug does for you:
Probenecid treats gout, an arthritis condition caused by too much uric acid in the blood, by reducing the amount of uric acid your body produces.

Probenecid is also used along with some antibiotics to make them more effective. It helps keep the blood levels of the antibiotics high.

Possible side effects of this drug:

- If you have an allergic reaction to this drug, you need to contact your doctor immediately. Some signs of an allergic reaction are swelling, rash, hives, and fever. Also call your doctor if you have blood in your urine, pain in your ribs or back, or yellow eyes and skin (jaundice).
- Other possible side effects are nausea, loss of appetite, headache, dizziness, flushing, sore gums, and frequent urination.
- You may experience a gout attack after you begin taking probenecid. This drug may also cause kidney stones.
- Even though it is very rare, probenecid can lower the number of blood cells you have. If you don't have enough white blood cells, your immunity is down, and you can get a fever, sore throat, or pneumonia. If you are lacking red blood cells, you can become anemic, and that makes you tired and weak. Not having enough blood platelets makes you bruise easily and keeps your blood from clotting properly when you're injured. Be on the lookout for any of these symptoms of bone marrow depression.

Special warnings:

- You shouldn't start taking probenecid during a gout attack.
- People with blood diseases or kidney stones should not take probenecid.
- Don't use probenecid with penicillin if you have poor kidney function.
- Take probenecid with caution if you have a history of ulcers or poor kidney function.

Pregnancy and nursing mothers:

This drug may not be safe to use while you are pregnant. Not known if safe to use while nursing.

Possible food and drug interactions:

- Probenecid may increase the effects of anesthetics.
- Probenecid may cause low blood sugar if used with anti-diabetic drugs.
- Probenecid may increase the risk of toxicity of nonsteroidal anti-inflammatory drugs (NSAIDs), acetaminophen, the anti-anxiety drug lorazepam, the cancer drug methotrexate and the tuberculosis drug rifampin.
- Effects of probenecid may be decreased by aspirin and the tuberculosis drug pyrazinamide.

Helpful hints:

- While you're taking this drug, drink 10 to 12 glasses of fluid per day to help prevent kidney stones.
- If the medicine upsets your stomach, you should let your doctor know. You may need a lower dose.

HEADACHE RELIEVERS

Butalbital with Acetaminophen and Caffeine

Brand name: *Fioricet*

What this drug does for you:

This combination drug is used to relieve mild to moderate pain, especially in tension (muscle contraction) headaches.

Possible side effects of this drug:

- This drug may cause dizziness, drowsiness, nausea, vomiting, stomach pain, and shortness of breath.
- Some less common side effects are shaky feeling, tingling, high energy, dry mouth, sweating, heartburn, rapid heartbeat, leg pain, ringing ears, confusion, and rash.
- Even though it is very rare, drugs containing acetaminophen can lower the number of blood cells you have. If you don't have enough white blood cells, your immunity is down, and you can get a fever, sore throat, or pneumonia. If you are lacking red blood cells, you can become anemic, and that makes you tired and weak. Not having enough blood platelets makes you bruise easily and keeps your blood from clotting properly when you're injured. Be on the lookout for any of these symptoms of bone marrow depression.
- Serious skin reactions are another rare side effect of this drug.

Special warnings:

- Don't take this drug if you are allergic to any of the ingredients or if you have the inherited metabolic disorder called porphyria.
- People with suicidal tendencies or depression should use this drug with caution.
- People with liver or kidney disease should have regular liver and kidney tests while taking this drug.

Pregnancy and nursing mothers:

Category C. See page 9 for a description of categories. Drug is present in mother's milk.

Possible food and drug interactions:

- If you take this drug along with alcohol or a drug that depresses your nervous system, such as tranquilizers, sedative-hypnotics, antihistamines, or muscle relaxants, the combination may dangerously depress your nervous system.
- Monoamine oxidase (MAO) inhibitors may cause this drug to further depress your nervous system.

Helpful hints:

- If you take this drug for a long time, you can become dependent on it, mentally and physically. It may take larger amounts to produce the same effects. When you stop taking the medicine, you may have withdrawal symptoms, such as rebound headaches.

- You shouldn't drive a car or operate heavy machinery until you are sure the medicine isn't making you drowsy or less than alert.

Butalbital with Acetaminophen, Caffeine, and Codeine

Brand name: *Fioricet with Codeine*

What this drug does for you:
This barbiturate and analgesic combination is used to relieve mild to moderate pain, especially in tension (muscle contraction) headaches.

Possible side effects of this drug:
- This drug may cause dizziness, drowsiness, nausea, vomiting, shortness of breath, and mental confusion.
- Some less common side effects are shaky feeling, tingling, high energy, dry mouth, sweating, heartburn, rapid heartbeat, leg pain, ringing ears, and rash.
- Even though it is very rare, drugs containing acetaminophen can lower the number of blood cells you have. If you don't have enough white blood cells, your immunity is down, and you can get a fever, sore throat, or pneumonia. If you are lacking red blood cells, you can become anemic, and that makes you tired and weak. Not having enough blood platelets makes you bruise easily and keeps your blood from clotting properly when you're injured. Be on the lookout for any of these symptoms of bone marrow depression.
- Serious skin reactions are another rare side effect of this drug.

Special warnings:
- Don't take this drug if you are allergic to any of the ingredients or if you have the inherited metabolic disorder called porphyria.
- People with suicidal tendencies or depression should use this drug with caution.

Pregnancy and nursing mothers:
Category C. See page 9 for a description of categories. Drug is present in mother's milk.

Possible food and drug interactions:
- If you take this drug along with a drug that depresses your nervous system, such as tranquilizers, alcohol, antihistamines, or muscle relaxants, the combination may dangerously depress your nervous system.
- This drug may decrease the effects of anticoagulants.

Helpful hints:
- If you take this drug for a long time, you can become dependent on it, mentally and physically. It may take larger amounts to produce the same effects. When you stop taking the medicine, you may have withdrawal symptoms, such as rebound headaches.
- You shouldn't drive a car or operate heavy machinery until you are sure the medicine isn't making you drowsy or less than alert.

Butalbital with Aspirin

Brand name: *Axotal*

What this drug does for you:
This barbiturate and analgesic combination relieves mild to moderate pain, especially in tension (muscle contraction) headaches.

Possible side effects of this drug:
- The most frequent reactions are drowsiness and dizziness. Less frequent reactions are lightheadedness, nausea, vomiting, and gas.
- Serious skin reactions are another rare side effect of this drug.

Special warnings:
- Don't use this drug if you are allergic to any of the ingredients (especially aspirin) or if you have the inherited metabolic disorder called porphyria.
- Take this drug with caution if you have peptic ulcer, blood clotting problems, suicidal tendencies, or depression.
- You may become physically and psychologically dependent on this drug if you take high doses for long periods of time.

Pregnancy and nursing mothers:
Not known if safe to use while you are pregnant. Drug is present in mother's milk.

Possible food and drug interactions:
- If you take this drug along with a drug that depresses your nervous system, such as tranquilizers, alcohol, antihistamines, or muscle relaxants, the combination may dangerously depress your nervous system.
- Butalbital may decrease blood levels of tricyclic antidepressants.

Helpful hints:
- You shouldn't drive a car or operate heavy machinery until you are sure the medicine isn't making you drowsy or less than alert.

Butalbital with Aspirin and Caffeine

Brand name: *Fiorinal*

What this drug does for you:
This barbiturate and analgesic combination relieves mild to moderate pain, especially in tension (muscle contraction) headaches.

Possible side effects of this drug:
- The most frequent reactions are drowsiness and dizziness. Less frequent reactions are lightheadedness, nausea, vomiting, and gas.
- Even though it is very rare, this drug may lower the number of blood cells you have. If you don't have enough white blood cells, your immunity is down, and you can get a fever, sore throat, or pneumonia. If you are lacking red blood cells, you can become anemic, and that makes you tired and weak. Not having enough blood platelets makes you bruise easily and

keeps your blood from clotting properly when you're injured. Be on the lookout for any of these symptoms of bone marrow depression.
- Serious skin reactions are another rare side effect of this drug.

Special warnings:
- Don't use this drug if you are allergic to any of the ingredients (especially aspirin) or if you have the inherited metabolic disorder called porphyria.
- Take this drug with caution if you have peptic ulcer, blood clotting problems, suicidal tendencies, or depression.
- You may become physically and psychologically dependent on this drug if you take high doses for long periods of time.

Pregnancy and nursing mothers:
Not known if safe to use while you are pregnant. Drug is present in mother's milk.

Possible food and drug interactions:
- If you take this drug along with a drug that depresses your nervous system, such as tranquilizers, alcohol, antihistamines, or muscle relaxants, the combination may dangerously depress your nervous system.

Helpful hint:
- You shouldn't drive a car or operate heavy machinery until you are sure the medicine isn't making you drowsy or less than alert.

Butalbital with Aspirin, Caffeine, and Codeine Phosphate

Brand name: *Fiorinal with Codeine*

What this drug does for you:
This barbiturate and analgesic combination relieves mild to moderate pain, especially in tension (muscle contraction) headaches.

Possible side effects of this drug:
- The most frequent reactions are drowsiness and dizziness. Less frequent reactions are lightheadedness, nausea, vomiting, and gas.
- Even though it is very rare, this drug may lower the number of blood cells you have. If you don't have enough white blood cells, your immunity is down, and you can get a fever, sore throat, or pneumonia. If you are lacking red blood cells, you can become anemic, and that makes you tired and weak. Not having enough blood platelets makes you bruise easily and keeps your blood from clotting properly when you're injured. Be on the lookout for any of these symptoms of bone marrow depression.
- Serious skin reactions are another rare side effect of this drug.

Special warnings:
- Don't use this drug if you are allergic to any of the ingredients (especially aspirin) or if you have the inherited metabolic disorder called porphyria.
- Don't use this drug if you have a stomach ulcer or blood clotting problems.

- If you have kidney or liver disease, your doctor should monitor you carefully while you take this drug.

Pregnancy and nursing mothers:
Not known if safe to use while you are pregnant. Drug is present in mother's milk.

Possible food and drug interactions:
- If you take this drug along with a drug that depresses your nervous system, such as tranquilizers, alcohol, antihistamines, or muscle relaxants, the combination may dangerously depress your nervous system.
- Monoamine oxidase (MAO) inhibitors may increase the side effects of this drug.
- This drug may increase the effects of anticoagulants, increasing your risk of bleeding.
- This drug may increase the toxic effects of methotrexate and 6-mercaptopurine.
- This drug may decrease the effects of probenecid and sulfinpyrazone, reducing their effectiveness in the treatment of gout.

Helpful hints:
- You shouldn't drive a car or operate heavy machinery until you are sure the medicine isn't making you drowsy or less than alert.
- You may become physically and psychologically dependent on this drug if you take high doses for long periods of time. Never take more medicine than you are prescribed.

Ergotamine Tartrate

Brand names: *Cafergot (contains caffeine), Ergomar, Ergostat, Wigraine (contains caffeine)*

What this drug does for you:
This drug is used to prevent or relieve throbbing migraine and cluster headaches. It seems to work by shrinking blood vessels in the head.

Possible side effects of this drug:
- Side effects may include nausea, vomiting, weakness in the legs, numbness and tingling in fingers and toes, muscle pain in extremities, slow or fast heartbeat, itching, and swelling.
- You can become dependent upon ergotamine if you take it for a long time. You may need increasingly larger amounts to relieve your headache. And, once you stop taking it, you may have "rebound headache" that is even more severe than your original headache.

Special warning:
- This drug should not be used by people with coronary artery disease, high blood pressure, poor liver or kidney function, severe itching, peripheral vascular disease (such as arteriosclerosis or Raynaud's disease), blood poisoning, or hypersensitivity to ergot alkaloids.

Pregnancy and nursing mothers:

Category X. See page 9 for description of categories. Drug is present in mother's milk.

Possible food and drug interaction:

- Taking ergotamine with other drugs that constrict blood vessels may result in dangerously high blood pressure.

Helpful hints:

- Take medicine at the first sign of headache. Place one 2-mg tablet under your tongue. If necessary, take another tablet in a half-hour, but don't take more than three tablets in 24 hours. You shouldn't take more than five tablets in one week.
- Don't take more than the recommended dose. Prolonged or excessive use can lead to ergotism (ergot poisoning).

Methysergide

Brand name: *Sansert*

What this drug does for you:

This drug is used to prevent migraine headaches, or, at least, reduce their frequency and intensity.

Possible side effects of this drug:

- Some common side effects are diarrhea, constipation, heartburn, dizziness (especially when you get up from a lying or seated position), drowsiness, nausea, vomiting, and insomnia.
- Call your doctor immediately if you have any of the following symptoms: leg cramps or swelling, chest pain, back pain, cold or numbness in hands or feet, or a change in the normal amount of urine.
- Other possible side effects are weight loss or gain, rapid heartbeat, joint or muscle pain, blood disorders, facial flushing, stomach pain, hair loss, rashes, lack of coordination, and weakness.
- A serious risk of using methysergide for long periods of time is scarring inside your chest, stomach, heart valves, lungs, kidneys, and major blood vessels.

Special warnings:

- Methysergide should only be used to treat frequent, severe migraines that don't respond to other treatments.
- Methysergide should not be used at the beginning of an attack.
- Methysergide should not be used by people with severe high blood pressure, coronary artery disease, severe arteriosclerosis, lung disease, poor liver or kidney function, peripheral vascular disease, disease of the heart valves, inflammation of the veins or connective tissues in the legs, collagen disease or fibrosis, or serious infections. Long-term treatment may cause fibrosis, which may affect the heart or lungs
- Use caution while driving.

Pregnancy and nursing mothers:

Category X. See page 9 for description of categories.

Possible food and drug interactions:

- If you take methysergide along with alcohol or a drug that depresses your nervous system, such as tranquilizers, antihistamines, or muscle relaxants, the combination may dangerously depress your nervous system.

Helpful hint:

- You shouldn't drive a car or operate heavy machinery until you are sure the medicine isn't making you drowsy or less than alert.

Sumatriptan Succinate

Brand name: *Imitrex*

What this drug does for you:

This drug is used to relieve a migraine attack. It constricts the blood vessels and relieves the swelling that is thought to cause migraines. Sumatriptan is not meant to prevent or reduce the number of attacks you experience.

Possible side effects of this drug:

- Common side effects are tingling, warm or hot sensation, flushing (redness of face lasting a short time), and heaviness.
- Another common side effect is chest, jaw, and neck tightness. If you have severe chest pain or it does not go away, call your doctor immediately. Although it is very rare, sumatriptan may cause heart problems, such as angina or transient ischemia (temporary deficiency of blood supply to a body part).
- Less common side effects are feeling drowsy, dizzy, tired, or sick. Tell your doctor about these side effects at your next visit. For the injection form, you may have pain or redness at the injection site.
- Tell your doctor immediately if you have any of these rare reactions: shortness of breath, wheezing, skin rash or lumps, heart throbbing, hives, or swelling of the eyelids, face, or lips.

Special warnings:

- People with angina, ischemia, or past heart attacks should not take sumatriptan.
- Sumatriptan can cause your blood pressure to go up, so people with uncontrolled high blood pressure shouldn't take it.
- You should not take sumatriptan within two weeks of taking the antidepressants called monoamine oxidase (MAO) inhibitors.
- Find out what kind of migraine you have before you take sumatriptan. It is not meant for people with basilar or hemiplegic migraines.
- People with poor liver or kidney function should take sumatriptan with caution.
- Sumatriptan may increase the risk of seizure for people with epilepsy.
- If you have had an allergic reaction to drugs before, you are more likely to be allergic to sumatriptan.

Pregnancy and nursing mothers:

Category C. See page 9 for a description of the categories. This drug is present in mother's milk.

Possible food and drug interactions:

- Don't use sumatriptan and any headache drugs containing ergotamine within 24 hours of each other.
- Store your medicine away from heat and light.

Helpful hint:

- You should take the medicine as soon as your migraine symptoms appear, but you can take it at any time during an attack. For the injection form, you can give yourself a second injection if you still have pain, but wait an hour after the first injection and talk to your doctor first.

MUSCLE RELAXANTS/STIMULANTS

Carisoprodol and Aspirin

Brand name: *Soma*

What this drug does for you:

This muscle relaxant is used to relax certain muscles in your body and relieve the pain caused by strains, sprains, or other muscle injuries.

Possible side effects of this drug:

- Drowsiness is the most common side effect. Less frequent reactions are dizziness and weakness.
- Rare reactions are shakiness, agitation, irritability, headache, fainting, and insomnia.
- Some people have an allergic reaction which includes extreme weakness, skin rash or lumps, itching, and confusion.
- Other possible side effects are rapid heartbeat, low blood pressure when you stand or sit up, facial flushing, nausea, hiccups, and stomach pain. Aspirin may cause nausea, constipation, diarrhea, stomach pain, swelling, asthma, rash, and hives.

Special warnings:

- People with kidney or liver problems should use this drug with caution.
- Use this drug with caution if you are prone to addiction.

Pregnancy and nursing mothers:

Category C. See page 9 for description of categories. Drug is present in mother's milk.

Possible food and drug interactions:

- If you take this drug along with alcohol or a drug that depresses your nervous system, such as tranquilizers, antihistamines, or muscle relaxants, the combination may dangerously depress your nervous system.
- Your doctor may need to adjust your dosage of gout, arthritis, or diabetes medicines.

- This drug may increase your risk of bleeding if you are taking anticoagulants.
- This drug may increase the toxic effects of methotrexate.
- This drug may reduce the effects of probenecid and sulfinpyrazone.
- If you take anti-diabetic drugs, your risk of hypoglycemia (low blood sugar) may be increased.
- Antacids may decrease the effectiveness of this drug.
- Corticosteroids may decrease the levels of this drug.

Helpful hints:
- You shouldn't drive a car or operate heavy machinery until you are sure the medicine isn't making you drowsy or less than alert.
- This drug can cause mild withdrawal symptoms if you stop taking it suddenly.

Chlorzoxazone

Brand names: *Paraflex, Parafon Forte DSC, Remular-S*

What this drug does for you:
Chlorzoxazone is a muscle relaxant used to treat severe muscular pain associated with spasms, strains, sprains, and bruises.

Possible side effects of this drug:
- Common side effects are upset stomach, drowsiness, dizziness, and lightheadedness.

Special warning:
- Call your doctor if you experience a rash or itching.

Pregnancy and nursing mothers:
Category C. See page 9 for description of categories. Not known if safe to use in pregnancy or while breast-feeding.

Possible food and drug interaction:
- If you take chlorzoxazone along with alcohol or a drug that depresses your nervous system, such as tranquilizers, antihistamines, or muscle relaxants, the combination may dangerously depress your nervous system.

Helpful hint:
- You shouldn't drive a car or operate heavy machinery until you are sure the medicine isn't making you drowsy or less than alert.

Cyclobenzaprine

Brand name: *Flexeril* **(Generic available)**

What this drug does for you:
Cyclobenzaprine relieves muscle spasms and the associated pain, tenderness, and tightness.

Possible side effects of this drug:
- The most common side effects are drowsiness, dry mouth, and dizziness.

Other possible side effects are tiredness, muscular weakness, nausea, constipation, indigestion, bad taste in mouth, blurred vision, headache, nervousness, and confusion.

- Rare side effects are fainting, rapid or irregular heartbeat, low blood pressure, loss of appetite, diarrhea, stomach pain, thirst, gas, swelling of the tongue, itching, rash, lack of coordination, tremors, difficulty talking, muscle twitching, insomnia, mental depression, hallucinations, excitement, tingling, double vision, sweating, ringing in the ears, and frequent urination or difficulty urinating. In rare instances, this drug may damage your liver and cause jaundice (yellow eyes and skin).

Special warnings:

- This drug should not be used by people with overactive thyroid, heart arrhythmias, congestive heart failure, heart block, or by people recovering from a heart attack.
- This drug should be used with caution by people with a history of urinary retention or certain kinds of glaucoma.

Pregnancy and nursing mothers:

Category B. See page 9 for description of categories. Not known if drug is present in mother's milk.

Possible food and drug interactions:

- Don't take cyclobenzaprine and the antidepressant drugs called monoamine oxidase (MAO) inhibitors at the same time. You should quit taking MAO inhibitors for at least two weeks before you begin taking cyclobenzaprine.
- Cyclobenzaprine may decrease the effectiveness of some high blood pressure drugs such as guanethidine.
- If you take cyclobenzaprine along with alcohol or a drug that depresses your nervous system, such as tranquilizers, antihistamines, or muscle relaxants, the combination may dangerously depress your nervous system.

Helpful hints:

- You shouldn't drive a car or operate heavy machinery until you are sure the medicine isn't making you drowsy or less than alert.
- If you suddenly stop taking this drug, you may have nausea, headache, and a tired, weak feeling.

Methocarbamol

Brand name: *Robaxin* **(Generic available)**

What this drug does for you:

This muscle relaxant is used to relieve painful muscles. It may also help control neuromuscular symptoms of tetanus.

Possible side effects of this drug:

- Side effects may include itching, rash, hives, blurred vision, stuffy nose, fever, headache, nausea, dizziness, drowsiness, and conjunctivitis (inflammation of the mucous membrane that lines the eyes).

Special warning:

- The injectable form should not be used by people with kidney problems.

Pregnancy and nursing mothers:

Not known if drug is safe to use while you are pregnant. Not known if drug is present in mother's milk.

Possible food and drug interactions:

- If you take methocarbamol along with alcohol or a drug that depresses your nervous system, such as tranquilizers, antihistamines, or muscle relaxants, the combination may dangerously depress your nervous system.

Helpful hint:

- You shouldn't drive a car or operate heavy machinery until you are sure the medicine isn't making you drowsy or less than alert.

Methocarbamol with Aspirin

Brand name: *Robaxisal* (Generic available)

What this drug does for you:

This muscle relaxant is combined with aspirin to relieve painful muscles.

Possible side effects of this drug:

- Common reactions to methocarbamol are dizziness and nausea. Less common side effects may include drowsiness, blurred vision, headache, fever, and allergic reactions such as hives and rash.
- Large doses of aspirin can cause nausea, ringing in the ears, vision and hearing problems, headache, dizziness, mental confusion, rapid heartbeat, sweating, and thirst. You can have an allergic reaction to aspirin that includes nausea, skin rashes or hives, asthma, swelling, and stomach pain. Some people have heartburn when they take aspirin.
- Even though it is very rare, large doses of aspirin may lower the number of blood cells you have. If you don't have enough white blood cells, your immunity is down, and you can get a fever, sore throat, or pneumonia. If you are lacking red blood cells, you can become anemic, and that makes you tired and weak. Not having enough blood platelets makes you bruise easily and keeps your blood from clotting properly when you're injured. Be on the lookout for any of these symptoms of bone marrow depression.

Special warning:

- Don't take this drug if you are allergic to aspirin or methocarbamol. You could have a severe allergic reaction.
- If you have any bleeding disorder, a vitamin K deficiency, a stomach ulcer, or severe liver damage, you should not take this drug.
- Don't use this drug to treat chickenpox or flu, as it could cause Reye's syndrome.
- People with the following conditions should use this drug with caution: liver or kidney damage, gallbladder disease or gallstones, breathing dif-

ficulties, irregular heartbeat, hypothyroidism, enlarged prostate, head injuries, or severe stomach problems. If you have liver or kidney damage, you should have regular liver and kidney tests while you take this drug.

Pregnancy and nursing mothers:

Not known if drug is safe to use while you are pregnant. Not known if methocarbamol is present in mother's milk. Aspirin is present in mother's milk.

Possible food and drug interactions:

- If you take methocarbamol along with alcohol or a drug that depresses your nervous system, such as tranquilizers, antihistamines, or muscle relaxants, the combination may dangerously depress your nervous system.
- You shouldn't take this drug if you are regularly taking anticoagulants. The combination could dangerously increase your bleeding time.

Helpful hint:

- You shouldn't drive a car or operate heavy machinery until you are sure the medicine isn't making you drowsy or less than alert.

Neostigmine

Brand name: *Prostigmin* **(Generic available)**

What this drug does for you:

This muscle stimulant is used to treat myasthenia gravis (nerve/muscle weakness disease). It is also used after surgery to prevent urinary retention and to reverse the effects of muscle relaxants used during surgery.

Possible side effects of this drug:

- Common side effects are increased watering of mouth, muscle twitching, stomach cramps, and diarrhea. You may also have an urge to urinate more often, small pupils, extra mucus in your lungs, increased sweating, gas, and watery eyes.
- Check with your doctor immediately if you have any of these less common side effects: nausea, vomiting, irregular heart rhythm, low blood pressure, fainting, wheezing or difficulty breathing, convulsions, extreme muscle weakness, dizziness, extreme drowsiness, vision disorders, hives, rash, and joint pain. In rare instances, the injectable form may cause a heart attack.

Special warnings:

- Neostigmine should not be used by people with allergies to bromides, with intestinal or urinary obstructions, or with peritonitis.
- Neostigmine should be used with caution by people with ulcers, asthma, slow or irregular heartbeat, epilepsy, overactive thyroid, hypersensitivity of the parasympathetic nervous system, or by people who have recently had a blood clot in the heart.

Pregnancy and nursing mothers:

Category C. See page 9 for description of categories. Not known if drug is present in mother's milk.

Possible food and drug interactions:

- Effects of neostigmine may be increased by the antibiotics neomycin, streptomycin, and kanamycin.
- Effects of neostigmine may be decreased by anesthetics, drugs that regulate heart rhythm, and drugs that relax muscles or relax the nervous system.

Helpful hint:

- If you are taking the drug for myasthenia gravis, you may want to keep a daily record of your condition (when you are the most tired, when you have the most energy, etc.) to help your doctor determine the best dosing schedule for you.

Orphenadrine

Brand name: *Norflex, Norgesic, Norgesic Forte* **(contains aspirin and caffeine)**

What this drug does for you:

This muscle relaxant is used to relieve mild to moderate pain and discomfort associated with muscle disorders such as sprains, strains, and other injuries.

Possible side effects of this drug:

- This drug may cause heart palpitations or a rapid heartbeat, dry mouth, blurred vision, dilated pupils, increased pressure in the eyes, difficulty urinating, nausea, vomiting, dizziness, hallucinations, tremors, and constipation.
- Rare side effects are hives and other skin problems and, especially in older people, confusion.

Special warnings:

- Don't take this drug if you have the nerve/muscle weakness disease called myasthenia gravis, glaucoma, enlarged prostate, stomach ulcers, difficulty swallowing because of dilation of the esophagus, or obstruction of the stomach, intestines, or bladder.
- Take this drug with caution if you have asthma, an irregular or rapid heartbeat, or heart failure.

Pregnancy and nursing mothers:

Category C. See page 9 for description of categories. Not known if drug is present in mother's milk.

Possible food and drug interaction:

- Taking orphenadrine with the pain reliever propoxyphene may cause confusion, anxiety, and tremors.

Helpful hints:

- This medicine should not take the place of rest, physical therapy, exercise, or any other treatment your doctor recommends.

- You shouldn't drive a car or operate heavy machinery until you are sure the medicine isn't making you drowsy or less than alert.
- If you use this medicine for a long time, you should have your blood, urine, and liver functions monitored periodically.

Pyridostigmine

Brand names: *Mestinon, Regonol*

What this drug does for you:
This muscle stimulant is used to treat myasthenia gravis (nerve/muscle weakness disease).

Possible side effects of this drug:
- Common side effects are increased watering of mouth, muscle twitching, stomach cramps, and diarrhea. You may also have an urge to urinate more often, small pupils, extra mucus in your lungs, increased sweating, gas, and watery eyes.
- Check with your doctor immediately if you have any of these less common side effects: nausea, vomiting, irregular heart rhythm, low blood pressure, fainting, wheezing or difficulty breathing, convulsions, extreme muscle weakness, dizziness, extreme drowsiness, vision disorders, hives, rash, and joint pain.

Special warnings:
- People with intestinal or urinary obstructions should not take this drug.
- Take this drug with caution if you have asthma.

Pregnancy and nursing mothers:
Not known if drug is safe to use while pregnant. Not known if drug is safe to use while nursing.

Possible food and drug interaction:
- The heartbeat regulators quinidine and atropine may decrease the effects of pyridostigmine.

Helpful hint:
- If you are taking the drug for myasthenia gravis, you may want to keep a daily record of your condition (when you are the most tired, when you have the most energy, etc.) to help your doctor determine the best dosing schedule for you.

Nonsteroidal Anti-Inflammatory Drugs

Aspirin with Codeine

Brand name: *Empirin with Codeine* (Generic available)

What this drug does for you:
This drug combines a narcotic painkiller with aspirin to relieve pain. Narcotics

relieve pain by depressing your central nervous system.

Possible side effects of this drug:

- Codeine most often causes dizziness, drowsiness, nausea, constipation, and slow breathing. Less common reactions to codeine include exaggerated feelings of excitement or depression and skin rashes.
- Large doses of aspirin can cause nausea, ringing in the ears, vision and hearing problems, headache, dizziness, mental confusion, rapid heartbeat, sweating, and thirst. You can have an allergic reaction to aspirin that includes nausea, skin rashes or hives, asthma, swelling, and stomach pain. Some people have heartburn when they take aspirin.
- Even though it is very rare, large doses of aspirin may lower the number of blood cells you have. If you don't have enough white blood cells, your immunity is down, and you can get a fever, sore throat, or pneumonia. If you are lacking red blood cells, you can become anemic, and that makes you tired and weak. Not having enough blood platelets makes you bruise easily and keeps your blood from clotting properly when you're injured. Be on the lookout for any of these symptoms of bone marrow depression.

Special warnings:

- Don't take this drug if you are allergic to aspirin or codeine. You could have a severe allergic reaction.
- If you have any bleeding disorder, a vitamin K deficiency, a stomach ulcer, or severe liver damage, you should not take this drug.
- Don't use this drug to treat chickenpox or flu, as it could cause Reye's syndrome.
- People with the following conditions should use this drug with caution: liver or kidney damage, gallbladder disease or gallstones, breathing difficulties, irregular heartbeat, hypothyroidism, enlarged prostate, head injuries, or severe stomach problems. If you have liver or kidney damage, you should have regular liver and kidney tests while you take this drug.

Pregnancy and nursing mothers:

Category C. See page 9 for description of categories. Drug is present in mother's milk.

Possible food and drug interactions:

- If you take drugs containing codeine along with alcohol or a drug that depresses your nervous system, such as tranquilizers, antihistamines, or muscle relaxants, the combination may dangerously depress your nervous system.
- This drug may increase the effects of diabetic drugs and insulin (causing hypoglycemia), penicillin and sulfonamide antibiotics, antidepressant drugs called monoamine oxidase (MAO) inhibitors, other nonsteroidal anti-inflammatory drugs (causing stomach ulcers), and steroids.
- You shouldn't take this drug if you are regularly taking anticoagulants. The combination could dangerously increase your bleeding time.
- This drug may decrease the effectiveness of the gout drugs probenecid

and sulfinpyrazone.
- Furosemide (a diuretic) and vitamin C may cause aspirin to accumulate to toxic levels in your body.

Helpful hints:
- You shouldn't drive a car or operate heavy machinery until you are sure the medicine isn't making you drowsy or less than alert.
- You may become physically and psychologically dependent on this drug if you take high doses for long periods of time. Never take more medicine than you are prescribed.
- Take your medicine with food or a full glass of milk or water so it won't irritate your stomach.

Aspirin with Drocode (Dihydrocodeine) Bitartrate and Caffeine

Brand name: *Synalgos-DC*

What this drug does for you:
This drug combines aspirin with a narcotic painkiller very similar to codeine. Narcotics relieve pain by depressing your central nervous system.

Possible side effects of this drug:
- Dihydrocodeine most often causes dizziness, drowsiness, nausea, constipation and slow breathing, and skin rashes.
- Large doses of aspirin can cause nausea, ringing in the ears, vision and hearing problems, headache, dizziness, mental confusion, rapid heartbeat, sweating, and thirst. You can have an allergic reaction to aspirin that includes nausea, skin rashes or hives, asthma, swelling, and stomach pain. Some people have heartburn when they take aspirin.
- Even though it is very rare, large doses of aspirin may lower the number of blood cells you have. If you don't have enough white blood cells, your immunity is down, and you can get a fever, sore throat, or pneumonia. If you are lacking red blood cells, you can become anemic, and that makes you tired and weak. Not having enough blood platelets makes you bruise easily and keeps your blood from clotting properly when you're injured. Be on the lookout for any of these symptoms of bone marrow depression.

Special warnings:
- Don't take this drug if you are allergic to aspirin or codeine. You could have a severe allergic reaction.
- If you have any bleeding disorder, a vitamin K deficiency, a stomach ulcer, or severe liver damage, you should not take this drug.
- Don't use this drug to treat chickenpox or flu, as it could cause Reye's syndrome.
- People with the following conditions should use this drug with caution: liver or kidney damage, gallbladder disease or gallstones, breathing difficulties, irregular heartbeat, hypothyroidism, enlarged prostate, head injuries, or severe stomach problems. If you have liver or kidney damage, you should have regular liver and kidney tests while you take this

drug.

Pregnancy and nursing mothers:

Category C. See page 9 for description of categories. Drug is present in mother's milk

Possible food and drug interactions:

- If you take this drug along with alcohol or a drug that depresses your nervous system, such as tranquilizers, antihistamines, or muscle relaxants, the combination may dangerously depress your nervous system.
- This drug may increase the effects of diabetic drugs and insulin (causing hypoglycemia), penicillin and sulfonamide antibiotics, antidepressant drugs called monoamine oxidase (MAO) inhibitors, other nonsteroidal anti-inflammatory drugs (causing stomach ulcers), and steroids.
- You shouldn't take this drug if you are regularly taking anticoagulants. The combination could dangerously increase your bleeding time.
- This drug may decrease the effectiveness of the gout drugs probenecid and sulfinpyrazone.
- Furosemide (a diuretic) and vitamin C may cause aspirin to accumulate to toxic levels in your body.

Helpful hints:

- You shouldn't drive a car or operate heavy machinery until you are sure the medicine isn't making you drowsy or less than alert.
- You may become physically and psychologically dependent on this drug if you take high doses for long periods of time. Never take more medicine than you are prescribed.
- Take your medicine with food or a full glass of milk or water so it won't irritate your stomach.

Aspirin with Hydrocodone Bitartrate

Brand names: *Azdone, Lortab ASA, Damason-P, Panasal*

What this drug does for you:

This drug combines aspirin with a narcotic painkiller very similar to codeine. Narcotics relieve pain by depressing your central nervous system.

Possible side effects of this drug:

- Hydrocodone most often causes dizziness, drowsiness, nausea, constipation, mood changes, and skin rashes. One of the most dangerous side effects of hydrocodone at high doses is slow or irregular breathing.
- Large doses of aspirin can cause nausea, ringing in the ears, vision and hearing problems, headache, dizziness, mental confusion, rapid heartbeat, sweating, and thirst. You can have an allergic reaction to aspirin that includes nausea, skin rashes or hives, asthma, swelling, and stomach pain. Some people have heartburn when they take aspirin.
- Even though it is very rare, large doses of aspirin may lower the number of blood cells you have. If you don't have enough white blood cells, your immunity is down, and you can get a fever, sore throat, or pneu-

monia. If you are lacking red blood cells, you can become anemic, and that makes you tired and weak. Not having enough blood platelets makes you bruise easily and keeps your blood from clotting properly when you're injured. Be on the lookout for any of these symptoms of bone marrow depression.

Special warnings:

- Don't take this drug if you are allergic to aspirin or codeine. You could have a severe allergic reaction.
- If you have any bleeding disorder, a vitamin K deficiency, a stomach ulcer, or severe liver damage, you should not take this drug.
- Don't use this drug to treat chickenpox or flu, as it could cause Reye's syndrome.
- People with the following conditions should use this drug with caution: liver or kidney damage, gallbladder disease or gallstones, breathing difficulties, irregular heartbeat, hypothyroidism, enlarged prostate, head injuries, or severe stomach problems. If you have liver or kidney damage, you should have regular liver and kidney tests while you take this drug.
- Hydrocodone suppresses the cough reflex, so people with lung disease should take this drug with caution.

Pregnancy and nursing mothers:

Category C. See page 9 for description of categories. Drug is present in mother's milk.

Possible food and drug interactions:

- If you take this drug along with alcohol or a drug that depresses your nervous system, such as tranquilizers, antihistamines, or muscle relaxants, the combination may dangerously depress your nervous system.
- This drug may increase the effects of diabetic drugs and insulin (causing hypoglycemia), penicillin and sulfonamide antibiotics, tricyclic antidepressants or antidepressant drugs called monoamine oxidase (MAO) inhibitors, other nonsteroidal anti-inflammatory drugs (causing stomach ulcers), and steroids.
- You shouldn't take this drug if you are regularly taking anticoagulants. The combination could dangerously increase your bleeding time.
- This drug may decrease the effectiveness of the gout drugs probenecid and sulfinpyrazone.
- Furosemide (a diuretic) and vitamin C may cause aspirin to accumulate to toxic levels in your body.

Helpful hints:

- You shouldn't drive a car or operate heavy machinery until you are sure the medicine isn't making you drowsy or less than alert.
- You may become physically and psychologically dependent on this drug if you take high doses for long periods of time. Never take more medicine than you are prescribed.
- Take your medicine with food or a full glass of milk or water so it won't irritate your stomach.

Aspirin with Oxycodone

Brand names: *Percodan, Roxiprin*

What this drug does for you:
This drug combines aspirin with a narcotic painkiller similar to morphine.

Possible side effects of this drug:
- The most common side effects are dizziness, sleepiness, and nausea.
- Large doses of aspirin can cause nausea, ringing in the ears, vision and hearing problems, headache, dizziness, mental confusion, rapid heartbeat, sweating, and thirst. You can have an allergic reaction to aspirin that includes nausea, skin rashes or hives, asthma, swelling, and stomach pain. Some people have heartburn when they take aspirin.
- Even though it is very rare, large doses of aspirin may lower the number of blood cells you have. If you don't have enough white blood cells, your immunity is down, and you can get a fever, sore throat, or pneumonia. If you are lacking red blood cells, you can become anemic, and that makes you tired and weak. Not having enough blood platelets makes you bruise easily and keeps your blood from clotting properly when you're injured. Be on the lookout for any of these symptoms of bone marrow depression.

Special warnings:
- Don't take this drug if you are allergic to aspirin or oxycodone. You could have a severe allergic reaction.
- Don't use this drug to treat chickenpox or flu, as it could cause Reye's syndrome.
- People with the following conditions should use this drug with caution: liver or kidney damage, gallbladder disease or gallstones, breathing difficulties, irregular heartbeat, hypothyroidism, enlarged prostate, head injuries, or severe stomach problems. If you have liver or kidney damage, you should have regular liver and kidney tests while you take this drug.

Pregnancy and nursing mothers:
Not known if safe to use in pregnancy or while breast-feeding.

Possible food and drug interactions:
- If you take this drug along with alcohol or a drug that depresses your nervous system, such as tranquilizers, antihistamines, or muscle relaxants, the combination may dangerously depress your nervous system.
- You shouldn't take this drug if you are regularly taking anticoagulants. The combination could dangerously increase your bleeding time.
- This drug may decrease the effectiveness of the gout drugs probenecid and sulfinpyrazone.

Helpful hints:
- You shouldn't drive a car or operate heavy machinery until you are sure the medicine isn't making you drowsy or less than alert.

- You may become physically and psychologically dependent on this drug if you take high doses for long periods of time. Never take more medicine than you are prescribed.

Aspirin with Pentazocine Hydrochloride

Brand name: *Talwin Compound*

What this drug does for you:

This drug combines aspirin with a narcotic painkiller very similar to codeine. Narcotics relieve pain by depressing your central nervous system.

Possible side effects of this drug:

- Possible side effects of this drug are nausea, dizziness, sleepiness, excitement, headache, confusion, and sweating. Less common side effects are constipation, weakness, disturbed dreams, insomnia, fainting, blurred vision, depression, low blood pressure, and flushing. Rare side effects are stomach pain, diarrhea, tremor, irritability, excitement, and chills.
- Some people experience hallucinations, disorientation, and confusion for a few hours after taking this drug.
- Large doses of aspirin can cause nausea, ringing in the ears, vision and hearing problems, headache, dizziness, confusion, rapid heartbeat, sweating, and thirst. You can have an allergic reaction to aspirin that includes nausea, skin rashes or hives, asthma, swelling, and stomach pain. Some people have heartburn when they take aspirin.
- Even though it is very rare, large doses of aspirin may lower the number of blood cells you have. If you don't have enough white blood cells, your immunity is down, and you can get a fever, sore throat, or pneumonia. If you are lacking red blood cells, you can become anemic, and that makes you tired and weak. Not having enough blood platelets makes you bruise easily and keeps your blood from clotting properly when you're injured. Be on the lookout for any of these symptoms of bone marrow depression.

Special warnings:

- Don't take this drug if you are allergic to pentazocine, aspirin, or other salicylates. You could have a severe allergic reaction.
- If you have any bleeding disorder, a vitamin K deficiency, a stomach ulcer, or severe liver damage, you should not take this drug.
- Don't use this drug to treat chickenpox or flu, as it could cause Reye's syndrome.
- People with the following conditions should use this drug with caution: liver or kidney damage, gallbladder disease or gallstones, breathing difficulties such as asthma, irregular heartbeat or heart attack, hypothyroidism, seizures, enlarged prostate, head injuries, or severe stomach problems. If you have liver or kidney damage, you should have regular liver and kidney tests while you take this drug.

Pregnancy and nursing mothers:

This drug may not be safe to use while you're pregnant. Drug is present in mother's milk.

Possible food and drug interactions:

- If you take this drug along with alcohol or a drug that depresses your nervous system, such as tranquilizers, antihistamines, or muscle relaxants, the combination may dangerously depress your nervous system.
- This drug may increase the effects of diabetic drugs and insulin (causing hypoglycemia), penicillin and sulfonamide antibiotics, tricyclic antidepressants or antidepressant drugs called monoamine oxidase (MAO) inhibitors, other nonsteroidal anti-inflammatory drugs (causing stomach ulcers), and steroids.
- You shouldn't take this drug if you are regularly taking anticoagulants. The combination could dangerously increase your bleeding time.
- This drug may decrease the effectiveness of the gout drugs probenecid and sulfinpyrazone.
- Furosemide (a diuretic) and vitamin C may cause aspirin to accumulate to toxic levels in your body.

Helpful hints:

- You shouldn't drive a car or operate heavy machinery until you are sure the medicine isn't making you drowsy or less than alert.
- You may become physically and psychologically dependent on this drug if you take high doses for long periods of time. Never take more medicine than you are prescribed.
- Take your medicine with food or a full glass of milk or water to help prevent stomach irritation.

Diclofenac

Brand names: *Cataflam* **(immediate-release tablets),** *Voltaren* **(delayed-release tablets)**

What this drug does for you:

Diclofenac relieves the symptoms of rheumatoid arthritis, osteoarthritis, and ankylosing spondylitis. The immediate-release tablets are also used for menstrual pain.

Possible side effects of this drug:

- Common side effects include stomach pain and cramps, headache, fluid retention, bloating, diarrhea, indigestion, nausea, constipation, gas, dizziness, rash, itching, and ringing in the ears.
- Bleeding stomach ulcers and liver damage are the most common serious reactions to diclofenac. Warning signs of liver damage include nausea, tiredness, red and itchy skin, yellow eyes and skin (jaundice), and flu-like symptoms.
- Rarely, people have an allergic reaction to nonsteroidal anti-inflammatory drugs (NSAIDs) like diclofenac. Signs of an allergic reaction are

hives, asthma, low blood pressure, and swelling of the eyelids, lips, and throat.

- Other rare side effects are sensitivity to light, high blood pressure, congestive heart failure, vomiting, black and tarry feces, inflammation of the mouth, dry mouth, bloody diarrhea, appetite change, insomnia, drowsiness, depression, double vision, anxiety, irritability, nosebleed, hair loss, blurred vision, taste disorder, temporary hearing loss, vision abnormalities, and kidney problems or failure.

- Even though it is very rare, large doses of diclofenac may lower the number of blood cells you have. If you don't have enough white blood cells, your immunity is down, and you can get a fever, sore throat, or pneumonia. If you are lacking red blood cells, you can become anemic, and that makes you tired and weak. Not having enough blood platelets makes you bruise easily and keeps your blood from clotting properly when you're injured. Be on the lookout for any of these symptoms of bone marrow depression.

Special warnings:

- Don't take diclofenac if you have ever had an allergic reaction such as asthma or hives to aspirin or other NSAIDs.

- High doses and long-term use of diclofenac may cause serious stomach problems such as ulcers or bleeding. People with stomach ulcers should not take this drug.

- Diclofenac may cause kidney problems, especially if you are elderly; if you are taking diuretics; or if you have lupus, heart failure, or poor liver or kidney function.

- Take diclofenac with caution if you have poor heart function, high blood pressure, or fluid retention.

Pregnancy and nursing mothers:

Category B. See page 9 for description of categories. Drug is present in mother's milk.

Possible food and drug interactions:

- Avoid alcohol and aspirin while taking NSAIDs including diclofenac.

- Avoid alcohol and other NSAIDs, including aspirin, when taking diclofenac.

- Diclofenac may prolong bleeding time if used with anticoagulants.

- Diclofenac may increase the levels or effects of the immunosuppressant cyclosporine, the psychosis drug lithium, the seizure drug phenytoin, and the anti-inflammatory methotrexate, possibly increasing toxicity of some of these drugs.

- Diclofenac may reduce the effects of beta-blockers and loop diuretics.

- The gout drug probenecid may increase levels of NSAIDs.

- Taking salicylates such as aspirin may decrease levels of diclofenac while increasing the risk of stomach problems.

- The ulcer drug cimetidine may increase or decrease blood levels of diclofenac.

Helpful hint:
- Take your medicine with food or a full glass of milk or water to help prevent stomach irritation.

Diflunisal

Brand name: *Dolobid* (Generic available)

What this drug does for you:
This drug is similar to aspirin. It relieves mild to moderate pain and treats the inflammation of osteoarthritis and rheumatoid arthritis.

Possible side effects of this drug:
- The most common side effects are nausea, indigestion, stomach pain, diarrhea, rash, and headache. You may also experience constipation, gas, insomnia, sleepiness, dizziness, ringing in the ears, and tiredness.
- Bleeding stomach ulcers and liver damage are the most common serious reactions to diflunisal. Warning signs of liver damage include nausea, tiredness, red and itchy skin, yellow eyes and skin (jaundice), and flu-like symptoms.
- Other rare side effects are various skin eruptions and disorders, itching, sweating, dry or inflamed mouth, loss of appetite, various kidney problems including kidney failure, nervousness, depression, hallucinations, confusion, tingling, and visual disturbances including blurred vision.
- Even though it is very rare, diflunisal may lower the number of blood cells you have. If you don't have enough white blood cells, your immunity is down, and you can get a fever, sore throat, or pneumonia. If you are lacking red blood cells, you can become anemic, and that makes you tired and weak. Not having enough blood platelets makes you bruise easily and keeps your blood from clotting properly when you're injured. Be on the lookout for any of these symptoms of bone marrow depression.

Special warnings:
- Diflunisal should not be used by people allergic to aspirin or other non-steroidal anti-inflammatory drugs (NSAIDs).
- Diflunisal should not be used to treat fever.
- Take diflunisal with caution if you have active gastrointestinal bleeding or active peptic ulcer, a history of gastrointestinal disease, poor heart function, high blood pressure, a low blood platelet count, or other conditions which may cause fluid retention.

Pregnancy and nursing mothers:
Category C. See page 9 for description of categories. Drug is present in mother's milk.

Possible food and drug interactions:
- Diflunisal should not be used with the NSAID indomethacin. The combination can cause dangerous stomach bleeding.
- Diflunisal may increase the effects of anticoagulants such as warfarin. Your doctor may need to adjust the dose of your anticoagulant.

- Diflunisal may increase the levels of the diuretic hydrochlorothiazide in the blood but decrease its effects.
- Diflunisal may increase levels of the analgesic acetaminophen.
- Diflunisal may decrease levels of the NSAID sulindac.
- Antacids may decrease levels of this drug in the blood.
- Diflunisal may increase levels of the anti-inflammatory drug methotrexate and the immunosuppressant cyclosporine.

Helpful hints:
- Swallow the tablets whole.
- Take your medicine with food or a full glass of milk or water to help prevent stomach irritation.

Etodolac

Brand name: *Lodine*

What this drug does for you:

This nonsteroidal anti-inflammatory drug (NSAID) is used to control the symptoms of osteoarthritis and to relieve pain.

Possible side effects of this drug:

- Common side effects include nausea, diarrhea, dizziness, constipation, stomach pain or cramps, indigestion, constipation, black and tarry feces, mental depression, weakness, nervousness, blurred vision, ringing in the ears, itching, rash, and frequent urination.
- Bleeding stomach ulcers and liver or kidney damage are the most common serious reactions to using etodolac for long periods of time. Warning signs of liver damage include nausea, tiredness, red and itchy skin, yellow eyes and skin (jaundice), and flu-like symptoms.
- Rare side effects are high blood pressure, fainting, palpitations, congestive heart failure, flushing, insomnia, sweating, fluid retention, rash, itching, changes in skin pigment, dry mouth, loss of appetite, mouth ulcers, and vision abnormalities.
- Even though it is very rare, etodolac may lower the number of blood cells you have. If you don't have enough white blood cells, your immunity is down, and you can get a fever, sore throat, or pneumonia. If you are lacking red blood cells, you can become anemic, and that makes you tired and weak. Not having enough blood platelets makes you bruise easily and keeps your blood from clotting properly when you're injured. Be on the lookout for any of these symptoms of bone marrow depression.

Special warnings:

- Don't use etodolac if you are allergic to aspirin or other nonsteroidal anti-inflammatory drugs.
- Taking etodolac is more likely to cause kidney problems if you are elderly, if you take diuretics, or if you have lupus, heart failure, or poor liver or kidney function.
- Take etodolac with caution if you have heart failure, high blood pressure, or clotting disorders.

Pregnancy and nursing mothers:

Category C. See page 9 for description of categories. Not known if drug is present in mother's milk.

Possible food and drug interactions:

- Avoid aspirin while taking NSAIDs such as etodolac.
- Etodolac may decrease the effectiveness of anticoagulants such as warfarin.
- Etodolac may increase the levels or effects of the heart drug digoxin, the immunosuppressant cyclosporine, the antipsychotic drug lithium, and the cancer drug methotrexate, possibly increasing the toxicity of some of these drugs.

Helpful hints:

- The usual adult dosage for pain is 200 to 400 mg every six to eight hours, not to exceed 1200 mg in one day.
- The usual adult dosage for osteoarthritis is 800 to 1200 mg a day in divided doses.

Fenoprofen Calcium

Brand name: *Nalfon* **(Generic available)**

What this drug does for you:

This nonsteroidal anti-inflammatory drug (NSAID) relieves mild to moderate pain associated with conditions such as rheumatoid arthritis and osteoarthritis.

Possible side effects of this drug:

- Side effects may include nausea, constipation, stomach pain or cramps, indigestion, gas, loss of appetite, diarrhea, headache, sleepiness, dizziness, confusion, itching, rash, sweating, ringing in the ears, difficulty hearing, blurred vision, palpitations, nervousness, difficulty breathing, and swelling of the hands or feet.
- Bleeding stomach ulcers and liver or kidney damage are the most common serious reactions to using fenoprofen for long periods of time. Warning signs of liver damage include nausea, tiredness, red and itchy skin, yellow eyes and skin (jaundice), and flu-like symptoms.
- Rare side effects are difficult or painful urination, blood in the urine or stools, hives, rapid heartbeat, and insomnia.
- Even though it is very rare, fenoprofen may lower the number of blood cells you have. If you don't have enough white blood cells, your immunity is down, and you can get a fever, sore throat, or pneumonia. If you are lacking red blood cells, you can become anemic, and that makes you tired and weak Not having enough blood platelets makes you bruise easily and keeps your blood from clotting properly when you're injured. Be on the lookout for any of these symptoms of bone marrow depression.

Special warnings:
- Don't use fenoprofen if you are allergic to aspirin or any NSAID.
- Take fenoprofen with caution if you have stomach ulcers, poor heart function, high blood pressure, or blood-clotting disorders.
- Taking fenoprofen is more likely to cause kidney problems if you are elderly, if you take diuretics, or if you have lupus, heart failure, or poor liver or kidney function.

Pregnancy and nursing mothers:
Not known if drug is safe to use while you are pregnant. Not known if drug is safe to use while you are nursing.

Possible food and drug interactions:
- Avoid alcohol and aspirin while taking NSAIDs such as fenoprofen.
- Fenoprofen may increase the effects of anticoagulants.
- Levels or effects of fenoprofen may be decreased by the sedative phenobarbital.

Helpful hints:
- Take your medicine with food or a full glass of milk or water to help prevent stomach irritation.
- You shouldn't drive a car or operate heavy machinery until you are sure the medicine isn't making you drowsy or less than alert.

Flurbiprofen

Brand name: *Ansaid* **(Generic available)**

What this drug does for you:
This nonsteroidal anti-inflammatory drug (NSAID) is used to relieve the symptoms of arthritis.

Possible side effects of this drug:
- Common side effects include water retention and stomach upsets such as nausea, diarrhea, constipation, stomach pain or cramps, indigestion, and gas. You may also experience headache, nervousness, rash, stuffy nose, tremors, ringing in the ears, dizziness, painful urination, depression, sleepiness, and memory problems. Let your doctor know about any side effects you experience.
- Bleeding stomach ulcers and liver or kidney damage are the most common serious reactions to using flurbiprofen for long periods of time. Warning signs of liver damage include nausea, tiredness, red and itchy skin, yellow eyes and skin (jaundice), and flu-like symptoms.
- Rare side effects are blood in stools, inflammation of the mouth, muscle twitching, lack of coordination, confusion, asthma, nosebleed, hives, itching, heart failure, and high blood pressure.
- Even though it is very rare, flurbiprofen may lower the number of blood cells you have. If you don't have enough white blood cells, your immunity is down, and you can get a fever, sore throat, or pneumonia. If you are lacking red blood cells, you can become anemic, and that makes you

tired and weak. Not having enough blood platelets makes you bruise easily and keeps your blood from clotting properly when you're injured. Be on the lookout for any of these symptoms of bone marrow depression.

Special warnings:

- Don't use flurbiprofen if you are allergic to aspirin or any NSAID.
- Take flurbiprofen with caution if you have stomach ulcers, poor heart function, high blood pressure, or blood-clotting disorders.
- Taking flurbiprofen is more likely to cause kidney problems if you are elderly, if you take diuretics, or if you have lupus, heart failure, or poor liver or kidney function.

Pregnancy and nursing mothers:

Category B. See page 9 for description of categories. Drug is present in mother's milk.

Possible food and drug interactions:

- Avoid alcohol and aspirin while taking flurbiprofen.
- Flurbiprofen may prolong bleeding time if used at the same time as anticoagulants.
- Flurbiprofen may decrease the effects of beta-blockers and diuretics.

Helpful hints:

- You shouldn't drive a car or operate heavy machinery until you are sure the medicine isn't making you drowsy or less than alert.

Ibuprofen

Brand names: *Children's Advil Suspension, Children's Motrin, IBU, IBU-TAB, Motrin* **(Generic available)**

What this drug does for you:

This nonsteroidal anti-inflammatory drug (NSAID) relieves the symptoms of arthritis, mild to moderate pain, and painful menstruation. Ibuprofen may not cause as many stomach problems as aspirin.

Possible side effects of this drug:

- Side effects may include water retention, loss of appetite, ringing in the ears, dizziness, headache, itching, and various stomach problems such as heartburn, nausea, stomach pain or cramps, diarrhea, constipation, gas, and bloating.
- Bleeding stomach ulcers and liver or kidney damage are rare but serious reactions to using ibuprofen for long periods of time. Warning signs of liver damage include nausea, tiredness, red and itchy skin, yellow eyes and skin (jaundice), and flu-like symptoms.
- Rare side effects may include blurred vision, hair loss, skin eruptions, hives, insomnia, depression, congestive heart failure, high blood pressure, heart palpitations, dry mouth, and stuffy nose.
- Even though it is very rare, ibuprofen may lower the number of blood cells you have. If you don't have enough white blood cells, your immunity is down, and you can get a fever, sore throat, or pneumonia. If you

are lacking red blood cells, you can become anemic, and that makes you tired and weak. Not having enough blood platelets makes you bruise easily and keeps your blood from clotting properly when you're injured. Be on the lookout for any of these symptoms of bone marrow depression.

- You should report any side effects you have to your doctor, especially signs of a stomach ulcer, skin rash, weight gain, blurred vision or other eye symptoms, or water retention.

Special warnings:
- Don't use ibuprofen if you are allergic to aspirin or any NSAID.
- Take ibuprofen with caution if you have stomach ulcers, poor liver or kidney function, heart problems, high blood pressure, or blood-clotting disorders.
- Taking ibuprofen is more likely to cause kidney problems if you are elderly, if you take diuretics, or if you have lupus, heart failure, or poor liver or kidney function.

Pregnancy and nursing mothers:
Not known if drug is safe to use while you are pregnant. Not known if drug is safe to use while you are nursing.

Possible food and drug interactions:
- Avoid alcohol while you're taking ibuprofen. Alcohol may increase your risk of internal bleeding.
- Ibuprofen may increase the effects of the cancer drug methotrexate.
- Ibuprofen may increase levels of the antipsychotic drug lithium.
- Ibuprofen may increase the effects of anticoagulants and the diuretic furosemide.
- Aspirin may decrease the anti-inflammatory effects of ibuprofen.
- If you need to stop taking corticosteroids while you're taking ibuprofen, be sure to withdraw slowly from the steroids instead of stopping suddenly.

Helpful hint:
- Take your medicine with food or a full glass of milk or water to help prevent stomach irritation.

Indomethacin

Brand names: *Indocin, Indocin SR* **(Generic available)**

What this drug does for you:
This nonsteroidal anti-inflammatory drug (NSAID) relieves the pain and inflammation of arthritis, gout, ankylosing spondylitis, and bursitis or tendinitis in the shoulder.

Possible side effects of this drug:
- Common side effects are nausea, indigestion, diarrhea, constipation, heartburn, ringing in the ears, dizziness, depression, tiredness, and headache.
- Bleeding stomach ulcers and liver or kidney damage are rare but serious

reactions to using indomethacin for long periods of time. Warning signs of liver damage include nausea, tiredness, red and itchy skin, yellow eyes and skin (jaundice), and flu-like symptoms.

- Other rare side effects may include bleeding from the rectum, vision changes, bloating, loss of appetite, itching, rash, hives, hair loss, high blood sugar, vaginal bleeding, enlargement of breasts in men and women, sudden decrease in blood pressure, fever, asthma, fluid retention, sweating, weight gain, high blood pressure, rapid heartbeat, and chest pain.
- Even though it is very rare, indomethacin may lower the number of blood cells you have. If you don't have enough white blood cells, your immunity is down, and you can get a fever, sore throat, or pneumonia. If you are lacking red blood cells, you can become anemic, and that makes you tired and weak. Not having enough blood platelets makes you bruise easily and keeps your blood from clotting properly when you're injured. Be on the lookout for any of these symptoms of bone marrow depression.

Special warnings:
- Don't use indomethacin if you are allergic to aspirin or any NSAID.
- Take indomethacin with caution if you have stomach ulcers, poor liver or kidney function, heart problems, high blood pressure, or blood-clotting disorders.
- Indomethacin may cause gastrointestinal bleeding.
- Taking indomethacin is more likely to cause kidney problems if you are elderly, if you take diuretics, or if you have lupus, heart failure, or poor liver or kidney function.
- Indomethacin may cause or worsen Parkinson's disease, epilepsy, and depression.

Pregnancy and nursing mothers:
Not recommended for use during pregnancy. Drug is present in mother's milk.

Possible food and drug interactions:
- Avoid alcohol and aspirin while taking NSAIDs such as indomethacin.
- Taking indomethacin and the arthritis drug diflunisal together could cause dangerous intestinal bleeding.

Helpful hint:
- Take with food, after meals, or with antacids to help prevent stomach irritation.

Ketorolac Tromethamine

Brand names: *Acular (for eyes), Toradol*

What this drug does for you:
The tablet form of this nonsteroidal anti-inflammatory drug (NSAID) is used to relieve short-term pain. Because of the risk of side effects, you should not use this drug on a long-term basis to treat chronic pain.

The ophthalmic solution is used to relieve itching eyes caused by seasonal allergies.

Possible side effects of this drug:

- The ophthalmic solution may cause burning and stinging, irritated eyes, allergic reactions, and eye infections or inflammations.
- The tablets may cause stomach or intestinal pain, headache, nausea, indigestion, gas, constipation, inflammation of the mouth, stuffy nose, hearing loss, rash, itching, fluid retention, high blood pressure, dizziness, drowsiness, and sweating.
- Bleeding stomach ulcers and liver or kidney damage are rare but serious reactions to using ketorolac tablets for long periods of time. Warning signs of liver damage include nausea, tiredness, red and itchy skin, yellow eyes and skin (jaundice), and flu-like symptoms.
- Rare side effects of the tablets may include asthma, loss of appetite, hallucinations, tremors, pain in the hip area, and fever. Allergic reactions to the drug include difficulty breathing, swelling of the tongue or throat, low blood pressure, and flushing.
- Even though it is very rare, ketorolac tablets may lower the number of blood cells you have. If you don't have enough white blood cells, your immunity is down, and you can get a fever, sore throat, or pneumonia. If you are lacking red blood cells, you can become anemic, and that makes you tired and weak. Not having enough blood platelets makes you bruise easily and keeps your blood from clotting properly when you're injured. Be on the lookout for any of these symptoms of bone marrow depression.

Special warnings:

- Don't use ketorolac tablets if you have an allergy to aspirin or other NSAIDs.
- People with nasal polyps, fluid retention, an active stomach ulcer, or asthma should not use ketorolac tablets.
- Take the tablets with caution if you have poor liver or kidney function, poor heart function, high blood pressure, blood clotting disorders, are taking diuretics, or are over 65.
- You should not use the ophthalmic solution while wearing soft contact lenses.

Pregnancy and nursing mothers:

Category C. See page 9 for description of categories. Drug is present in mother's milk.

Possible food and drug interactions:

- Ketorolac tablets may increase the levels or effects of the antipsychotic drug lithium and the cancer drug methotrexate, possibly increasing them to toxic levels.
- Ketorolac tablets may increase the effectiveness of diuretics and the anticoagulant warfarin.
- The gout drug probenecid may increase levels of ketorolac.

Helpful hints:
- The usual adult dose of the ophthalmic solution is one drop four times a day.
- The maximum recommended daily dose of the tablets is 150 mg for the first day and 120 mg a day thereafter.

Meclofenamate Sodium

Brand names: *None available* **(Generic available)**

What this drug does for you:
This nonsteroidal anti-inflammatory drug (NSAID) relieves mild to moderate pain associated with arthritis and menstrual cramps.

Possible side effects of this drug:
- Side effects may include nausea, diarrhea, constipation, stomach pain or cramps, heartburn, gas, dizziness, headache, rash, hives, itching, loss of appetite, constipation, inflammation of the mouth, ringing in the ears, and fluid retention and swelling.
- Bleeding stomach ulcers and liver or kidney damage are rare but serious reactions to using meclofenamate for long periods of time. Warning signs of liver damage include nausea, tiredness, red and itchy skin, yellow eyes and skin (jaundice), and flu-like symptoms.
- Rare side effects may include skin eruptions and lupus.
- Even though it is very rare, meclofenamate may lower the number of blood cells you have. If you don't have enough white blood cells, your immunity is down, and you can get a fever, sore throat, or pneumonia. If you are lacking red blood cells, you can become anemic, and that makes you tired and weak. Not having enough blood platelets makes you bruise easily and keeps your blood from clotting properly when you're injured. Be on the lookout for any of these symptoms of bone marrow depression.

Special warnings:
- This drug should not be used by people with allergies to aspirin or other aspirin substitutes such as NSAIDs.
- People with stomach ulcer should not take this drug.
- Taking meclofenamate is more likely to cause kidney problems if you are elderly, if you take diuretics, or if you have lupus, heart failure, or poor liver or kidney function.

Pregnancy and nursing mothers:
Category D in first and third trimesters; Category B in second trimester. See page 9 for description of categories. Drug is present in mother's milk.

Possible food and drug interactions:
- Avoid alcohol and any products containing aspirin while taking meclofenamate.
- Meclofenamate may increase the effects of the anticoagulant warfarin.

Helpful hint:
- Take with food, after meals, or with antacids to help prevent stomach

irritation.

Nabumetone

Brand name: *Relafen*

What this drug does for you:

This nonsteroidal anti-inflammatory drug (NSAID) is used to relieve the pain and inflammation associated with arthritis.

Possible side effects of this drug:

- This drug may cause nausea, diarrhea, constipation, stomach pain or cramps, blood in the stool, indigestion, gas, loss of appetite, fluid retention, ringing in the ears, itching, rash, dizziness, fatigue, headache, dry mouth, and insomnia.
- Bleeding stomach ulcers and liver or kidney damage are rare but serious reactions to using nabumetone for long periods of time. Warning signs of liver damage include nausea, tiredness, red and itchy skin, yellow eyes and skin (jaundice), and flu-like symptoms.
- Rare side effects may include anxiety, confusion, depression, skin eruptions, weight gain, vision abnormalities, and sensitivity to light.
- Even though it is very rare, nabumetone may lower the number of blood cells you have. If you don't have enough white blood cells, your immunity is down, and you can get a fever, sore throat, or pneumonia. If you are lacking red blood cells, you can become anemic, and that makes you tired and weak. Not having enough blood platelets makes you bruise easily and keeps your blood from clotting properly when you're injured. Be on the lookout for any of these symptoms of bone marrow depression.

Special warnings:

- This drug should not be used by people with allergies to aspirin or other aspirin substitutes such as NSAIDs.
- People with stomach ulcer should not take this drug. This drug may cause gastrointestinal bleeding.
- Taking nabumetone is more likely to cause kidney problems if you are elderly, if you take diuretics, or if you have lupus, heart failure, or poor liver or kidney function.
- Take this drug with caution if you have liver abnormalities, high blood pressure, or heart failure.

Pregnancy and nursing mothers:

Category C. See page 9 for description of categories. Not known if drug is present in mother's milk.

Possible food and drug interactions:

- Avoid alcohol and any products containing aspirin while taking nabumetone.
- Nabumetone may increase the effects of the anticoagulant warfarin.

Helpful hint:

- Take with food, after meals, or with antacids to help prevent stomach irritation.

Naproxen

Brand name: *Anaprox, Anaprox DS, Aflaxen, Naprosyn* (Generic available)

What this drug does for you:

This nonsteroidal anti-inflammatory drug (NSAID) relieves the pain and symptoms of rheumatoid arthritis, juvenile arthritis, osteoarthritis, tendinitis, bursitis, gout, and ankylosing spondylitis. It is also used to relieve painful menstruation and mild to moderate pain from other conditions.

Naproxen sodium has been developed as a painkiller because it is more rapidly absorbed than napoxen.

Possible side effects of this drug:

- This drug may cause nausea, diarrhea, constipation, stomach pain or cramps, indigestion, inflammation of the mouth or tongue, headache, dizziness, heart palpitations, drowsiness, itching, sweating, skin eruptions, bleeding under the skin, ringing in the ears, vision abnormalities, thirst, and water retention.
- Bleeding stomach ulcers and liver or kidney damage are rare but serious reactions to using naproxen for long periods of time. Warning signs of liver damage include nausea, tiredness, red and itchy skin, yellow eyes and skin (jaundice), and flu-like symptoms.
- Rare side effects may include hair loss, rash, sensitivity to light, fever, chills, muscle pain and weakness, depression, unusual dreams, and heart failure.
- Even though it is very rare, naproxen may lower the number of blood cells you have. If you don't have enough white blood cells, your immunity is down, and you can get a fever, sore throat, or pneumonia. If you are lacking red blood cells, you can become anemic, and that makes you tired and weak. Not having enough blood platelets makes you bruise easily and keeps your blood from clotting properly when you're injured. Be on the lookout for any of these symptoms of bone marrow depression.

Special warnings:

- This drug should not be used by people with allergies to aspirin or other aspirin substitutes such as NSAIDs.
- People with stomach ulcer should not take this drug. This drug may cause gastrointestinal bleeding.
- Taking naproxen is more likely to cause kidney problems if you are elderly, if you take diuretics, or if you have lupus, heart failure, or poor liver or kidney function.
- Take this drug with caution if you have liver abnormalities, high blood pressure, or heart failure.

Pregnancy and nursing mothers:

Category B. See page 9 for description of categories. Drug is present in mother's milk.

Possible food and drug interactions:

- Naproxen should not be taken with the related drug naproxen sodium.
- Avoid alcohol and any products containing aspirin while taking naproxen.
- Naproxen may increase the risk of bleeding if taken with the anticoagulant warfarin.
- Naproxen may increase the levels or effects of the antipsychotic drug lithium and the cancer drug methotrexate, possibly increasing them to toxic levels.
- Naproxen may decrease the effects of the diuretic furosemide and the beta-blocker propanolol.
- The gout drug probenecid may increase the effects of naproxen, which may increase the risk of intestinal problems.

Helpful hint:

- You shouldn't drive a car or operate heavy machinery until you are sure the medicine isn't making you drowsy or less than alert.

Oxaprozin

Brand name: *Daypro*

What this drug does for you:

This nonsteroidal anti-inflammatory drug (NSAID) relieves the pain and symptoms of arthritis.

Possible side effects of this drug:

- The most common side effects are nausea and indigestion. Also common are stomach pain, weight loss, constipation, diarrhea, gas, depression, sleepiness, insomnia, rash, ringing in the ears, and frequent urination.
- Bleeding stomach ulcers and liver or kidney damage are rare but serious reactions to using oxaprozin for long periods of time. Warning signs of liver damage include nausea, tiredness, red and itchy skin, yellow eyes and skin (jaundice), and flu-like symptoms.
- Rare side effects may include inflammation of the mouth, bleeding from the rectum, itching, rash, sensitivity to light, blurred vision, swelling or fluid retention, and allergic shock reaction.
- Even though it is very rare, oxaprozin may lower the number of blood cells you have. If you don't have enough white blood cells, your immunity is down, and you can get a fever, sore throat, or pneumonia. If you are lacking red blood cells, you can become anemic, and that makes you tired and weak. Not having enough blood platelets makes you bruise easily and keeps your blood from clotting properly when you're injured. Be on the lookout for any of these symptoms of bone marrow depression.

Special warnings:

- This drug should not be used by people with nasal polyps, with water retention or swelling, or with allergies to aspirin or other aspirin substitutes such as NSAIDs.
- People with stomach ulcer should not take this drug. Alcoholics and

smokers also have an increased risk of stomach and intestinal problems.
- Taking oxaprozin is more likely to cause kidney problems if you are elderly, if you take diuretics, or if you have lupus, heart failure, or poor liver or kidney function.
- Take this drug with caution if you have liver abnormalities, high blood pressure, blood clotting disorders, or poor heart function.

Pregnancy and nursing mothers:
Category C. See page 9 for description of categories. Not known if drug is present in mother's milk.

Possible food and drug interactions:
- Avoid aspirin while taking this drug.
- Oxaprozin may increase the risk of bleeding if taken with the anticoagulant warfarin.
- Oxaprozin may decrease the effects of the beta-blocker metoprolol.
- Levels or effects of oxaprozin may be increased by the ulcer drugs cimetidine and ranitidine.
- Antacids don't seem to interfere with the absorption of this drug.

Helpful hint:
- This drug may make your skin extra-sensitive to sunlight, so protect your skin if you'll be outdoors in sunny weather.

Piroxicam

Brand name: *Feldene* (Generic available)

What this drug does for you:
This nonsteroidal anti-inflammatory drug (NSAID) is used to relieve the symptoms of arthritis.

Possible side effects of this drug:
- Common side effects include nausea, stomach pain, loss of appetite, constipation, indigestion, diarrhea, inflammation of the mouth, headache, ringing in the ears, dizziness, sleepiness, and water retention.
- Signs that you are having an allergic reaction to piroxicam include rash, skin eruptions, itching, joint pain, and fever.
- Bleeding stomach ulcers and liver or kidney damage are rare but serious reactions to using piroxicam for long periods of time. Warning signs of liver damage include nausea, tiredness, red and itchy skin, yellow eyes and skin (jaundice), and flu-like symptoms.
- Rare side effects may include sweating, blurred vision, worsening of angina or heart failure, wheezing, and sensitivity to light.
- Even though it is very rare, piroxicam may lower the number of blood cells you have. If you don't have enough white blood cells, your immunity is down, and you can get a fever, sore throat, or pneumonia. If you are lacking red blood cells, you can become anemic, and that makes you tired and weak. Not having enough blood platelets makes you bruise easily and keeps your blood from clotting properly when you're injured.

Be on the lookout for any of these symptoms of bone marrow depression.

Special warnings:
- Don't take this drug if you are allergic to aspirin or other NSAIDs.
- Take this drug with caution if you have low platelet counts, poor kidney or liver function, heart failure, high blood pressure, or any disorder that causes fluid retention.

Pregnancy and nursing mothers:
Not known if safe to use while you are pregnant. Not known if safe to use while you are nursing.

Possible food and drug interactions:
- Avoid alcohol while taking NSAIDs including piroxicam.
- Piroxicam may increase the antipsychotic drug lithium to toxic levels.
- Piroxicam may interact with anticoagulants.
- Effects of this drug may be decreased by aspirin.
- Antacids don't seem to interfere with the absorption of this drug.
- If you need to stop taking corticosteroids while you're taking piroxicam, be sure to withdraw slowly from the steroids instead of stopping suddenly.

Helpful hint:
- You shouldn't drive a car or operate heavy machinery until you are sure the medicine isn't making you drowsy or less than alert.

Sulindac

Brand name: *Clinoril* **(Generic available)**

What this drug does for you:
This nonsteroidal anti-inflammatory drug (NSAID) relieves the symptoms of arthritis, bursitis, gout, and ankylosing spondylitis.

Possible side effects of this drug:
- Common side effects include nausea, diarrhea, constipation, gas, stomach cramps, loss of appetite, ringing in the ears, itching, rash, water retention or swelling, headache, nervousness, and dizziness.
- Bleeding stomach ulcers and liver or kidney damage are rare but serious reactions to using sulindac for long periods of time. Warning signs of liver damage include nausea, tiredness, red and itchy skin, yellow eyes and skin (jaundice), and flu-like symptoms.
- Rare side effects may include inflammation of the tongue or mouth, inflammation of the pancreas, sensitivity to light, heart failure, heart palpitations, high blood pressure, abnormal sense of taste, allergic reaction, blurred vision and serious eye disorders, muscle weakness, vertigo, convulsions, and prickling or tingling sensation in hands or feet.
- Even though it is very rare, sulindac may lower the number of blood cells you have. If you don't have enough white blood cells, your immunity is down, and you can get a fever, sore throat, or pneumonia. If you are lacking red blood cells, you can become anemic, and that makes you

tired and weak. Not having enough blood platelets makes you bruise easily and keeps your blood from clotting properly when you're injured. Be on the lookout for any of these symptoms of bone marrow depression.

Special warnings:
- Don't take this drug if you are allergic to aspirin or other NSAIDs.
- Take this drug with caution if you have intestinal disease, poor liver or kidney function, poor heart function, high blood pressure, fluid retention, diabetes, or kidney stones.

Pregnancy and nursing mothers:
Not known if safe to use while you are pregnant. Not known if safe to use while you are nursing.

Possible food and drug interactions:
- Avoid alcohol and aspirin while taking NSAIDs such as sulindac.
- Sulindac may prolong bleeding time if used at the same time as anticoagulants.
- Sulindac may increase levels of the cancer drug methotrexate and the immunosuppressant cyclosporine to toxic levels.
- Effects of this drug may be decreased by the arthritis drug diflunisal.
- If you need to stop taking corticosteroids while you're taking sulindac, be sure to withdraw slowly from the steroids instead of stopping suddenly.

Helpful hint:
- Take with food, after meals, or with antacids to help prevent stomach irritation.

Tolmetin

Brand names: *Tolectin, Tolectin DS* **(Generic available)**

What this drug does for you:
This nonsteroidal anti-inflammatory drug (NSAID) relieves the symptoms of rheumatoid arthritis, osteoarthritis, and juvenile rheumatoid arthritis.

Possible side effects of this drug:
- This drug may cause headache, increase in blood pressure, fluid retention and swelling, dizziness, nausea, diarrhea, indigestion, constipation, gas, ulcer, ringing in the ears, skin irritation, and inflammation of the mouth or tongue.
- Bleeding stomach ulcers and liver or kidney damage are rare but serious reactions to using tolmetin for long periods of time. Warning signs of liver damage include nausea, tiredness, red and itchy skin, yellow eyes and skin (jaundice), and flu-like symptoms.
- Rare side effects may include itching and skin eruptions, fever, and heart failure.
- Even though it is very rare, tolmetin may lower the number of blood cells you have. If you don't have enough white blood cells, your immunity is down, and you can get a fever, sore throat, or pneumonia. If you are

lacking red blood cells, you can become anemic, and that makes you tired and weak. Not having enough blood platelets makes you bruise easily and keeps your blood from clotting properly when you're injured. Be on the lookout for any of these symptoms of bone marrow depression.

Special warnings:

- Don't take this drug if you are allergic to aspirin or other NSAIDs.
- People with stomach ulcer should not take this drug. This drug may cause gastrointestinal bleeding.
- Taking tolmetin is more likely to cause kidney problems if you are elderly, if you take diuretics, or if you have lupus, heart failure, or poor liver or kidney function.
- Take this drug with caution if you have liver abnormalities, high blood pressure, blood clotting disorders, or poor heart function.

Pregnancy and nursing mothers:

Category C. See page 9 for description of categories. Drug is present in mother's milk.

Possible food and drug interactions:

- Avoid alcohol and aspirin while taking NSAIDs such as tolmetin.
- Tolmetin may increase the effects of the anticoagulant warfarin.
- Tolmetin may increase levels of the cancer drug methotrexate, possibly to toxic levels.
- If you need to stop taking corticosteroids while you're taking tolmetin, be sure to withdraw slowly from the steroids instead of stopping suddenly.

Helpful hints:

- You may not get the full effect of this drug until you've been taking it for two to four weeks.
- If you are having stomach trouble, you can take antacids other than sodium bicarbonate along with tolmetin.

OTHER PAINKILLERS

Acetaminophen

Brand names: *Feverall, APAP, Redutemp* **(Generic available)**

What this drug does for you:

Acetaminophen temporarily relieves fever, minor aches and pains, and headaches.

Possible side effects of this drug:

- If you use high doses of acetaminophen for a long time, you could have severe liver damage. Warning signs of liver damage include nausea, tiredness, red and itchy skin, yellow eyes and skin (jaundice), and flu-like symptoms.
- Even though it is very rare, acetaminophen may lower the number of

blood cells you have. If you don't have enough white blood cells, your immunity is down, and you can get a fever, sore throat, or pneumonia. If you are lacking red blood cells, you can become anemic, and that makes you tired and weak. Not having enough blood platelets makes you bruise easily and keeps your blood from clotting properly when you're injured. Be on the lookout for any of these symptoms of bone marrow depression.

● Other rare side effects are rash, hives, and low blood sugar.

Special warnings:
● Don't take acetaminophen repeatedly if you have anemia or kidney or liver disease.
● Because of possible liver damage, take acetaminophen cautiously if you have a history of chronic alcohol abuse.
● Consult a doctor before giving acetaminophen to a child under 2 years old.

Pregnancy and nursing mothers:
Category B. See page 9 for description of categories. Drug is present in mother's milk, but breast-feeding mothers can use it safely in low doses for short periods of time.

Possible food and drug interactions:
● Don't use acetaminophen along with high doses of barbiturates, carbamazepine, hydantoins, rifampin, or sulfinpyrazone. These drugs can reduce the effects of acetaminophen and increase the possibility of liver damage.
● Caffeine may increase the pain-relieving effects of acetaminophen.
● Diflunisal may increase blood levels of acetaminophen.
● Taking ethanol and acetaminophen together increases your risk of liver damage.
● If you take this drug along with the tuberculosis drug isoniazid, the combination may cause liver damage.
● Taking zidovudine and acetaminophen together may increase your risk of bone marrow suppression.
● Alcohol increases the risk of liver damage from acetaminophen.

Helpful hints:
● If your fever is over 103.1 degrees Fahrenheit or it lasts for more than three days, you may have a serious illness. Call your doctor.
● This drug should begin working within 10 minutes to one hour.
● Acetaminophen will not significantly reduce inflammation.

Acetaminophen with Codeine

Brand names: *Capital and Codeine, Phenaphen with Codeine, Tylenol with Codeine* **(Generic available)**

What this drug does for you:
This drug combines a narcotic painkiller with acetaminophen to relieve pain. Narcotics relieve pain by depressing your central nervous system.

Possible side effects of this drug:

- This drug most often causes dizziness, drowsiness, shortness of breath, and nausea. Less common reactions include constipation, exaggerated feelings of excitement or depression, stomach pain, and skin rashes. At high doses, codeine can depress your respiratory system, causing slow or irregular breathing.

Special warnings:

- This drug should be used with caution by people with head injuries, as it may increase fluid pressure on the brain.
- This drug should be used with caution by people who have stomach pain, kidney or liver disorders, underactive thyroid, or narrowing of the urethra.

Pregnancy and nursing mothers:

Category C. See page 9 for description of categories. Not known if drug is present in mother's milk.

Possible food and drug interactions:

- If you take drugs containing codeine along with alcohol or a drug that depresses your nervous system, such as tranquilizers, antihistamines, or muscle relaxants, the combination may dangerously depress your nervous system.
- If you take this drug along with the tuberculosis drug isoniazid, the combination may cause liver damage.
- If you take this drug along with the antiparkinson drug benztropine mesylate, the combination may cause paralysis of the intestines.

Helpful hints:

- You shouldn't drive a car or operate heavy machinery until you are sure the medicine isn't making you drowsy or less than alert.
- You may become physically and psychologically dependent on this drug if you take high doses for long periods of time. Never take more medicine than you are prescribed.

Acetaminophen with Hydrocodone Bitartrate

Brand names: *Anexsia, Bancap HC, Hydrocet, Lorcet, Lorcet Plus, Lortab, Panacet, Vicodin, Vicodin ES* **(Generic available)**

What this drug does for you:

This drug combines acetaminophen with a narcotic painkiller very similar to codeine. Narcotics relieve pain by depressing your central nervous system.

Possible side effects of this drug:

- This drug most often causes dizziness, drowsiness, and nausea. It can also cause constipation, mood changes, mental clouding, and difficulty urinating. One of the most dangerous side effects of hydrocodone at high doses is slow or irregular breathing.

Special warnings:

- Hydrocodone suppresses the cough reflex, so people with lung disease should take this drug with caution.
- This drug should be used with caution by people with head injuries, as it may increase fluid pressure on the brain.
- Older people and people with liver or kidney damage, an underactive thyroid, Addison's disease, or an enlarged prostate should take this drug with caution.

Pregnancy and nursing mothers:

Category C. See page 9 for description of categories. It is not known whether drug is present in mother's milk.

Possible food and drug interactions:

- If you take this drug along with alcohol or a drug that depresses your nervous system, such as tranquilizers, antihistamines, or muscle relaxants, the combination may dangerously depress your nervous system.
- Taking monoamine oxidase (MAO) inhibitors or tricyclic antidepressants with this drug can increase the effects of either the antidepressant or this drug.
- If you take this drug along with the antiparkinson drug benztropine mesylate, the combination may cause paralysis of the intestines.
- If you take this drug along with the tuberculosis drug isoniazid, the combination may cause liver damage.

Helpful hints:

- You shouldn't drive a car or operate heavy machinery until you are sure the medicine isn't making you drowsy or less than alert.
- You may become physically and psychologically dependent on this drug if you take high doses for long periods of time. Never take more medicine than you are prescribed.

Acetaminophen with Oxycodone

Brand names: *Percocet, Tylox, Roxicet*

What this drug does for you:

This drug combines acetaminophen with a narcotic painkiller similar to morphine.

Possible side effects of this drug:

- Side effects include dizziness, sleepiness, nausea, rash, itching, constipation, and mood changes. Large doses may cause slow or irregular breathing.

Special warnings:

- This drug should be used with caution by people with head injuries, as it may increase fluid pressure on the brain.
- Older people and people with liver or kidney damage, an underactive thyroid, Addison's disease, or an enlarged prostate should take this drug with caution.

Pregnancy and nursing mothers:

Category C. See page 9 for description of categories. Not known if drug is present in mother's milk.

Possible food and drug interactions:

- If you take this drug along with alcohol or a drug that depresses your nervous system, such as tranquilizers, antihistamines, or muscle relaxants, the combination may dangerously depress your nervous system.
- Taking monoamine oxidase (MAO) inhibitors or tricyclic antidepressants with this drug can increase the effects of either the antidepressant or this drug.
- If you take this drug along with the antiparkinson drug benztropine mesylate, the combination may cause paralysis of the intestines.
- If you take this drug along with the tuberculosis drug isoniazid, the combination may cause liver damage.

Helpful hints:

- You shouldn't drive a car or operate heavy machinery until you are sure the medicine isn't making you drowsy or less than alert.
- You may become physically and psychologically dependent on this drug if you take high doses for long periods of time. Never take more medicine than you are prescribed.

Acetaminophen with Propoxyphene

Brand name: *Darvocet-N* (Generic available)

What this drug does for you:

This drug combines acetaminophen with a narcotic painkiller similar to morphine to relieve pain and fever.

Possible side effects of this drug:

- The most common side effects are dizziness, sleepiness, and nausea. Other side effects include headache, constipation, hallucinations, liver damage, exaggerated feelings of depression or anxiety, rash, dangerously low blood pressure, and stomach pain.

Special warnings:

- High doses or long-term use of propoxyphene can lead to drug dependence. Take this drug with caution if you are prone to addiction or if you are taking other depressants.
- People with liver or kidney problems may need a reduced dose.

Pregnancy and nursing mothers:

Not known if drug is safe to use in pregnancy. Drug is present in mother's milk.

Possible food and drug interactions:

- If you take propoxyphene along with alcohol or a drug that depresses your nervous system, such as tranquilizers, antihistamines, or muscle relaxants, the combination may dangerously depress your nervous system.

- Propoxyphene may increase the effects of anticoagulants and anticonvulsants.
- If you take propoxyphene with high doses of aspirin, the combination may cause kidney damage.

Helpful hints:

- You shouldn't drive a car or operate heavy machinery until you are sure the medicine isn't making you drowsy or less than alert.
- You may avoid some of the side effects if you lie down after taking this drug.
- You may become physically and psychologically dependent on this drug if you take high doses for long periods of time. Never take more medicine than you are prescribed.

Meperidine

Brand name: *Demerol* **(Generic available)**

What this drug does for you:

This drug is a narcotic pain reliever.

Possible side effects of this drug:

- The major risks of taking this drug are slowed or irregular breathing (some people have stopped breathing) and slowed circulation (some people have had cardiac arrest, which means their circulation has stopped).
- The most common side effects are dizziness, sleepiness, nausea, and sweating. Other side effects include constipation, headache, convulsions, agitation, hallucinations, visual abnormalities, dry mouth, flushing, rash, itching, hives, rapid or irregular heartbeat, low blood pressure, and fainting.

Special warnings:

- You should take meperidine with extreme caution if you have head injuries, asthma, or other respiratory diseases.
- People with a history of convulsions, kidney or liver problems, Addison's disease, underactive thyroid, enlarged prostate, or irregular heartbeat should take meperidine with caution.

Pregnancy and nursing mothers:

Not known if drug is safe to use in pregnancy. Drug is present in mother's milk.

Possible food and drug interactions:

- If you take meperidine along with alcohol or a drug that depresses your nervous system, such as tranquilizers, antihistamines, or muscle relaxants, the combination may dangerously depress your nervous system.
- Don't take meperidine and the antidepressant drugs called monoamine oxidase (MAO) inhibitors at the same time. You should quit taking MAO inhibitors for at least two weeks before you begin taking meperidine.

Helpful hints:

- You shouldn't drive a car or operate heavy machinery until you are sure

the medicine isn't making you drowsy or less than alert.
- You may become physically and psychologically dependent on this drug if you take high doses for long periods of time. Never take more medicine than you are prescribed.

Methadone

Brand name: *Dolophine* (Generic available)

What this drug does for you:
This narcotic painkiller is used to relieve severe pain and to treat drug addiction.

Possible side effects of this drug:
- The major risks of taking this drug are slowed or irregular breathing (some people have stopped breathing) and slowed circulation (some people have had cardiac arrest, which means their circulation has stopped).
- The most common side effects are dizziness, sleepiness, nausea, and sweating. Other side effects include weakness, insomnia, headache, loss of appetite, constipation, dry mouth, difficulty urinating, rash, itching, hives, water retention, flushing, heart palpitations, and fainting.

Special warnings:
- You should take this drug with caution if you have head injuries, asthma, underactive thyroid, poor kidney or liver function, enlarged prostate, or low blood pressure.

Pregnancy and nursing mothers:
Not known if drug is safe to use in pregnancy. Not known if drug is safe to use while nursing.

Possible food and drug interactions:
- If you take methadone along with alcohol or a drug that depresses your nervous system, such as tranquilizers, antihistamines, or muscle relaxants, the combination may dangerously depress your nervous system.
- Methadone may increase the effects of the antidepressant desipramine.
- Levels or effects of methadone may be decreased by the tuberculosis drug rifampin.
- Methadone and the antidepressant drugs called monoamine oxidase (MAO) inhibitors should be taken together very cautiously. Your doctor may want to give you small doses of the drugs and observe you for side effects.

Helpful hints:
- You shouldn't drive a car or operate heavy machinery until you are sure the medicine isn't making you drowsy or less than alert.
- You may become physically and psychologically dependent on this drug. Never take more medicine than you are prescribed.
- This drug can cause very low blood pressure. Be careful when you stand or sit up quickly — you may feel lightheaded and dizzy.

Morphine

Brand names: *Astramorph/PF, Duramorph, MS Contin, MSIR, Roxanol, Oramorph SR, Rescudose, MS/L, MS/S, OMS, RMS* **(Generic available)**

What this drug does for you:

This narcotic analgesic relieves moderate to severe pain.

Possible side effects of this drug:

- The major risks of taking this drug are slowed or irregular breathing (some people have stopped breathing) and slowed circulation (some people have had cardiac arrest, which means their circulation has stopped).
- The most common side effects are constipation, dizziness, sleepiness, nausea, sweating, and mood changes. Other side effects may include insomnia, weakness, tremors, prickling or tingling sensation, loss of appetite, headache, difficulty urinating, itching, hives, rash, water retention, dry mouth, vision abnormalities, fainting, and heart palpitations.

Special warnings:

- Morphine should not be used by people with allergies to narcotics, asthma, breathing difficulty, or paralysis of the intestines.
- Morphine should be used with extreme caution by people with head injuries, lesions or increased pressure in the skull, or respiratory depression.
- Use morphine with caution if you have any of the following conditions: inflammation of the pancreas, swelling and fluid retention associated with underactive thyroid, alcoholism or alcohol withdrawal, Addison's disease (progressive weakening of the adrenal gland), enlarged prostate, psychosis resulting from exposure to a toxic substance, coma, curvature of the spine, or liver, kidney, or lung disease.

Pregnancy and nursing mothers:

Category C. See page 9 for description of categories. Drug is present in mother's milk.

Possible food and drug interactions:

- If you take morphine along with alcohol or a drug that depresses your nervous system, such as tranquilizers, antihistamines, or muscle relaxants, the combination may dangerously depress your nervous system.

Helpful hints:

- Don't crush or break the morphine tablets as it may lead to rapid absorption and possible overdose.
- You shouldn't drive a car or operate heavy machinery until you are sure the medicine isn't making you drowsy or less than alert.
- You may become physically and psychologically dependent on this drug. Never take more medicine than you are prescribed.
- This drug can cause very low blood pressure. Be careful when you stand or sit up quickly — you may feel lightheaded and dizzy. You may want

to lie down for a while after you take the morphine to help prevent some of the side effects.

Oxycodone

Brand name: *Roxicodone*

What this drug does for you:
This drug is a narcotic painkiller similar to morphine.

Possible side effects of this drug:
- Side effects include dizziness, sleepiness, nausea, rash, itching, constipation, and mood changes. Large doses may cause slow or irregular breathing.

Special warnings:
- This drug should be used with caution by people with head injuries, as it may increase fluid pressure on the brain.
- Older people and people with liver or kidney damage, an underactive thyroid, Addison's disease, or an enlarged prostate should take this drug with caution.

Pregnancy and nursing mothers:
Not known if drug is safe to use while you're pregnant. Not known if drug is present in mother's milk.

Possible food and drug interactions:
- If you take this drug along with alcohol or a drug that depresses your nervous system, such as tranquilizers, antihistamines, or muscle relaxants, the combination may dangerously depress your nervous system.

Helpful hints:
- You shouldn't drive a car or operate heavy machinery until you are sure the medicine isn't causing blurred vision or making you drowsy, dizzy, or less than alert.
- You may become physically and psychologically dependent on this drug if you take high doses for long periods of time. Never take more medicine than you are prescribed.
- You may want to lie down for a while after you take the oxycodone to help prevent some of the side effects.

Propoxyphene

Brand names: *Darvon, PP-CAP* (Generic available)

What this drug does for you:
This narcotic analgesic is used to relieve mild to moderate pain.

Possible side effects of this drug:
- The most common side effects are dizziness, sleepiness, and nausea. Other side effects include headache, constipation, hallucinations, liver damage, exaggerated feelings of depression or anxiety, rash, dangerous-

ly low blood pressure, and stomach pain.

Special warnings:
- High doses or long-term use of propoxyphene can lead to drug dependence. Take this drug with caution if you are prone to addiction or if you are taking other depressants.
- People with liver or kidney problems may need a reduced dose.

Pregnancy and nursing mothers:
Not known if drug is safe to use in pregnancy. Drug is present in mother's milk.

Possible food and drug interactions:
- If you take propoxyphene along with alcohol or a drug that depresses your nervous system, such as tranquilizers, antihistamines, or muscle relaxants, the combination may dangerously depress your nervous system.
- Propoxyphene may increase the effects of anticoagulants and anticonvulsants.
- If you take propoxyphene with high doses of aspirin, the combination may cause kidney damage.

Helpful hints:
- You shouldn't drive a car or operate heavy machinery until you are sure the medicine isn't making you drowsy or less than alert.
- You may avoid some of the side effects if you lie down after taking this drug.
- You may become physically and psychologically dependent on this drug if you take high doses for long periods of time. Never take more medicine than you are prescribed.

Natural Alternatives 🍎

ARTHRITIS

◄ Joint pain or stiffness
◄ Redness, warmth, or tenderness in joints
◄ Swelling of joints, especially fingers
◄ Limited movement in affected joints

Ace arthritis
According to an old Yiddish proverb, "People can be divided into three groups: Those who make things happen, those who watch things happen, and those who wonder what happened." Traditional medicine has not yet found a cure for arthritis, or for many conditions that cause long-lasting pain. So if you have any form of arthritis or chronic pain, you can't afford to be in any group except the one that makes things happen. That means taking an active role in developing a plan to lessen your arthritis pain.

Exercise! Before the 1980s, doctors didn't advise people with arthritis to exercise because they thought that too much activity would make arthritis worse. But studies have shown that moderate, carefully planned exercise programs really help most people with arthritis. Exercise can reduce the amount of pain medication you need and can increase strength and flexibility by making the muscles around joints stronger. If your joints are swollen and inflamed, you must exercise gently and cautiously. Avoid exercises that are jarring or put strong pressure on joints. If you feel intense pain for several hours after exercising or if your joints feel stiffer than before, you may need to reevaluate your exercise program and cut back the intensity.

The best arthritis program includes three types of exercise:
◁ *Range of motion exercises* move a joint through its full range of motion and just to the point where you start to feel pain or discomfort. They reduce pain and keep joints mobile.
◁ *Strengthening exercises* improve muscle strength and increase endurance. Exercises that are isometric (using the muscle without moving the joint) and isotonic (using the muscle and moving the joint fully) fall into this category. They improve the ability to bear weight, move easily, and lift objects.
◁ *Endurance exercises* such as walking, swimming, and stationary bicycling improve your overall physical fitness and endurance.

Be sure to check with your doctor before you begin exercising. Once he gives his OK, work with a certified physical therapist, or look for a book at your local library that illustrates these different exercises.

Take steps to make your life more comfortable. A big part of your plan for living with arthritis should be finding new, less painful ways to accomplish your daily activities. Try these ways to organize yourself and your day.
◁ Each morning, plan out your day. List all the things you need to do in order of importance. Get the most important things done earlier in the day in case you get tired early.
◁ Organize your work space so all of your "tools" are nearby. Keep the television remote control in the same place so you can always find it. Store sewing supplies or cooking utensils in waist-level cabinets or shelves. Keep a notepad and pen on a table beside the telephone.
◁ Arrange chairs so that you can sit instead of stand while cooking, talking on the phone, ironing, cleaning, etc. That will take pressure off your joints. A high stool is useful in the kitchen for cooking or washing dishes.
◁ Avoid soft, deep-cushioned chairs. They can be hard to get out of, putting unnecessary strain on your arms and shoulders. Even in someone else's home, look for a chair that will allow you to sit down and get up easily.

Plan your moves to prevent excess stress on your joints.
◁ Avoid tight grasping motions that may strain your hands. Install larger handles on household objects. One simple way is to use soft foam rubber and wide tape to build up handles with foam padding, so you don't have to grip as tightly.
◁ Use your strongest joints and muscles to do a task. You could carry a

small backpack or fanny pack instead of a purse with a handle. Start pushing open doors with your arm or shoulder rather than your hand.

◁ Always use good posture to avoid unnecessary strain. Make sure work-tables are the correct height. You should be able to work on a table with your arms comfortably at your sides, with your forearms at 90 degree angles from your upper arms. When lifting an object off the floor, bend your knees, rather than your back, and keep your back straight as you go down and back up.

◁ Don't sit in the same position for a long time. Get up and move around every once in a while so you don't become stiff. Do a few range-of-motion exercises to loosen up again.

◁ Find a balance between activity and rest. Rotate periods of work with periods of light activity or rest. Rest is just as important as keeping active, but both should be done in moderation.

Put pressure on pain. Try acupressure. With this method, you use your hands to put pressure on 12 pressure points (located on or near certain joints) on each side of your body, to strengthen joints and relieve pain. To find out more about acupressure, read *Arthritis Pain at Your Fingertips: The Complete Self-Care Guide to Easing Aches and Pains without Drugs* by Michael Reed Gach (Warner Books, New York, 1989).

Fight arthritis with food

The role of diet in arthritis is controversial, and studies on this subject are ongoing. Some doctors believe that it is an important factor, and some do not think it has any effect at all. As long as the diet changes you make are healthy ones, you don't have anything to lose by trying them, and you could have a lot

---

Miracle cures aren't all they're cracked up to be, but real cures could be right around the corner

Be cautious of trying new "cures" for arthritis. It's best to check with your doctor before trying anything that sounds unlikely or dangerous.

On the other hand, researchers are studying new treatments every day. Some scientists predict that within five years, doctors will be transplanting new cartilage into joints damaged by osteoarthritis.

Research on animals has shown that collagen is a promising new treatment for rheumatoid arthritis. Collagen treatments in humans may begin soon.

Studies of the immune system are also bringing to light new information about how inflammation starts in rheumatoid arthritis. If researchers can figure out how it starts, they may be able to develop ways to stop it. And that would be the first step toward a cure.

So keep an eye toward new treatments and keep a positive attitude. But don't let your enthusiasm get you too carried away by miracle cures. Read, study, think for yourself, and then talk to your doctor.

Source —
Unproven Remedies, Arthritis Foundation, P.O. Box 19000, Atlanta, Ga. 30326, 1987

to gain.

Forgo saturated fat. Recently, scientists fed a diet high in saturated fat to a group of mice and fed a second group a diet high in unsaturated fat. The group that ate saturated fat developed more severe cases of osteoarthritis.

Saturated fat is found in meat and dairy products and in palm and coconut oils. Eliminating saturated fat from your diet is important for your overall health too.

Go vegetarian. Changing to a vegetarian diet may improve your symptoms of rheumatoid arthritis. In one study, participants fasted for a week and then ate a carefully controlled diet for about five months.

The first phase of the diet was limited to vegetables and juices. Then other foods were gradually added one at a time. But the dieters continued to avoid meat, fish, eggs, dairy products, citrus fruits, refined sugar, alcoholic beverages, coffee, tea, and foods containing gluten such as wheat, oats, barley, and rye.

As a result, pain and swelling decreased, and grip strength increased. The diet seemed very successful, since the participants' symptoms were still improved a year later.

Use the right oil. A recent Australian study has shown that using oils and spreads rich in linoleic acid can fight the pain and swelling of arthritis. Linoleic acid is found in flaxseed, corn, safflower, sunflower, and canola oil. Look for the cold-pressed versions of these oils.

Evening primrose oil is a natural supplement high in linoleic acid. Taking fish oil supplements or adding more fish to your diet may also help your arthritis.

Beat arthritis with B vitamins. Vitamin B supplements can offer you the pain relief of traditional prescription arthritis medicines at a fraction of the cost. Researchers at the University of Missouri in Columbia found that taking a daily supplement of 6,400 mcg of folic acid and 20 mcg of cobalamin (two common B vitamins) can relieve the pain and tenderness of osteoarthritis.

Unlike nonsteroidal anti-inflammatory drugs (NSAIDs), the vitamin supplements do not usually cause side effects, and they are much less expensive to use. You will need to get your doctor to write a prescription for the supplements and have him supervise your treatment. A doctor can prescribe larger doses of the vitamins in a more compact form, so that you don't have to take a lot of pills.

Expose arthritis impostors

Sometimes joint pain that seems like arthritis is actually caused by something else entirely. That is why it's called "false" arthritis. A doctor can do specific tests to determine whether you have real arthritis or an imposter.

It could be a food allergy. A recent study seems to suggest that food allergies may be a cause of rheumatoid arthritis. About half the study participants believed they had certain food allergies. Most of them actually felt better while they were fasting, and they got worse when they started eating again.

If you have arthritis, pay particular attention to foods you don't digest well or that cause any unusual symptoms. Here are the top arthritis triggers, listed in order of most common trigger to least: corn, wheat, pork, oranges, milk, oats, rye, eggs, beef, coffee, malt, cheese, grapefruit, tomatoes, peanuts, sugar, butter, lamb, lemon, and soybeans.

To test a food you suspect may be causing you problems, eliminate that food from your diet for one week. If your symptoms subside, you may have identified one of your food triggers. You can double-check by reintroducing the suspect food into your diet to see if your symptoms return.

It could be a curable illness. Another arthritis imposter is the tiny human parvovirus. It causes a curable illness that seems like arthritis. The illness is called "chronic arthropathy" to distinguish it from arthritis.

Symptoms include a flulike sickness and stiff joints. Those most vulnerable to getting human parvovirus are people with AIDS, chronic anemia, or sickle cell anemia.

It could be food poisoning. The food poisoning illness called "salmonella," which is caused by bacteria, can also cause joint inflammation. But the arthritis-like symptoms may not appear until after the salmonella illness is over.

Doctors can diagnose it because of the presence of antibodies, which are produced by the body in response to an attack by a foreign organism.

It could be a drug reaction. A number of prescription drugs can cause joint pain that seems like arthritis. If you are taking any prescription drug and begin to get symptoms of arthritis, see your doctor. It may be true arthritis, or it may be a drug reaction.

Sources —

American Journal of Clinical Nutrition (50,2:353 and 61,2:320)

Arthritis Relief at Your Fingertips: The Complete Self-Care Guide to Easing Aches and Pains Without Drugs, Warner Books, New York, 1989

Arthritis, Farmers, and Ranchers, Arthritis Foundation, P.O. Box 19000, Atlanta, Ga. 30326, 1993

British Journal of Rheumatology (32,6:507)

Food, Nutrition and Health (18,5:3)

Journal of the American College of Nutrition (13,4:351)

Medical Tribune (36,7:18)

National Institute of Arthritis and Musculoskeletal and Skin Diseases, Box AMS, 9000 Rockville Pike, Bethesda, Md. 20892

Science News (138,19:294)

The Doctor's Complete Guide to Vitamins and Minerals, Dell Publishing, New York, 1994

The Lancet (338,8772:899 and 344,8930:1125)

Using Your Joints Wisely, Arthritis Foundation, P.O. Box 19000, Atlanta, Ga. 30326, 1992

BACK PAIN

◄ **Low backache or sharp back pain**
◄ **Pain radiating from the back down into the legs**

Beat back attacks

Back pain got you down for the count?

Don't let yourself be beaten by a bad back. Harness your own healing powers and knock out back pain forever.

Take a painkiller and take it easy. Aspirin or ibuprofen, gentle massage, and bed rest may the best treatment the first couple of days after you hurt your back. Lie in bed on your back with a pillow under your knees or on your side with a pillow between your knees. Relax and think positive thoughts. Remind yourself that this is only temporary.

Don't get too comfortable. Too much bed rest may make your road to recovery longer than necessary. Get out of bed and move around as soon as you can — even if it's just for short periods of time.

Pack on ice or heat. Freeze water in a paper cup to make yourself a cheap and convenient massage tool. Once the ice is solid, peel away the paper from one end of the cup. Have a spouse or friend use the icy end of the cup to massage the painful area of your back for seven to 10 minutes. You can repeat the ice massage once an hour if you need it.

If you normally get more pain relief from warmth, try an electric heating pad. Place it against the painful area of your back, but be sure not to burn yourself with too much heat or fall asleep with it turned on.

Lose weight. Carrying those extra pounds around your waist is a constant strain on your back. Excess weight is easier to lose if you exercise as well as eat a low-fat and low-calorie diet.

Snuff out those cigarettes. If you are a smoker, you may be worsening your back pain. Some researchers think that smoking decreases blood flow to the backbone. Less blood flow means more risk of injury. Others think that "smoker's cough" strains the muscles in your back.

Get your aerobic exercise. Try for at least 30 minutes of aerobic exercise three or four times a week, stretching before and after you exercise to prevent injury and strengthen your back.

Walking is an excellent exercise. It gives you the same benefits as running without the high-impact movements that compress disks or twist ligaments. Bike riding and swimming are also back-friendly aerobic exercises.

Don't bend and twist your back when you rake, vacuum, or mop. Keep your back straight, and move your arms and legs smoothly. Your job may take longer, but your back will appreciate it. Buy lightweight gardening tools and cleaning equipment with long handles.

When unloading your dishwasher, pivot on your feet so that you keep your hips and shoulders in line and bend at the knees and hips.

To reach a high shelf, put your feet in a staggered stance (one foot in

Strike out sciatica

Many people think back pain is only caused by lifting heavy objects or somehow injuring your back, but you can develop sciatica — pain in the lower back, buttocks, and legs — during pregnancy or just from sitting at your desk all day.

The sciatic nerve runs from the lower back through the buttocks and down the back of your leg. Pressure on this nerve can shoot pain from the lower back to the feet. You may feel some numbness or tingling along the nerve too.

For most sciatica sufferers, treatment is not far away. Everyday pain relievers, such as aspirin and ibuprofen, can ease your discomfort, and bed rest will get you in the groove again quickly.

Sudden attacks of pain can be soothed by lying flat on your back for a while. Gentle stretches can also take the pain away. You should see your doctor if your pain doesn't go away after a couple of days.

To prevent future sciatica attacks, remember to take regular breaks if you have to stand or sit for long periods of time.

Sources —

Complete Guide to Symptoms, Illness and Surgery, The Putnam Berkeley Group, New York, 1995

The American Medical Association Encyclopedia of Medicine, Random House, New York, 1989

---

front of the other), then push off your back foot onto your front foot as you reach up, keeping your hips and shoulders in line. Don't lift heavy objects above your shoulders. Stand on a stool or sturdy chair instead.

Sleep on your side with your legs drawn up slightly toward your chest. You can use a pillow under your head and between your knees. Make sure your mattress is firm and in good condition.

If you absolutely must sleep on your stomach, tuck a small pillow under your tummy to keep your back straight. If you sleep on your back, put a pillow under your knees to relieve strain on your back.

Lift with your knees. When lifting things from the ground, squat with a straight back while bending your knees. Let your legs do the lifting instead of your back.

Kick the high heel habit. Wear comfortable, flat shoes with good support.

Say no to surgery. Most people with back pain improve without surgery. In fact, the long-term results of people who have surgery are the same as those who don't.

In a study of 126 people with ruptured disks, half the group underwent surgery and the other half were treated without surgery. Four years later, the two groups showed very little — if any — difference.

The number of surgeries done on the lower back increases with the growth of new imaging techniques, such as MRI. When an MRI reveals a ruptured disk, doctors are likely to point to that as the cause of your back pain. They will probably suggest surgery as a cure.

But interpretations of an MRI scan can vary from doctor to doctor. So if your doctor suggests back surgery based on the results of imaging testing, get a second opinion.

And keep in mind that 96 percent of all back injuries will heal with rest and rehabilitative exercises.

Exercise to build a strong back

The better your overall health is, the less likely you are to have a back injury. By strengthening the muscles that affect your back you are taking out your own insurance policy against back injury. Plus, you'll often relieve your back pain in the process. Being in good physical shape can prevent future back attacks too.

Stretch your back gently. Stretching will control muscle spasms and relieve muscle tightness. You can do these easy stretches at home or work:

◁ Push back into your chair's back support to stretch. Straighten your legs and flex your ankles and feet.

◁ Stretch like a cat. Stand up and place your hands about shoulder width apart on a table. Arch your back like a cat, looking at the floor, then push your back downward, looking at the ceiling.

◁ Sit on the floor and draw your knees to your chest. Hold this position for 10 seconds, then relax. Repeat the exercise two or three times to stretch out your muscles.

◁ Relaxing your entire body is a great way to ease back muscle pain. Close your eyes and try to feel yourself contracting and relaxing each muscle in your body. Begin with your face muscles and work your way down to your toes.

◁ Lie on your back on a firm surface with your knees bent. Place your

---

Work a miracle with your mind

In his book *Mind Over Back Pain*, Dr. John Sarno discusses his revolutionary approach of allowing your mind to work with your body to heal back pain. He believes that tension and your body's physical response to it are at the root of most chronic back pain, instead of injury or abnormal structure of the spine.

Tension, followed by pain and then fear, begins a vicious cycle. You feel pain, then fear more pain and physical limitation, causing even more tension to continue the cycle.

Dr. Sarno believes that you can break this cycle by understanding the process of the pain, being aware of it, and accepting it. When you feel in control, instead of feeling helpless and victimized by some outside force, you can bring about your own healing. Most people get relief from Dr. Sarno's program in four to eight weeks.

Neck and shoulder pain; sciatica; and tendinitis of the knee, ankle, Achilles tendon, and elbow ("tennis elbow") may respond well to this same type of therapy.

Source —
Mind Over Back Pain, Berkeley Books, New York, 1986

hands beneath the small of your back. Let your back rest on your hands while you tilt your pelvis upward. Hold for several seconds and relax. Repeat four or five times.

◁ Sit up straight in a chair. Raise both feet about one inch off the floor at the same time. Hold for several seconds. Repeat.

◁ Lie on your back with your rear end close to the wall, and your legs and heels placed against the wall. Do not bend your legs at the knee. If your legs bend, move farther back from the wall. Hold this position about 15 minutes. Repeat every day. As your hamstrings loosen, you will be able to move closer to the wall.

Stand up straight. Standing and sitting properly help more than just your looks. Good posture strengthens your bones, muscles, and ligaments and helps keep your back healthy.

To learn what good standing posture feels like, get to work on the following exercise. Repeat the entire exercise three times a day.

Stand with your back against a wall, heels three inches from the wall, feet about six inches apart. Let your arms hang at your sides, palms facing forward. Keep your ankles straight, knees facing front, and lower back close to the wall. Straighten your upper back, lifting your chest and placing your shoulders against the wall. Lean your head against the wall and tuck your chin in toward your chest.

Now, pull up and in with your lower abdominal muscles, trying to flatten your stomach. Hold this position for 10 seconds, breathing normally. Relax and repeat three or four times.

Strike a kingly pose. To improve your sitting posture, try the previous exercise sitting in a straight-back, armless chair with both feet flat on the floor. Repeat the entire exercise three times a day.

Pay attention to your posture at all times. At work or home, keep your head up while typing or writing, and keep your chair close to the desk. If you feel your back begin to arch forward, put your feet on a stool.

Tighten your tummy. Poor posture weakens the lower stomach muscles, but you can improve your posture by doing the following tummy tightener three times a day:

Stand comfortably. Clasp your hands and cup them around your lower abdomen. Pull up and in with your lower stomach muscles, drawing in your abdomen.

Hold this position for 10 seconds. Relax and repeat four or five times.

Sources —

American Family Physician (49,1:171)
Back Works, BookPartners, Seattle, 1993
Geriatrics (49,2:22)
Managing Back Pain, We Care for You, Baylor College of Medicine, Houston, Texas
Medical Tribune (34,10:10)
Medical Update (16,9:4)
No More Aching Back, Villard Books, New York, 1990
Surgical Neurology (1993,39:5)
The New England Journal of Medicine (331,2:69)

The Physician and Sportsmedicine (21,3:183)
The Secret of Good Posture, American Physical Therapy Association, 1111 North
Fairfax Street, Alexandria, Va., 22314, 1985

BURSITIS

◀ Severe pain in the joints of the hip, knee, elbow, groin, or foot
◀ Severe shoulder pain with movement of the arm

Five ways to beat bursitis

A sharp blow or too much exercise can bring on an attack of bursitis. The
shoulder and the hip are the most common sites of pain, but other vulnerable
spots are the knee, elbow, groin, and foot joints (bunions are a form of bursitis). You usually bring on the pain by overusing or straining your joints and
muscles.

Here are some things you can do for bursitis pain:

Rest to avoid further damage. Stop the activity that caused the problem
until the pain is gone and the inflammation heals. Try to find alternatives to
activities that irritate the inflamed area.

Ice it. For the first 48 hours of treatment, use ice or cold packs to stop the
swelling. After that, you can use a heating pad to stimulate blood flow and
ease the pain.

Give it support. You may want to use a splint or sling to keep your shoulder or elbow still, or add padding to protect from bumps. An elastic bandage
may help decrease swelling and provide support to the area. You may also
want to try using an elbow, wrist, ankle, or knee brace for support.

Aspirin can help. Any anti-inflammatory, such as aspirin or ibuprofen, can
help ease pain and speed healing.

Gentle exercises promote healing. As the pain subsides, you can begin
gentle range-of-motion exercises. Exercise slowly, and stop if you feel pain.

Sources —
Exercise and Your Arthritis, Arthritis Foundation, P.O. Box 19000, Atlanta, Ga. 30326,
1994
U.S. Pharmacist (20,1:33)

GOUT

◀ Fever
◀ Red, hot, swollen, and very tender joints

◀ Red and shiny skin over joints
◀ Sudden, severe, throbbing pain
  in a joint, especially the big toe

Get rid of gout

Some people may not be aware that gout is a type of arthritis. It mostly
strikes men over the age of 40, and occurs when too much uric acid builds up
in the blood and then lodges in a joint. The result is usually a very sore,

swollen big toe.

The symptoms can come on suddenly, virtually overnight, and can last for just a few days and go away. But the gout may come back and be worse the next time. Gout can attack other areas, including the shoulders, elbows, wrists, fingers, spine, pelvis, and some organs of the body. Here's how to help your gout:

Lose weight and eliminate alcohol. The causes of gout are easy to pinpoint. Being overweight and drinking too much alcohol on a regular basis are known to contribute to uric acid buildup.

Go on a low-purine diet. Eating too many foods high in a substance called "purines" could cause gout or worsen its symptoms. The body converts purines into uric acid. Foods high in purines include liver, kidneys, brains, anchovies, sardines, scallops, peas, dried beans, asparagus, cauliflower, mushrooms, and spinach.

Drink six to eight glasses of water a day. Water dilutes uric acid and helps the kidneys remove it.

Check your blood pressure drugs. In some cases, gout may be caused by thiazide diuretics — drugs used to treat high blood pressure. This form of gout usually attacks joints in the hands and knees of older women who may have poor kidney function.

If you are taking a thiazide diuretic and you get severe pain in your hands or knees, you should be checked for gout.

Sources —
Bowes and Church's Food Values of Portions Commonly Used, 15th ed., Harper-Collins Publishers, New York, 1989
FDA Consumer (29,2:19)
Western Journal of Medicine (150,4:419)

HEADACHES

◀ Drooping eyelid

◀ Irritated, teary eyes

◀ Light and noise sensitivity

◀ Nausea

◀ Vomiting

◀ Intense pain in the head, neck, and shoulders

◀ Nasal congestion

◀ Throbbing pain in the head

Head off headaches

It's been said that two heads are better than one. When you have a raging headache, don't you sometimes wish you had an extra head you could switch for the hurting one?

It would be nice, but medical technology hasn't progressed that far just yet. They have, however, managed to classify headaches into three basic types:

Migraine headaches throb intensely on one or both sides of your head. They are often accompanied by nausea, vomiting, light and noise sensitivity, and the inability to carry out normal activities.

Cluster headaches begin with sudden and excruciating pain on one side of the head, usually around the eye or temple, accompanied by an irritated, teary eye, drooping eyelid, and nasal congestion. They occur in a series, or cluster, that may happen several times a day for a short or extended period of time. There is no known cause or cure although stopping smoking and not napping may help.

Tension-type headaches feel like a band tightening around your head, with additional pain sometimes occurring in your scalp, face, neck, and shoulder muscles. Tension headaches often develop in response to stress and anxiety.

Nine out of 10 headaches are the "tension-type," says The National Headache

Superhighway to a headache

For some people, certain foods, situations, and sounds are just a superhighway to a superheadache — a migraine.

Learn what triggers your migraines and try to avoid those things, so you can stay off the headache highway.

Common culprits include:

◁ Anxiety, depression, and fatigue
◁ Bright or flashing lights, loud noises, smoke, and strong odors
◁ Little or irregular physical activity; the motion of trains, cars, or planes; eyestrain; or head injury
◁ Too much or too little sleep
◁ Hormonal influences, such as premenstrual tension, estrogen supplements, or contraceptives
◁ Overuse of over-the-counter pain medicines
◁ Skipping meals
◁ Alcohol (especially red wine)
◁ Reactions to the following foods:
  Aspartame — artificial sweetener used to sweeten diet drinks and low-calorie foods
  Caffeine — chocolate, coffee, tea, and colas
  Dairy products — milk, buttermilk, cream, ice cream, yogurt, and processed and aged cheeses
  Fruits — citrus fruits, bananas, figs, raisins, papaya, kiwi, plums, and pineapples
  Meats with nitrites and nitrates — preserved meats and deli meats
  Monosodium glutamate (MSG) — a flavor enhancer often included in Chinese food
  Nicotine
  Nuts
  Sulfites — found in salad bar foods, shrimp, and soft drinks
  Vegetables — most peas, onions, olives, pickles, and sauerkraut
  Yeast products — fresh breads, doughnuts, and yeast extract

Source —
The National Headache Foundation, 5252 N. Western Avenue, Chicago, Ill. 60625

Foundation. But when you have a headache, you don't really care what kind you have. You just want relief right then and there.

Here's how to get it:

Take breaks during stressful situations. To win the headache battle, look for these warning signs: pressure in your temples, tightness in your neck and shoulders, and irritability. When you see these signs, take a break, relax for a while, and give your mind and body a rest. Stop worrying. Don't let stress or circumstances you can't control trigger a migraine or tension headache. Breathing slowly and deeply (concentrate on moving your stomach in and out) can help to get rid of the tension in your body and prevent headaches. Gentle music, pleasant scents, or low lighting may also help you relax.

Don't pass up a vacation or a day off work. When headaches become a daily trial, you need to give yourself some time off.

Go to bed and get up at the same time every day, so that you get the right amount of sleep. Get enough sleep so you don't feel tired during the day. But don't overdose yourself on sleep during weekends. You're more likely to wake up with a headache.

Don't skip meals. Make sure you eat something for each meal of the day, even if it's just a quick snack. If your blood sugar falls too low, it can cause a migraine.

Exercise regularly. Try for three times a week, at least 30 minutes a session. For some migraine sufferers, exercise will stop a mild migraine even after it's begun.

Check your magnesium level. Researchers are now zeroing in on how pain in the head from a migraine or cluster headache could result from too little magnesium in the body. In one study of several hundred people, nearly half of those with migraine and cluster headaches were suspected of having a lack of active magnesium. This lack of magnesium seems to affect the constriction of blood vessels in your head, which can bring on a migraine attack.

Be sure to get your Recommended Daily Allowance for magnesium (350 mg for men 18 years and older and 280 mg for women 11 years and older). But check with your doctor before taking a magnesium supplement. Too much can be dangerous, and it can react badly with certain medicines.

Put riboflavin to the test. Riboflavin, also known as vitamin B2, may help with migraines. In a recent Belgian study, migraine sufferers who took a 400 mg supplement of riboflavin daily experienced less severe headache symptoms. More research needs to be done, but this vitamin may turn out to be an effective weapon against migraine pain.

Give two other nutrients a try — calcium and vitamin D. Supplements of these two nutrients recently helped provide relief to four women who suffered from migraines. Two of the women had migraines related to their menstrual periods. The other two women had passed menopause.

All the women originally had low blood levels of vitamin D. If you suspect you may have low vitamin D levels, taking a daily multivitamin that contains calcium and vitamin D may help your headaches.

Put your head on ice or be a little hot-headed. Keep an ice pack or a hot pack at the office so you can place it on your head or neck at the first sign of pain. A long, hot shower will also help ease tension and an aching head.

Eat a healthy diet. Emphasize fresh vegetables and fruits, whole grains, and low-fat foods.

Keep tabs on your caffeine intake. A caffeine-withdrawal headache feels just like a tension headache. If you normally drink several cups of coffee, tea, and soda a day, your head will probably ache dully when you miss your regular dose of caffeine.

Too much caffeine can give you a headache too. Your best bet is to try and give up caffeine gradually. If you must consume caffeine, spread it out evenly during the day. That way, you won't get too much at one time, and you'll have less chance of a reaction.

Headaches and depression go hand in hand. Depression may be the cause of a daily tension headache that hits the moment you wake up or early in the morning. If your headache falls into this pattern, you may have a chemical imbalance that could be improved with medication or you may need to work with friends, family members, a local support group, or a counselor to pull yourself out of the dumps.

Don't pop a pain reliever every day. For chronic headaches that occur more than 15 times a month, don't keep taking over-the-counter pain relievers without visiting your doctor. Pain relievers that you can buy without a prescription are generally less harmful than prescription medications, but they do have their side effects .

Aspirin, ibuprofen, and acetaminophen, especially those products that contain caffeine, can lead to a "rebound effect." Your body adapts to the pain reliever being in your system, and you become extra sensitive to pain when the medicine starts to wear off.

See your doctor if you're taking a large number of pain relievers, if frequent headaches are interfering with your daily life, or if a severe or constant headache is accompanied by weakness, dizziness, numbness, or other unusual physical sensations.

Sources —

American Family Physician (47,4:799 and 49,3:633)
Complete Guide to Vitamins, Minerals & Supplements, Fisher Books, Tucson, Ariz., 1988
Emergency Medicine (27,1:45)
Head Lines (Spring 1995, 92:3)
Headache (34,9:544 and 34,10:590)
National Headache Foundation Newsletter (86:14 and 87:6)
National Institute of Neurological Disorders and Stroke, Office of Scientific and Health Reports, Building 13 Room 8A16, 31 Center Dr. MSC 2540, Bethesda, Md. 20814
Pharmacy Times (61,9:34)
The National Headache Foundation, 5252 N. Western Avenue, Chicago, Ill. 60625

Nature's powerful painkillers

More and more scientific research supports what home healers have known for a long time. The same foods that please your palate can sometimes put a stop to your pain. Take a look at five of Mother Nature's most powerful painkillers.

Ginger — This savory spice is a food remedy for relieving arthritis and headaches. To relieve arthritis, take about 1/3 teaspoon of ginger three times a day. Dissolve the ginger in liquid or mix with food. Straight ginger can burn your mouth. At the first sign of headache, mix 1/3 teaspoon of powdered ginger into a glass of water and drink. If you have headaches frequently, especially migraines, you may benefit from including ginger in your diet regularly.

Peppermint — Peppermint tea works wonders for relieving headaches, especially migraines. To make peppermint tea, boil 1 pint of water. Remove from heat and add 2 tablespoons of fresh or dried peppermint leaves. Cover mixture and let steep for 50 minutes; strain. Drink one or two cups of tea.

You may also obtain relief by rubbing a little peppermint oil on your forehead, temples, and back of your neck.

Fish — This is a long-term cure, which means that a bite of fish when you have a headache won't relieve the pain right away. However, regularly including fish such as mackerel, sardines, salmon, and tuna in your diet can help lessen the frequency of migraine headaches. Eating fish may also prevent or relieve rheumatoid arthritis and osteoarthritis symptoms.

Turmeric — To relieve arthritis, add 1 teaspoon of turmeric to some juice. Drink this mixture in the morning and evening. You can also mix 2 tablespoons of turmeric with 1 tablespoon of lime juice and enough boiling water to make a warm paste. Apply mixture to sore area. Cover with plastic wrap to retain heat.

Hot peppers — Researchers have found that the active ingredient in red peppers, capsaicin, effectively relieves discomfort caused by arthritis, diabetes, and shingles. Made from dried cayenne peppers, capsaicin is available as a nonprescription cream. It is absorbed through your skin and works by deadening local nerves.

Sources —

Food — Your Miracle Medicine: How Food Can Prevent and Cure Over 100 Symptoms and Problems, HarperCollins Publishers, New York, 1993
Heinerman's Encyclopedia of Fruits, Herbs and Vegetables, Parker Publishing, West Nyack, N.Y., 1988

Heel Spurs

◄ Discomfort and numbness with walking
◄ Stabbing pain in the bottom of the heel

Put your foot down on heel pain

One of the most aggravating — and very common — causes of foot pain is a group of problems collectively referred to as "heel spur syndrome." One of its most characteristic symptoms is intense pain on the bottom of your heel when you first step out of bed in the morning. After a half-hour of walking, the pain subsides, but it returns when you sit for long periods and then stand up.

Although the name implies that a spur or growth on your heel is causing the pain, that isn't necessarily the case. Heel pain usually comes from inflammation of the large connective plantar tissue that runs along the bottom of your foot. Your heel hurts when the tissue loses its flexibility or is strained or injured.

You can probably treat a heel spur yourself, but you should see your doctor in case other more serious conditions are causing your heel pain. Fortunately, you don't have to resort to surgery to get almost complete relief from heel spurs. Here are some ways to help the pain.

Be particular about shoes. Wear shoes with low, but slightly raised, heels — not flat or extremely high heels. The shoes should have cushioning across the entire sole. Use donut-shaped heel inserts in your shoe to protect the sore area from impact. Insert arch supports in your shoes to even out the pressure on your foot.

Reduce inflammation of the tissue around your heel. Try ice packs on the affected area, or take nonsteroidal anti-inflammatory medications such as aspirin or ibuprofen.

Stretch the plantar tissues on the bottom of your feet to keep them flexible. Before you walk in the morning, flex your toes up toward your head, then relax your foot. Do this several times.

After you stand up, stand two feet from a wall and put your hands on the wall. Bend your elbows and lean into the wall. Keep your feet flat on the ground.

Check with your doctor. If you don't get relief from these techniques, ask your doctor about custom-designed orthotic inserts for your shoes, foot taping, or steroid injections for your heel.

Sources —
   American Health (13,3:77)
   Journal of the American Podiatric Medical Association (81,2:68)
   One Hundred Orthopaedic Conditions Every Doctor Should Understand by Roy A. Meals, Quality Medical Publishers, St. Louis, Mo., 1992

KNEE PAIN

◀ Dull ache in the knee
◀ Sharp pain with movement of the knee joint

Knock out knee pain

Tape your kneecap. Studies have shown that pulling your kneecap to the inside of your leg with a piece of tape can lessen your discomfort and give you a safe, inexpensive way to make climbing stairs and walking a little easier. While not a substitute for a doctor's advice or a physical therapy routine, moving the kneecap to one side can decrease leg pain for a while.

According to researchers, taping is a safe method of treatment for knee pain in older people as well as in young athletes, when it's combined with the proper exercises. The tape helps relieve pain so that you can exercise and build your thigh muscles. Strong thigh muscles will help hold your kneecap in place and relieve your pain permanently. The proper way to tape your knee is to pull the kneecap toward the inner part of your leg. The two ends of a piece of 2-inch-wide tape should be on the outer side of your leg, not touching each other. A physical therapist can give you a simple training lesson.

Wear knee braces by prescription only. If the ligaments in your knee are extremely loose and your knee is so weak that it could give way easily, it is safer to wear a brace when exercising. It could also help you avoid a lot of pain. Your doctor can prescribe a specific brace for your needs.

However, don't use a knee brace just because you think it might be a good idea. Extensive tests in Sweden and California have shown that because the blood flow to the knee is reduced when wearing a knee brace, muscular strength in the braced leg is reduced by as much as 35 percent, causing fatigue in a shorter time.

The result is more pressure being placed on ankle and foot muscles to compensate for tiredness in the knee, and the possibility of injuring those lower muscle groups. So, wear a knee brace only if your doctor prescribes one for you.

Sources —

American Family Physician (50,3:676)
British Medical Journal (308,6931:753)
Medicine and Science in Sports and Exercise (25,9:989)
The American Journal of Sports Medicine (22,6:830)

LEG CRAMPS

◀ Sudden, intense pain in the muscles of the legs

Let go of leg cramps

When muscle pain strikes suddenly in the form of a "charley horse," grab your leg, massage it, and use heat or ice if it helps. Stretch the muscle by standing on the affected leg and leaning forward.

You also can relieve a muscle cramp by sitting on the ground, stretching your legs straight out in front of you, and gently pulling your toes and the ball of your foot toward your kneecap.

Here are some other tips to help you rein in those charley horse nightmares:

Stretch your calf muscles every day. Try this quick and easy calf stretch. With your shoes off, stand two to three feet from a wall. Place your hands on the wall and lean forward, being sure to keep your legs and back straight.

Press your heels into the floor. You should feel a pulling sensation in the back of your lower legs. Hold this position for 10 seconds, relax five seconds, and do the exercise once more. Repeat exercise three times daily.

Drink at least eight glasses of water a day. You'll need to drink more if you've been physically active. Dehydration (lack of fluids) is probably the biggest contributor to muscle cramping.

Control cramps with minerals. Sometimes you may develop leg cramps because you have too little potassium, calcium, or magnesium in your body.

For potassium, eat plenty of oranges and bananas. Include lots of calcium-rich foods in your diet, such as milk, yogurt, salmon, sardines, shrimp, dark-green leafy vegetables, and dried peas and beans. Eat foods high in magnesium, such as almonds, cashews, apricots, whole grains, dark-green leafy vegetables, and soybeans.

Expect muscle soreness. Don't be alarmed if your muscle is a little sore for a few days. This is very common.

If your leg cramps occur frequently, are accompanied by other symptoms, or aren't relieved by stretching and massaging, see your doctor to make sure it isn't something more serious.

Sources —
Postgraduate Medicine (96,1:155)
The Physician and Sportsmedicine (21,7:115)
U.S. Pharmacist (17,6:23)

NECK PAIN

◀ Stiff, sore neck
◀ Throbbing pain in neck and shoulders

Head off neck pain

A pain in the neck usually comes from not keeping a straight head on your shoulders. The more you lean your head forward or sideways to work, drive, or read, the harder your neck muscles have to work. Eventually, your tired muscles will become strained, tight, and painful. You can prevent most neck pain by keeping your head in a straight, natural position as much as possible.

Ice it, then warm it. Over-the-counter pain relievers and ice can help relieve neck pain. Hold an ice pack over the painful area for 20 minutes. Wait two hours, then use the ice again. After a few days, when the muscle spasms in your neck have stopped, you can use a heating pad. Apply it for 20 minutes at a time two or three times a day.

Wear a cervical collar. A cervical collar, available at medical supply stores, can help when your neck pain is severe. It rests the muscles and relieves spasms. But wearing a collar too long can make your neck weak and stiff. When your pain stops, take the collar off and begin neck exercises.

Exercise your options. Neck exercises can help you get rid of pain and will strengthen your neck — preventing strained muscles in the future. The following exercises will help you regain mobility and strength after an injury, once the severe pain has gone away.

◁ Lie on your back on the floor or on a firm mattress. Tilt your left ear toward your left shoulder until you feel a gentle stretch, but no pain. Hold for 10 to 30 seconds. Repeat on the right side. Do this exercise two or three times to each side, once or twice a day. If you feel tingling in your arms or an increase in pain, stop and see a doctor.

◁ While lying on your back, turn your head to the left (left cheek toward the floor), until you feel a gentle stretch. Hold for 10 to 30 seconds. Repeat on the right side. Do this exercise two or three times to each side, once or twice a day. If you feel tingling or pain, stop and see a doctor.

◁ Sit and place your palm firmly against your forehead. Push your head against your hand. Hold for 10 seconds. Rest and repeat three times.

◁ Next, put your hand behind your head. Push your head back against your hand for 10 seconds. Repeat three times.

◁ Place your hand over your right ear and push. Repeat for three times, then switch to your left ear.

If you choose to sit and exercise, make sure you don't roll your head in full circles. Rolling your head backward strains your neck.

Source —
The Physician and Sportsmedicine (22,9:35)

RAYNAUD'S SYNDROME

◀ Throbbing, painful fingers and toes when exposed to cold

Resist Raynaud's syndrome

If you have Raynaud's (pronounced Ray-nose), you know the symptoms — your fingers (or toes, nose, or ears) first turn white when exposed to the cold. That's when the blood supply is cut off. Then they turn blue and numb because they are starved for oxygen. Then finally they grow red and painful as the blood comes flowing back.

Cold isn't the only thing that brings on the symptoms; vibration, such as mowing the lawn or typing a report, can have the same painful effect. There's no cure for Raynaud's syndrome, but most attacks can be warded off simply by keeping warm, especially your hands and feet. Here are some ways to deal with Raynaud's:

Dress in layers. Wear woolen socks and mittens, plus a hat, when you go out. When it's chilly, keep your wrists and neck covered, even indoors.

You may want to stay warm with chemical hand-warmers, available in most sporting goods or camping supply stores. Slip them in your pockets or shoes. Or try reflective insoles.

Take mittens or gloves to the supermarket. You can slip them on before reaching for a carton of milk or frozen vegetables.

Embark on a home cold patrol. Don't forget the simple remedies that can make your own home more comfortable for you.

◁ Keep a pot holder or oven mitt beside the refrigerator.

◁ Rinse food and dishes in lukewarm water instead of cold.

◁ Use stemware or insulated picnic tumblers. (Or, if you're away from home, put your glass in a foam rubber holder, or wrap several napkins around it.)

◁ Cover your cold metal doorknobs and keys with rubber caps.

Warm your engine. Start the engine and turn on the car heater for 10 minutes before driving in the cold. Cover the steering wheel with sheepskin or insulated leather. If the seat is plastic or leather, sit on a fabric cushion.

Pick your cold medicines carefully. You should avoid over-the-counter cold remedies and diet pills that contain the drug phenylpropanolamine.

Think your fingers warm. Some people have actually learned to raise their fingers' temperature just by concentrating on it. One reason this technique may work is that the act of concentrating itself can help you relax.

Stress can trigger Raynaud's, so any relaxation technique you enjoy, such as deep breathing or imagining the sights and sounds of a deserted beach, may help.

Condition yourself to the cold. You can help your body adapt to colder temperatures. Every other day, spend some time outdoors in cool weather or in a cool room. Try for 10 minutes at a time, several times a day. After three to four weeks of this treatment, you should have a more comfortable winter.

Don't smoke. Need another reason to quit? The nicotine in cigarettes is a big contributor to Raynaud's.

Prepare your resume. Since vibration can bring on attacks, the condition is common for typists, musicians, meat cutters, and those who use vibrating tools such as jack hammers and chain saws. Normally, an attack won't end until the offending activity is stopped, so it could require retraining for a different job.

Mention it during your yearly checkup. Raynaud's can occur by itself, or as a symptom of another health problem. It's best to have it checked by your doctor to rule out such diseases as lupus, scleroderma, and rheumatoid arthritis.

Sources —
   Nurse Practitioner (18,3:18)
   The New York Times (Dec. 14, 1989)

SHINSPLINTS

◀ Sharp, stabbing pain in the lower legs

Keep shinsplints at bay

Once you've made the decision to start exercising regularly, you don't need any barriers to stand in your way. Shinsplints can stop a successful exercise program in its tracks. The pain in the front of your lower leg can keep you from exercising, or even working, for several days or longer if you don't treat it correctly. Here's what you can do to help shinsplints:

Ease into exercise. You should never have a problem with shinsplints if you begin an exercise program slowly and carefully. Shinsplints are usually caused when you overuse and strain the muscles of your lower legs.

Step out in style with new shoes. Worn-out shoes are a common shinsplint culprit. Some people who run regularly believe the shock-absorbing power of running shoes wears out by about 300 miles of use.

Don't work out on hard surfaces. You should always do aerobics on a floor with a little give to it. Cement floors are too hard. And don't run on asphalt if you can avoid it.

Fix flat feet. Fallen arches can cause shinsplints. If you have flat feet, you may need shoe inserts to get your legs correctly balanced.

Never push through the pain. If you start to feel pain in your lower legs while you are exercising, stop! If you keep going, you'll probably make the injury worse. For the next three days, ice the area for 15 minutes twice a day. If the pain doesn't go away, apply moist heat for the next week. A hot shower or bath, along with gentle massage for five to 10 minutes, can help ease shinsplints.

When the shinsplints go away, you can begin exercise again. Start with half the workout you were doing before the shinsplints. Work up to your normal level over the next week or so.

Be sure to apply ice to the injured shin after you exercise, at least until the 10th day after the injury. (If you still have pain after 10 days, you should see a doctor.)

Stretch and strengthen. Lack of flexibility causes many cases of shinsplints. Stretching should be a part of every workout.

Stretching and strengthening exercises will also help heal your injury once you have shinsplints. Begin these exercises the third day after the injury:

◁ *Calf muscle stretch:* Lean against a wall with your arms outstretched at shoulder height. Place one foot forward, keeping your back leg straight with the heel down. Bend your front knee and push into the wall. This should not cause pain, but you should feel tightness in the back of your calf. Hold the position for 10 seconds, then repeat with the other leg forward. Stretch each leg five to 10 times. Repeat two or three times a day.

◁ *Lower calf muscle and Achilles tendon stretch:* Start in the same position as previous stretch (one foot forward). Bend both knees and keep your heels on the floor. You should feel tightness in the sides of your calf, but this should not be painful. Hold the position for 10 seconds, then stretch with the other leg forward. Stretch each leg five to 10 times. Repeat two or three times a day.

◁ *Calf raises (for strength):* Stand straight, holding onto something that will support you, like a table. Rise up on your toes for five seconds. Repeat 10 times, two or three times a day. If you don't feel pain, work your way up to 30 calf raises at a time.

As an alternative, you may want to ride a stationary bike for five to 10 minutes a day. Set the tension at low to medium. Work your way up to 20 minutes a day. Or try running in a pool to strengthen your calves.

Source —
The Physician and Sportsmedicine (22,4:31)

SORE SHOULDER

◀ Pain and stiffness of the shoulder

Shrug off a sore shoulder

Whether your shoulders ache from carrying the weight of the world or just from swinging your tennis racquet too many times, there are ways to ease the pain. First, remember the old joke, "Doctor, it hurts when I do this"? Well, you have to try to stop doing what hurts. You can't quit using or exercising your arm, but you don't want to do anything that is painful.

You should also put ice packs on your shoulder for 20 minutes three or four times a day.

Finally, you need to do these stretching and strengthening exercises twice a day (but only if they don't cause pain).

Draw circles in the air. While standing, lean over and look at the floor. Let the arm with the sore shoulder hang straight down. You may want to hold a pocketbook or other light object in your hand. Now let your arm swing in circles for about a minute. Start with small circles, and then swing in wider ones.

Stretch with a broomstick. Lie on your back and hold a broomstick in both hands. Use your uninjured arm to pull your injured arm through a complete range of motion. Continue for three to five minutes.

Pull your arm across your chest. Grasp the bent elbow of your sore arm with your other hand. Gently pull the sore arm by the elbow across your chest until you feel a stretch in your shoulder muscles. If it hurts, don't pull the arm so far across your chest. Hold for 10 seconds. Repeat three times.

Run your fingers up the wall. Stand near a wall and walk your fingers up and down the wall. When your shoulder starts hurting, don't go any higher and hold for 10 seconds. Repeat three times. You can do this both facing the wall and with your side toward the wall.

Give yourself a pat on the back. Reach one palm over your shoulder to pat your back and place the back of your other hand on your lower back. Slide your hands toward each other, trying to touch your fingertips. Hold for 10 seconds. Alternate arms.

Try a soup-can workout. For these exercises, use either hand weights or a 15- or 16-ounce can of soup. If you do have weights, start with a low weight and increase the weight as you become comfortable. Don't use weights heavier than 5 pounds.

◁ Lie on your back with your elbows on the floor touching your sides. Put your hands in the air like you're holding a steering wheel. With a weight in your hand, lower your forearm to the side, then raise it.

◁ Lie on your side with your top elbow tucked into your waist. With a weight in your hand, lower your forearm across your stomach, then raise your forearm into the air. Keep your elbow at your side.

◁ Standing with your arms hanging loosely, lift your arm out to the side — 90 degrees from your body. Hold it there, then lift above your head (unless it hurts). Pause, then lower your arm. Next, turn your palms backward with your thumbs pointed down, and lift your arms to the side.

Source —
American Family Physician (51,7:1677)

SPRAINED ANKLE

◀ Sudden pain and swelling of the ankle

How to relieve the pain of a sprain

If you've ever sprained your ankle, you are familiar with the sudden rush of pain and the feeling of helplessness it brings. Fortunately, a sprained ankle is usually something you can take care of at home.

For the first two days, stay off your feet as much as possible. If you have to walk, use a cane or a crutch on the side that's not injured. That way, you can lean away and take weight off the hurt foot. Here are other ways to treat your sore ankle:

Ice it. Put an ice pack on your ankle for about 20 minutes three or four times a day.

Do a figure-eight wrap. Wrap your ankle in an elastic bandage to control swelling and to support and protect it, especially if you must walk around. Start wrapping at your toes, make a figure eight at the ankle, and continue wrapping loosely about six inches up the leg.

Don't wrap so tightly that your toes go numb or turn red. Wear the bandage as long as your ankle hurts when you try to walk.

Put your ankle above your heart. You need to keep your swollen ankle propped above the level of your heart if you can. Stretch out on your sofa with your foot on a pillow.

Take a "contrast bath." If your ankle is still swollen after a few days, try a contrast bath twice a day. Put your foot in a tub of cold water for one minute, then move to a tub of warm water for two minutes. Do this for 15 minutes, gently moving your foot up and down in the water all the while.

Give it support. Since you risk another sprain as long as your ankle is weak, continue to support it with sturdy shoes or boots even after the pain is gone. Wear a bandage or brace when you plan to walk or exercise vigorously.

Stand like a stork. For an easy strengthening exercise, put all your weight on the sore leg, keeping the other foot slightly raised above the floor. Maintain this position for a few minutes. A good time to do this is when you brush your teeth in the morning and evening.

Repeat this exercise for seven to 10 days, then practice it with your eyes closed. Continue the exercise until you can easily maintain your balance on your injured leg.

Roll your foot five to 10 times a day. This exercise will strengthen the muscles that support your ankle. First, remove any bandage or brace and let your leg hang freely off a bench, sturdy table or tall chair. Roll your foot in a circle at least three or four times. Make both clockwise and counterclockwise circles.

Don't push so hard. Some people spend half their lives in an ankle brace because they sprain it again and again. If you have a chronic ankle sprain, you may be pushing too hard and too long when you exercise.

If you walk or work out until you're exhausted or suddenly start to run faster than you normally do, you're putting yourself at risk for a sprain. The muscles that support the ankle are particularly vulnerable to fatigue.

Sources —
Postgraduate Medicine (94,2:091)
The American Journal of Sports Medicine (21,6:805 and 22,6:830)
The Physician and Sportsmedicine (21,11:43)

TMJ

◀ Headache
◀ Jaw pain radiating to the head and ears
◀ Sensitive teeth

Turn off the pain of TMJ

Temporomandibular joint syndrome, usually called TMJ, is a joint disorder of the jaw that often leads to severe headaches. Teeth grinding, called bruxism, and teeth clenching are common causes of TMJ.

In addition to headaches, an aching, tired, or tender jaw; a clicking in your jaw; sharp pain when you yawn, talk, or chew; pain in your neck or shoulders or near your ears; sensitive teeth and toothache can all be symptoms of TMJ.

You can buy a specially fitted appliance from your dentist to hold your jaw in place while you sleep. But you might want to try these simpler remedies first.

Think calm. Many people grind their teeth unconsciously in response to stress. Anything you can do to make your life less stressful will probably help you quit grinding your teeth. Give yourself an hour to relax before bedtime. You may want to seek counseling if you feel stressful circumstances are out of your control.

Examine your psyche. Bruxism may be a subconscious outlet for anxiety or anger. If you are very achievement-oriented and compulsively punctual, you're more likely to grind your teeth. Even a stressful event late in life, such as the loss of a spouse, can trigger bruxism.

Ask your sleeping partner to wake you up. Sleeping partners don't have to grit their teeth and bear it when they hear you grinding your teeth. Waking you up will help you break the habit.

Close your lips, hold your teeth apart, and relax your jaw. Do this as often as 50 times a day. When you are comfortable with this exercise, picture yourself sleeping with your mouth in this relaxed position.

Clench your teeth for five seconds, then relax your jaw for five seconds. Do this exercise five times in a row, six times a day, for two weeks.

Change your sleeping position. Lying on your back with a pillow under your neck and knees may help relax your lower jaw. If you must sleep on your side, try piling pillows so that they support your shoulder and arm as well as your head. That position should take some of the strain off your neck and pressure off your teeth.

Create a stress-free home environment for child tooth grinders. Have a relaxed and enjoyable bedtime ritual. Talk about what happened during the day, especially about anything that may have scared or worried your child.

Get rid of allergy triggers. People with allergies, especially children, have a tendency to grind their teeth. It somehow helps relieve itching, sneezing and coughing. See the ***Breathing Problems*** chapter for hints on how to control your allergies.

Be nice to your jaws. If your tooth grinding is causing your jaw to ache, try eating soft foods for a while, take aspirin or ibuprofen, and hold a heating pad to your jaw. Stop chewing gum, and avoid hard, chewy foods like caramels, tough meats, raw carrots, and celery. Don't open your mouth too wide when you yawn.

Sources —
American Family Physician (49,7:1617)
Pain and the TMJ, American Academy of Otolaryngology, Alexandria, Va. 22312

WRIST PAIN

◀ Sudden swelling or pain in wrist

Wrestle away wrist pain
If you experience pain in your wrists from overuse, pay attention to your body's warning signs. Catching an injury early and dealing with it quickly can

prevent more serious problems.

In most cases, controlling the pain and getting your wrist back up to par should only take several days. But if your wrist, hand or forearm is swollen or if it feels warm, tender, or numb, see your doctor.

If you've simply overdone it, try these tips, and you'll be back in the swing of things in a hurry.

◁ Stop doing what hurts, and try to find what's causing your pain.

◁ Check out your sports equipment and your form to help identify the cause of your problem. Your racket or clubs may be worn out, or you may need more instruction on the proper grip. The right equipment and the proper form will improve performance and enhance your enjoyment of the activity.

◁ Treat the pain with over-the-counter painkillers like ibuprofen or aspirin.

◁ Apply ice to the painful area.

◁ Try this exercise. Keeping your hand and palm face down, place your wrist over the edge of a table. Holding a 1 to 2 lb. weight, bend your wrist as far down as possible. Slowly lift the weight. Continue moving your wrist up and down without stopping. See if you can do three sets of 10 once or twice a day. Try it with your palm up too.

If you are overweight, you may have more wrist problems. The heavier you are, the more stress there is on your wrists, and injuries are more likely. Now you have another good reason to lose a few pounds.

Source —
The Physician and Sportsmedicine (22,2:41)

Please check with your doctor for approval before taking or discontinuing any prescription drug or using a natural healing alternative.

SKIN CONDITIONS

Prescription Drugs

Natural Alternatives

Prescription Drugs ℞

ACNE DRUGS

Isotretinoin

Brand name: *Accutane*

What this drug does for you:

This metabolite of vitamin A is used to treat severe acne that does not respond to other treatments.

Possible side effects of this drug:

- Nine out of 10 isotretinoin users experience swollen lips. Also very common is conjunctivitis — inflammation of the mucous membrane that lines the eyelids. Many people experience muscle pain and chest pain.
- Less than one out of 10 isotretinoin users experiences dry skin, itching, rash, dandruff, and thinning of hair.
- About one out of 20 users experiences peeling of palms and soles, skin infections, upset stomach, headache, fatigue, and an increased risk of sunburn.
- Isotretinoin may cause increased pressure on the brain in adults. Signs of this high pressure include headache, nausea, and visual disturbances. Let your doctor know immediately if you develop these symptoms.
- Rare side effects include depression and eye problems such as clouding of the cornea, dry eyes, and difficulty seeing at night.
- Isotretinoin may also raise your cholesterol and triglyceride levels and lower your red and white blood cell count. A low red blood cell count could cause anemia and a low white blood cell count could lower your resistance to infection.
- Very rarely, isotretinoin may cause hepatitis or inflammatory bowel disease. If you experience stomach pain, bleeding from the rectum, or severe diarrhea, you should contact your doctor immediately.

Special warning:

- Treatment with this drug should be stopped if hepatitis, inflammatory bowel disease, or visual disorders develop.

Pregnancy and nursing mothers:

Category X. See page 9 for description of categories. This drug must not be taken by pregnant women. Even small doses for short periods can cause serious birth defects. Women of childbearing age should use effective contraception from at least one month before until one month after treatment. If you become pregnant while you are taking this drug, notify your doctor immediately. Not known if drug is present in mother's milk, but it should not be used by nursing women.

Possible food and drug interactions:

- Don't take vitamin supplements containing vitamin A while you are taking this drug.
- Avoid alcohol while taking this drug because it may cause very high triglyceride levels.
- Taking this drug with the antibiotic tetracycline may cause increased pressure in the brain.

Helpful hints:

- Be extra careful when driving at night since this drug may cause a decrease in night vision.
- If you miss a dose, take it as soon as possible. If several hours have passed or it's almost time for your next dose, don't try to catch up by doubling the dose (unless your doctor tells you to).
- Take this drug with meals.
- Do not crush the capsules.
- Your acne may get worse when you first begin taking isotretinoin. That doesn't mean you should stop taking the drug.
- This drug may make your skin extra-sensitive to sunlight, so protect your skin if you'll be outdoors in sunny weather.
- Do not donate blood while you are taking this drug or for 30 days after you quit taking this drug.

Tretinoin

Brand name: *Retin-A*

What this drug does for you:

This vitamin A acid is used to treat common acne. It comes as a cream, gel, or liquid.

Possible side effects of this drug:

- This drug may cause redness, blistering, peeling, crusting, swelling, abnormal skin pigmentation, and sensitivity to light. If your skin becomes excessively red or irritated, call your doctor.

Special warnings:

- If you work outdoors or are naturally sensitive to sunlight, use this drug with caution.
- Use this drug with caution if you have eczema. Excessive use may irritate your skin, and it will not improve the condition.

Pregnancy and nursing mothers:

Category C. See page 9 for description of categories. Not known if drug is present in mother's milk.

Possible food and drug interactions:

- Any of the following may increase the side effects of tretinoin: medicated or abrasive soaps; products with a strong skin-drying effect; high levels of alcohol, lime, astringents or spices; and topical products containing salicylic acid, sulfur, benzoyl peroxide, or resorcinol. If you've been using these products, wait a few days before beginning tretinoin.

Helpful hints:

- Wash your skin with warm water and a mild soap. Gently pat dry with a clean towel. Wait until your skin is completely dry before applying this medication.
- Avoid exposure to sunlight or sunlamps, and don't use this drug on sunburned skin.
- This drug may make your skin more sensitive to wind and cold temperatures. Be sure to wear clothing that will protect your skin.
- Lightly apply at bedtime, avoiding the eyes, mouth, and angles of the nose. Wash your hands immediately after applying.
- You can use makeup while using tretinoin, but thoroughly remove makeup before applying the drug.
- Your acne may appear worse when you first begin using tretinoin. It may take many weeks before you see positive effects.

DRUGS FOR FUNGAL INFECTIONS OF THE SKIN

Clotrimazole and Betamethasone Dipropionate

Brand name: *Lotrisone*

What this drug does for you:

This drug combines an antifungal with a corticosteroid to treat skin infections caused by fungus. It treats athlete's foot, fungus of the genital and anal areas, and whole body fungus.

Possible side effects of this drug:

- This drug may cause itching, blisters, hives, irritated skin, peeling, reddened skin, and swelling caused by fluid retention. Call your doctor if your skin becomes more irritated than before.

Special warning:

- Don't use this drug if you are sensitive to clotrimazole, betamethasone dipropionate, other corticosteroids, or imidazoles.

Pregnancy and nursing mothers:

Category C. See page 9 for description of categories. Not known if drug is present in mother's milk.

Helpful hints:
- With clean hands, gently massage this cream into the affected and surrounding area.
- Apply this cream twice a day, in the morning and evening.
- Do not wrap or bandage the area after you apply the medicine (unless your doctor tells you to).
- Use the full course of treatment even if symptoms improve.
- When you're treating a fungus in the groin area, you should wear loose-fitting clothing and you should apply the cream sparingly for two weeks only. Let your doctor know if the fungus hasn't disappeared after two weeks.
- For athlete's foot, you should let your doctor know if the fungus hasn't improved in two weeks. For other types of fungus, you should let your doctor know if you haven't seen any improvement after one week.

Griseofulvin

Brand names: *Fulvicin P/G, Grifulvin V, Grisactin, Gris-PEG*

What this drug does for you:
This drug is an antibiotic used to treat fungal infections such as ringworm and athlete's foot.

Possible side effects of this drug:
- This drug may cause hives, rashes, nausea, diarrhea, upset stomach, oral thrush (yeast infection in the mouth), headache, fatigue, confusion, dizziness, and insomnia.
- Rare side effects include bleeding in the stomach and intestines, kidney and urinary problems, liver toxicity, menstrual problems, decreased white blood cell count (lowered resistance to infection), and numbness or tingling in your hands and feet (this could be an indication of nerve damage, so be sure to tell your doctor about it).

Special warnings:
- This drug should not be used by people with liver disease or the metabolic disorder called porphyria.
- If you are allergic to penicillin, you may be allergic to this drug.

Pregnancy and nursing mothers:
Category X. See page 9 for description of categories. Discuss any plans for pregnancy with your doctor. Not known if drug is present in mother's milk.

Possible food and drug interactions:
- Griseofulvin may increase the effects of alcohol and cause rapid heartbeat and flushing.
- This drug may decrease the effects of oral contraceptives and anti-coagulants.
- Barbiturates may decrease the effectiveness of griseofulvin.

Helpful hints:
- Good hygiene and skin care is important during treatment.

- This drug may make your skin extra-sensitive to sunlight, so protect your skin if you'll be outdoors in sunny weather.
- If you will be taking this drug for a long period of time, be sure your doctor orders regular liver, kidney, and bone marrow tests.
- Ringworm of the body may require only two weeks of treatment, but most cases of ringworm will require at least four. Athlete's foot can take two months of treatment to cure, and ringworm at the toenails takes at least six months.
- You may need an ointment or cream in addition to griseofulvin, especially for athlete's foot.

Miconazole

Brand names: *Fungoid Tincture, Monistat-Derm, Monistat Dual-Pak, Monistat 3, Ony-Clear* (Generic available)

What this drug does for you:

This drug is used to treat fungal infections such as athlete's foot, jock itch, ringworm, tinea versicolor, and yeast infections. It is available as a cream, powder, solution, and spray. The vaginal cream and suppositories treat vaginal yeast infections.

Possible side effects of this drug:

- This drug may cause burning, rash, hives, irritation, and itching. Any of these symptoms may indicate that you're having an allergic reaction to the drug.
- If the vaginal cream causes burning or irritation, contact your doctor.

Special warnings:

- Use miconazole cautiously if your skin is blistered, raw, or oozing.
- Contact your doctor if ringworm, jock itch, or yeast infections have not improved within two weeks or if athlete's foot has not improved after four weeks.

Pregnancy and nursing mothers:

This drug should not be used in the first trimester of pregnancy. Not known if drug is present in mother's milk.

Helpful hints:

- Avoid contact with your eyes, nose, and mouth.
- Use the full course of treatment even if symptoms improve. Contact your doctor if you haven't seen any improvement after four weeks.
- Do not wrap or bandage the area after you apply the medicine (unless your doctor tells you to).
- Clean and dry the infected area before applying the medicine.
- For the vaginal cream, insert the cream high into the vagina. Continue taking this drug during menstruation, but wear a sanitary napkin instead of a tampon. If you have sexual intercourse during treatment, the male partner should use a condom.

Nystatin

Brand names: *Mycostatin, Mycostatin Pastilles, Pedi-Dri* **(Generic available)**

What this drug does for you:
This drug is used to treat yeast infections of the skin and mucous membranes. It is available as tablets, oral suspension, powder, troches, cream, or ointment. Nystatin usually relieves your symptoms within 24 to 72 hours.

Possible side effects of this drug:
- This drug may cause irritation at treatment site. Large oral doses of nystatin may cause stomachache, nausea, and, rarely, rash.

Special warning:
- Use nystatin cautiously if your skin is blistered, raw, or oozing.

Pregnancy and nursing mothers:
Category C. See page 9 for description of categories. Not known if drug is present in mother's milk.

Helpful hints:
- Hold the oral suspension, troches, and lozenges in your mouth as long as possible. Do not chew or swallow the lozenges.
- Avoid contact with your eyes, nose, and mouth.
- Continue using the medicine for at least two days after your symptoms have disappeared (or as long as your doctor prescribes).
- Do not wrap or bandage the area after you apply the medicine (unless your doctor tells you to).
- Clean and dry the infected area before applying the medicine. Apply the cream and ointment twice a day or as directed. For fungal infections of the feet, the powder should be dusted on the feet and in shoes and socks.

IMPETIGO DRUGS

Mupirocin

Brand name: *Bactroban*

What this drug does for you:
This antibiotic ointment is used to treat the symptoms of the skin disease impetigo.

Possible side effects of this drug:
- This drug may cause burning, stinging, itching, pain, contact dermatitis, swelling, rash, dry skin, and nausea.

Special warning:
- People with kidney problems should use this drug with caution.

Pregnancy and nursing mothers:
Category B. See page 9 for description of categories. Not known if drug is present in mother's milk.

Helpful hints:
- If you haven't seen any improvement in three to five days, contact your doctor.
- Apply a small amount of ointment to the affected area three times a day. You can cover the area with a loose gauze dressing.
- Avoid contact with your eyes.

DRUGS FOR INFLAMED OR IRRITATED SKIN

Betamethasone Dipropionate

Brand names: *Alphatrex, Diprolene, Diprolene AF* (Generic available)

What this drug does for you:
This corticosteroid drug is used to treat itching, inflamed, and irritated skin. It comes as an ointment, cream, and lotion.

Possible side effects of this drug:
- Side effects are very rare, but this drug may cause stinging, itching, burning, irritated skin, skin lesions, changes in skin pigment, skin wasting, inflammation of the skin around the mouth, stretch marks, and prickly heat.
- Very high doses or long-term use, especially in children, may cause Cushing's syndrome, a disease of the adrenal gland. Signs of this disease include weight gain and slow growth. Children are also at risk for increased pressure in the brain. Signs are headache and bulging "soft spots."

Special warning:
- You should not use this drug if you are allergic to other steroid creams.

Pregnancy and nursing mothers:
Category C. See page 9 for description of categories. Drug is present in mother's milk.

Helpful hints:
- Do not wrap or bandage the area after you apply the medicine (unless your doctor tells you to).
- Avoid contact with your eyes.
- Don't use this drug for longer than prescribed. The high-potency formulations shouldn't be used for longer than two weeks.
- Apply a thin film and rub in gently and completely.
- If you are covering a very large area of your skin and therefore using lots of medicine, you should be tested regularly for hypothalamic-pituitary-adrenal axis suppression. Regular testing could prevent severe side effects and withdrawal symptoms associated with steroids.

Desonide

Brand names: *DesOwen, Tridesilon* **(Generic available)**

What this drug does for you:

This drug is used to relieve and heal inflamed or irritated skin conditions including eczema, dermatitis, psoriasis, severe diaper rash, insect bites, minor burns, and sunburn. It is a corticosteroid, and it is available as an ointment or cream.

Possible side effects of this drug:

- This drug may cause burning, itching, irritation, dryness, inflammation of hair follicles, excess hair growth, pimples, skin wasting, loss of skin pigment, inflammation of the skin, mild infection, streaks on the skin, and obstruction of sweat glands. If your skin becomes irritated, contact your doctor.
- Very high doses or long-term use in children may cause Cushing's syndrome, a disease of the adrenal gland. Signs of this disease include weight gain and slow growth. Children are also at risk for increased pressure in the brain. Signs are headache and bulging "soft spots."

Special warning:

- You should not use this drug if you are allergic to other steroid creams.

Pregnancy and nursing mothers:

Category C. See page 9 for description of categories. Not known if drug is present in mother's milk.

Helpful hints:

- Do not wrap or bandage the area after you apply the medicine unless your doctor tells you to. For diaper rash, you should not use tight-fitting diapers or plastic pants after applying this medicine.
- Avoid contact with your eyes.
- Don't use this drug for longer than prescribed.
- Apply a thin film and rub in gently and completely.
- If your skin is infected, you'll also need an antifungal or antibacterial medicine.
- If you are covering a very large area of your skin and therefore using lots of medicine, you should be tested regularly for hypothalamic-pituitary-adrenal axis suppression. Regular testing could prevent severe side effects and withdrawal symptoms associated with steroids.

Desoximetasone

Brand name: *Topicort* **(Generic available)**

What this drug does for you:

This drug is used to relieve and heal inflamed or irritated skin conditions including eczema, dermatitis, psoriasis, severe diaper rash, insect bites, minor burns, and sunburn. It is a corticosteroid, and it is available as an ointment, cream, and gel.

Possible side effects of this drug:

- Side effects are rare, but this drug may cause burning, itching, irritation, dryness, inflammation of hair follicles, excess hair growth, pimples, loss of skin pigment, skin wasting, inflammation of the skin, mild infection, streaks on the skin, and obstruction of sweat glands. If your skin becomes irritated, contact your doctor.
- Very high doses or long-term use in children may cause Cushing's syndrome, a disease of the adrenal gland. Signs of this disease include weight gain and slow growth. Children are also at risk for increased pressure in the brain. Signs are headache and bulging "soft spots."

Special warning:

- You should not use this drug if you are allergic to other steroid creams.

Pregnancy and nursing mothers:

Category C. See page 9 for description of categories. Not known if drug is present in mother's milk.

Helpful hints:

- Do not wrap or bandage the area after you apply the medicine unless your doctor tells you to. For diaper rash, you should not use tight-fitting diapers or plastic pants after applying this medicine.
- Avoid contact with your eyes.
- Don't use this drug for longer than prescribed.
- Apply a thin film and rub in gently and completely.
- If your skin is infected, you'll also need an antifungal or antibacterial medicine.
- If you are covering a very large area of your skin and therefore using lots of medicine, you should be tested regularly for hypothalamic-pituitary-adrenal axis suppression. Regular testing could prevent severe side effects and withdrawal symptoms associated with steroids.

Fluocinolone

Brand names: *Derma-Smooth/FS, Fluonid, FS Shampoo, Synalar, Synemol* (Generic available)

What this drug does for you:

This drug is used to relieve and heal inflamed or irritated skin conditions including eczema, dermatitis, psoriasis, severe diaper rash, insect bites, minor burns, and sunburn. It is a corticosteroid, and it is available as an ointment, cream, solution, and powder.

Possible side effects of this drug:

- Side effects are rare, but this drug may cause burning, itching, irritation, dryness, inflammation of hair follicles, excess hair growth, pimples, loss of skin pigment, skin wasting, inflammation of the skin, mild infection, streaks on the skin, and obstruction of sweat glands. If your skin becomes irritated, contact your doctor.

- Very high doses or long-term use in children may cause Cushing's syndrome, a disease of the adrenal gland. Signs of this disease include weight gain and slow growth. Children are also at risk for increased pressure in the brain. Signs are headache and bulging "soft spots."

Special warning:

- You should not use this drug if you are allergic to other steroid creams.

Pregnancy and nursing mothers:

Category C. See page 9 for description of categories. Not known if drug is present in mother's milk.

Helpful hints:

- Do not wrap or bandage the area after you apply the medicine unless your doctor tells you to. For diaper rash, you should not use tight-fitting diapers or plastic pants after applying this medicine.
- Avoid contact with your eyes.
- Don't use this drug for longer than prescribed.
- Apply a thin film and rub in gently and completely.
- If your skin is infected, you'll also need an antifungal or antibacterial medicine.
- If you are covering a very large area of your skin and therefore using lots of medicine, you should be tested regularly for hypothalamic-pituitary-adrenal axis suppression. Regular testing could prevent severe side effects and withdrawal symptoms associated with steroids.

Fluocinonide

Brand names: *Dermacin, Fluocinonide E, Lidex, Lidex-E* **(Generic available)**

What this drug does for you:

This drug is used to relieve and heal inflamed or irritated skin conditions including eczema, dermatitis, psoriasis, severe diaper rash, insect bites, minor burns, and sunburn. It is a corticosteroid, and it is available as an ointment, cream, solution, and gel.

Possible side effects of this drug:

- Side effects are rare, but this drug may cause burning, itching, irritation, dryness, inflammation of hair follicles, excess hair growth, pimples, loss of skin pigment, skin wasting, inflammation of the skin, mild infection, streaks on the skin, and obstruction of sweat glands. If your skin becomes irritated, contact your doctor.
- Very high doses or long-term use in children may cause Cushing's syndrome, a disease of the adrenal gland. Signs of this disease include weight gain and slow growth. Children are also at risk for increased pressure in the brain. Signs are headache and bulging "soft spots."

Special warning:

- You should not use this drug if you are allergic to other steroid creams.

Pregnancy and nursing mothers:

Category C. See page 9 for description of categories. Not known if drug is

present in mother's milk.

Helpful hints:

- Do not wrap or bandage the area after you apply the medicine unless your doctor tells you to. For diaper rash, you should not use tight-fitting diapers or plastic pants after applying this medicine.
- Avoid contact with your eyes.
- Don't use this drug for longer than prescribed.
- Apply a thin film and rub in gently and completely.
- If your skin is infected, you'll also need an antifungal or antibacterial medicine.
- If you are covering a very large area of your skin and therefore using lots of medicine, you should be tested regularly for hypothalamic-pituitary-adrenal axis suppression. Regular testing could prevent severe side effects and withdrawal symptoms associated with steroids.

Flurandrenolide

Brand name: *Cordran*

What this drug does for you:

This drug is used to relieve and heal inflamed or irritated skin conditions including eczema, dermatitis, psoriasis, insect bites, and minor burns. It is a corticosteroid, and it is available as an ointment, cream, lotion, and tape.

Possible side effects of this drug:

- This drug may cause irritation, acne-like breakout, dryness, itching, burning, skin discoloration, mild infection, excessive hair growth, dry and itching skin around the mouth, inflammation of hair follicles, blocked sweat glands, skin wasting, and streaks on the skin.
- Very high doses or long-term use in children may cause Cushing's syndrome, a disease of the adrenal gland. Signs of this disease include weight gain and slow growth. Children are also at risk for increased pressure in the brain. Signs are headache and bulging "soft spots."

Special warning:

- You should not use this drug if you are allergic to other steroid creams.

Pregnancy and nursing mothers:

Category C. See page 9 for description of categories. Not known if drug is present in mother's milk.

Helpful hints:

- Apply a thin film one to four times a day and rub in gently and completely.
- Avoid contact with your eyes.
- Do not wrap or bandage the area after you apply the medicine unless your doctor tells you to. For diaper rash, you should not use tight-fitting diapers or plastic pants after applying this medicine.
- If you have psoriasis or a similar skin condition and your doctor has told you to wrap or bandage the area, you may want to follow these steps:

1) Soak in a bath and remove as much of the scaling skin as possible.
2) Rub the lotion in thoroughly.
3) Place moist gauze or a dampened cloth over the area and cover with a plastic wrap.
4) Seal the edges with tape.
- Don't use this drug for longer than prescribed.
- If your skin is infected, you'll also need an antifungal or antibacterial medicine.
- If you are covering a very large area of your skin and therefore using lots of medicine, you should be tested regularly for hypothalamic-pituitary-adrenal axis suppression. Regular testing could prevent severe side effects and withdrawal symptoms associated with steroids.

Halcinonide

Brand names: *Halog, Halog-E*

What this drug does for you:

This drug is used to relieve and heal inflamed or irritated skin conditions including eczema, dermatitis, psoriasis, severe diaper rash, insect bites, minor burns, and sunburn. It is a corticosteroid, and it is available as an ointment, cream, and solution.

Possible side effects of this drug:

- This drug may cause irritation, burning, itching, dryness, acne-like breakout, skin discoloration, infection, weakening and wasting of the skin, excessive hair growth, dermatitis around the mouth, blockage of sweat glands, and streaks on the skin.
- Very high doses or long-term use in children may cause Cushing's syndrome, a disease of the adrenal gland. Signs of this disease include weight gain and slow growth. Children are also at risk for increased pressure in the brain. Signs are headache and bulging "soft spots."

Special warning:

- You should not use this drug if you are allergic to other steroid creams.

Pregnancy and nursing mothers:

Category C. See page 9 for description of categories. Not known if drug is present in mother's milk.

Helpful hints:

- Apply a thin film one to four times a day and rub in gently and completely.
- Avoid contact with your eyes.
- Do not wrap or bandage the area after you apply the medicine unless your doctor tells you to. For diaper rash, you should not use tight-fitting diapers or plastic pants after applying this medicine.
- If you have psoriasis or a similar skin condition and your doctor has told you to wrap or bandage the area, you may want to follow these steps:
    1) Rub a small amount of cream in thoroughly. Then add a thin coat-

    ing of cream.

    2) Wet the area or place a dampened cloth over the area and cover with a plastic wrap.

    3) Seal the edges with tape.

- Don't use this drug for longer than prescribed.
- If your skin is infected, you'll also need an antifungal or antibacterial medicine.
- If you are covering a very large area of your skin and therefore using lots of medicine, you should be tested regularly for hypothalamic-pituitary-adrenal axis suppression. Regular testing could prevent severe side effects and withdrawal symptoms associated with steroids.

Mometasone

Brand name: *Elocon*

What this drug does for you:

This drug is used to relieve and heal inflamed or irritated skin conditions including eczema, dermatitis, psoriasis, severe diaper rash, insect bites, minor burns, and sunburn. It is a corticosteroid, and it is available as an ointment, cream, and lotion.

Possible side effects of this drug:

- This drug may cause irritation, burning, itching, dryness, acne-like breakout, skin discoloration, infection, weakening and wasting of the skin, excessive hair growth, dermatitis around the mouth, blockage of sweat glands, and streaks on the skin.
- Very high doses or long-term use in children may cause Cushing's syndrome, a disease of the adrenal gland. Signs of this disease include weight gain and slow growth. Children are also at risk for increased pressure in the brain. Signs are headache and bulging "soft spots."

Special warning:

- You should not use this drug if you are allergic to other steroid creams.

Pregnancy and nursing mothers:

Category C. See page 9 for description of categories. Not known if drug is present in mother's milk.

Helpful hints:

- Apply a thin film of the cream or ointment once a day. Also apply the lotion once a day and massage lightly until it disappears. You won't waste any lotion if you'll hold the nozzle of the bottle very close to the affected area and gently squeeze.
- Avoid contact with your eyes.
- Do not wrap or bandage the area after you apply the medicine unless your doctor tells you to. For diaper rash, you should not use tight-fitting diapers or plastic pants after applying this medicine.
- Don't use this drug for longer than prescribed.
- If your skin is infected, you'll also need an antifungal or antibacterial medicine.

- If you are covering a very large area of your skin and therefore using lots of medicine, you should be tested regularly for hypothalamic-pituitary-adrenal axis suppression. Regular testing could prevent severe side effects and withdrawal symptoms associated with steroids.

Psoriasis Drugs

Etretinate

Brand name: *Tegison*

What this drug does for you:

This drug is used to treat severe psoriasis in people who cannot use other drugs (perhaps because they are allergic to them).

Possible side effects of this drug:

- Etretinate has many side effects. The most common are dry nose, chapped lips, hair loss, peeling of the hands and feet, thickening of bones, thirstiness, sore mouth, dry and fragile skin, itching, rash, red and scaly face, bone and joint pain, and tiredness.
- Some people also experience nosebleeds, bruising, sunburn, muscle cramps, headache, eye pain, stomach pain, and changes in appetite. Almost one-quarter of the people taking etretinate may experience inflamed and swollen lips, sore tongue, fingernail and toenail deformities, fever, and nausea.
- Etretinate commonly raises triglyceride and cholesterol levels.
- This drug may cause eye and vision disorders. For instance, it may cause eye irritation, double vision, or blurred vision or affect the corneas of your eyes, making contact lenses difficult to wear.
- Two common risks of taking etretinate for long periods of time are liver damage (including hepatitis and cirrhosis) and increased pressure on the brain. Signs of this high pressure include headache, nausea, fluid retention, and visual disturbances. Let your doctor know immediately if you develop these symptoms.
- Etretinate may make your psoriasis worse when you first begin taking it. That doesn't mean you should stop taking the drug.
- Less common side effects include bleeding gums, blister-like skin eruptions, infected skin around the fingernails, loosening of the fingernails, difficulty breathing, cold and clammy skin, fluid retention, muscle pain, dizziness, and dry eyes, nose, or mouth.
- Rare side effects include frequent urination, kidney stones, diarrhea, constipation, gas, mouth ulcers, sore throat, anxiety, mental depression, faintness, low blood pressure, chest pain, and irregular heartbeats.

Special warnings:

- Don't use this drug if you are allergic to vitamin A.
- You should have a liver function test before you begin taking etretinate.
- If you are diabetic, obese, or drink alcohol, or have a family history of

these conditions, you should use this drug with caution.

Pregnancy and nursing mothers:

Category X. See page 9 for description of categories. Drug may remain in the blood for a long time after treatment is finished, so if you are planning to become pregnant, talk with your doctor. Not known if drug is present in mother's milk. However, women should not nurse during treatment.

Possible food and drug interactions:

- Don't take vitamin supplements containing vitamin A while you are taking this drug.
- Avoid alcohol while taking this drug because it may cause very high triglyceride levels.

Helpful hints:

- Take etretinate with food or milk to increase absorption of the drug.
- Use a moisturizer to help relieve dry skin. Apply one hour after using etretinate.
- This drug may make your skin extra-sensitive to sunlight, so protect your skin if you'll be outdoors in sunny weather.
- Be careful when driving because this drug may cause vision problems, including decreased night vision.
- Don't drive or operate dangerous appliances or machinery until you are sure the drug isn't making you drowsy or less than alert.
- Usually, you quit taking etretinate (under your doctor's supervision) when your psoriasis clears up.

Natural Alternatives

ACNE

◀ Blackheads
◀ Pimples
◀ Whiteheads

◀ Inflammation of skin
◀ Redness

Avoid adult acne attacks

Acne — it seems appropriate that this nasty little word falls into the same section of the dictionary as words like awful, abominable, atrocious, and appalling.

Those may be just a few of the feelings you have as you look in the mirror and experience a frightening flashback to your teen-age years. Thankfully, hopeless is not a word that's near or even associated with acne — because there's plenty you can do to ace adult acne starting right now.

Eat a healthy diet, but chocolate is OK! You've probably heard that you should not eat chocolate if you're acne-prone. But clinical studies have shown no scientific evidence linking certain foods and acne. It's important to eat a well-balanced diet, however. You'll not only feel healthier, but your skin will look healthier as well.

Clean your face gently. Scrubbing your skin can make the acne worse. Wash oily skin with water and a mild, unscented soap one to three times a day. Don't use deodorant soaps or abrasive sponges.

Keep your hands off your face. Squeezing and picking at your pimples can lead to more redness and swelling. Don't lean on your hands or rub your face either.

Be aware of your environment. Avoid polluted and humid conditions whenever possible. Heavy sweating can aggravate your acne. Also, getting out in the sun will make acne worse for some people. Wear a hat to shade your face.

Make sure your makeup is water-based. Oil-based products will aggravate your skin condition. Also, watch out for suntan oils, hair gels, and sprays.

Shampoo daily if your hair is oily. This will keep excess oil off your face.

Reduce emotional stress and tension. Stress triggers acne.

If you make these simple changes, you should see results within two months. Don't give up too soon.

Source —
American Family Physician (50,1:89)

ATHLETE'S FOOT

◀ Inflammation of the skin, especially between the toes
◀ Itching, especially between the toes
◀ Redness

Sidestep athlete's foot

When you're experiencing the all-consuming itch of athlete's foot, you think how pleasant life was when you were footloose and fungal-free.

Yes, there is a fungus among us, and that's what is causing your annoying itch. If you can, take comfort in the thought that you're not alone. As the most common fungal infection, about 10 percent of the population is scratching away at athlete's foot at any given time. The fungus can grow in any warm, dark, moist place, like your bathroom. You increase your chances of athlete's foot by simply wearing shoes, especially without socks, wearing the same pair of shoes all the time, or forgetting to wash your socks often enough.

Don't scratch your irritated feet, and be especially careful if you're diabetic, have impaired circulation, have AIDS, or are on medication for cancer therapy. Here's how you can stamp out athlete's foot forever:

Try Epsom salt soaks. When you have athlete's foot, try soaking your feet in Epsom salt for 10 to 15 minutes, three times a day, for three to five days. Or soak your feet in a gallon of warm water with two capfuls of bleach. After toweling your feet dry, take a cotton ball and completely dry your feet with rubbing alcohol. This really burns, but it's a good antiseptic.

Sprinkle with cornstarch. You can sprinkle some cornstarch on your feet to help keep them dry when you have athlete's foot, but don't use talc or baking soda if the fungus is weeping.

Keep it clean and dry. The easiest way to prevent athlete's foot is to wash your feet often with soap and water, keep your feet dry, and change your socks often. You can use a foot powder, but make sure it's medicated. Talcum powder smells nice, but it won't kill the fungus on your feet.

Soak your feet in warm tea. Feet that sweat a lot are at risk for a fungus. Try putting a couple of tea bags in hot water just long enough to turn the water brown. Let it cool until it's warm, then soak your feet for five to 10 minutes. Tea contains tannins, natural chemicals that help pull excess moisture from your feet. A solution of one part vinegar to 10 parts water also works well. Dry your feet thoroughly after soaking. You also can spray your feet with an antiperspirant deodorant spray. If your case of athlete's foot lasts for more than five to seven days, or seems to be affecting a toenail, go see your doctor.

Sources —

Bryant Stamford, Ph.D., director of the Health Promotion and Wellness Center and professor of allied health, School of Medicine, University of Louisville, Louisville, Ky.

Dr. Chet Evans, dean of the School of Podiatric Medicine, Barry University, Miami, Fla.

The Physician and Sportsmedicine (22,7:79)

BURNS

◀ Painful red or white blisters
◀ Wet or waxy dry blisters
◀ Charred, painless blisters

Self-care or doctor's care for burns?

Sometimes it's hard to know if a burn is superficial or if it's deeper and more damaging than it appears. You can treat first-degree burns and most second-degree burns at home. Third-degree burns should be treated professionally. Here's how to determine if your burn is serious enough to see a doctor:

First-degree burns involve only the top layers of skin and usually leave no scars. The skin is red and turns white when touched.

Second-degree burns look white or white with some redness, and they feel wet or waxy dry. Flames, oil, or grease are often the cause of second-degree burns, and they usually do scar.

You might not be able to tell the difference between a second-degree burn and a third-degree burn. If you're not sure, go ahead and see your doctor. He'll treat the burn in the office and show you how to care for it at home.

Third-degree burns usually look white or charred. You will only be able to feel deep pressure in a third-degree burn. The nerves are destroyed so you can't feel pain.

You definitely need to see a doctor for a burn if:

◁ The burn is from electricity or from a chemical. Burns from electricity can cause heart problems and damage that you may not see to tissues deep in the body. Chemicals such as hydrofluoric acid, commonly used in the semiconductor industry, cause burns that are initially painless, but can severely injure deep tissues.

◁ The burn goes all the way around your neck, trunk, leg, or arm, or covers a large area.

◁ You are burned on the eyes, ears, or genital area.

◁ You have diabetes, heart disease, or an immune system disorder.

◁ The burn is on a baby under 2 years old or on a person over 60.

◁ You have inhaled enough smoke to damage your lungs.

How to care for burns at home

When you stumble into a hot iron or spill boiling water on yourself, your first instinct should be to head for cool water. That's smart — the sooner you get the temperature of your skin back to normal, the less damage you'll have. You can soak the area in cool water or use cool, wet towels. You should keep the burned area in cool water until the pain stops.

For first-degree burns, just dry the burn off and for the next day or two keep it covered loosely with some gauze. After the first day, you can use something like aloe vera cream to relieve the stinging.

For second-degree burns, smooth on a layer of antibiotic cream, preferably silver sulfadiazine ointment. Use something sterile instead of your bare hands to apply the cream (such as a cotton swab). Then cover the burn with a dressing like a Telfa pad and wrap the burned area loosely with gauze. Completely wash off and reapply the antibiotic cream every day. Repeat this process until your wound begins to heal.

Sources —
American Family Physician (45,3:1321)
U.S. Pharmacist (17,4:28)

CONTACT DERMATITIS

◀ Bright red blisters, sometimes weeping   ◀ Inflammation of the skin after
◀ Itching   touching an irritating substance
◀ Redness

Cosmetics can be culprits

From the lotions on your squeaky-clean hair to your pedicured toes, any grooming aid can be the culprit behind a skin reaction.

An allergic reaction to a cosmetic can be triggered by ingredients such as fragrances and preservatives. Your reaction may not occur overnight. You can become sensitized to some ingredient in a cosmetic you've used for years and suddenly develop an allergy to it. Even sticking to natural products from plant or animal sources is no guarantee of safety. Allergies to such substances as lanolin (made from sheep's wool) are fairly common.

If you have a skin reaction to a cosmetic, follow these guidelines:

◁ Stop using the product you most recently began using. If that doesn't help, limit or discontinue use of all cosmetics to give the reaction time to clear up.

◁ Gradually reintroduce one cosmetic at a time into your grooming routine.

◁ If a cosmetic has changed color or developed an odor, the preservatives may no longer be working, and bacteria may be lurking within. Stop using the product immediately and throw it away.

◁ Read labels of all skin-care products that you use. You may find that cosmetics containing a certain ingredient cause you an allergic reaction.

◁ Call your doctor if the reaction persists.

You can develop an allergic reaction to plenty of other products besides cosmetics. Common sources of contact dermatitis are:

◁ Medicated creams and ointments. Ingredients you may be allergic to are antibiotics, antihistamines, antiseptics, and stabilizers.

◁ Tanning agents in shoes.

◁ Rubber accelerators and antioxidants in gloves, shoes, underpants, bras, and other clothes.

◁ Dyes and metal compounds such as nickel and mercury.

Recent studies show that taking vitamins C and E may help prevent skin allergies.

Sources —
Cutis (52,5:316)
FDA Consumer (27,9:32)
The Atlanta Journal/Constitution (Dec. 8, 1993, B4)
The Complete Book of Natural Cosmetics, Simon and Schuster, New York, 1974

CUTS AND SCRAPES

◀ Bleeding
◀ Broken skin

First aid for cuts and scrapes

Some wounds need more than a Band-Aid, but don't need a doctor's attention. Most cuts and scrapes get well without much outside help, but here are a few tips to get better faster:

Clean the wound. It's important to clean the wound with mild soap and water to remove any dirt or other foreign materials that might cause infection. If the pressure of running water isn't enough to remove all the dirt and debris, use a sterile pad to gently brush the dirt out.

For easy cleaning of dirty wounds, keep a can of aerosol saline solution in your first-aid kit. You'll find it in the contact-lens section of the drugstore. The preservative-free saline for sensitive eyes is safest.

Stop the bleeding. Many minor wounds stop bleeding on their own. If it is still bleeding after you clean it, apply pressure directly to the wound for a couple of minutes. If you can't easily stop the bleeding, you should see a doctor.

Kill the germs. You can help prevent infection in wounds by applying antiseptic to kill the germs as soon as possible after the wound occurs. Isopropyl alcohol or hydrogen peroxide are excellent antiseptics, but they may sting. You can find nonstinging antiseptic ointments, creams, and sprays at your pharmacy.

Iodine is also used as an antiseptic, but it burns and discolors the surrounding skin. Iodine and hydrogen peroxide can be dangerous if used on large areas. Decolorized iodine does not kill germs.

Several antibiotic creams are available without a prescription. Apply a small amount (enough to cover your fingertip) one to three times a day. If your wound is too large to be covered by a fingertip's worth of antibiotic cream, you probably should see a doctor.

Heal yourself with honey. Using honey as first aid for cuts and scrapes is a practice as old as ancient Egypt. Today, it is thought that honey acts much like hydrogen peroxide when applied to a surface wound. Honey may have antibacterial properties taken from the many plants a bee visits in making his rounds.

Act quickly with aloe vera. Studies suggest that aloe gel can ease pain, reduce swelling, prevent blistering, and combat bacteria and fungi. Because aloe gel seems to regenerate damaged skin tissues, it prevents scarring in many cases.

Aloe will stop minor cuts from bleeding. If you apply it directly to your cut, the aloe will dry immediately and slow the escape of blood.

Stick with fresh aloe for best results. The aloe plant is inexpensive, easy to maintain, and looks great in a kitchen window. It's handy too. When you need it, just break off a leaf segment and squeeze the sap onto your injury.

If you don't want to grow your own aloe, you can pick up an aloe-based ointment at a natural-foods store. Just read the labels carefully and be sure the product contains at least 70 percent aloe vera gel.

Cover the wound. Dressings help stop bleeding, they absorb fluid that may ooze from the wound later, and they protect the wound from dirt and further damage.

Most minor wounds should be covered with a dressing that won't stick. First-aid kits usually contain this kind of dressing, and it is readily available at any pharmacy.

Wounds that drain may require additional absorbent dressing on top of the nonstick dressing. Don't put gauze directly on a wound because it might stick. Change the dressing daily, or more often if the wound is draining.

Secure the dressing. Use tape to firmly secure all four sides of the dressing. You can choose from several kinds of first-aid tapes. Cloth tape won't cause allergic reactions, and it is very strong. Use cloth tape if the dressing is bulky.

Plastic tape stretches with the skin. Paper tape isn't as sticky, so it doesn't irritate the skin as much as the other kinds, but it may come loose in areas where the skin moves.

Try a high-tech bandage option. Older skin tears more easily than young skin because it isn't anchored as securely (the top layer can easily pull away from lower layers). Plus, once aging skin is injured, it takes longer to heal.

For these reasons, researchers have been working for decades on more effective bandages for aging skin. In recent years they've come up with a totally new kind of bandage that can actually speed healing and cut down on scarring.

Much better than the old cotton gauze, hydrocolloid bandages are made from a chemical called calcium alginate which is found in seaweed. This special gift from the sea stimulates the natural healing process and helps fight off infection like no adhesive bandage ever could.

These high-tech bandages can be used for all kinds of surface wounds as well as deep wounds. Instead of several times a day, hydrocolloid bandages only need to be changed about once a week on some kinds of wounds.

Hydrocolloid bandages are available through home medical care suppliers. The cost is usually higher than a typical gauze bandage. But when you consider the time and money saved in faster healing, less scarring, and significantly less pain, it's worth the extra cost.

Eat a scar-free diet. The American Academy of Cosmetic Surgery warns health-conscious Americans to make sure their diets contain wound-healing nutrients. Your body requires certain nutrients in order to heal quickly without ugly scars.

If you're a vegetarian or a chronic dieter, make sure your diet isn't hindering your body's ability to heal. It takes less than one week on a poor diet to lower the production of essential wound healers in your body.

Your diet must include albumin (contained in proteins); glucose (in carbohydrates); essential fatty acids; vitamins A, B complex, C, and K; and the minerals zinc, copper, iron, and manganese.

All these nutrients are essential to help you avoid scars that last a lifetime.

Sources —
American Journal of Surgery (167,1:21S)
British Journal of Surgery (77,5:568)
Drug Topics (138,22:40)
Emergency Medicine (25,7:45)
Harvard Health Letter (20,10:6)
Heinerman's Encyclopedia of Fruits, Vegetables and Herbs, Parker Publishing Company, West Nyack, N.Y., 1988
Herbal Medicine, Beaconsfield Publishers, Beaconsfield, England, 1991
Herbs, The Reader's Digest Association, Pleasantville, N.Y., 1990
Miracle Medicine Herbs, Parker Publishing, West Nyack, N.Y., 1991
Nursing Homes (43,1:27)
Science News (145,13:206)
The American Medical Association Family Medical Guide, Random House, New York, 1982
The Compass in Your Nose and Other Astonishing Facts About Humans, Jeremy P. Tarcher, Inc., Los Angeles, Calif., 1989
The Honest Herbal, Pharmaceutical Products Press, Binghamton, N.Y., 1993
The Journal of the American Medical Association (273,12:910)
The Lancet (341,8837:90)
U.S. Pharmacist (19,10:1 Supplement)

DANDRUFF

◀ Dry, flaking scalp
◀ Itching of the scalp

Down with dandruff

If you're getting a reputation for being flaky because of all the dandruff on your shoulders, you need to take action. A flaky pastry is preferred, but a flaky person is not.

Here's what to do:

Make an herbal oil treatment. Mix together two tablespoons of plain vegetable oil with six drops of burdock root oil. Warm the mixture and then gently massage it into your scalp and hair.

Put a shower cap over your head. Soak a towel in hot water, wring it out, and wrap your head with it. Keep the towel and shower cap in place for 20 minutes.

Then wash your hair with a mild shampoo. Rinse thoroughly, two to three times. Style as usual. Other herbal oils that may be mixed with vegetable oil to treat dandruff include rosemary, parsley, chamomile, and licorice.

Rinse with bay laurel tea. You've probably cooked with sweet bay or bay laurel. For dandruff shampoo, the thick, aromatic leaves should be dried and crushed. Mix three teaspoons of the crushed leaves into a quart of boiling water. Cover the pot and let the leaves soak for about a half-hour. Strain the leaves and pour the "tea" into a plastic container.

After shampooing, rinse your hair well and then slowly pour about a cup of the mixture over your head. Distribute it well, all through the hair and over the entire scalp. Rinse out after one hour. If used regularly, the bay mixture should control common dandruff. Keep the "tea" in your refrigerator for external use.

If at first you don't succeed … If dandruff is a frequent uninvited guest, you may have eczema or psoriasis. You should probably try one of the "medicated" dandruff shampoos.

They contain ingredients like salicylic acid or coal tar. A dandruff shampoo will loosen those dry flakes and cleanse your scalp and hair. Always rinse thoroughly, two to three times, and follow up with a hair conditioner.

But use these stronger shampoos with caution: Shampoos containing coal tar can discolor lighter hair. They shouldn't be left on your skin for long periods, and they can make your skin and hair sensitive to sunlight.

Wash your hair every day. Dandruff occurs more often in people with oily hair, not dry hair. Frequent washings will help remove the oil.

Alternate your dandruff shampoo with a regular shampoo. Keep both in the shower. Leave the cap flipped up or turn the bottle upside-down to show which one you used last, in case you forget.

If regular use of a dandruff shampoo doesn't control your flaky scalp or if your head really itches, make an appointment with a dermatologist. You may need a prescription drug to control your dandruff. And meanwhile, resist the urge to scratch. You should even keep your fingernails trimmed so that you won't break the skin of your scalp.

Sources —
FDA Consumer (28,8:25)
The Lawrence Review of Natural Products, Facts and Comparisons, St. Louis, Mo., 1991

DIAPER RASH

◀ Red, irritated, blistered skin in baby's diaper area

Don't neglect diaper duty

A dirty diaper left on your baby can cause diaper rash, so frequent changes are extremely important. But parents frustrated with dirty diapers should take heart! Your baby will grow older, will need less frequent diaper changes, and diaper rash will become a thing of the past. Meanwhile, here are some other tips for keeping diaper rash out of the family picture.

Keep 'em dry with disposables. Whatever their environmental impact, disposable diapers do a better job of keeping moisture away from your baby's skin. Babies in reusable cloth diapers get diaper rash more often and more severely.

Give rubber panties a rest. Avoid the use of plastic or rubber pants, since these trap moisture against the baby's skin. Not only does the moisture irritate the skin, it also lets irritants enter the skin more easily.

Ask your doctor about zinc. One study showed that infants who often get diaper rash have lower than normal levels of zinc in their bodies. In another study, babies given 10 mg of oral zinc gluconate crushed and mixed with milk had less diaper rash than babies who didn't get the zinc.

Breast-feed if possible. For pregnant women debating breast-feeding vs. the bottle: You may want to know that breast-fed babies have fewer diaper rashes because their urine and stool are more acidic.

Blot or blow your baby dry. If your baby has already developed diaper rash, your major focus should be on keeping his skin dry. Don't wash the diaper area when your baby is only wet. Simply blot the urine dry. You can also use a blow dryer set on its coolest temperature. Hold it so that you can just barely feel the air against your baby's skin.

Wash with a mild soap. After a bowel movement, when washing is necessary, use a mild soap (such as Dove, Tone, or Caress) and water instead of baby wipes, since the wipes may contain irritating chemicals.

Watch out for these harmful products. Cornstarch can help keep a baby dry, but don't use talcum powder. It's so light that it can be inhaled by your baby and cause chemical pneumonia. When using any kind of powder, be sure to keep it away from your baby's face.

Other harmful products you should never use are boric acid, baking soda, egg whites (an old home remedy), and ointments such as Vaseline or A & D ointment. These ointments don't allow moisture to evaporate.

Don't use antibiotic ointments, products containing hydrocortisone, or non-prescription antifungal products until you've checked with your doctor.

Source —
    U.S. Pharmacist (19,3:27)

DRY SKIN

◀ Dry, rough, peeling, cracking skin
◀ Intense itching
◀ Pain and stinging

Dry-skin cures for winter woes

For many people with dry skin, cold weather means "winter itch," that dry, scaly, itching, irritating condition that plagues you every year. This year, fight it with these simple self-help tips.

◁ Use warm water, rather than hot, to bathe.

◁ Use a very mild, moisturizing soap, and use it sparingly.

◁ Don't scrub with a washcloth or a towel. Gently pat your skin dry.

◁ While skin is still slightly damp, apply a thick lotion to seal in the moisture. White petroleum jelly is an excellent soothing and softening agent.

◁ Don't wear rough, scratchy clothing. Go for soft, natural fibers.

◁ Use a humidifier in your home, and keep the heat turned as low as you can comfortably stand it.

◁ Check to see if your bath soap or laundry detergent is causing your itching. If so, switch to another brand.

◁ Be sure you drink eight glasses of water a day.

◁ Try taking three flaxseed-oil capsules a day for healthy skin. They are a vegetable source for omega-3 fatty acids.

◁ Take your vitamins. The most important ones for your skin are A, B-complex, C, and E.

◁ Ask your pharmacist to recommend one of the new over-the-counter products made with ammonium lactate or alpha-hydroxy acids.

◁ To temporarily relieve itching, fill a plastic bag with ice and apply to the itchy area.

If your itchy skin cannot be conquered, see your doctor to be sure there isn't some other cause for it and to get prescription medication to knock out the itch. But keep on using the tips above, and be sure to protect your skin when you're out in the winter weather.

Sources —
    Cutis (54,4:229)
    Medical Tribune (32,20:14)
    The Physician and Sportsmedicine (23,1:53)

INGROWN NAILS AND FUNGUS NAILS

◀ Painful, red skin at edge of nails
◀ Thick and dull-looking nails

Nurture your nails

Nails can be an attractive ending to fingers and toes, but they can also be painful and troublesome. Take good care of your nails to keep them healthy and pain-free. Here are a few tips.

◁ Always trim your nails straight across. You don't want the edge to curve down into the skin. When it grows, the nail can become ingrown. This gets even more important as you get older because your nails tend to grow wider.

◁ Clip nails when they're damp and soft. Try clipping your nails immediately after bathing.

◁ Keep your nails short, but never trim them deeper than the tip of your fingers or toes. File down any rough edges that may catch on a surface and cause your nail to tear.

◁ Use moisturizers on hands and feet to keep your nails from breaking, splintering, and cracking. Nails become more brittle as you age.

◁ For nails infected with fungus, put 4 to 6 ounces of boric acid in a jar and fill with water. Paint this mixture on your nails twice a day. This method takes a long time to work, but is less expensive than prescription drugs.

Your nails can also serve as a warning signal that you need medical treatment. If a nail becomes thick and dull-looking, you may have a fungal infection or a more serious condition. A nail with a black or brown streak in it could be cancerous. If you notice a change in one or more of your nails, make sure you ask your doctor about it.

Sources —
American Family Physician (50,2:322)
Geriatrics (49,3:21)

POISON IVY

◀ Streaks or patches of redness and blisters
◀ Itching
◀ Pus or soft yellow scabs when infected

Put off poison ivy

One spring or summer camping trip or nature walk can be all it takes to give you a case of poison ivy. Here's how to cope:

◁ Immediately wash your hands and exposed areas with rubbing alcohol and rinse with clean water.

◁ Wash the clothes you were wearing when you were exposed to the poison ivy. Anything with oil or sap from the plant can spread the rash even more. This includes the family pet. Wash clothes and pets with soap and water. Clean shoes with equal parts of rubbing alcohol and water.

◁ Soak the rash in cool water and colloidal oatmeal for 20 minutes, or massage with an ice cube as often as necessary to help relieve itching.

◁ Apply a cool compress of equal parts milk and water.

◁ To avoid infection, don't scratch. Scratching the blisters does not spread the rash, but it can make the skin condition worse and lead to infection.

◁ Apply calamine lotion or over-the-counter hydrocortisone cream or gel to relieve itching and dry the blisters.

◁ Consider taking an over-the-counter oral antihistamine to relieve itching, especially at night.

◁ Stay out of the sun. The rash is aggravated by sunlight.

Sources —
Child Health Alert (June 1995, 13:2)

PSORIASIS

◀ **Red areas with silvery scales**
◀ **Usually affects scalp, elbows, knees, and lower back**
◀ **Cracking, itching, and thickening of skin**

Stamp out psoriasis

Every day your body has to shed an incredible amount of old, dead surface skin tissue just to make room for new cells. New cells are constantly pushing their way out from deeper skin layers. But for some people, that balanced rate of skin replacement goes haywire, and new cells develop much faster than the old are shed. The result is itchy, red, scaly patches of thickened skin — the most common sign of psoriasis.

Get it diagnosed. Since there are other skin problems that may look like psoriasis, first get your condition diagnosed by a specialist. Also, since psoriasis comes in several forms, you need to identify the type you have before starting treatment.

Treatment focuses on removing the buildup of skin cells and slowing the rate of new skin growth. Although psoriasis is triggered by internal, biological mechanisms, you can help prevent flare-ups. Here are some ways to enhance your doctor's prescribed treatments:

Lay off the bad habits. Several studies reveal that alcohol triggers psoriasis flare-ups. And smoking may account for one-quarter of all cases of a certain type of psoriasis, one study suggests.

Get yourself in shape. If you're overweight, try to lose a few pounds. Maintaining a normal weight should improve your psoriasis.

Exercise is one of the greatest natural healers, even for psoriasis. Skin, like all the other body organs, will be healthier if you exercise and eat a healthy diet. Good nutrition and exercise habits will keep your immune system functioning well too.

Keep your skin moist and supple. Buy a humidifier for your home. Your skin won't get so dry if the air is moist. Stay away from harsh soaps, cleaners, and long, hot baths. A warm bath with an oatmeal bath product will help heal your skin.

Water- or oil-based moisturizers will soften your skin and help control flaking and bleeding. Use moisturizers with alpha-hydroxy skin exfoliants. Find a concentration that doesn't burn.

Ask your doctor about your medications. Some medicines such as steroids, certain heart regulators, lithium, and blood pressure medications aggravate psoriasis.

Treat your skin gently. Buy soft clothes so that you don't chafe your skin with rough clothing, and don't scratch or pick at affected areas.

Get over-the-counter relief. Two psoriasis healers you can buy without a prescription are topical corticosteroid creams and coal tar preparations. You can buy coal tar soaps, shampoos, and ointments. Make sure you follow the manufacturer's directions carefully. You don't want to make your problem worse instead of better.

Try mineral baths. Some people believe in the healing powers of natural mineral waters, such as Soap Lake in Washington state and the Dead Sea between Israel and Jordan.

Have fun in the sun. Sunbathing may help, but sun with care. You cer tainly don't want to burn your skin.

Sources —
> *British Medical Journal* (308,2:428)
> *Cutis* (53,1:21)
> *Journal of the American Academy of Dermatologists* (28,4:632)
> *Pharmacy News*, National Psoriasis Foundation (5,1:8)
> *The New England Journal of Medicine* (322,9:581 and 322,16:1449)

RINGWORM

◀ Itchy, scaly rash
◀ Red, circular, flat skin eruptions

Relieve your ringworm

Surprisingly, ringworm is not caused by a worm at all, but by a very small fungus! The characteristic ring-shaped rash spreads out from a central spot, leaving dry, itchy skin behind.

Ringworm rashes should be kept clean and dry and should be treated with miconazole, which is available in an over-the-counter cream. Other nonprescription treatments include clotrimazole and tolnaftate.

To hasten the healing process:

◁ After bathing, carefully dry the rash with a towel and then a blow dryer on a cool setting.

◁ Wear absorbent cotton clothing over the area rather than synthetic fabrics.

◁ Sometimes the rash may "weep" liquid. In this case, apply a wet compress. The water in the compress will actually help to dry up the rash.

Since ringworm is very contagious, avoid close contact with other people and animals.

Source —
Before You Call the Doctor, Fawcett Columbine, New York, 1992

ROSACEA

◀ Redness, flushing, and inflammation of the nose and cheeks
◀ Small, visible blood vessels (sometimes a small red dot surrounded by tiny lines)
◀ Pimples or cysts
◀ Itching or burning

Reduce facial flushing of rosacea

W.C. Fields was famous for saying, "It ain't a fit night out for man nor beast." Looking at his ruddy complexion and bulbous red nose, you might have thought he coined that phrase after he'd been caught in some mighty bad weather — a sandstorm perhaps.

Actually, Fields suffered from rosacea, a skin disorder that most often affects fair-skinned women between the ages of 30 and 50.

Rosacea can cause the blood vessels of the face to enlarge, until you have a reddened face and a bulging red nose. It can also cause a burning and irritation of the eyes known as conjunctivitis. Rosacea can get worse and worse if you don't get it diagnosed and treated early on.

Here are some other tips to help you deal with this condition:

◁ Don't rub or massage your face; it will irritate inflamed skin.

◁ Avoid irritating cosmetics, and keep hair sprays off your face.

◁ Limit your exposure to sunlight, extreme heat, and very cold weather. Apply sunscreen daily. Choose a sunscreen with a minimum Sun Protection Factor (SPF) of 15. This will limit the damaging effects of sunlight.

◁ Don't smoke, and avoid alcoholic beverages, hot liquids, and spicy foods. These can all trigger or worsen the redness by causing blood to rush to the affected areas.

◁ Bypass saunas, hot showers, whirlpool baths, and steam rooms since extreme heat can force blood vessels to dilate.

◁ Use mild soaps and gentle moisturizers instead of abrasive cleaners and harsh astringents.

◁ Certain drugs can worsen rosacea. Ask your doctor about this if you are taking nitroglycerin or theophylline.

◁ Try to avoid stressful situations. Repressed anger, fear, or other strong emotions can trigger an attack. Use relaxation techniques when stressful situations can't be avoided.

◁ Use green-tinted makeup to cover bouts of inflammation. It's specially designed to tone down skin redness. You can find this makeup in department stores.

Sources —
National Institute of Arthritis and Musculoskeletal and Skin Diseases Information Clearinghouse, 1 AMS Circle, Bethesda, Md., 20892-2350
Rosacea, American Academy of Dermatology, P.O. Box 3116, Evanston, Ill. 60204-3116, 1993

SUNBURN

◀ Blistering
◀ Peeling
◀ Red, painful, burned areas of skin

Sunburn solutions

You spent more time in the sun than you planned to, your sunscreen stopped working hours ago, and now you have a sunburn. Try the tips below for some soothing relief.

◁ Put a cool compress of water on the sunburned area. Or add a half-cup of baking soda or colloidal oatmeal to a tub of cool water and soak.

◁ Drink lots of water. Your skin's ability to keep fluids inside the body is

---

When a sunburn is not a sunburn

Certain food additives, medicines, and skin-care products contain drugs that cause you to be more sensitive to sunlight. These can cause two types of reactions:

Photoallergic reactions usually result from substances you apply to your skin. Within 20 seconds of exposure to natural sunlight or artificial light from a tanning booth, skin rashes can appear, spreading to parts of the body that are not exposed. But sometimes reactions can take up to three months to develop.

Phototoxic reactions are more common, and can result from substances injected, taken orally, or applied to the skin. They cause sunburnlike symptoms to occur only on parts of the body exposed to light. This can happen within a few minutes or several hours after sun exposure. The resulting skin damage can last from six months to 20 years.

The results of photosensitivity can look like a bad case of sunburn, a rash, or an allergic reaction, so you may not always recognize the cause. However, you should be wary and check with your doctor if you suspect photosensitivity.

Newer sunscreen products that contain titanium dioxide will protect you better if you are photosensitive. Also, be sure to cover yourself with dark glasses, a hat, and a long-sleeved shirt when you go out in the sun.

Source —
Pharmacy Times (61,6:23)

damaged by sunburn.

◁ Don't cover up the burn while you're indoors.

◁ Apply vitamin E to the burned areas to prevent damage and decrease swelling and sensitivity.

◁ Apply a light moisturizer to the burned areas. Wait 24 hours before applying petroleum jelly or medicated creams, such as hydrocortisone and benzocaine. The medicated creams can irritate the skin and the jelly can cause your skin to retain heat.

◁ Stay out of the sun until the burn heals. It takes a week to 10 days for this to happen.

◁ Call your doctor if you develop fever, severe chills, dizziness, or blisters.

Sources —
Parents Magazine (70,5:26 and 70,7:20)
Scanning Microscopy (7,1994:1269)

> Please check with your doctor for approval before taking or discontinuing any prescription drug or using a natural healing alternative.

Smoking and Alcohol Addiction

Prescription Drugs

Natural Alternatives

Prescription Drugs ℞

Alcohol Addiction Drugs

Disulfiram

Brand name: *Antabuse*

What this drug does for you:

This drug is used to treat certain chronic alcoholics who want to remain sober. It doesn't stop the craving or impulse to drink, but it almost forces you to stay sober because the consequences of drinking are so terrible. Disulfiram causes an alcohol intolerance with effects such as flushing, a throbbing headache, vomiting, difficult breathing, blurred vision, and confusion when you drink alcohol.

Possible side effects of this drug:

- This drug may cause drowsiness, restlessness, weakness, headache, impotence, joint disease, metallic or garlic-like aftertaste, liver problems, psychotic reaction, and skin eruptions.
- Disulfiram may also cause nerve disorders including inflammation of the nerves, particularly of the eyes, which may cause poor vision, poor color perception, and blindness.

Special warnings:

- Don't use alcohol in any form while you are taking this drug. Even in small amounts, it may produce a severe reaction that can cause slowed breathing, irregular heart rhythms, heart attack, unconsciousness, convulsions, and death. Ask your pharmacist about the alcohol content of any medications you intend to buy, including over-the-counter products. Also avoid vinegar, some sauces, aftershave lotions, colognes, and ointments.
- This drug should not be used by people with an allergy to any thiuram derivatives, which are used in the production of rubber and pesticides. It should also not be used by people with psychoses, severe heart disease, or coronary thrombosis.
- People with brain damage, epilepsy, diabetes, kidney or liver disease, or underactive thyroid should use this drug with caution.

Pregnancy and nursing mothers:

Not known if safe to use in pregnancy. Not known if drug is present in mother's milk, but either avoid this drug or don't breast-feed.

Possible food and drug interactions:

- You should not take disulfiram with the antibiotic metronidazole because a dangerous psychotic reaction can occur.
- If you take disulfiram while taking the seizure drug phenytoin, toxic levels of phenytoin may accumulate in the blood.
- Disulfiram may increase levels of some tranquilizers, including chlordiazepoxide and diazepam.
- Disulfiram may increase the actions or effects of the anticoagulant warfarin.
- Difficulty walking or changes in behavior may occur if you use the tuberculosis drug isoniazid while taking disulfiram.

Helpful hints:

- Take disulfiram at bedtime if it makes you drowsy.
- You shouldn't drive a car or operate heavy machinery until you are sure the medicine isn't making you drowsy or less than alert.

SMOKING DETERRENTS

Nicotine

Brand names: *Habitrol, Nicoderm, Nicotrol, Prostep*

What this drug does for you:

This drug is used to help reduce nicotine withdrawal symptoms in people trying to quit smoking cigarettes.

Possible side effects of this drug:

- The most common side effects are rash, itching, or burning at the site of the patch. This drug may also cause local swelling and an allergic reaction, nausea, vomiting, diarrhea, constipation, stomach pain, indigestion, dry mouth, inflamed sinuses, sore throat, cough, chest pain, weakness, back pain, headache, muscle pain or tenderness, joint pain, painful menstruation, poor concentration, numbness or tingling, sleepiness, nervousness, dizziness, insomnia, abnormal dreams, sweating, high blood pressure, and abnormal taste.

Special warnings:

- This drug should not be used by people with an allergy to nicotine or to any component of the transdermal patch, such as adhesive material. If skin irritation develops at the patch site, call your doctor.
- The use of this drug may seriously aggravate the following medical conditions: angina, heart attack, high blood pressure, diabetes, kidney or liver disease, overactive thyroid, stomach ulcer, and irregular heartbeat.
- Don't use any form of tobacco while you are being treated with this drug.

Pregnancy and nursing mothers:

Category D. See page 9 for description of categories. Effective birth control should be used during treatment. Drug is present in mother's milk.

Possible food and drug interactions:

- This drug may increase levels of the pain reliever acetaminophen, the asthma drug theophylline, the blood pressure drug propranolol, the alcohol withdrawal drug oxazepam, the stimulant caffeine, the antidepressant imipramine, and the pain reliever pentazocine.
- For diabetics who use insulin, this drug may increase insulin levels, requiring a decrease in dose.
- Levels of the beta-blocker labetalol and the blood pressure drug prazosin may also be increased while taking this drug.
- This drug may decrease levels or effects of the nervous system stimulant phenylephrine and the beta-blocker/asthma drug isoproterenol.

Helpful hints:

- Dispose of used patches carefully. There is still enough nicotine in a used patch to poison a child or a pet.
- When you apply a new patch, choose a different area on your skin. Don't apply the patch to a previously used area for at least a week.

Natural Alternatives

SMOKING ADDICTION

◀ Automatic desire for a cigarette upon waking, after meals, during any stressful time

◀ Feelings of irritation and even panic when a cigarette is not available

◀ Realization that smoking is one of the top priorities of your life

◀ Structuring your life and activities to accommodate smoking

You can quit smoking: Here's how

You wake up with a hacking cough. And, let's be frank, your hair, breath, and clothes smell awful. Each time you inhale, you increase your risk of mouth, larynx, esophagus, pancreas, kidney, and bladder cancer. You also have a higher risk of heart disease, stroke, osteoporosis, and emphysema.

You know you should quit, and it's not as if you don't want to. You just can't seem to shake the smoking habit. The good news is you can quit — even if you've been hooked on cigarette for decades. The key is to find several strategies that work for you. Researchers have found that the methods listed below are some of the best ways to help conquer the urge to smoke.

Educate yourself. Contact your doctor's office and local chapters of the American Lung Association for information on smoking's dangers and tips on how to break the habit.

Talk to friends who have quit to learn what to expect. While it's true that you may experience unpleasant withdrawal symptoms for a while — like anxiety, drowsiness, inability to concentrate, and digestive problems — remember that some people report no withdrawal symptoms at all.

Postpone dieting. Worried about gaining extra pounds? Don't put yourself on a strict diet at the same time you're breaking away from cigarettes. To keep weight down, munch on healthy snacks like fresh fruit and veggies. When you are cigarette-free, your stamina will increase so you can exercise more. That will also help keep your weight stable.

Know what triggers your need to smoke. By figuring out when you smoke, you can change your behavior so you won't light up automatically. Keep a smoking diary, or try wrapping a piece of paper around your cigarette pack and securing it with a rubber band. Then jot down every time you take out a cigarette.

Do you smoke when you first get up? When you're anxious? Once you've identified the times you're most likely to smoke, find an activity to substitute for cigarettes. If you usually smoke after dinner, for example, take a stroll around the block instead.

Set a date. Pick a date to completely stop smoking a few weeks from now. In the meantime, taper off by switching to cigarettes with lower nicotine levels and gradually smoking fewer cigarettes. This can reduce symptoms of nicotine withdrawal.

Not everyone can taper off cigarettes, however. The most severely addicted smokers — chain smokers — may have to go "cold turkey" and cut out cigarettes completely. That's because cutting down can be almost impossible if you continuously crave cigarettes. While it's difficult to stop smoking all at once, it will help to remember you are giving up something harmful and taking control of your life and health.

When your day to quit arrives, throw away your cigarettes and get smoking accessories like ashtrays and lighters out of your house.

Make a list of reasons to stop. The early part of quitting is the hardest, and researchers say it may help to write down the reasons you want to stop smoking. Be specific. For instance, you might include, "I don't want my chil-

---

A powerful anti-smoking combination:
Nicotine patch plus nicotine gum

Want to quit smoking yet avoid the agony of withdrawal? Try the gum/patch combo.

Australian researchers have found that combining nicotine gum with a nicotine patch works better than either method alone. They studied 83 people who had smoked heavily for over two decades and were trying to quit using a variety of approaches, from counseling to nicotine gum or patches.

After six months, 16 percent of those who used nicotine patches and 36 percent of those on nicotine gum were still cigarette-free. But 70 percent using the patch plus gum had quit smoking. Why? Dr. Joy Petrie of Sydney's St. Vincent's Hospital thinks the combination probably raises nicotine levels in the body just enough to banish withdrawal symptoms.

For maximum effectiveness, chew your nicotine gum very slowly when you crave a cigarette. Chewing quickly releases nicotine too fast, producing side effects like lightheadedness and nausea.

After about 15 chews, you'll notice a tingling or pepperlike taste. "Park" the gum between your cheek and gum until those sensations subside. Chew again until the tingling/peppery taste returns, then "park" the gum again. Keep this up for about 30 minutes. By then, the nicotine will be gone. After two or three weeks, you'll gradually reduce your use of the gum, and may soon be able to get by without any nicotine.

The nicotine patch, worn 24 hours a day, sends nicotine into your body through your skin. You start with a high-nicotine-level patch and switch to a lighter-dosage patch in four to eight weeks. To avoid skin irritation, change the spot where you place the patch each day. Nicotine gum and patches must be prescribed by your doctor, who'll decide if they are safe for you. Remember, you must give up smoking while using the gum and patches or risk serious illness from nicotine overdose.

The gum and patch combo could be the one-two punch you need to knock out your cigarette habit for good.

Sources —
  FDA Consumer reprint, Publication No. (FDA) 94-3203, 1994
  Geriatrics (49,5:16)

dren to smoke because I do," or "I have bad breath." When that old craving kicks in, get out your list and read how downright unappealing smoking is.

Focus on the benefits. Remind yourself of the immediate benefits of not smoking. You may soon find yourself without that morning cough, for example, and there will be no more dirty ashtrays littering your house. You'll auto matically have some extra money when you stop buying cigarettes, so enjoy it. Be good to yourself. Buy a new best-selling novel or indulge in fresh flowers.

Learn to say no. How do you deal with a tempting offer of a cigarette? Politely, but firmly, say no. Tell family and friends you are no longer smoking and ask them not to smoke in your home.

Chug some soda water. Dissolve 1/2 teaspoon of bicarbonate of soda into a glass of water. Drink two to three glasses of soda water daily.

Find a friend you can share with. Find a buddy you can call for encourage-ment when you're fighting the urge to light up. In fact, several studies show that for long-term success in breaking free from nicotine addiction, it's important to find someone — other smokers who are determined to quit, a counselor, or your doctor — to share your ups and downs face to face.

Get help if you need it. While quitting smoking on your own is the cheapest approach and has worked for millions, if you need extra help, there's plenty available. Commercial programs and treatment centers are listed in the phone book and low-cost smoking cessation programs are offered by the American Cancer Society, the American Lung Association, and local hospitals. Ask your doctor for a recommendation. An organized program can help with group support, individual counseling, and hypnosis techniques. Studies show that when smokers who want to quit use these combined approaches, 50 to nearly 70 percent give up cigarettes within six months.

If other methods fail, ask your doctor if you're a candidate for nicotine gum or nicotine patches, which can help wean you from nicotine. The high blood pressure drug clonidine is also prescribed sometimes for its ability to block withdrawal symptoms in people who stop smoking.

What happens when you've given up cigarettes ... only to light up again? Does that mean you're hopelessly addicted? Not at all. Keep on trying. Think of each attempt as a learning process that's bringing you closer and closer to your long-term goal — a smoke-free, healthier lifestyle.

Sources —
National Institute of Aging "Age Page," U.S. Department of Health and Human Services, 1991
The Columbia University College of Physicians and Surgeons Complete Home Medical Guide, Crown Publishers, 1989
U.S. Pharmacist (20,6:84)

ALCOHOLISM

◀ Feel angry or guilty if someone suggests you drink too much
◀ Miss work due to hangovers
◀ Need a drink early in the day
◀ Have blackouts
◀ Hide your drinking from family and friends
◀ Need a drink when you're stressed

Problem drinking: How to stop

Magazines feature glitzy wine and beer ads. The latest James Bond movie has our hero still ordering his martini "shaken, not stirred." Medical researchers say a drink or two a day may reduce the risk of heart disease.

But for millions of people, there's nothing glamorous or healthy about alcohol. If you're a problem drinker, you may have already learned the hard way: Alcohol can have devastating social consequences and deadly health repercussions.

If you think you have a problem with alcohol, the good news is you can stop drinking. In fact, if you've quit denying you are a problem drinker, you've already made a first step toward sobriety. The tips below will guide you to success.

Rev up your motivation. Ask your doctor for advice and get a checkup to see if you have any alcohol-related health problems that need treatment.

If you are severely addicted to alcohol, your physician may recommend a brief stay (3-10 days) at a detoxification center, or prescribe the drug Antabuse, which causes violent illness if you have just a sip of alcohol.

For others who need less intense extra help, outpatient care is available. Recent studies show that just one to four sessions with a counselor trained to help problem drinkers can help reinforce your reasons for quitting alcohol and keep you on the road to sobriety. Researchers have found that 20 percent or more of problem drinkers are able to quit on their own without any formal treatment. The key seems to be strong family and peer support. So enlist the aid of friends and loved ones to help you through the early rough times when you first stop drinking.

Remember, withdrawal from alcohol can result in unpleasant side effects like anxiety, mood swings, and insomnia. But they will pass. The first three months are the most difficult; the urge to drink decreases over time.

Seek support. Attending support groups like Alcoholics Anonymous (AA) or Rational Recovery (RR), both of which you can find listed in your local telephone directory, can help boost your resolve, as can helping someone else stay sober. Studies show that 91 percent of alcoholics who become sponsors in Alcoholics Anonymous, aiding other recovering drinkers, are living alcohol-free lifestyles at ten-year follow-ups.

Expect ups and downs. The downs, of course, include times of relapse. Don't think of yourself as hopeless if you take a drink. It took courage to stay off alcohol. You did it before, so you know you can do it again. Call support group members for help and encouragement at these times.

Think about situations and cues that may trigger the urge to drink,

Mastering the five steps of change

Change — probably the most resisted word in the English language. It's also one of the most important when it comes to health. The problem is, there isn't a magical way to change habits like smoking or problem drinking.

But researcher James Prochaska, Director of Rhode Island's Cancer Prevention Center, has documented specific stages people go through when making a health change. Understanding them may help you reach your goal of altering unhealthy habits.

1) **Precontemplation** - You think you need to stop drinking or smoking, but you're not quite ready to do it. You may need to learn more about the health risks of your current behavior.

2) **Contemplation** - Convinced you have to change, you may still be resisting throwing out those cigarettes or attending an AA meeting. It may take a warning from your doctor about your health to send you to the next stage.

3) **Preparation** - You think about the reasons you need to stop drinking or smoking and you start to make some changes like switching to a lower nicotine cigarette or asking your doctor for more information.

4) **Action** - After about six months of getting ready to change (far longer than most people expect), you take decisive action.

5) **Maintenance** - Here's where the hardest work begins — maintaining your new healthier lifestyle.

If you relapse, don't give up. Dr. Prochaska's research shows that most people who quit smoking, for example, try three or four times — over seven to ten years — before they successfully boot nicotine from their lives. But eventually they succeed.

And so can you.

Source —
Medical Tribune (35,10:19)

---

like parties and other social events, and avoid them, especially when you first give up alcohol. Eventually, however, you want to be able to be in these tempting situations without drinking.

Do your homework. Keep a small notebook handy to write down situations that make you long for a drink. Record your thoughts and feelings as well as ways you can cope with these scenarios. Come up with a plan of action. Think about how you will feel. What will be the likely consequences? What, exactly, will you say if offered a drink? Do you feel confident to carry out your plan?

In the early stages of breaking free from alcohol, give yourself fairly easy assignments and avoid very risky situations, like bars. Stick to a task that is challenging, like an office party where you would have probably gotten drunk in the past, and use it to practice new behaviors. For example, you can order your favorite mixer (minus the alcohol) complete with garnish. By demonstrating personal control you will gain a confidence-building victory.

Remind yourself why you want to quit. Your determination to stop drinking may change from day to day. But you can renew your motivation by reminding yourself frequently just why you need to give up alcohol: how your problem drinking affected your career, your health, your spouse and children.

Another way to stay motivated is to remember that although you are giving up something, drinking and getting high, you are gaining much more. Living sober requires changes in your values and lifestyle that can be exciting and positive.

Beware of "magical thinking." Don't fantasize that all your problems will disappear now that you're determined to stop drinking. Indeed, you may be faced with family members still angry at your previous drunken antics, and there may be other problems to deal with, at home and at work, that your drinking has obscured.

Look for new, healthy outlets for your anxieties and energies. For example, walking, jogging, and other exercise can stimulate your brain to release calming chemicals, providing a kind of "natural tranquilizer."

Make new friends that share interests not centered around booze and bars. Consider taking up new hobbies or returning to school.

Without the health-robbing, mind-numbing effects of alcohol, you'll soon be on your way to a healthier, happier lifestyle.

Choosing a support group

For countless alcoholics, support groups — offering compassion, understanding, and advice — have made the difference between a life ruled by alcohol and one of sobriety and health.

Founded in 1935, Alcoholics Anonymous (AA) is the best-known group, with 1.5 million members in 92 countries. (There are also subgroups: AlAnon for family members of alcoholics and Alateen for teenage children of alcoholics.) AA's famous 12-step program is based on the healing power of God. Although AA does have spiritual aspects, it is not affiliated with any particular religion, and it was developed with a strong emphasis on social psychology and group support. In fact, several studies have shown that attending AA meetings is a good sign that a person will beat an alcohol problem. Many mental health professionals and physicians consider AA the core of any alcoholic therapy.

Membership is free and open to anyone. There are two kinds of meetings. Open meetings allow anyone, including the problem drinker's family, to attend and hear speakers describe their struggles with alcohol and how AA has helped them regain sobriety. At closed meetings, only members attend. This helps new members talk openly about their drinking problems and discuss specific ways to recover.

While AA is the most widely used resource for kicking alcohol addiction in the United States, it's not the only support group. Rational Recovery (RR) may be useful for people who feel uncomfortable with AA's approach.

While RR is fairly new and chapters may be harder to find than AA, the support group has a high success rate. In one study, about 75 percent of RR members who attended meetings for three months or more became free of alcohol and/or drug abuse. RR is based on the observation that many people quit drinking on their own, so getting problem drinking under control must be a natural response. RR strengthens this natural ability by the use of Addictive Voice Recognition Technique (AVRT).

Simply put, RR believes that the problem drinker needs to recognize the "addictive voice" inside that keeps coming up with excuses like "I'm depressed," or "My parents were drunks," to justify their abuse of alcohol. Dubbed "the Beast," this addictive voice comes from the part of the brain (the subcortex) that controls appetites for survival. The Beast believes it needs alcohol to survive. RR members are taught to use the rational part of their mind to fend off the demands of the Beast. RR emphasizes that you may think about drinking for years without relapsing. The key is to give up attempting to reason with the ruthless Beast and make a conscious decision to remain sober.

Unlike AA's "one day of sobriety at a time" approach, RR believes you can adopt a plan for lifelong abstinence. Also different from AA, RR recognizes the possibility that some problem drinkers may eventually learn to drink moderately without problems.

AA and RR both zero in on negative thinking and use education to overcome it. Likewise, both organizations encourage members to use statements like "I can stop and stay stopped." Both consider recovery a lifelong process and emphasize self-help and active homework. Neither support group believes in rehashing past bad experiences.

While support groups don't work for everyone, they are free. So there's no risk involved — and you may find that the understanding and strategies offered are just what you need to solve your problem drinking.

Sources —
Behavioral Health Management (14,1:30)
Complete Guide to Symptoms, Illness and Surgery, Putnam/Berkeley Group, New York, 1995
"If You Drink Alcoholic Beverages, Do So in Moderation," Home and Garden Bulletin Number 253-8, Human Nutrition Information Service, July 1993
Psychology Today (25,6:64 and 27,5:46)
The Addiction Letter (10,7:S1 and 10,11:S1)
The American Medical Association Encyclopedia of Medicine, Random House, New York, 1989
The Columbia University College of Physicians and Surgeons Complete Home Medical Guide, Crown Publishers, 1989
The Complete Life Encyclopedia, Thomas Nelson Publishers, Nashville, Tenn., 1995
The Western Journal of Medicine (60,1:53)

URINARY, VAGINAL, AND PROSTATE PROBLEMS

Prescription Drugs ℞

Nitrofurantoin

Brand names: *Macrobid, Macrodantin* **(Generic available)**

What this drug does for you:
This antibacterial drug is used to treat urinary tract infections.

Possible side effects of this drug:
- This drug commonly causes headache, nausea, and gas.
- Rare side effects include diarrhea, constipation, indigestion, stomach pain, weakened vision, dizziness, drowsiness, hair loss, itching, hives, inflammation of the pancreas, inflammation of the optic nerve, weakness, depression, confusion, and liver problems such as hepatitis and jaundice. Tell your doctor if you develop a rash, yellow skin or eyes, or severely upset stomach.
- Taking an antibiotic for a long time can cause bacteria or fungus to overgrow, leading to another infection (such as a yeast infection of the mouth or skin). If you get one of these "superinfections," you may need to stop taking nitrofurantoin and start taking another antibiotic for the second infection.
- Nitrofurantoin may cause increased pressure on the brain. Signs of this high pressure include headache, nausea, and blurred vision. Let your doctor know immediately if you develop these symptoms.
- If you take nitrofurantoin for many months, you may be at risk for lung complications. Report any unusual tiredness, chest pain, difficulty breathing, fever, chills, or cough to your doctor.
- Even though it is very rare, nitrofurantoin can lower the number of blood cells you have. If you don't have enough white blood cells, your immunity is down, and you can get a fever, sore throat, or pneumonia. If you are lacking red blood cells, you can become anemic, and that makes you tired and weak. Not having enough blood platelets makes you bruise easily and keeps your blood from clotting properly when you're injured. Report

any of these symptoms of bone marrow depression to your doctor.

Special warnings:
- People with poor kidney function, hemolytic anemia, or decreased urine output should not use this drug.
- This drug may cause hemolysis, a destruction of red blood cells, particularly in people with G6PD deficiency. Your doctor will stop your drug treatment if you have this side effect.
- People with poor liver function should use this drug with caution.

Pregnancy and nursing mothers:
Category B. See page 9 for description of categories. Drug is present in mother's milk.

Possible food and drug interactions:
- Antacids that contain magnesium trisilicate may increase the effects of this drug.
- Probenecid and sulfinpyrazone, drugs used to treat gout, may increase the effects of nitrofurantoin.

Helpful hints:
- Take with food or milk to help prevent upset stomach and to help your body absorb the drug.
- The usual adult dose is one 100 mg capsule every 12 hours for seven days.
- Don't be alarmed if the color of your urine becomes brownish.

Norfloxacin

Brand names: *Chibroxin (eye ointment), Noroxin (tablets)*

What this drug does for you:
The tablet form of this antibacterial drug is used to treat urinary tract infections, sexually transmitted diseases, and inflammation of the prostate. The ointment is used to treat eye infections.

Possible side effects of this drug:
- This drug may cause dizziness, nausea, stomach pain or cramping, loss of appetite, fatigue, rash, and sweating.
- Rare side effects include constipation, gas, heartburn, bad taste in the mouth, mental depression, weakness, dry mouth, fever, vomiting, diarrhea, back pain, and itching.
- Serious, sometimes fatal, allergic reactions can occur, causing symptoms such as swelling of the face or throat, difficulty breathing, itching, hives, tingling or loss of consciousness.
- Taking an antibiotic for a long time can cause bacteria or fungus to overgrow, leading to another infection. If you get one of these "superinfections," you may need to quit taking norfloxacin and start taking another antibiotic for the second infection.
- The eye ointment may cause your eyes to burn, sting, itch, redden, water, or dry out. It may also cause your pupils to dilate and your eye-

lids to swell or become crusty. Quit using the eye ointment and call your doctor if your eyes become very irritated or if you develop a skin rash or another sign of allergic reaction.

Special warnings:

- This drug should not be taken by people with allergies to fluoroquinolones or quinolone antibacterials, anyone under 18 years of age, pregnant women, or nursing mothers.
- If you have any disorders of the central nervous system, such as epilepsy, which may increase your risk of seizures, you should use this drug with caution.
- Kidney and liver functions should be checked and blood tests done periodically while you are taking this drug.

Pregnancy and nursing mothers:

Category C. See page 9 for description of categories. Not known if drug is present in mother's milk; however, do not take the drug while you are breast-feeding.

Possible food and drug interactions:

- This drug may increase the effects of caffeine, the anticoagulant warfarin, the immunosuppressant cyclosporine, and the asthma drug theophylline.
- Levels of this drug may be increased by probenecid, a drug used to treat gout.
- Levels or effects of this drug may be decreased by the antibacterial drug nitrofurantoin.
- Take antacids, vitamins or any products containing iron or zinc four hours before or two hours after taking norfloxacin.

Helpful hints:

- Take norfloxacin on an empty stomach — one hour before or two hours after meals.
- Drink plenty of fluids while you are taking this drug.
- This drug may make your skin extra-sensitive to sunlight, so protect your skin if you'll be outdoors in sunny weather.
- You shouldn't drive a car or operate heavy machinery until you are sure the medicine isn't making you drowsy, dizzy, or less than alert.
- If you miss a dose, take it as soon as possible. If several hours have passed or it is nearing time for the next dose, don't try to catch up by doubling up your dose unless your doctor tells you to.
- When applying the eye ointment, don't let the container touch your eye.

Phenazopyridine Hydrochloride

Brand names: *Azo-Standard, Prodium, Pyridium*

What this drug does for you:

This drug is used to relieve urinary tract pain, burning and frequent urination caused by infection, illness, or medical procedures affecting the urinary tract. This drug does not treat urinary tract infections.

Possible side effects of this drug:
- Phenazopyridine may cause itching, rash, upset stomach, allergic reaction, or headache.
- If your skin or the whites of your eyes become yellow, call your doctor. Your kidneys may be allowing the drug to accumulate in your body.

Special warning:
- People with decreased kidney function should not take this drug.

Pregnancy and nursing mothers:
Category B. See page 9 for description of categories. Not known if drug is present in mother's milk.

Helpful hints:
- Take this drug after meals since it may upset your stomach.
- Phenazopyridine may cause your urine to become a red-orange color. It could also stain soft contact lenses.
- If you have a urinary tract infection, you should only use this drug for two days.

Terconazole

Brand name: *Terazol*

What this drug does for you:
This vaginal suppository or cream is used to treat yeast infections of the vagina.

Possible side effects of this drug:
- This drug may cause headache, menstrual cycle abnormalities, stomach pain, and vaginal burning or itching. If irritation occurs, call your doctor.

Special warning:
- Don't get this drug in your eyes or mouth.

Pregnancy and nursing mothers:
Category C. See page 9 for description of categories. Not known if drug is present in mother's milk.

Helpful hints:
- Continue taking this drug during menstruation, but wear a sanitary napkin instead of a tampon.
- Insert the cream or suppository high into the vagina.
- If you have sexual intercourse during treatment, the male partner should use a condom.

Trimethoprim

Brand names: *Proloprim, Trimpex* **(Generic available)**

What this drug does for you:
These antibacterial tablets are used to treat urinary tract infections.

Possible side effects of this drug:
- This drug may cause rash, itching, skin eruptions, fever, nausea, inflammation of the tongue, and upset stomach.
- Even though it is rare, trimethoprim can lower the number of blood cells you have. If you don't have enough white blood cells, your immunity is down, and you can get a fever, sore throat or pneumonia. If you are lacking red blood cells, you can become anemic, and that makes you tired and weak. Not having enough blood platelets makes you bruise easily and keeps your blood from clotting properly when you're injured. Be on the lookout for any of these symptoms of bone marrow depression.
- Taking an antibiotic for a long time can cause bacteria or fungus to overgrow, leading to another infection (such as a yeast infection of the mouth or vagina). If you get one of these "superinfections," you may need to quit taking trimethoprim and start taking another antibiotic for the second infection.

Special warnings:
- This drug should not be taken by people with megaloblastic anemia, a folic acid deficiency.
- Blood counts should be done if sore throat, unusual bleeding or bruising, fever, or other signs of infection occur.
- People who have poor liver or kidney functions should use with caution.

Pregnancy and nursing mothers:
Category C. See page 9 for description of categories. Drug is present in mother's milk.

Possible food and drug interaction:
- This drug may increase the effects of the seizure drug phenytoin.

Helpful hints:
- Take this drug with food or milk if it upsets your stomach.
- Take all of the prescribed medication.

Natural Alternatives

PROSTATITIS

- ◀ Bloody or cloudy urine
- ◀ Fever, chills
- ◀ Impotence (sometimes)
- ◀ Low back pain

- ◀ Difficulty urinating
- ◀ Frequent urination with burning sensation
- ◀ Pain between the scrotum and rectum

Don't panic over prostatitis

If you're like most men, "prostate trouble" is one problem you'd prefer to keep private. But if you're having difficulty urinating, or any of the other symptoms above, you don't have to panic but you should see your doctor. A checkup could reveal prostatitis, a simple inflammation or infection of the prostate, common among men of all ages, and usually caused by bacteria.

Your doctor may treat you with antibiotics to knock out the infection, since you don't want it to become chronic and cause complications such as kidney infection. But in addition to your doctor's treatment, here are some simple measures you can take to help recover from prostatitis, and to prevent its recurrence.

Add zinc to your diet. Pumpkin seeds contain lots of healing nutrients for your prostate, especially zinc and magnesium. Brewer's yeast is also a good source of zinc.

Drink plenty of water. Increase your fluid intake to at least eight cups of water a day. This will help prevent kidney infection.

Exercise. Keep up your fitness program, but don't ride a bike; it could cause irritation. Walking is a good alternative.

Try parsley, asparagus, and natural herbal treatments. (See *Seven ways to cleanse your urinary tract* under **Urinary Tract Infection.**)

Eat low-fat. A diet high in fat and cholesterol is particularly unhealthy for your prostate.

Take your vitamins. Vitamins C and E are especially important for fighting an infection.

Avoid irritants in your diet. Alcohol, coffee, spicy foods, chocolate, and tomato products may irritate your prostate.

Try hydrotherapy. Three times a day, sit in a tub of six to eight inches of warm water for 15 minutes. A whirlpool bath is also helpful.

Strike out stress. Just as in every other health problem, it seems, stress is an aggravating factor in prostatitis.

Postpone sex. While your prostate is infected and irritated, sexual intercourse may delay your recovery, and it may spread infection to your partner. Wait until you're well.

Once you've established that your symptoms mean prostatitis, you can use your doctor's help and the tips above to get well. And those words "prostate trouble" never need to cause panic again.

Sources —
Alternative Medicine, Future Medicine Publishing Group, Puyallup, Washington, 1993
Prescription for Nutritional Healing, Avery Publishing Group, New York, 1990
Super Healing Foods, Parker Publishing Company, New York, 1995

URINARY TRACT INFECTION (UTI)

◄ Bladder that feels full even when empty   ◄ Burning sensation when urinating
◄ Cloudy urine   ◄ Frequent urge to urinate
◄ Pain above the bladder or in the low-to-mid back

Seven ways to cleanse your urinary tract

Infections of the urinary tract are among the most common in the human body — so common, in fact, that only respiratory infections occur more often. One woman in five and most men with prostate problems visit their urologists at least once a year with urinary tract infections. For 25 percent of women, infections will recur.

Most UTIs require antibiotics prescribed by your doctor. However, promptly applied home remedies can sometimes prevent a urinary tract infection while it's still in its early stages. Here are seven good things to try:

Add asparagus. This delectable bright green vegetable is a powerful diuretic (increasing the flow of urine) and detoxifying substance.

Go for some goldenrod. A cup or two of goldenrod tea may help relieve irritation of the urinary tract. Bring one cup of water to a boil, add one or two teaspoons of dried goldenrod, and steep two minutes. Strain and drink. Don't use this remedy, however, if you have a respiratory allergy to goldenrod.

Pick parsley. Eating parsley leaves helps to suppress the inflammation of UTI, and you can get a delicious dose of them in a serving of tabbouleh, a Middle Eastern salad. Use caution, however, if you have kidney disease or if your skin is extra-sensitive to sunlight.

Brew some buchu tea. The dried leaves of buchu, a South African flowering shrub, have long been used as a urinary antiseptic and diuretic. Look for it in your local health food store.

Enjoy your fruits and veggies. Watermelon, cantaloupe, celery, and artichokes are natural diuretics, and nutritious too.

Utilize uva ursi. This herb, also known as bearberry, is effective as an antibacterial treatment for UTIs. To keep it from tasting bitter when brewed as a tea, place the dried leaves in cold, not hot, water and allow them to steep overnight. Uva ursi is also available over-the-counter in powder or capsules. Eating a diet rich in milk, tomatoes, and other fruits and vegetables will give you the maximum benefit from uva ursi.

Cleanse with water and baking soda. By drinking water, you may be able to flush the infection from your system before it gets a good grip. If your urine is a pale yellow when you go to the bathroom, you'll know you're drinking enough water. Go for at least eight cups of water a day.

Add a teaspoon of baking soda to a full glass of water to help relieve the painful burning sensation. But don't use baking soda for a long period of time or if you have high blood pressure.

Other natural helpers for UTI

Chug some cranberry juice. For decades people have believed that cranberry juice can ward off or treat a bladder infection because of its acid content. While it's true that bacteria cannot grow very well in an acidic environment, that's not how cranberry juice works.

Cranberry juice actually prevents bacteria from clinging to the walls of the urinary tract. It makes your urinary walls too slippery for bacteria. Since the bacteria cannot hold on inside the body, they are less likely to cause an infection or make an existing infection worse.

Drink at least two 8-ounce glasses of cranberry juice at the first sign of a bladder infection to give bacteria the slip. Be sure, however, that the juice you're getting is the real thing. The cranberry cocktail sold in groceries may not contain enough pure juice to do you any good. Look for pure cranberry juice in the natural foods section or in a specialty store. Don't use baking soda in your water and drink cranberry juice at the same time. The two remedies cancel each other out.

Add more vitamin C. It helps to provide an acid environment that is hostile to bacteria. Try taking 1000 mg three or four times daily.

Cut back on sugar. A sugar-filled diet increases your risk of urinary tract infections. If you suffer frequent infections, reduce your intake of sugar, corn syrup, molasses, and the products made with them. You can even get cranberry juice that is artificially sweetened.

Dabble with dandelion. Extract of dandelion and dandelion tea act as natural diuretics and help relieve bladder discomfort.

Don't eat citrus fruits. They cause your body to produce alkaline urine, which encourages bacterial growth.

Avoid irritants such as coffee, tea, caffeine, chocolate, carbonated beverages, and spicy food.

Don't smoke. Women who smoke now or have in the past are at greater risk for incontinence than nonsmokers. A smoker's excessive coughing places a great amount of stress on the bladder, resulting in urine leakage. The tobacco smoke also negatively affects the bladder and urethra, and diseases associated with smoking (asthma, blood circulation diseases, etc.) affect your bladder, too

Stop using a diaphragm for birth control. Diaphragms have been shown to be one of the causes of recurrent UTIs.

Turn on the heat. A heating pad placed on the lower abdomen may help relieve some of the pain.

Go when nature calls. Many people resist the urge to go to the bathroom when they have a bladder infection because of the painful burning they experience.

But the more you go to the bathroom, the quicker you'll be rid of those bothersome bacteria.

Wear loose, comfortable clothing. Pantyhose and tight pants can irritate tissue and make it easier for bacteria to invade your urinary tract.

Head off future infections. If you've had one UTI, you know you never want another one.

Here's what you can do to keep your urinary system running smoothly in the future.

◁ Drink at least eight glasses of water a day.

◁ Go to the bathroom every two to three hours and after sexual intercourse.

◁ Wipe from front to back. Wiping from back to front pulls bacteria from the rectum up towards the urethral opening and increases the risk of infection.

◁ Wash yourself and your undergarments with a mild soap.

◁ Cleanse the genital area before sexual intercourse

◁ Avoid using feminine hygiene sprays and scented douches.

If your symptoms don't improve within 24 hours or if you have bloody urine, pain in your lower back, fever, nausea, or vomiting, see your doctor immediately. Urinary tract infections that are not treated properly can cause permanent kidney damage.

Sources —

American Journal of Obstetrics and Gynecology (167,5:1213)

Before You Call the Doctor, Random-Ballantine, New York, 1992

Family Urology, Fall 1995, American Foundation for Urologic Disease

Geriatrics (48,5:86)

Herbs of Choice: The Therapeutic Use of Phytomedicinals by Varro E. Tyler, PhD, ScD, Haworth Press, New York, 1994

National Institute of Diabetes & Digestive & Kidney Disease, NIH Publication No. 88-2097, 1988

Prescription for Nutritional Healing, Avery Publishing Group, New York, 1990

Super Healing Foods, Parker Publishing Company, New York, 1995

The American Medical Association Encyclopedia of Medicine, Random House, New York, 1989

The Doctor's Complete Guide to Vitamins and Minerals, Dell Publishing, New York, 1994

The Honest Herbal by Varro E. Tyler, PhD, Haworth Press, Binghamton, New York, 1993

The Journal of the American Medical Association (271,10:751)

VAGINAL YEAST INFECTION (VAGINITIS)

◀ **Pain during urination or intercourse**　　　◀ **Thick, milky discharge**
◀ **Vaginal itch, soreness, or rash**

How to keep the yeast away

At any given time, different areas of your body may be harboring colonies of *Candida albicans,* the tiny fungus cells responsible for yeast infections. When you're healthy, your body's defense systems are quite capable of handling these little organisms.

But when your immune system is weakened by physical or mental stress, hormonal changes, or illness, fungus cells can quickly launch an invasion, especially in the genital tract, where there's plenty of warmth and moisture. Women who are pregnant or have diabetes are particularly susceptible to yeast infections. So are those taking antibiotics, which can upset the balance of good and bad bacteria in the body.

Once you've had a yeast infection, you'll know if you get one again. But if you have the symptoms above for the first time, don't make the mistake of self-diagnosis. More serious conditions, like sexually transmitted diseases, can have some of the same symptoms. See your doctor for a laboratory test to be sure.

If you do have a vaginal yeast infection, take your doctor's advice and any medication she gives you. Then try some of these natural methods to help you through the infection and help prevent another one.

Blow it dry. Yeast thrives in warm, damp places, so keep the area around your thighs and crotch as dry as possible. Take extra time to towel off after a shower, especially in the summer. You may want to use your blow dryer on a low setting to help dry your genital area after you bathe or shower.

Change clothes after swimming. Don't sit around in a damp bathing suit and give yeast infection a friendly place to start. As soon as possible, put on some dry clothes.

Dress loose and cool. Summer or winter, the right clothes can help prevent yeast infection. Try to avoid fabrics that keep moisture trapped against your skin. Wear cotton panties for better ventilation; nylon panties trap heat and moisture. And don't wear pantyhose or tight clothes every day. Synthetic fibers in panty hose and underwear, and even the heavy fibers in very tight-fitting jeans, hold dampness next to your body.

Wipe from front to back. Wiping front to back when you use the toilet will help keep the bacteria in your rectum away from your vagina.

Don't douche. And don't use feminine hygiene sprays, deodorant sanitary pads or tampons, bubble bath, or colored or perfumed toilet paper. All of these products can change the acidic environment in your vagina, and that allows the yeast to grow.

Eat yogurt to ward off bacteria. Some studies suggest that eating live bacteria found in yogurt might ward off fungal growth. More research needs to be done, but meanwhile yogurt is a healthy addition to your diet.

Buy an over-the-counter anti-fungal medicine. Inexpensive, non-prescription, anti-fungal drugs usually destroy most yeast cells in just a few days. To make sure the infection is really cleared up, you should use the full supply of medicated inserts or suppositories as directed. See your doctor if symptoms don't clear up in a few days.

Vaginal yeast infections are pretty miserable things to have. But with good medicine and natural preventive care, yours should be cleared up soon.

Sources —
American Family Physician (51,7:1723)
FDA Consumer (27,10:10)
Medical Tribune (33,6:25)

> Please check with your doctor for approval before taking or discontinuing
> any prescription drug or using a natural healing alternative.

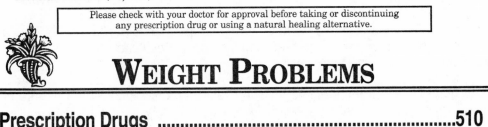

WEIGHT PROBLEMS

Prescription Drugs ℞

Fenfluramine

Brand name: *Pondimin*

What this drug does for you:
This drug is used to reduce appetite and aid in weight loss.

Possible side effects of this drug:
- Fenfluramine may cause dry mouth, drowsiness, diarrhea, nausea, stomach pain or discomfort, constipation, eye irritation, flushing, fever, chills, excessive sweating, urinary problems, impotence, changes in sex drive, menstrual problems, blood disorders, rash, hives, hair loss, skin problems, muscle pain or tenderness, chest pain, palpitations, abnormal heart rhythms, fainting, high or low blood pressure, nervousness, dizziness, weakness, insomnia, agitation, confusion, tension, headache, drowsiness, lack of coordination, depression, and anxiety.

Special warnings:
- Fenfluramine should not be taken by people with high blood pressure, heart disease, glaucoma, alcoholism, or psychotic disorders such as schizophrenia.
- Don't take this drug if you have a history of drug abuse or if you are planning to have general anesthesia for surgery.

- Fenfluramine should not be used within 14 days of taking monoamine oxidase (MAO) inhibitors.

Pregnancy and nursing mothers:
Category C. See page 9 for description of categories. Drug may be present in mother's milk.

Possible food and drug interactions:
- Avoid alcohol while taking fenfluramine.
- This drug may increase the effects of high blood pressure drugs such as guanethidine, methyldopa, and reserpine.
- If you take this drug along with any drug that depresses your nervous system, such as tranquilizers, antihistamines, or muscle relaxants, the combination may dangerously depress your nervous system.

Helpful hints:
- You shouldn't drive a car or operate heavy machinery until you are sure the medicine isn't causing blurred vision or making you drowsy or less than alert.
- This drug may cause insomnia, so don't take it late in the day.
- Take the drug on an empty stomach.
- Appetite suppressants are no substitute for a healthy diet and exercise.

Phentermine

Brand names: *Adipex-P, Fastin, Ionamin (Phentermine Resin), Obenix, Oby-Cap, Oby-Trim, Zantryl*

What this drug does for you:
This drug is used to reduce appetite and aid in weight loss over short periods of time.

Possible side effects of this drug:
- Phentermine may cause high blood pressure, heart palpitations, rapid heartbeat, dizziness, overstimulation, headache, tremors, restlessness, insomnia, exaggerated feelings of depression or anxiety, hives, impotence, dry mouth, bad taste in mouth, constipation, and diarrhea.
- Psychosis is a rare side effect.

Special warnings:
- Don't take this drug if you have a history of drug abuse.
- Phentermine should not be taken by people with high blood pressure, arteriosclerosis or heart disease, overactive thyroid, glaucoma, alcoholism, or psychotic disorders such as schizophrenia.
- Phentermine should not be used within 14 days of taking monoamine oxidase (MAO) inhibitors.

Pregnancy and nursing mothers:
Not known if safe to use while you are pregnant or nursing.

Possible food and drug interactions:
- Avoid alcohol while taking this drug.

- Phentermine may increase the effects of insulin. Insulin dosage may need to be adjusted.
- This drug may decrease the effects of the blood pressure drug guanethidine.

Helpful hints:
- You shouldn't drive a car or operate heavy machinery until you are sure the medicine isn't causing blurred vision or making you drowsy or less than alert.
- This drug may cause insomnia, so don't take it late in the day.
- Take the drug on an empty stomach.
- Appetite suppressants are no substitute for a healthy diet and exercise.

Natural Alternatives

WEIGHT PROBLEMS

◀ Cycles of strict dieting followed by overeating
◀ Difficulty moving or exercising
◀ Excess fat on the body
◀ Fatigue
◀ Shortness of breath during exercise
◀ Uncontrolled eating
◀ Weigh 20 percent or more over ideal weight

Weight and calorie calculator helps you lose pounds

George Bernard Shaw claimed that "There is no love sincerer than the love of food." Unfortunately, his statement seems to be supported by statistics.

Today in the U.S., over one-third of women and almost one-third of men age 20 or older are considered obese, along with one-fourth of children and adolescents.

If you are 20 percent or more over the suggested weight for your height, you are considered obese. If you are heavier than your recommended weight, but by less than 20 percent, you are considered overweight.

The problem is actually much more complex than just loving food. But eating more calories than your body can use is at the heart of obesity. However, this is one disease in which self-care usually provides the cure.

Maintaining a healthy weight is one of the most important things you can do for yourself. Your weight affects your health, your self-image, and your personal comfort. It can also have a big effect on how well you feel and how active a lifestyle you're able to enjoy. Use the weight calculator and calorie calculators below to help you reach and maintain your ideal weight.

The weight calculator. Dr. Richard Freeman, vice-chairman of medicine at the University of Wisconsin in Madison, has developed a simple formula for calculating ideal weight. Dr. Freeman's formula has two steps. First you figure your ideal weight based on your height, then you adjust that number to match your frame size.

Don't consider the number you come up with to be carved in stone. You may weigh a little more or less depending on your age and activity level.

Weight for women: The ideal weight for a woman who is exactly five feet tall is 100 pounds. For every additional inch above five feet, add five pounds. If you are shorter than 5 feet tall, subtract five pounds for every inch you measure below 5 feet.

Next, determine whether you have a small, medium, or large frame. Using a measuring tape, measure your wrist at the point where your hand and arm connect.

If your wrist measures exactly 6 inches, you have a medium frame, and the weight number that you calculated earlier does not need to be adjusted.

If your wrist measures less than 6 inches, subtract 10 percent from your ideal weight.

If your wrist measures more than 6 inches, add 10 percent to your ideal weight.

Weight for men: The ideal weight for a man who is exactly 5 feet tall is 106 pounds. For every additional inch above 5 feet, add six pounds.

To determine whether you have a small, medium, or large frame, measure your wrist at the point where your hand and arm connect.

If your wrist measures exactly 7 inches, you have a medium frame, and you don't need to adjust your ideal weight.

If your wrist is smaller than 7 inches, you have a small frame, and you should subtract 10 percent from your ideal weight.

If your wrist is larger than 7 inches, you have a large frame, and you should add 10 percent to your ideal weight.

Here's an example. If you're a five-foot-eleven-inch man, your ideal weight would be 172 pounds. 106+ (11x6) = 172. If you have a large frame, you should add 10 percent to 172 to determine your adjusted ideal weight. 10 percent of 172 is a little over 17 pounds. Add that to your ideal weight of 172 for an adjusted ideal weight of 189 pounds.

The calorie calculator. Once you've determined your ideal weight, you can easily calculate how many calories you need each day. To get an accurate estimate, you need to take into account how active you are.

◁ If you are totally inactive and usually get no exercise, multiply your ideal weight by 11.

◁ If you get regular exercise two to three times a week, multiply your ideal weight by 13.

◁ If you get regular exercise four to five times a week, multiply your ideal weight by 15.

◁ If you get regular exercise six to seven times a week, multiply your ideal weight by 18.

On average, healthy adult men need between 2,000 and 3,900 calories a day and women need 1,200 to 3,000.

Lose a pound a week with the 500-calorie solution. You can easily lose a pound a week by cutting 500 calories a day out of your diet. You can burn

150 of those calories with about 30 minutes of daily aerobic exercise, such as bicycling, dancing, or walking. To get rid of the other 350, look for high-calorie foods you can easily eliminate from your diet like mayonnaise, doughnuts, and alcoholic drinks.

Keep track of your daily calories for a couple of days. This will give you a better idea of where you can cut calories you don't really want or need. You'll be surprised at how quickly little things add up.

You also want to make sure you don't let your calorie intake fall too low. Fewer than 1,200 calories for men and 900 for women can cause your metabolic rate to drop and make losing weight even harder.

Figure your fat grams. When you know how many calories you need each day, you can easily figure out how much fat you can eat. Nutrition experts say that most people should limit their daily fat calories to about 30 percent of their total calories. If you want to lose weight or if you have a history of heart disease or cancer, you should limit your daily fat intake to 20 percent of your total calories.

For example, if you're a five-foot-four-inch woman with a medium frame, your ideal weight would be 120 pounds. If you're trying to lose weight, you'll want to keep your fat calories down to about 20 percent. If you exercise two to three times a week, you would multiply your ideal weight by the number that matches your activity level, which in this case would be 13. Now you know that the total calories you need each day are 1,560. Take 20 percent of 1,560 (1,560 multiplied by .20) to figure how many fat calories you can have, and you get 312.

If you translate fat calories into fat grams, it will be very helpful when you're checking food labels. Simply divide your fat calories by 9 (the number of calories that one gram of fat contains). You could eat approximately 35 grams of fat a day.

If your ideal weight and your present weight don't match up, you'll have to adjust your total calorie consumption. In order to lose one pound, you need to eliminate 3,500 calories.

Sources —
Atherosclerosis and Thrombosis (14,11:1751)
Choices for a Healthy Heart, Workman Publishing, New York, 1987
Controlling Your Fat Tooth, Workman Publishing, New York, 1991
Healthy Weight Journal (9,3:45 and 8,5:86)
Journal of the American Dietetic Association (95,4:417)
Science News (146,4:53 and 146,13:195)
The Physician and Sportsmedicine (23,3:15)

An eating plan that works

Having a plan is the first step to healthy weight loss. The nine suggestions below will start you on the road to success.

◁ Eat a healthy breakfast, a hearty lunch, and a small dinner. You'll lose weight if you eat one 2,000-calorie meal a day in the morning, but you'll gain weight if you eat that meal at night.

◁ Don't feel that you must eat three large meals. Satisfy your hunger

Fat substitutes save the day

For people on the weight loss wagon, fat substitutes are a real sanity saver. You get to enjoy the taste of fat without suffering guilt sensations.

Here's the scoop on the most popular stand-ins for fat:

Simplesse is a fat substitute that's been in use since 1989. It has already made its way into a number of foods including baked goods, butter, cheese, cheesecake, dips, frozen desserts, ice cream, margarine, mayonnaise, puddings, sour cream, salad dressings, and yogurt.

Simplesse is made up of tiny particles of protein that give foods the creamy taste of real fat. However, it only contains 1 1/2 calories per gram compared to 9 calories per gram of fat.

The major drawback of many fat substitutes, including Simplesse, is that they cannot withstand intense heat. Simplesse, for example, gels when exposed to high heat levels, so it can't be used for frying or baking.

Oatrim, one of the newest fat substitutes to hit supermarket shelves, has an unusual advantage over other fat substitutes — it lowers cholesterol. Preliminary studies also indicate that it lowers blood pressure and helps keep blood sugar levels constant, a big plus for diabetics and others who have trouble controlling their blood sugar.

Both Quaker Oats and ConAgra have been licensed to use Oatrim in their products. ConAgra is already using Oatrim in some of its Healthy Choice cheeses and ground beef. Oatrim is also being used in breads, brownies, cakes, cookies, and muffins.

Consumers can also buy Oatrim in its powdered form to use for cooking at home, including baking. Some health food stores carry it.

Olestra is another new fat substitute which has just been approved by the Food and Drug Administration. Olestra looks and tastes like real fat, and it can be used for frying or baking. However, the use of Olestra is controversial because it leaches vitamins A, D, E, and K from your body. It may also remove beta-carotenes from your body and cause gastrointestinal distress.

So, go ahead, indulge yourself in some low-fat taste sensations. Just remember — low-fat or not, calories still count.

Sources —

Interview with Dr. George Inglett, creator of Oatrim, Agricultural Research Service
Nutrition Concepts and Controversies, West Publishing, St. Paul, Minn., 1994
Science News (145,19:296)

pangs with a small, healthy snack midmorning and when you get home from work, and eat smaller portions for dinner. Let your kids eat a healthy snack when they're starving (usually right after school), and don't force them to clean their plates at mealtimes.

◁ Use whole-grain breads, cereal, rice, and pasta to get your fiber and B vitamins.

◁ Eat five to six servings of fruits and vegetables a day for vitamin A, vitamin C, and fiber.

◁ For proteins, choose lean meat, poultry without skin, fish, tofu, and dried beans. You should get no more than five or six ounces of meat a day. (A three-ounce serving of meat looks about like a stacked deck of cards.)

◁ Choose skim or low-fat dairy products only — no whole milk or high-fat cheese.

◁ Make low-fat cooking choices: Steam your vegetables or sauté them in chicken broth instead of butter or oil. Bake or broil your meat instead of frying it.

◁ Flavor food with lemon or lime juice and herbs instead of butter or margarine. Try mustard instead of catsup.

◁ Get all the candy, potato chips, and gooey cinnamon rolls out of your house and don't buy any more. Fill your refrigerator with tasty fruits and vegetables to snack on instead. If you decide to eat a cookie or a cup of ice cream every once in a while, buy a single serving.

The fat factor in weight loss

You know that eating too much fat raises your risk of heart disease and certain types of cancer. So you've sworn off fatty foods, but you still have trouble controlling your cravings for fats and maintaining the weight you want. Wondering what to do? Try these suggestions:

Remind yourself that you don't need to cut out all fats, just learn to eat them in moderation. In fact, your body needs a certain amount of fat to function properly. Fat provides the energy you need to exercise, protects your internal organs against jarring or repetitive actions such as exercise or motorcycle riding, helps control your body temperature, and aids in several other body processes as well.

Some researchers even believe eating small amounts of fat can actually keep you from overindulging on too many total calories. Ohio State University nutrition scientist John Allred points out that dietary fat causes your body to produce a hormone that tells your intestines to slow down the emptying process. You feel full and are less likely to overeat.

This could explain why adding a little peanut butter to your rice cake may satisfy your hunger longer and prevent you from wolfing down the whole bag of rice cakes later.

Certain fats, like olive oil and the omega-3 fatty acids found in salmon, may help prevent heart disease. And most people say a little fat simply makes food taste, look, and smell more appetizing.

Make a commitment to eliminate excess fat from your diet. The U.S. Department of Health and Human Services recommends that you limit the fat in your diet to 30 percent or less of total calories.

One way to figure this is to make sure that all of the foods you eat meet this 30-percent guideline. No food that you choose to eat should have more than 3 grams of fat for every 100 calories. If you decide to splurge on a favorite high-fat food, you can compensate for that by limiting your fat calories for the rest of the day or week.

Learn to recognize which fats are OK. The easiest rule to remember is to stay away from saturated fats such as those in cheese, butter, and meat

Less than 10 percent of your calories should come from saturated fats.

You should also limit the polyunsaturated fats you eat to less than 10 percent of your calories. Common sources are safflower oil, soybean oil, sunflower oil, and hydrogenated or partially hydrogenated margarines. Hydrogenated fats may be changed into trans fatty acids, which have much the same effec on the body as saturated fats.

Finally, you may find that as you reduce the amount of fats you eat, your cravings for them will decline. Researchers at the Fred Hutchinson Cancer Research Center in Seattle found that people who switch from high-fat to low-fat foods soon develop a preference for lower-fat foods.

Substitute other foods for fat in baking. Use monounsaturated fats, such as olive and canola oils, in place of saturated or polyunsaturated fats whenever possible. These are the healthiest of the three types of fats.

Replace stick margarines with soft margarine spreads, which are usually less hydrogenated. If you buy stick margarine, look for a brand that lists liquid oil as the first ingredient. These margarines are less hydrogenated than other types.

The latest stand-in for butter or margarine is prune puree. To save lots of fat and calories, just mix up your favorite brownie, cake, cookie, or bread recipe and substitute prune puree for the exact amount of butter, shortening, or oil the recipe recommends.

The real skinny on food portions

You're doing everything you can to cut down on fat and calories, you're exercising regularly, but your weight just isn't going down. It could be a portion problem.

A New York hospital conducted a study on overweight people who were considered "diet resistant" because they had been unable to lose weight in the past. Doctors found that the dieters were actually consuming many more calories than they thought they were.

It's easy to misjudge the size of the portions you are eating and underestimate the amount of fat and calories. Here are some tips to help you get control of the food you eat:

◁ Measure the amount of food your favorite serving utensils hold and post the amounts in your kitchen.

◁ Serve food with a measuring cup. You'll have exact portions without extra effort.

◁ Once a month, get in touch with portion size by weighing and measuring everything you eat for the day.

◁ For leftovers, buy containers that have size markings on the side.

◁ For times when you're eating out, learn some basic rules of size. For example, three to four ounces of meat is about the size of a deck of cards. A restaurant pat of butter is 1 1/2 teaspoons.

Sources —
NCRR Reporter (17,3:1)
The Diabetes Advisor (2,3:18)

Applesauce and apricot purees are also good substitutes for butter and margarine in baked goods recipes. But in some cases, you may only be able to replace three-quarters of the butter or margarine. The other drawback to using applesauce and apricots as fat substitutes is that these baked goods tend to become soggy and moldy within a day or two.

When baking with fat substitutes, use cake flour instead of all-purpose flour. This will help keep your baked goods tender. Also, be careful not to overbake fat-reduced recipes, since they dry out more quickly than traditional variations that call for butter or oil.

Remember that calories still count, even if they're low-fat. Although Americans have significantly reduced their fat intake in recent years, they're still packing on extra pounds. Thinking that low-fat or fat-free means low-calorie, Americans are eating too many calories. And anytime you eat more calories than you need — whether from fat or carbohydrates — your body stores them as fat.

More bulge busters

Here are some other weapons you can use to fight excess weight in the "battle of the bulge."

Eat at the right time. A good time to eat the majority of your calories is in the morning. Adults who eat breakfast every day tend to weigh less and have lower cholesterol levels.

The body's ability to burn calories is greater in the morning than in the afternoon or evening. People who skip breakfast tend to eat more high-fat snacks too.

Don't eat when you're distracted by television or a book. The average person eats eight times more food watching prime time TV than any other time. Concentrating on your food will help you be satisfied with smaller, better quality meals instead of just eating until your stomach feels full.

Don't skip meals. Meal-skipping is a big factor in falling off the diet bandwagon and into an eating binge. Giving your body fuel at regular intervals keeps blood sugar levels stable and helps your body burn calories more efficiently.

Tailor your diet to your style of eating. If you are a constant nibbler, plan healthy snacks and meals ahead of time to meet your calorie goals. If you eat more when you're bored or frustrated, plan pleasant activities to distract you from overeating. If the vending machines at your office are a constant temptation, take healthy snacks with you from home.

Try a structured eating plan. In a study in Baton Rouge, Louisiana, a group of women given a detailed eating plan and shopping list lost 50 percent more weight than a similar group without the structured plan.

Try to plan your meals ahead of time so that you get the right number of calories and all the proper foods for your good health.

Be careful of eating socially. People eat more when they are with other people, says a study at Georgia State University. So if you are counting your calories. be a little more careful when you are eating in a group.

Suppress your appetite naturally. Drink a glass of orange juice a half-hour to one hour before a meal. You'll eat fewer calories during the meal and still feel comfortably full. Just don't forget to include that glass of orange juice when figuring total calories for the day.

Make your cheddar better. Don't want to give up your favorite high-fat cheese? Make a low-fat version by zapping it in the microwave for a minute or two. Heating will make the fat separate somewhat from the cheese. Any oil you can pour or blot off will significantly reduce the cheese's fat content. This method also works well for pizza, fajitas, cheese sandwiches, or cheese toppings on casseroles.

Fill up on fiber. Eating foods high in natural fiber slows down digestion and makes you feel full. Whole grains, fresh fruits, and vegetables are good sources of fiber.

Give chromium a chance. The dietary supplement chromium picolinate may help reduce body fat even without cutting calories. Chromium works with insulin in the body to keep blood sugar levels even, so your energy level remains stable and you burn food more efficiently.

Research indicates that supplementing your diet with chromium picolinate is safe, but consult your doctor before trying it.

Sources —
Controlling Your Fat Tooth, Workman Publishing, New York, 1991
Dairy Council Digest (64,2:7)
Dietary Guidelines for Americans, United States Department of Agriculture, 1993
Eat Smart for a Healthy Heart Cookbook, Baron's Educational Series, New York, 1987
ESHA Research Issues (8,4:5)
Food and Nutrition News (66,4:29)
Food, Nutrition and Health (17,4:1)
Journal of Nutrition for the Elderly (13,2:66)
Medical Tribune (34,2:4)
Medical Tribune for the Family Physician (35,10:19)
Methods for Voluntary Weight Loss and Control, National Institutes of Health, Federal Building, Room 618, Bethesda, Md. 20892
The American Journal of Clinical Nutrition (51,3:428 and 51,6:963)
The Atlanta Journal/Constitution (Jan. 6, 1994, H9)
The Newnan Times-Herald (Oct. 25, 1995, 7B)
USA Today (Oct. 26, 1995, 1D)

Eating and exercising: How to get the timing right

Whether you should eat before you exercise or after you exercise is a dilemma for many people. For one thing, it depends on whether or not you're hungry. But if you want a little more guidance than just your stomach, let your health condition be your guide. Here's how to decide:

Very overweight people who exercise to burn calories would get the most benefits from eating first. Your body has to work harder to digest food when you exercise on a full stomach. You use more calories during and just after exercising on a full stomach than during and just after exercising on an empty stomach. On the other hand, don't worry if you'd rather exercise before you eat.

Metabolism matters

Eat next to nothing and still can't lose weight?

You could be energy efficient. Energy efficiency is a great trait if you're a house (you'll save your owners lots of money), but it can be a real drawback if you're trying to lose weight.

Being energy efficient means that your metabolism is always in high gear, burning calories very efficiently. Your body is trying to preserve a constant amount of body fat at all times by squeezing every bit of energy out of the calories you take in. This makes it difficult to work off any extra fat you may be carrying around.

If you have a low heart rate, a low energy level, and often feel cold when others around you are warm, there's a good chance you're energy efficient. If so, you're going to have a tougher time losing weight than other people. Still, it's not impossible.

Boost your metabolism into high gear by eating a well-balanced, low-fat diet and exercising (such as brisk walking) every day for at least 30 minutes. Three 10-minute workouts are actually just as effective as a single 30-minute workout, and may be even better.

Since metabolic rate is directly linked to your muscle mass, as you increase your muscle mass, you'll increase your metabolic rate. It's also important to boost your intake of lean protein since low-fat meals may not be supplying all you need. Great sources of lean protein include beans, chicken, low-fat cottage cheese, and skim milk.

Source —
  The Physician and Sportsmedicine (22,1:29,33)

If you have heart disease, you should exercise before you eat. Aerobic exercise before a meal will get the blood flowing to your heart most effectively. Also, vigorous exercise after you eat a large meal can dangerously decrease the oxygen flow to your heart. But a short, brisk walk after a meal is fine.

Diabetics should exercise after they eat, within two hours of a meal. If you wait three or more hours after a meal or exercise in the morning, your blood sugar will be too low. Exercise can lower a diabetic's blood sugar for eight hours.

Eat a snack before exercising and take a snack with you if you plan to exercise for over an hour.

If you don't have a special health condition, waiting until after exercising to eat has its advantages. You burn extra calories for at least an hour and sometimes several hours after exercising.

This is called "afterburn" or "excess postexercise oxygen consumption." (People who are obese don't get the same "afterburn" benefits as people who are not obese.)

For about two hours after you exercise, your tired muscles need glycogen — their energy source. Carbohydrates and even candy bars eaten after exercising will be more easily converted to glycogen instead of being stored as fat.

Exercising after a meal can cause a stomachache because your digestive system just doesn't get enough blood flow. Keep post-meal exercise moderate.

The most important point is that your eating schedule should never keep you from exercising. Experiment to see what time is best for you, but keep exercising!

Beat the potbelly blahs

If you're tired of people teasing you about your "Buddha" belly or asking when the baby is due and you're not even pregnant, take heart.

Here are four ways you can avoid the potbelly blahs.

◁ Don't eat a lot of food at once, especially in the evening. Too much food in your stomach puts pressure on your stomach muscles and pushes them out. When you eat a lot and then go to bed, your abdominal muscles relax, making it easy for the food to exert pressure on your tummy muscles. Do this enough times and you're likely to be the not-so-proud owner of a perfect potbelly.

◁ Suck it in. Consciously holding in your stomach whenever you think of it is one of the best stomach exercises. It also helps you to sit and stand straighter and avoid back pain. Remember to hold your stomach muscles in even when you're running or walking.

◁ Be sure to stretch your hamstrings (muscles on the backs of your thighs) after you run or walk for exercise. Tight hamstrings can cause you to develop a slight swayback and make your potbelly all the more notice-

---

Exercise: Just do it!

Even without weight loss, exercise benefits your body. It raises the good cholesterol in your body and increases lean muscle mass, allowing you to burn calories better.

As part of a weight loss program, exercise helps you lose weight faster and keep it off longer.

The minimum recommended cardiovascular exercise for adults is at least 20 minutes at a time, three or more times a week. However, only 37 percent of us are exercising this much, and the numbers are declining. The age groups with the lowest participation in regular strenuous exercise are 40-to-49-year-olds (30 percent) and people over 65 (26 percent).

A 1995 study by a group of doctors and nutritionists in Georgia and Washington state found that fat loss is related more to total energy used than to the intensity of your workout. You can exercise at high intensity for a short time, or at low intensity for a long time, and get the same benefits from your workout.

So, it doesn't matter if you have a lot of time to work out, or just a little time to work out harder. If you want to lose fat and get fit, the important thing is to exercise. Your body will thank you for it, and you'll be very pleased with the results.

Source —

Methods for Voluntary Weight Loss and Control, National Institutes of Health, Federal Building, Room 618, Bethesda, Md. 20892

able.

◁ Exercise your stomach and lower back muscles regularly. Exercise improves posture and helps prevent your stomach from sticking out.

Here are two good exercises for your stomach muscles:

Sit-ups: Lie on the floor with your arms folded across your chest. Bend your knees, keeping feet and back pressed to the floor. Lift only your head and shoulders off the floor. Be careful not to raise all the way up. You won't do your stomach muscles any good, and you're likely to hurt your back. Repeat exercise 10 times.

Pelvic tilt: Lie on your back with your knees bent and your hands at your sides. Put a folded towel under your head and a rolled up towel under your neck. Inhale. Press your back to the floor and pull in your stomach. Hold position for 10 to 20 seconds. Exhale. Slowly repeat exercise 10 times.

These back exercises will also have a positive effect on your stomach:

Cat stretch: Get on your hands and knees on the floor. Keep your back straight. Arch your back. Hold for two seconds. Return to starting position and repeat exercise 10 times.

Pseudo swim: Lie face down on the floor. Place a plump pillow under your stomach and hips. At the same time, raise your right arm and your left leg until you feel the muscles in your lower back and buttocks tighten. Hold two seconds. Repeat with your left arm and right leg. Do exercise 10 times.

Try to work at least 30 minutes of strength training exercises like the ones described above into your routine three or four times a week. Push-ups and pull-ups are also good exercise choices.

Walk your way to a healthy weight

Walking is one of the easiest, most accessible forms of exercise. It is suitable for almost everyone, and has the lowest dropout rate of any form of exercise. The only equipment it requires is a pair of sturdy walking shoes, and it doesn't cost anything to participate.

Some of the benefits of walking include improvement in the efficiency of your heart and lungs, lower blood pressure, and the burning of excess calories. And walking burns as many calories per mile as running.

Here are some tips for walking as exercise:

◁ Hold your head up, back straight, and stomach in. Your toes should point straight ahead, and your arms should swing loosely at your sides.

◁ When you step, land on your heel and roll forward to push off from the ball of your foot.

◁ Take smooth, easy strides. When walking uphill or at a rapid pace, lean slightly forward.

◁ Breathe deeply as you walk.

◁ Begin by walking 20 minutes at a time, four or five times a week. After about a month of this schedule, start walking 30 minutes at a time. Eventually, try to work up to walking three miles in 45 minutes.

◁ If you are elderly or ill, you may want to begin by walking two minutes, then resting a minute. Repeat this cycle until you begin to feel fatigued.

Don't be discouraged; improvement may take time, but it will happen.
◁ Walk as often as you can. Three times a week are necessary for maintenance. For faster improvement, walk more often.

Sources —
American Demographics (November 1995, 17)
Journal of the American Dietetic Association (94,4:409)
The American Journal of Clinical Nutrition (61,5:1013)
The Journal of the American Dietetic Association (95,6:661)
The Journal of the American Medical Association (273,6:503)
The Physician and Sportsmedicine (20,12:141; 21,2:177; 21,3:187; 21,11:89; 22,1:29 and 23,4:16)
Walking for Exercise and Pleasure, The President's Council on Physical Fitness and Sports, U.S. Government Printing Office, SSOP, Washington, D.C. 20402-9328

Dieting suggestions for seniors

As you get older, it often gets harder to keep off those pesky pounds. You know you're not eating any more than you used to, but you keep putting on weight.

Understand why so you can fight back effectively. There are three reasons it gets harder to lose weight as you get older:
1) The rate your body burns calories (your metabolic rate) decreases about 2 percent every 10 years.
2) Your body makes less protein as you get older. Protein burns calories, so your body doesn't need as many calories as before.
3) You are probably less active and get less exercise than when you were younger.

As stubborn as your body can be, you can still win the weight loss war, no matter what your age. Here's how:

Calculate your calorie needs. You can lose weight safely eating about 1,200 calories a day. (To get a more precise estimate of the calories you need each day, use the weight calculator at the beginning of this chapter.)

Don't neglect needed nutrients. Ask your pharmacist to help you choose a good multivitamin/mineral supplement so you'll be sure to get all your needed nutrients.

Shoot for 70 grams of protein a day. You can get this much from five or six ounces of lean meat and two large glasses of skim milk. You also get some protein from grains, fruits, and vegetables.

Count your calcium. Make sure you take in 1,200 to 1,500 milligrams of calcium a day. The body has more trouble absorbing calcium after women turn 60 and men turn 70. Older people often avoid dairy products because of lactose intolerance (milk products causing stomach cramps or diarrhea). You may need lactase-treated milk or Lactaid tablets. You probably should take a cal cium supplement if your multivitamin doesn't provide calcium.

Buy dairy with D — vitamin D that is. Look for dairy products that have vitamin D added to them, or help your body produce vitamin D by spending 15 minutes a day in the sun. (Vitamin D helps your body absorb calcium.)

Fill up with fluids. Drink plenty of fluids while dieting, especially if you're taking diuretics (water pills).

Stay active and exercise. No matter what you may have heard, you don't automatically lose muscle and gain fat as you get older. You just need to exercise to keep your muscles toned and your weight down.

Good exercises for seniors include stretching exercises, walking, low-impact aerobics, water aerobics, swimming, and cycling. If you can't move very well, do leg lifts and arm exercises while you are sitting or lying down. Even if one arm or leg is painful to move, exercise the other one.

It's best to exercise at your target heart rate for 20 minutes with a 10-minute warm-up and 10-minute cool-down. To get your target heart rate, subtract your age from 220 and multiply the result by 0.6. Check with your doctor before you start exercising.

And tell your body to get ready because you're going to win at weight loss once and for all!

Sources —
   American Family Physician (47,5:1187)
   Geriatrics (48,9:88)

Glossary

acanthosis nigricans — a rare inflammatory disorder of the skin that involves growths and abnormal pigmentation. It is sometimes associated with cancer of an internal organ.

ACE (angiotensin converting enzyme) inhibitor — a category of heart drugs that are used in the treatment of high blood pressure and heart failure.

acute — a severe condition or illness, of short duration but intense; opposite of "chronic."

adrenocorticosteroid — a category of drugs used to treat a variety of conditions including allergic reactions, inflammation, swelling, and poor adrenal gland function.

aminoglycosides — a category of antibiotic drugs that may be produced synthetically or from living organisms.

amphetamine — a category of drugs that act as a stimulant to the central nervous system of the body.

anaphylaxis — a kind of allergic reaction that can be life-threatening. It can be caused by exposure to many different substances including drugs, foods, dust, pollen and exercise.

anemia — a condition in which the number of red blood cells in the blood decreases. It can be caused by many different diseases as well as a lack of iron in the diet.

angina — a painful cramping attack in the left side of chest area over the heart. It may extend down the left arm or up to the left side of the face. It means that the heart is not getting enough oxygen. Attacks may last only a minute or as much as several hours.

ankylosing spondylitis — an inflammatory condition involving the bones and joints.

anorexiant — a substance that causes loss of appetite.

antiarrhythmic — a category of drugs that regulate the rhythm of the heart.

antibacterial — a category of drugs that kill bacteria or slow down their growth.

anticholinergic — a category of drugs that block impulses from part of the autonomic nervous system. This system controls various involuntary actions in the body such as digestion, breathing and heartbeat.

anticoagulant — a category of drugs that prevent the formation of blood clots.

anticonvulsant — a category of drugs that prevent or relieve convulsions.

antiemetic — a category of drugs that relieve nausea and vomiting.

antigen — a type of cell in the body that signals that an immune response is needed.

antihistamine — a category of drugs that works against the histamine response. Histamines are released in the nasal passages when a person has allergies, resulting in a stuffy nose.

antihyperlipidemic — a category of drugs that help to lower the amount of fats in the blood.

anti-inflammatory — a category of drugs that reduce inflammation at the site of an injury or tissue damage.

antineoplastic — a category of drugs that prevent the growth of cancerous cells.

antiparkinson — a category of drugs that control the symptoms of Parkinson's disease.

antipsoriatic — a category of drugs that control the symptoms of psoriasis.

antipsychotic — a category of drugs that control the symptoms of psychosis.

antiviral — a category of drugs that control the growth of viruses.

arteriosclerosis — a condition involving hardening of the arteries.

arthritis — a condition of the inflammation of the joints involving pain, swelling and difficult movement.

atrial fibrillation — a condition of the heart characterized by a rapid quivering of the heart instead of its normal regular beating.

attention deficit disorder (ADD) — a disorder that affects children involving the inability to keep the attention focused on a task. It may also include hyperactivity.

barbiturate — a category of drugs that depress the central nervous system.

benign — a condition of stability, with no recurrence and no worsening; opposite of malignant.

bile — yellow liquid that the liver secretes into the intestines to aid in digestion.

bladder neck obstruction — a physical blockage of the tube leading away from the bladder.

"black" tongue — a discoloration of the tongue that occurs with some illnesses and as a result of some drugs.

blood count — a measure of the various components of the blood such as white and red blood cells and platelets.

bone loss — a diminishing of the density of bones as a result of aging, illness or medication.

bone marrow suppression — a decrease in the bone marrow's ability to produce blood components.

bromides — a category of drugs that suppress the central nervous system.

cardiogenic shock — the inability of the heart to pump strongly enough to supply all of the body with blood.

cerebral infarction — a condition in which not enough blood gets to the cerebellum of the brain, resulting in the death of brain tissue.

cestodiasis — a condition in which the body is infested with tapeworms.

cholesterol — a substance in the blood that comes from food and is also manufactured by the body. Too much fat in the diet can cause high levels of this substance to accumulate in the blood, where it sticks to the walls of blood vessels. This condition can lead to a variety of health problems, particularly involving the heart.

cholinergic crisis — a dangerous condition that can result from overdose of certain drugs such as neostigmine. It is characterized by a general weakening of all of the muscles in the body and can affect the ability of the respiratory system to maintain breathing. It may be confused with a similar condition called a "myasthenic crisis," which is actually a worsening of the disease called myasthenia gravis. The two conditions are treated very differently, so correct diagnosis is very important.

chronic — long-term condition or lingering of an illness; opposite of "acute."

cirrhosis — a disease of the liver in which liver tissue gradually dies and the liver cannot continue to perform its function. It can be caused by diet, alcohol abuse, poisons, bacteria, and viruses.

colitis — a condition in which the tissue of the colon (large intestine) becomes inflamed and cannot function normally. It can be caused by antibiotic treatment as well as microorganisms. Symptoms include diarrhea, mucus in the stools, stomach cramping, and bleeding.

collagen-vascular disease — also called "diffuse connective tissue disease," this is a syndrome involving inflammation of the joints, especially of the legs and arms. Symptoms include pain, stiffness that lasts 30 minutes or more upon arising from sleeping, tiredness in the afternoons, and low-grade fever. Joints may gradually become deformed and deteriorate until normal movement is no longer possible.

congestive heart failure — a dangerous condition in which the heart fails to provide an adequate supply of blood to all body parts, causing pain, fluid retention and difficulty breathing.

conjunctivitis — the inflammation of the tissue at the inside corner of the eyes. It can be caused by many different things including bacterial infection, viruses, chemicals, ultraviolet radiation, and allergies.

Coombs' test — a blood test used to diagnose various forms of anemia.

coordination — the combined effort of a group of muscles to accomplish a certain movement such as walking.

cornea — the clear, gel-like coating over the eye that protects the eye and aids in vision.

cryptococcal meningitis — a fungal disease of the central nervous system in which deterioration can be gradual or rapid. Symptoms may include fever, nerve abnormalities, backache, headache, and swelling on the brain. It is often caused by other diseases in the body including cancer and AIDS and by treatment with immunosuppressive or steroidal drugs.

cyst — an abnormal fluid-filled sac or pouch that can develop in the skin or internal organs. Cysts can be caused by a large variety of factors. Some can be removed easily and some require more invasive procedures.

cystitis — an inflammation of the bladder. Symptoms include fever, frequent urination, pain upon urination, bladder spasms, and cloudy urine.

depressant — a category of drugs that slow down the functions of the body, particularly breathing and muscle movement.

diabetes — a group of diseases characterized by excessive urination, some of which are caused by hormonal abnormalities and some by metabolic abnormalities. The term usually refers to diabetes mellitus, a disorder in which your body doesn't metabolize carbohydrates properly because it doesn't produce or use insulin properly.

diuretic — a category of drugs that speed up the formation and elimination of urine.

drug fever — a fever that is caused by some drugs, rather than by an illness.

drug rash — an allergic response that is caused by some drugs, taking different forms depending on the type of drug.

Duchenne's muscular dystrophy — a disease of the muscles that usually affects children and is fatal. Symptoms include a long period of weakening and wasting of the muscle and loss of movement of the spinal cord.

eczema — a skin condition, also called dermatitis, with symptoms that include inflammation, eruptions, peeling, scabs, itching, and burning.

electrolytes — a group of salts that may be composed of sodium, chloride, or potassium. Because they are vitally important to certain body functions, they must be replenished if they are lost through vomiting, diarrhea, or sweating.

embolism — a blockage of a blood vessel by an object such as a blood clot.

endocarditis — inflammation of the tissue around the heart or heart valves, sometimes caused by a bacterial infection.

endocrine system — a group of glands that function together to produce and distribute hormones that affect a number of body functions, including metabolism, resistance to disease, sexual function, and growth.

endometriosis — a condition in which tissue that should be confined to the inside of the uterus spreads outside the uterus. Symptoms include severe stomach pain, infertility, and heavy menstrual flow.

enteric coating — a special coating applied to the surface of many drug tablets that keeps them from dissolving before they reach the intestines.

enzymes — a specialized group of proteins, each of which stimulates a specific reaction in the body, such as the breakdown of food in digestion.

epilepsy — a disorder of the brain with symptoms that include various types of seizures and abnormal brain activity. It can be caused by injury to the brain, brain tumors, or diseases of the nervous system.

esophagus — the tube that carries food and liquid from the throat to the stomach.

estrogen — female sex hormones produced by the ovaries. Prescription drugs which include estrogen are used to treat menopause and other conditions and to prevent pregnancy.

euphoria — an exaggerated sense of well-being and good health.

extremities — the parts of the body that extend out from the trunk, including the legs and arms.

fatal — causing death.

fluoroquinolones — a category of antibacterial drugs that fight a variety of infections including urinary tract infections, bacterial diarrhea, and venereal diseases.

folic acid — one of the B vitamins that naturally occurs in green plants and liver.

fungus — a plant-like organism that may live as a single cell, as in yeast, or in a colony, as in mushrooms. Some forms can cause illness and disease in people.

G6PD deficiency — a metabolic condition in which a certain enzyme is missing or improperly formed and cannot perform its normal function. It is most common in blacks and in whites from the Mediterranean region.

gastroesophageal reflux disease (GERD) — a condition that occurs when the valve at the top of the stomach does not close properly and allows food to flow back up toward the throat.

general anesthesia — a type of drug treatment that results in a sleep-like state, allowing surgery to be performed without inflicting pain.

giardiasis — an intestinal infection by a microorganism called Giardia lamblia.

glaucoma — a disease of the eye in which pressure builds in the eye and the optic nerve no longer performs correctly. Symptoms include poor night vision and seeing rings around lights. It eventually may result in blindness.

Goodpasture's syndrome — a hypersensitivity disease of the lungs and kidneys that is generally fatal. Symptoms include chronic inflammation of the kidneys, spitting up blood, and blood in the urine.

gout — a hereditary form of arthritis that involves inflammation of the joints, often in the feet or knees. It is caused by too much uric acid in the blood. Symptoms include pain in the joints that may begin at night. People with gout often develop kidney stones.

heart block — a heart condition that involves improper conduction of nerve impulses through the tissues of the heart chambers, causing irregular heartbeat.

hemolysis — the destruction of red blood cells by disease or exposure to toxins such as snake venom. It causes the hemoglobin to be released from the damaged red blood cells into the blood and eventually the urine, making it red.

hemolytic anemia — a form of anemia that results from hemolysis. It may be either hereditary or from exposure to toxic substances.

hepatic coma — a condition resulting from the inability of the liver to remove waste products such as ammonia from the blood. Symptoms include confusion, abnormal nerve or muscle activity, difficulty speaking, and loss of consciousness.

hiatal hernia — an abnormal protrusion of the stomach up into the esophagus that can allow stomach contents to flow back up toward the throat.

histamine blockers — a category of drugs that interfere with the actions of histamines. Histamines produce the redness and swelling around a bug bite, cause some of the constriction of the lungs during an asthma attack, and promote the secretion of stomach acids. An example of a histamine blocker is the ulcer drug ranitidine.

HIV — human immunodeficiency virus, which is the virus that leads to AIDS, acquired immune deficiency syndrome. HIV destroys cells by altering their genetic material.

hives — an allergic reaction that produces red, itchy skin eruptions.

hypercalcemia — a condition in which too much calcium accumulates in the blood.

hyperglycinemia — a disease in which too much of the amino acid glycine accumulates in the blood.

hypersensitivity — an allergic response to a substance that causes itching, hives, rash, swelling, and fluid retention and can be dangerous if swelling occurs in the throat.

hypertension — higher than normal blood pressure, usually because blood vessels are too narrow.

hypnotic — a category of sedative drugs that cause sleepiness, kill pain, or cause a loss of consciousness.

hypoglycemia — a condition in which there is not enough sugar (glucose) in the blood. Symptoms include weakness, irritability, dizziness, and confusion.

hypotension — lower than normal blood pressure, usually because blood vessels are expanded. Postural hypotension is a temporary form that may occur upon standing up from a sitting or lying position.

immunosuppressant — a category of drugs which prevent a normal immune response in order to allow certain other vital processes to take place.

impotence — a condition in which a man cannot maintain an erection and thus perform sexually.

indigestion — a condition of improper or incomplete digestion of certain foods that causes pain, bloating, heartburn, gas, or belching.

infertility — inability or reduced ability to produce offspring.

inflammation — an immune response to a substance that invades or injures body tissue. It consists of redness, swelling, pain, and warmth at the site

insulin — a hormone secreted by the pancreas or produced synthetically for injection in diabetics. It functions in the metabolism of sugar and maintains the level of sugar in the blood.

interaction — a reaction that occurs between two substances such as drugs that causes unwanted effects. The reaction can raise or lower the level of one of the two drugs or affect another body process.

iodides — a category of drugs that thin the mucus in congestive conditions such as bronchitis.

iron-deficiency anemia — a condition in which the body lacks the iron it needs to make enough hemoglobin for the red blood cells.

irritable bowel syndrome — a condition of the intestines in which the bowels do not function normally, resulting in constipation, cramping, gas and bloating.

ketoacidosis — an abnormal acidity of the blood caused by too many ketones, which are produced by the metabolism of fat.

lactation — the process of producing and accumulating milk in the breasts.

lesion — a general term for an eruption or wound occurring on the skin or other tissue.

libido — the natural sexual drive.

lupus — a complex skin and tissue disease that ranges from mild to severe, attacking mostly young women, with no known cause.

lymphoma — a malignant form of cancer that grows in a specific area of bone, tissue, or organ.

magnesium — a mineral that is essential to health. It is available from many foods including vegetables and fruits and is stored in the bones and muscles.

malaria — an infectious disease gotten from the bite of infected female mosquitoes. Symptoms include chills, fever, and sweating. It can be prevented by taking the drug chloroquine before being exposed.

malignant — a worsening or continued spreading of a cancerous tumor.

MAO inhibitor — a category of drugs used to treat mental depression by acting on a chemical called monoamine oxidase.

meningitis — a condition in which the tissues of the spinal cord or the brain become inflamed; can be very serious to fatal.

metabolism — the breakdown and transformation of food into energy for use by the body.

methyltestosterone — a hormone that is used to treat male and female menopause as well as malfunctions of sexual organs.

mononucleosis — an infection caused by the Epstein-Barr virus that attacks the lymph system. Symptoms include skin rash, fever, swollen and sore lymph nodes, and enlargement of the spleen.

myasthenia gravis — a disease of the nerves and muscles that causes extreme fatigue and weakness. Symptoms include a gradual weakening of the muscles of the face and neck, making it hard to chew and swallow. Treatment with drugs can restore the normal actions of the nerves on muscles.

myasthenic crisis — a sudden worsening of the symptoms of myasthenia gravis. The symptoms can progress to respiratory failure and death. Similar to a "cholinergic crisis," which can be brought on by certain drugs. The two conditions are treated very differently, so correct diagnosis is very important.

narcolepsy — a disease of sudden attacks of sleepiness in the daytime, which may occur even while eating or talking.

narcotic — a category of drugs that cause sleepiness or relieve pain; they are generally habit-forming, and overdose can cause coma and death.

nasal polyp — a small tumor that grows in the nasal passages and interferes with breathing.

Neuroleptic Malignant Syndrome (NMS) — a rare, sometimes fatal reaction to antipsychotic drugs. Symptoms include variable blood pressure, sweating, fever, rigid muscles, and difficulty breathing.

neurosis — a mental state marked by confusion and conflict that give rise to defensive behaviors in order to cope.

nonsteroidal anti-inflammatory drug (NSAID) — a category of drugs that reduce inflammation and fever and relieve pain. They are used to treat a variety of conditions such as arthritis and muscle aches.

obsessive-compulsive disorder (OCD) — a neurosis that involves an irresistible urge to perform certain actions or behaviors in a repetitive, specific manner. If something interferes with this pattern, it causes the person anxiety.

obstruction — a blockage of an organ or passageway that stops normal functioning.

osteoarthritis — a condition involving chronic inflammation of weight-bearing joints. Bones gradually grow spurs and cartilage disintegrates so that movement is more and more difficult.

osteoporosis — a condition in which the bones continually lose density and mass, progressing until the bone can no longer provide support and breaks easily.

palpitation — a rapid fluttering or pounding of the heart.

paranoia — imagined feelings of persecution or harassment.

parasympathetic nervous system — part of the autonomic nervous system that controls some involuntary movements of organs such as the heart, intestines, glands, and lungs.

peritonitis — a condition involving inflammation of the lining of the body cavity that surrounds the organs.

platelets — the components of blood that bond together to form clots over wounds. They can cause problems in some forms of heart disease.

pneumocystis pneumonia (PCP) — a form of pneumonia caused by an unknown microorganism, characterized by little if any fever, rapid shallow breathing, and coughing. Often occurs in people with weakened immune systems.

pneumonia — a condition of the lungs involving inflammation, fluid buildup, fever, and coughing. Can be fatal, especially in the elderly, if not treated correctly.

porphyria — a general term for a group of hereditary illnesses that involve the metabolism of porphyrin. (One type of porphyrin is a component of hemoglobin, the pigment of red blood cells.) Symptoms often involve the skin, liver and spleen.

psychosis — a mental condition in which the person loses contact with reality and creates an alternative version. Major personality changes occur and may be accompanied by hallucinations or hearing voices.

pylorus — the valve at the end of the stomach through which food flows to the intestines.

quinolone — a category of antibiotics that treat a variety of infections and illnesses.

reflux — a condition in which digestive juices from the stomach flow back up the esophagus and throat, causing pain and burning.

respiratory depression — a slowing and weakening of breathing caused by illness or drugs such as sedatives.

Reye's syndrome — a condition that results from a viral infection, mainly in children who have been treated with aspirin incorrectly. It can be fatal. Symptoms include vomiting, nausea, mental confusion, and abnormal liver function.

rhabdomyolysis — a disease that involves the destruction of muscles; it can be caused by very strenuous exercise followed by a sedative drug such as heroin or cocaine.

rheumatism — a general name for a group of conditions that affect the muscles and joints. Symptoms include stiffness, pain, and inflammation.

rheumatoid arthritis — a form of arthritis in which the immune system attacks the joints and cartilage. It can advance to the point where movement is limited and very painful.

rhinitis — a condition in which the nasal passages become inflamed and congested. Allergic rhinitis is also known as hay fever. Treatment includes antihistamines but not antibiotics.

salivary glands — a group of glands around the mouth that contribute saliva during the eating process. They can also be stimulated by smells and thoughts of food.

schizophrenia — a group of mental disorders characterized by disturbed thinking, an altered sense of reality, hallucinations, and personality changes.

sedative — a category of drugs that relax and relieve tension in different muscles or areas of the body.

sepsis — a group of infections in the bloodstream that affect the whole body through the blood or the lymph system. One form is also known as blood poisoning. Symptoms include fever, chills, and pain in an affected area.

sick sinus syndrome — a particular form of abnormal heartbeat that originates from the right side of the heart. Symptoms include irregular heartbeat, fainting, dizziness, and angina. Treatment may include a pacemaker.

sleep apnea — a condition in which breathing stops during sleep for more than 10 seconds at a time. Can be caused by blockage of breathing passages, physical weakness, or medication.

smooth muscle — a kind of muscle that is found around organs and is not under conscious control.

steroid — a category of drugs that suppress the function of the adrenal gland in the treatment of various conditions and illnesses.

sudden infant death syndrome (SIDS) — a general name for the sudden, unexplained death of an infant who was not ill. Also called "crib death."

sulfonamides — a category of drugs that are antibacterial; they are used to treat a variety of conditions including urinary tract infections, genital infections, and colitis.

sympathicolytic — a substance that inhibits the actions of the sympathetic nervous system, which controls many different involuntary muscles.

syndrome — a group of symptoms that go together to describe a condition but not do not name its cause.

tardive dyskinesia — a disorder of the nerves and muscles brought on by certain drugs. Symptoms include involuntary movements of muscles in the face, mouth, tongue, neck, shoulders, hands, and hips.

thrush — an fungal infection of the mouth or throat. Symptoms include white ulcers, fever, and inflamed intestines.

tic — abnormal muscle movement or involuntary sound, also known as "habit spasms." They occur most often in children.

tolerance — a condition that results from taking a drug for a long time; gradually it takes more of the drug to achieve the desired result.

Tourette's syndrome — a rare childhood disease that can last into adulthood. Symptoms include uncontrollable speech, muscle twitches, and tics.

toxic — poisonous to the body.

tranquilizer — a category of drugs that relieve tension and anxiety and slow physical activities without affecting mental abilities.

transdermal patch — a method of delivering drugs through the skin by means of an adhesive material. Drugs available in patch form include nicotine, nitroglycerin, and estrogen.

tricyclic antidepressants — a category of drugs used to treat mental depression.

tryptophan — a substance that occurs naturally in the body and is found in certain foods. It induces relaxation and sleepiness. It can interact with certain drugs.

ulcerative colitis — a condition of the large intestine involving inflammation and abnormal bowel activity. Symptoms include constipation, diarrhea, bloody stools, and stomach pain.

urethra — the tube that conveys urine from the bladder to the outside of the body.

urinary retention — the inability to urinate when the urge is present. It can be caused by drugs, obstruction, illness, or aging.

vascular headache — a headache thought to be caused by sudden constriction or relaxation of the blood vessels in the head.

vascular system — the group of organs and tissues that convey the blood through the body.

vertigo — a form of dizziness in which either the victim or other objects seem to be spinning around in space. May be caused by a variety of illnesses and drugs.

white blood cells — the infection-fighting cells of the blood.

yeast infection — a fungal infection that can attack many different areas of the body including the mouth and the vagina. May also attack the whole body by getting into the blood.

General Index

Drug index is located at front of book. See page ix.

Drug index is located at front of book. See page ix.

Drug index is located at front of book. See page ix.

Drug index is located at front of book. See page ix.

Drug index is located at front of book. See page ix.

Drug index is located at front of book. See page ix.

Drug index is located at front of book. See page ix.

Drug index is located at front of book. See page ix.

Drug index is located at front of book. See page ix.